Preventive Management
for Children with Genetic Conditions: Providing a Medical Home

Second Edition

Golder N. Wilson

Texas Tech University Health Sciences Center,
KinderGenome^{SM} Private Practice, Dallas, Texas

and

W. Carl Cooley

Crotched Mountain Rehabilitation Center, Greenfield,
New Hampshire and Dartmouth-Hitchcock Medical Center,
Hanover, New Hampshire

Golder N. Wilson

Texas Tech University Health Sciences Center,
KinderGenome^{SM} Private Practice, Dallas, Texas

and

W. Carl Cooley

Crotched Mountain Rehabilitation Center, Greenfield,
New Hampshire and Dartmouth-Hitchcock Medical Center,
Hanover, New Hampshire

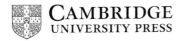

CAMBRIDGE
UNIVERSITY PRESS

CAMBRIDGE UNIVERSITY PRESS
Cambridge, New York, Melbourne, Madrid, Cape Town, Singapore, São Paulo

CAMBRIDGE UNIVERSITY PRESS
The Edinburgh Building, Cambridge CB2 2RU, UK

Published in the United States of America by Cambridge University Press, New York

www.cambridge.org
Information on this title: www.cambridge.org/9780521617345

First published 2006

Printed in the United Kingdom at the University Press, Cambridge

A catalogue record for this publication is available from the British Library

Library of Congress Cataloguing in Publication data

ISBN-13 978-0-521-61734-5 paperback
ISBN-10 0-521-61734-0 paperback

For SHAMUS WILSON and the physicians who care for special children.

GNW

For my wife, SEDDON SAVAGE, who is, among other more important things, the best physician I know.

WCC

Contents

Preface   ix
Glossary of genetic and molecular terms   xv

Part I   Approach to the child with special needs

1   Approach to the child with genetic disease   3

2   Providing a primary care medical home for the child with a developmental disability   21

3   Approach to preventive management   33

Part II   The management of selected single congenital anomalies and associations

4   Congenital anomalies associated with developmental disability   61

5   Single anomalies, sequences, and associations   90

6   Teratogenic syndromes   116

Part III   Chromosomal syndromes

7   Autosomal aneuploidy syndromes   151

8   Sex chromosome aneuploidy and X-linked mental retardation syndromes   194

9   Chromosome microdeletion syndromes   230

Part IV   Syndromes remarkable for altered growth

10   Syndromes with proportionate growth failure as a primary manifestation   265

11   Syndromes with disproportionate growth failure (dwarfism)   293

12   Overgrowth syndromes   326

13   Hamartosis syndromes   346

Part V   Management of craniofacial syndromes

14   Craniosynostosis syndromes   375

15   Branchial arch and face/limb syndromes   388

Part VI   Management of connective tissue and integumentary syndromes

16   Connective tissue disorders   413

17   Integumentary syndromes   437

Part VII The management of neurologic and neurodegenerative syndromes

18   Neurologic syndromes including the arthrogryposes   457

Part VIII Management of neurodegenerative metabolic disorders

19   Organellar and miscellaneous neurodegenerative disorders   477

20   Metabolic dysplasias susceptible to dietary treatment   506

      References   524
      Index   549

Preface

How to use this book

This book is designed as a reference in which health professionals can review complications and design preventive management for common congenital anomalies or syndromes. Over 250 disorders are discussed, including 29 disorders and 3 syndrome families that are described in detail with standardized flow sheets for preventive care (e.g., see the general checklist at the end of this preface). These preventive management checklists are meant to be copied and placed in the medical record. By checking off the appropriate boxes and entering notes, the practitioner can assemble an ongoing record of key concerns, evaluations, and referral/counseling measures. The appended general checklist can be used for less common disorders summarized in this book or elsewhere; complications can be listed and management considerations written in as the child is followed.

A new checklist format of four pages is provided for this second edition. The first page includes a succinct description of the disease and summarizes its complications in a standardized organ-system format. The second and third pages include age-specific recommendations with evaluations and key concerns in the first column and management considerations in the second. The third column has room for physician notes, with occasional reminders for high-risk problems. Below the columns are succinct summaries of disease-specific risks as well as general genetic or social risk factors for that child (e.g., coronary artery disease, prematurity, nutritional deprivation). The presence of general and disease-specific risks on the same flow sheet provides the practitioner with a comprehensive, on-going summary of patient care. The last page contains parent-oriented information on the disorder that may be copied and provided to families.

The more common disorders have longer discussions organized as sections on terminology, etiology, differential diagnosis, genetic/family counseling, complications, and preventive management strategies. The less common disorders have a more succinct format listing complications by region/organ system with management considerations. It is envisioned that most users will turn to the book with a specific disorder in mind and focus on the relevant medical problems and management suggestions. A detailed table of contents and index are available for this purpose.

Since the first edition, an enormous amount of general and disease-specific information about disabilities has appeared on the Internet. With each disorder are included Internet addresses for parent support groups or medical information sites with physician- and parent-oriented information. This wealth of web information has allowed condensation of references to standard textbooks for background – particularly Gorlin et al. (2001) and Jones (1997) – and a few recent articles. The *Online Mendelian Inheritance in Man* database (search on OMIM or go to www.ncbi.nlm.nih.gov/entrez), plus its linked *Entrez* databases like *PubMed*, will provide updated references on most of the disorders in this book. Searching on disease names like cerebral palsy or Down syndrome will provide information on conditions that are not caused by single genes.

Another use of the book is to read more broadly about the approach to children with developmental disabilities and genetic disease. Because of rapid progress in the field of medical genetics, certain terms or concepts encountered in the chapters may be unfamiliar. For this reason, introductory chapters on the approach to genetic disease and developmental disabilities have been provided (Part I, Chapters 1 and 2). These sections review categories of disease and the specialized tests that are available for diagnosis of syndromes and congenital anomalies. Familiarity with the diagnostic approach allows generalists to be informed participants in the evaluation and management of congenital disorders. A glossary is also provided to aid with specialized terminology.

Which disorders are included?

The more common congenital anomalies and syndromes were selected for detailed discussion, with emphasis on those requiring chronic management due to mental and physical disability. To qualify as a "more common" disorder, an incidence above 1 in 25,000 births was required, since that number makes it probable that the disorder will come to the attention of the average pediatric practitioner. If the disorder is rarely encountered by practitioners, or if there are limited strategies for preventive care, then the discussion is limited to a succinct summary without inclusion of a checklist. The general checklist in this preface can be used for these rarer disorders after appropriate entry of their disease-specific complications. The rationale for preventive management strategies is discussed in Chapter 3.

It should be noted that hydrocephalus and spina bifida are isolated anomalies rather than syndromes, and that cerebral palsy is a functional description of brain injury or developmental anomaly. However, their congenital origin and requirements for chronic management justify coverage in this book. It is expected that the developmental pediatrician will provide specialty expertise for the latter disorders, while the pediatric geneticist will be more actively involved with patients having malformation syndromes.

Some common metabolic disorders are also discussed in this book, although it is recommended that metabolic specialists be continuously involved in their care. The frequent laboratory measurements and dietary modifications required by acute metabolic disorders are not adequately conveyed by a checklist approach, but the frequency of developmental disabilities in these children justifies attention to preventive management in other areas. Checklists are definitely useful for some chronic metabolic conditions, exemplified by the mucopolysaccharidoses discussed in Chapter 19.

Rationale for preventive guidelines

For those interested in the rationale for particular management guidelines, reading of Chapter 3 is recommended. The central rationale is that each syndrome or anomaly places the patient at higher risk for particular complications as compared to the general population; preventive screening or evaluation for these complications is then justified by criteria of efficiency (selection of high-risk patients) and ethics (improved quality of life). This strategy of ameliorating complications is one of secondary or tertiary rather than primary prevention, since few congenital disorders can be prevented or cured (see Chapter 3). A list of complications is the basis for preventive management guidelines, and is rendered in a standard format according to anatomic location or organ system. General complications are listed first (e.g., increased mortality, feeding problems), followed by a standard sequence of body regions and systems.

The Committee on Genetics, American Academy of Pediatrics (1995a, b, 1996a, b, 2001a, b) has published consensus recommendations for the health care supervision of children with, achondroplasia, neurofibromatosis-1, Marfan, fragile X syndrome, Turner, and Down syndrome. These recommendations are certainly followed in this book, and their spirit is extrapolated to other disorders for which consensus guidelines are not yet formulated.

Although there is a clear rationale for alerting practitioners to the complications of a disorder, the nature and timing of intervention often require clinical judgment. Some children with severe dysfunction may benefit more from palliative care than the inconveniences of medical intervention. Decisions about screening measures become particularly difficult when anesthesia is required (e.g., brain imaging), or when a positive result has controversial significance (e.g., cervical spine radiographs for atlantoaxial instability in Down syndrome). Such recommendations are often footnoted in the checklists, with the reminder that clinical judgment must always be used.

Types of preventive guidelines

The United States Surgeon General has recommended that all families know their family history, and columns for risk factors ascertained from family background or prenatal history are included on the checklists. Social and environmental concerns can also be listed, providing a summary of general and disease-specific risks that will remind practitioners of age-related concerns. In Chapter 3, the effectiveness of checklists in improving preventive care is documented.

"Family Support" appears frequently under management considerations in the second column of the checklists. This is a prompt to the primary care physician to inquire about the general impact of the child's condition on family life. Questions should routinely be raised about specific family stresses, school issues, the status of siblings, access to information, contact with others affected by the same condition, and financial pressures. Eligibility for benefits such as Medicaid, Supplemental Security Income (SSI), Title V, and respite care should be considered and followed with appropriate referrals. Some families may need to consider the financial planning issues related to income taxes, trusts, and estate planning when individuals with developmental disabilities are involved. Many states have family support programs for families of children with disabilities which may include the services of a family support coordinator. All eligible families should be referred to such programs. Birthdays, anniversaries of the initial diagnosis, and life transitions (e.g., preschool to elementary school; school to work/adult life) are particularly difficult times for families during which extra support may be needed. Included on the checklists and with text discussions are websites for parent support groups and parent information that can be invaluable for negotiating times of crisis.

Validation of preventive management guidelines

Having stated that the preventive management guidelines are based on disease complications, it must again be emphasized that the invasiveness and frequency of preventive screening may be subject to dispute. Judgments about screens (e.g., echocardiography for all infants with Down syndrome) versus a wait for symptoms (e.g., echocardiography for a heart murmur) are often difficult, and practitioners should keep in mind that consensus guidelines are available for few disorders. Certainly practitioners should feel free to modify the guidelines based on their experience and style.

In summary, this book should be used to enhance the health care of patients with congenital anomalies and syndromes by considering preventive management guidelines. It is certainly not intended to impose unwanted advice on experienced physicians or to add new burdens to the already busy routines of those involved in patient care. However, anyone observing the improved outcomes for patients with Down syndrome over the past few decades must award some merit to preventive management. While congenital disorders may not be cured, the attentive physician can almost always heal by enhancing the quality of life of children with developmental or genetic disorders.

Acknowledgements

The authors wish to thank John C. Carey MD, MPH, James W. Hansen MD, Michael Msall MD, and Joel Steinberg MD for their insights as advisors for the first edition.

Congenital anomalies

General preventive medical checklist for congenital anomalies or syndromes

Patient Name_____ **Birth date** __ / __ / ____ **Number**_____

Patient has following diagnosis(es): _____ with
potential concerns listed below, taken from Wilson/Cooley, p.____; other source: _____

Age	Evaluations: key concerns	Management considerations		Notes
New-born ↓ 9 months	Neurologic problems, anomalies Hearing, vision, feeding[2] Airway, jaw, neck: obstruction, mobility Other:	❏ Imaging;[3] specialists;[1,3] family support[4] ❏ ABR; ophthalmology;[3] video swallow[3] ❏ Radiology;[3] ENT;[3] anesthesia precautions[3] ❏	❏ ❏ ❏ ❏	
1 year ↓ 3 years	Growth, development:[1] feeding Hearing, vision, feeding, sleep[2,7] Internal defects: heart, kidneys, gut Airway, jaw, neck: obstruction, mobility Other:	❏ Consider ECI;[3,5] family support[4] ❏ ABR;[3] ophthalmology;[3] sleep study[3] ❏ Cardiology;[3] urology;[3] GI[3] ❏ Radiology;[3] ENT;[3] anesthesia precautions[3] ❏	❏ ❏ ❏ ❏ ❏	
4 years ↓ 9 years	Growth, development:[1] school transition[6] Hearing;[2] vision;[2] sleep[2,7] Airway:[2] anesthesia precautions Other:	❏ Family support;[4] IEP[6] ❏ Audiology;[3] ophthalmology[3] ❏ Radiology;[3] ENT[3] ❏	❏ ❏ ❏ ❏	
10 years ↓ 15 years	Growth, hearing, vision[2] Diet, activity, exercise, sleep[2,7] Puberty, behavior Other:	❏ ENT;[3] ophthalmology;[3] school progress, IEP[6] ❏ Dietician;[3] sleep study[3] ❏ Vocational, behavioral counseling[3] ❏	❏ ❏ ❏ ❏	
16 years ↓ 18 years	Growth, hearing, vision[2] Diet, activity, exercise, sleep[2,7] Puberty, behavior Other:	❏ ENT;[3] ophthalmology;[3] school progress, IEP[6] ❏ Dietician;[3] sleep study[3] ❏ ❏	❏ ❏ ❏ ❏	
19 years ↓ 23 years	Adult care transition[6] Hearing;[2] vision;[2] sleep[2,7] Diet, activity, exercise, behavior Other:	❏ Vocational, behavioral counseling[3] ❏ ENT;[3] ophthalmology;[3] sleep study[3] ❏ Dietician;[3] behavior therapy[3] ❏	❏ ❏ ❏ ❏	
Adult	Adult care transition[6] Hearing;[2] vision;[2] sleep[2,7] Diet, activity, exercise Other:	❏ Vocational, behavioral counseling[3] ❏ ENT;[3] ophthalmology;[3] sleep study[3] ❏ Dietician[3] ❏	❏ ❏ ❏ ❏	

Disease-specific concerns		Other concerns from history	
		Family history/prenatal	Social/environmental
_____	_____	_____	_____
_____	_____	_____	_____
_____	_____	_____	_____
_____	_____	_____	_____
_____	_____	_____	_____

Guidelines for the neonatal period should be undertaken *at whatever age* the diagnosis is made; ABR, auditory brainstem evoked response; ECI, early childhood intervention; IEP, individualized educational plan; GI, gastrointestinal; [1]infants with unexplained delays or multiple anomalies should have pediatric developmental, genetic, and neurologic assessment; consider karyotype and/or cranial sonogram/head MRI for anomalies; [2]by practitioner; [3]as dictated by clinical findings; [4]if suspected disability, consider parent group, family/sib, financial, and behavioral issues; [5]if disability, early intervention and preschool program; [6]monitor individual education plan, educational testing, balance of special education and inclusion, academic progress, behavioral differences, later vocational planning; [7]snoring, pause in breathing, daytime sleepiness, unusual sleep positioning.

Glossary of genetic and molecular terms

These brief definitions should be supplemented by consulting the texts recommended in the Preface.

Acrocentric chromosome: Chromosome with small short (p) arms as opposed to metacentric chromosomes with approximately equal short and long (q) arms.

Allele: Alternative gene structure (e.g., S and A alleles of the β-globin gene).

Agenesis: Absence of a part of the body caused by an absent anlage.

Aneuploidy: Abnormal chromosome number that is not an even multiple of the haploid karyotype (i.e., 47,XX,+21 or 90,XX).

Anlage, primordium, blastema: Embryonic precursor to a tissue, organ or region.

Anomaly: Any deviation from the expected or average type in structure, form and/or function which is interpreted as abnormal.

Anticipation: Worsening of phenotype with subsequent generations.

Aplasia: The absence of a body part resulting from a failure of the anlage to develop.

ASO: Allele-specific oligonucleotides used for DNA diagnosis.

Association: Any non-random occurrence in one or more individuals of several morphologic defects not identified as a sequence or syndrome. Associations represent the idiopathic occurrence of multiple congenital anomalies during blastogenesis.

Atavism: A developmental state that is normal in phylogenetic ancestors, but abnormal in their descendants.

Atrophy: Decrease in a normally developed mass of tissue(s) or organ(s) due to decrease in cell size and/or cell number.

Base pairs (bp): Adenine–thymine (A–T) or guanine–cytosine (G–C) pairing in DNA; also the basic unit for DNA strand length.

Blastogenesis: Stages of development from karyogamy and the first cell division to the end of gastrulation (stage 12, days 27–28).

Candidate gene: A gene implicated in pathogenesis based on protein function, chromosomal location, or sequence homology.

Chromosomal rearrangements: Aberration where chromosomes are broken and rejoined as opposed to numerical excess or deficiency.

Chromosome painting: Use of repetitive DNA FISH probes to fluoresce entire chromosomes or chromosome regions.

Contiguous gene deletions: Deletion encompassing neighboring genes to produce a composite phenotype.

Crossover: Breakage and reunion of chromosomes that realign parental loci.

Cytogenetic notation: Formal nomenclature describing karyotypes and chromosome location, that is:

47,XY+11: Extra chromosome 11 (Trisomy 11)

45,XY−11: Absent chromosome 11 (Monosomy 11)

46,XY,11q−: Terminal deletion of chromosome 11

46,XY,11q+: Extra material of unknown origin on 11q

46,XY,del(11p11p13): Interstitial deletion between bands p11 and p13 of chromosome 11

46,XY,dup(3q): Extra material derived from the long arm of chromosome 3.

Dysmorphogenesis: Abnormal development leading to abnormal shape of one or more body parts (dysmorphology).

DNA cloning: Isolation of a DNA segment by insertion into a simple genome (plasmid, bacteriophage) and production of multiple copies.

DNA diagnostic techniques: Use of DNA modifying enzymes, hybridization, and size separation technologies for diagnosis of identity, genetic disease, or predisposition.

DNA hybridization: Rejoining (reannealing) of complementary DNA or RNA stands.

DNA marker: DNA segment, often anonymous, that exhibits sufficient sequence variation to be useful in genetic linkage and DNA diagnosis.

DNA sequence: Order of nucleotides in a DNA segment, usually displayed from the 5′-triphosphate (5′ end) to the 3′-hydroxyl (3′ end) nucleotides.

Empiric risks: Recurrence risk based on epidemiologic survey of affected families.

Exon: Portion of gene that encodes protein.

First-degree relative: Those with 50% of genes in common (child, parent, sibs).

FISH: Fluorescent *in situ* hybridization, a technique by which flourochromes are attached to DNA probes and hybridized with cytogenetic or cell preparations.

Functional cloning: Isolation of gene segments based on gene function; that is, using antibodies to a characterized protein or expression assays where traits are deleted or restored to cultured cells.

Gene map: Order of genes within a chromosome or entire genome.

Genetic heterogeneity: Multiple loci where mutations can produce a similar phenotype, such as autosomal-dominant or X-linked Charcot–Marie–Tooth disease.

Genetic mapping: Use of genetic linkage to produce a relative gene order based on recombination distances (centimorgan = approximately 1 megabase).

Genome: Complete set of genes (DNA) in an organism.

Genomic DNA: DNA isolated from an organism or tissue, containing transcription signals and introns that will be absent from cDNA.

Genomics: The study of function and disease based on gene structure and organization.

Genotype: Genetic constitution, often with reference to particular alleles at a locus.

Germinal mosaicism: Mosaicism within the germ line, whereby a fraction of eggs or sperm may contain a particular mutation or chromosome aberration.

Heteroplasmy: Different mitochondrial genomes in the same cell, a mechanism by which the proportions of altered mitochondria may increase in specific tissues to cause disease.

Heterozygote: Individual with different alleles at a locus.

Homeobox: A DNA sequence shared by several Drosophila segmentation genes.

Homeotic mutations: Mutations altering segment identity in *Drosophila*. In a broader sense, a developmental switch analogous to that replacing one homologous insect segment with another.

HOX, hox: Gene clusters in humans and mice that exhibit homology to the structure and expression of *Drosophila* homeotic loci.

Hyperplasia: Overdevelopment of an organism, organ, or tissue resulting from a decreased or increased number of cells.

Hypertrophy: Increase in size of cells, tissue, or organ.

Hypoplasia: Underdevelopment and overdevelopment of an organism, organ, or tissue resulting from a decreased or increased number of cells.

Hypotrophy: Decrease in size of cells, tissue, or organ.

IGF: Insulin-like growth factor.

Incomplete penetrance: Absence of phenotypic expression in a person known from a pedigree to have an abnormal genotype.

Interstitial deletions: Chromosomal deletion removing regions between termini.

Isochromosomes: Duplicate long or short chromosome arms that result in deficiency (i.e., Turner syndrome patients with i(Xq) are monosomic for Xp).

Karyotype: A standard number and arrangement of chromosomes as obtained from human blood or tissue specimens. A normal karyotype is 46,XX for females and 46,XY for males.

Kilobases (kb): Unit of DNA/RNA length = 1000 bp; megabase = 1 million bp.

L1CAM: L1 cell adhesion molecule implicated in X-linked hydrocephalus.

Linkage: The tendency for neighboring genes to segregate together in families.

Locus: Unique location of a gene on a chromosome.

Major anomaly: Anomaly with cosmetic or surgical consequences.

Malformation: A morphologic defect of an organ, or larger region of the body, resulting from an intrinsically abnormal developmental process.

Maternal inheritance: Inheritance mechanisms that exhibit maternal transmission based on abnormal mitochondria or maternal RNAs.

Meiosis: The process of germ cell division that randomly allots one chromosome of each pair to gametes.

Mendelian inheritance: The classical autosomal dominant, autosomal recessive, and X-linked inheritance mechanisms derived from Mendel's observations in peas.

Microdeletions: Chromosome deletions requiring prometaphase banding for visualization.

Minor anomaly: Anomaly of no medical but considerable diagnostic significance.

Mitosis: The process of somatic cell division that produces identical genomes in daughter cells.

Morphogenesis: A developmental process that includes the stages of blastogenesis and organogenesis.

Morphology: Discipline of zoology that concerns itself at once with the form, formation, and transformation of living beings.

Mosaicism: Variation in DNA sequence or chromosome constitution among different cells of an organism.

Multifactorial determination: Dependence of traits on multiple genes plus the environment.

Multipoint linkage: Linkage analysis that examines multiple traits or markers in a pedigree and orders them relative to one another.

Normal variant: Deviation from expected or average type in structure, form or function that is more frequent (arbitrarily >4% of population) and more innocuous than an anomaly.

Obligate carrier: Carrier deduced by pedigree structure.

Oligonucleotide: Short nucleotide sequence often obtained by chemical synthesis.

Organogenesis: A developmental process that extends from late stage 13 (day 28) until the end of stage 23 (day 56) when the major organs and body parts are formed.

Paired box: A DNA sequence motif found in the *paired* gene of the fruit fly.

PAX: Genes in mice and humans containing *paired* boxes.

PCR: Polymerase chain reaction by which individual gene segments are amplified through sequential cycles of polymerization, heat denaturation, and reannealing.

Phenotype: Individual traits or characters.

Physical mapping: Gene order based on actual physical measurements in terms of chromosome bands or DNA base pairs.

Pleiotropy: Multiple traits determined by a single cause, often a gene mutation.

Point mutations: Nucleotide substitutions.

Polymorphism: Multiple alleles at a locus, producing amino acid or DNA sequence variation.

Polypeptide chains: Proteins or, in the case of multiple subunits, components of proteins formed by peptide bonds between amino acids.

Polyploidy: Abnormal chromosome number that is a multiple of the haploid karyotype (e.g., 69,XXY or 92,XXXX).

Positional cloning: Isolation of gene segments based on chromosome location.

Primary relative: First-degree relative (i.e., those sharing 50% of genes).

Primer: Oligonucleotide used to begin nucleic acid polymerization at a particular site on a DNA strand (e.g., with PCR or reverse transcriptase).

Proband: Individual bringing family to attention, indicated by arrow in pedigrees.

Prometaphase analysis: Karyotype prepared from synchronized cells arrested in early prophase; these studies require prior notice to the laboratory.

Propositus: Same as proband.

Protein polymorphism: Products of alternate alleles at a locus exemplified by the ABO or HLA systems.

Quantitative traits: Incremental phenotypes such as height or blood pressure.

Recombinant DNA: Chimeric DNA molecules produced by joining of segments from different species, often using the complementary "sticky ends" produced by restriction endonucleases.

Recombination: Breakage and reunion of DNA strands.

Repetitive DNA: DNA sequences that have multiple copies in a genome.

Restriction endonuclease: A bacterial enzyme designed for defense against bacteriophage that recognizes and cleaves at specific nucleotide sequences.

Reverse genetics: Genetic analysis proceeding from chromosomal location to cloned gene; positional cloning is now the preferred term.

Robertsonian translocations: Joining of two acrocentric chromosomes at their short arms to produce a single translocation chromosome.

Sequence: A cascade of primary and secondary events that are consequences of a single primary malformation or a disruption.

Somatic mosaicism: Variation in DNA sequence or karyotype among different somatic cells of an organism.

Sporadic: Isolated case, often implying lack of inheritance or genetic causation.

Submicroscopic deletion: Small chromosome deletions that can be visualized only by DNA analysis.

Syndrome: Multiple anomalies thought to be pathogenetically related and not representing a sequence.

Syndrome variability: Differing phenotypic manifestations among individuals with the same syndrome.

Targeting sequences: Amino acid regions that direct proteins to particular cellular locations.

Teratology: The study of abnormal development, particularly with regard to the disruptive influence of drugs, chemicals, and physical agents.

Threshold: A theoretical barrier at which an individual's combination of genes and environmental exposure crosses from predisposition to actual defect.

Translocation breakpoint: The region of recombination between two chromosomes.

Translocation carriers: Individuals with "balanced" translocations that have no extra or missing chromosome material.

Triplet repeat amplification: Increased number of tandemly repeating 3-bp units that can alter gene expression, as in Fragile X syndrome or mytonic dystrophy.

Trisomies/monosomies: Karyotypes with extra or missing entire chromosomes.

Uninformative: Genetic linkage study where parental alleles and therefore the risk for disease transmission cannot be distinguished.

Uniparental disomy: Two copies of a chromosome pair derived from one parent.

Variable expressivity: Variable symptoms among affected individuals in a family.

Zygotic expression: Synthesis of gene products from zygotic DNA rather than maternal RNA molecules.

Part I

Approach to the child with special needs

Children with special health care needs account for a substantial proportion of pediatric hospital and outpatient visits. While the individual disorders causing chronic disease may be rare, the aggregate impact of chronic care occupies a significant fraction of the health professional's time. It is often cited that the sickest 1% of the population consumes 30% of the health care resources while the sickest 5% consumes 50%. The impact of chronic illness is similarly exaggerated in pediatric practice, with disproportionate demands on practitioners. Preventive management offers an important opportunity to minimize complications in children with special health care needs, and the key to preventive management is a specific diagnosis and approach.

This section previews those on specific disorders by outlining general approaches to the child with genetic disease and developmental disability. The practitioner should realize that the many rare genetic and developmental disorders can be grouped into disease categories, providing general guidelines for specialty referral and preventive management. Rather than being overwhelmed by long lists of eponyms or symptoms, the primary care provider can recognize categories such as multiple defect syndromes or increased muscle tone and use these introductory chapters to refine their approach to the diagnosis and management or congenital disorders.

Chapter 2 examines different causes of developmental disability, with an overview of assessment and therapy. Early recognition of developmental disabilities is emphasized, so that a *Chronic Condition Management* protocol can be instituted that optimizes pivotal functions like hearing and vision. Chapter 3 reviews the rationale for preventive management and applies these principles to the child with special health care needs. The chapter concludes with an overview of the preventive measures used in this book, and highlights common strategies that can be used for children with disabilities but without a specific diagnosis.

Approach to the child with genetic disease

Medical genetics is a harlequin specialty. One side is bright with the power of DNA diagnosis and genotyping; the other is darkened by ignorance of complex phenotypes. Fortunately, the molecular revolution is proceeding so rapidly that even complex syndromes are being drawn into the light of genetic analysis. For a growing number of developmental and/or metabolic disorders, proper recognition and referral can lead to definitive diagnostic testing. It is thus extremely important for practitioners to be familiar with common presentations of genetic and developmental diseases, allowing affected children and their families to receive the benefits of informed management and genetic counseling.

A correct diagnosis is the gateway to anticipatory guidance and case management. Although the primary care physician may not be the first practitioner to establish the correct diagnosis, it is essential that he or she be able to incorporate specialty opinions and laboratory data into a comprehensive care plan. It is not necessary for practitioners to know long lists of eponymic disorders, but it is necessary that they recognize the possibility of genetic or congenital disease so that appropriate referrals and information can be obtained. Computerized databases such as Online Mendelian Inheritance in Man (OMIM – www.ncbi.nlm.nih.gov/entrez) with links to genome and literature databases of the National Institutes of Health, *Recognizable Patterns of Human Malformation* (Jones, 1997), *Syndromes of the Head and Neck* (Gorlin et al., 2001), and *The Metabolic and Molecular Bases of Inherited Disease* (Scriver et al., 2001) are available to provide details on particular diseases. This chapter will review the clinical approach to children with morphologic and/or metabolic alterations, beginning with the important component of family history and presenting for management based on categories of disease. Italicized terms are defined in the glossary at the end of the book.

The family history: A preventive measure for all children

The documentation of a family history is a key first step in the care of all children, especially for those with developmental disabilities. The family history is important for two reasons: first, for recognizing general risk factors that can apply to any child and second for revealing specific genetic disease that explains or affects a particular child. This latter use of family history is less common, but recognition of a Mendelian or chromosomal inheritance pattern is essential for early referral and diagnosis of at-risk families.

The general use of family history in defining risk factors is receiving increased attention as advances in genetic technology accumulates DNA markers for risk modification. DNA testing is increasingly available to identify individuals with higher risks for disorders such as coronary artery disease, breast cancer, auto-immune disease, learning disabilities, or mental illness. The American surgeon general has recently emphasized the need for all individuals to know their family history as a guide to disease susceptibility and prevention.

A more traditional use of the family history is to determine if a particular medical disease or disability is inherited. This step is particularly crucial for congenital anomalies and syndromes, since every parent has anxiety and guilt that they have contributed to their child's illness by their habits or genes. Education of the parents that the majority of disabilities are inborn allows the practitioner to allay fears about prior habits or pregnancy exposures. When a disorder is clearly genetic, as in chromosomal disorders like Down syndrome, the cause is often a spontaneous mutation that was not inherited and thus is not the fault of either parent. A key finding of the human genome project is that every individual carries numerous genetic changes that are not inherited (spontaneous mutations), and conveying this information to parents when appropriate is simple and powerful information.

Documenting a family history

Figure 1.1a provides an easily understandable template that can be used by parents or prospective parents to record their family history. An excellent time to present this form is during the prenatal conference with pediatricians and family practitioners, and it can supplement the information already collected during obstetric visits. The history is taken from the perspective of an affected child or patient that has attracted medical attention, but the form could also be used as a general screening measure in pediatrics. The family should be told that the form gives them a template for tracking down necessary information, and that confusion or incomplete information will be clarified by later interview with their health care provider. The family will at least have knowledge of the types of information needed, allowing them to contact informed relatives and gather records preparatory to a more formal pedigree at a later visit.

Figure 1.1b provides a template for health care professionals to convert the family history into a more formal pedigree. Pedigree symbols are listed as a reminder, and the scheme for numbering generations and individuals allows documentation

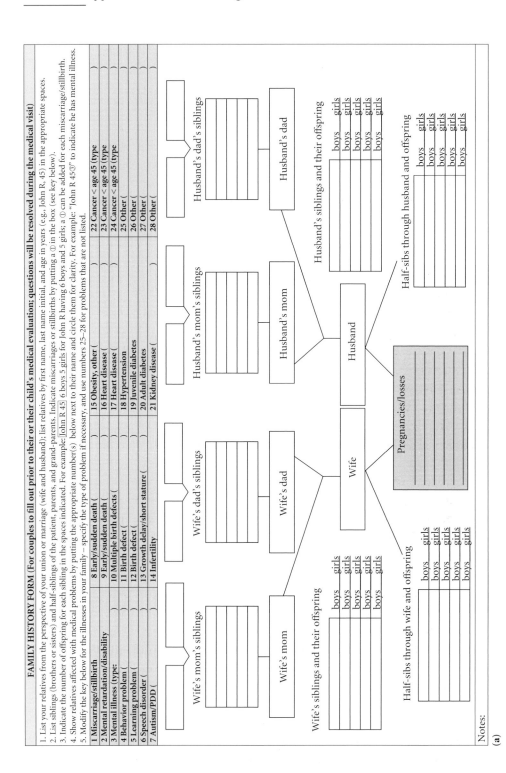

Fig. 1.1   (a) Family history form for patients to fill out.

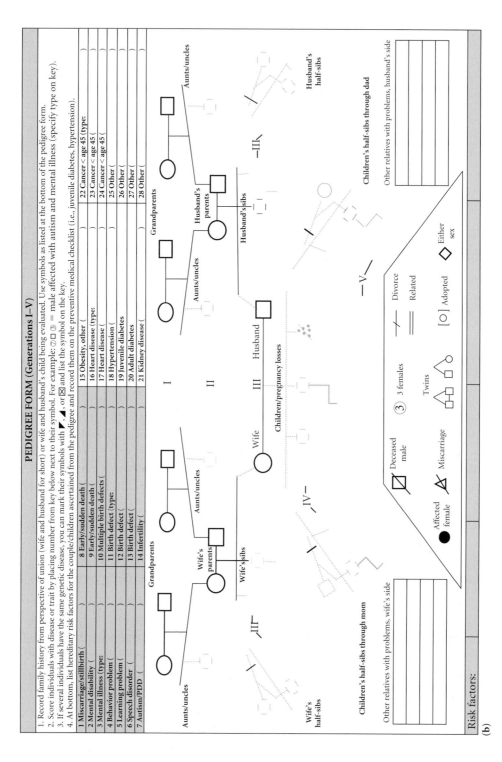

PEDIGREE FORM (Generations I–V)

1. Record family history from perspective of union (wife and husband for short) or wife and husband's child being evaluated. Use symbols as listed at the bottom of the pedigree form.
2. Score individuals with disease or trait by placing number from key next to their symbol. For example: ⊘□ ③ = male affected with autism and mental illness (specify type on key).
3. If several individuals have the same genetic disease, you can mark their symbols with ▼, ▲, or ⊠ and list the symbol on the key.
4. At bottom, list hereditary risk factors for the couple/children ascertained from the pedigree and record them on the preventive medical checklist (i.e., juvenile diabetes, hypertension).

1 Miscarriage/stillbirth (	8 Early/sudden death (	15 Obesity, other (
2 Mental disability (	9 Early/sudden death (	16 Heart disease (type:
3 Mental illness (type:	10 Multiple birth defects (	17 Heart disease (
4 Behavior problem (	11 Birth defect (type:	18 Hypertension (
5 Learning problem (	12 Birth defect (	19 Juvenile diabetes
6 Speech disorder (	13 Birth defect (	20 Adult diabetes
7 Autism/PDD (	14 Infertility (	21 Kidney disease (

22 Cancer < age 45 (type:
23 Cancer < age 45
24 Cancer < age 45 (
25 Other (
26 Other (
27 Other (
28 Other (

Risk factors:

(b)

Fig. 1.1   (b) Pedigree form for health professionals.

of diseases above the diagram without cluttering the body of the pedigree. Health care providers should not focus unduly on the "correctness" of pedigree symbols, and individuals can be numbered as they are discussed during interview rather than worrying about the formal numbering by pedigree position that is listed in textbooks. The template facilitates conversion of family information into a readable and permanent document that is available for all care providers.

Once the pedigree is documented, multiple instances of common diseases like diabetes or heart disease can be recognized and entered on the bottom line as risk factors for the particular child. These risk factors can then be entered on the appropriate preventive checklist for the child, allowing consideration of glucose or blood cholesterol testing in children with positive family histories. These general risk factors are particularly important for children with special health care needs, because co-morbidities can be so devastating for fragile patients. Note that Fig. 1.1b emphasizes cancers with onset before age 45, an arbitrary limit that encourages focus on premature illness rather than common afflictions of the aged. As a general rule, earlier onset and increased severity reflects greater contribution of genes (e.g., juvenile versus adult diabetes mellitus or multifactorial coronary artery disease versus that due to familial hypercholesterolemia).

If a specific genetic disorder like Marfan syndrome is encountered in a pedigree, symbols for the affected individuals can be scored to help with recognition of a particular inheritance pattern. The correlation of pedigree patterns and inheritance mechanisms is discussed below, but this special aspect of family history taking is too-often emphasized and very little used (less than 5% of family histories are positive for a specific genetic disorder even in a genetic specialty practice). Practitioners certainly need to recognize pedigrees with specific medical disorders, but their main and most important role will be to highlight risk factors due to common, multifactorial diseases (see below).

Categories of genetic disease

Hereditary factors are involved in more than 5000 diseases. The hereditary contribution may be partial, as with *multifactorial inheritance* of cleft palate, or major, as with *Mendelian inheritance* of sickle cell anemia. Because they are congenital disorders, malformation syndromes are included within the specialty of pediatric genetics even though many, including fetal alcohol syndrome, are caused by environmental factors. Table 1.1 summarizes the number, frequency, morbidity, and mortality of genetic diseases and syndromes classified according to their mode of inheritance (Wilson, 1990, 1992, 2000). Several studies have suggested that genetic disorders are estimated to account for 15–25% of admissions in a general pediatric hospital. Yoon et al. (1996) reported that 12% of hospital admissions in the states

Table 1.1. Numerology of genetic disease

Category	Number	Frequency (%)	Mortality (%)	Morbidity (%)
Mendelian				
Autosomal dominant	2557	0.7	34	61
Autosomal recessive	1477	0.25	74	87
X-linked	310	0.5	62	85
Multifactorial	>100	3–5	>50	>50
Chromosomal	>100	0.5	95	98
Syndromal	>1000	0.8	>90	98

Source: Wilson (1992, 2000).

of California and South Carolina were related to birth defects and genetic diseases, generating about twice the charges per patient compared to other diseases.

Table 1.2 indicates that patients with genetic diseases come to attention in three ways: those requiring genetic counseling, those with congenital anomalies, and those with metabolic disorders. Each patient category is associated with particular inheritance mechanisms and laboratory evaluations (Table 1.2). Individuals requiring genetic counseling represent the largest category, since genetic diseases can affect any organ system. The patient with cystic fibrosis or the patient with sickle cell anemia is usually not managed by geneticists, but these patients share a need for genetic counseling. Because genetic counseling is frequently a complex process, it will often involve individuals with specialized training. Nevertheless, the key role of practitioners in bringing families to attention mandates that they be aware of risk factors such as the multiple miscarriages, consanguinity, or advanced parental age listed in Table 1.2.

A second category of patients referred for genetic evaluation is the child with congenital anomalies (*dysmorphology*). This category includes children with single anomalies, multiple anomaly syndromes, or chromosomal disorders and accounts for 3–5% of all births. The third category of referral consists of inborn errors of metabolism, which affect an estimated 1 in 600 births. Metabolic disorders may present in the neonatal period, but often become evident in later infancy or childhood when symptoms of episodic illness, visceromegaly, and/or neurodegeneration become evident.

The categories of morphologic and metabolic disease present with different signs and symptoms, and their diagnosis requires different laboratory measurements (Table 1.2). Intrauterine growth retardation and breech presentation frequently accompany congenital malformations and syndromes, as do altered head size, delayed or accelerated growth, and skeletal disproportion. Subtle (minor) anomalies such as epicanthal folds or single palmar creases raise questions of a syndrome pattern, particularly when several are detected. Observation of a surgically or cosmetically

Table 1.2. Categories of pediatric genetic disease

Category	Characteristics	Laboratory evaluations
Genetic counseling	Relative with genetic disorder	DNA testing
	Parental consanguinity	Parental chromosomal studies
	Advanced maternal age (>35 years)	
	Advanced paternal age (>40 years)	
	Multiple miscarriages	
Dysmorphology	Breech presentation	Routine karyotype
	Intrauterine growth retardation	FISH studies
	Major and minor anomalies	Skeletal radiographs
	Microcephaly, macrocephaly	DNA testing
	Skeletal disproportion	
	Developmental and/or growth delay	
	Growth acceleration	
Acute metabolic disease	Lethargy, coma	Blood glucose, ammonia
	Developmental delay, seizures	Blood pH, lactate
	Hypoglycemia, particularly when no ketosis	Blood amino acids
		Blood carnitine
	Acidosis with increased anion gap	Blood acylcarnitine profile
	Lactic acidosis	Urinary ketones
	Neutropenia, thrombocytopenia	Urinary reducing substances
	Unusual odors	Urinary organic acids
Chronic metabolic disease	Hypotonia, seizures,	Skin, liver, muscle biopsy
	Developmental delay, regression	Leukocyte preparations
	Retinal or corneal changes	Enzyme assays
	Visceromegaly	Skeletal radiographs
	Skeletal changes	DNA diagnosis

Note:
FISH: fluorescent *in situ* hybridization.
Source: Wilson (2000).

significant (major) anomaly should always initiate a search for other anomalies, so the different prognoses for children with isolated versus multiple anomalies are correctly assigned. Since the nervous system is affected in at least 55% of hereditary syndromes (Wilson, 1992), developmental delay is also an indication for syndrome evaluation. Chromosomal and skeletal radiographic studies are important laboratory considerations in a child with growth and/or developmental delay.

Inborn errors of metabolism may occasionally present with congenital malformations, but maternal metabolic compensation will usually protect fetal morphogenesis. A common scenario is the normal newborn who becomes irritable, lethargic, and comatose after feeding, often with accelerated physiologic jaundice or unusual odors. Hypoglycemia and acidosis are also frequent accompaniments of metabolic disease, particularly when the hypoglycemia is not combined with the appropriate ketotic response. Other presentations for metabolic disease include visceromegaly, bone marrow suppression, developmental delay or regression, and episodic vomiting or hypoglycemia.

Approach to genetic counseling

Genetic counseling is an educational process that provides individuals with information about a genetic disease and their recurrence risks. To paraphrase its definition by the American Society of Human Genetics, genetic counseling is a communication process which deals with the occurrence, or the risk of occurrence, of a genetic disorder in a family. During this communication process, appropriately trained individuals assist the family to understand:

1 the diagnosis and management options for the disorder;
2 the contribution of heredity to the disorder and how this translates to recurrence risks among family members;
3 the alternatives (i.e., prenatal diagnosis) for dealing with these recurrence risks.

The counseling process should also assist the family choose a course of action based on their particular family goals or ethical/religious background and to make the best possible adjustment to the presence and future implications of a genetic disorder.

The need for genetic counseling often arises from a family history, which should be part of every medical evaluation. A pedigree is simply a codified family history, with generations, individuals, and the presenting patient (*proband* or *propositus*) diagrammed in a standard format as discussed above regarding the template in Fig. 1.1. Numbering of the generations (Roman numerals) and individuals (Arabic numerals) facilitates documentation of a clear pedigree diagram.

Once a pedigree is constructed, inheritance mechanisms are often evident from the pattern of affected individuals (Fig. 1.2). Autosomal dominant or X-linked inheritance often exhibits a vertical inheritance pattern, with male-to-male transmission ruling out the possibility of X-linked inheritance. Horizontal patterns of affected individuals (i.e., siblings) suggest the operation of autosomal recessive inheritance, and this mechanism is sometimes made more plausible by parental consanguinity (inbreeding).

In order to begin the process of genetic counseling, the physician must document the family history, inspect the pedigree for evidence of inherited diseases, and understand the genetic risks implied by particular inheritance mechanisms. The Online Mendelian Inheritance in Man database (www.ncbi.nlm.nih.gov/entrez) provides a useful resource for deciding which, if any, inheritance mechanism has

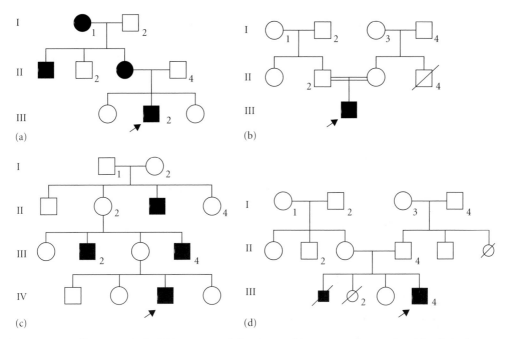

Fig. 1.2   Pedigrees typical of (a) autosomal dominant; (b) autosomal recessive; (c) X-linked recessive; and (d) chromosomal inheritance displaying symbols for males (squares), females (circles), affected individuals (filled symbols), consanguinity or inbreeding (double line), abortions (small symbols), death (diagonal line), and individuals coming to medical attention (arrows).

been established for a pediatric disease. Since diseases may exhibit genetic heterogeneity with several possible inheritance mechanisms (e.g., Charcot–Marie–Tooth disease, retinitis pigmentosa, cleft palate), referral to a genetic specialist is often necessary for accurate genetic counseling. Practitioners can then review this specialty counseling with the family, utilizing their rapport and knowledge of the family to place the genetic information in context.

It is important to avoid a judgmental attitude towards reproductive options or disabilities, since overly negative portrayals of disorders such as Down syndrome can rupture the parent–physician relationship. In the case of prenatal diagnosis, anticipation, adoption or foster care should be mentioned as alternatives to abortion. Parent support groups are very useful in arranging contact with affected individuals so at-risk families can become familiar with disease manifestations.

For a growing number of diseases, genetic counseling can include the provision of DNA diagnosis for at-risk family members. Some understanding of the methods and requirements for DNA diagnosis are useful for practitioners, and these are summarized below. It is important that pediatricians be attuned to genetic risks in parents (or other relatives) that result from a child's diagnosis.

Table 1.3. Types of congenital anomalies

Category	Subcategory	Definition	Example
Isolated defects			
Normal variant		Present in >4% of population, not abnormal	Mongolian spot
Anomaly		Deviation from expected or average type in structure, form and/or function which is interpreted as abnormal	
	Major anomaly	Anomaly of surgical or cosmetic consequence	Cleft palate
	Minor anomaly	Little impact on individual well-being	Bifid uvula
	Malformation	Morphological defect resulting from an intrinsically abnormal developmental process	Radial aplasia
	Sequence	Pattern of anomalies derived from a single known or presumed prior anomaly or mechanical factor	Robin sequence
Multiple defects	Syndrome	Multiple anomalies thought to be pathogenetically related and not representing a sequence	Zellweger syndrome
	Association	Non-random occurrence in one or more individuals of several morphologic defects not identified as a sequence or syndrome	VATER association

Note:

VATER: *V*ertebral, *A*norectal, *c*ardiac, *T*racheo-*E*sophageal, *R*enal.

Diagnostic approach to the child with congenital anomalies

The term dysmorphology literally means painful or abnormal shape, and its presence orients the physician toward abnormalities of embryonic and fetal development. Until better laboratory measures of morphogenesis are available, the physical examination is paramount in the evaluation of children with congenital anomalies. The recognition of subtle anomalies often guides the diagnostic and management plan.

Table 1.3 summarizes the categories of single and multiple anomaly disorders (Opitz & Wilson, 1997). As emphasized previously, isolated anomalies (cleft palate, spina bifida) affect a single body region and commonly are associated with multifactorial determination. When a child has multiple anomalies affecting different organ systems, the underlying cause is more likely to involve chromosomal or Mendelian disease. Genetic causation is, particularly, likely if the pattern of minor and major anomalies is associated with the recognizable facial appearance that characterizes a *syndrome*. Although exceptions such as the fetal alcohol syndrome certainly occur, more than 75% of the syndromes listed in Jones (1997) are due to Mendelian or chromosomal disease.

The first principle of evaluation is to ask whether a child has a single or multiple anomalies. Children with isolated anomalies will usually have normal mental development (unless the anomaly involves the brain), while the child with multiple congenital anomalies is at high risk for mental disability. Single anomalies such as cleft palate, pyloric stenosis, congenital heart disease, or congenital hip dislocation are usually amenable to surgical correction and imply a low (2–3%) recurrence risk for parents. When several anomalies occur together, concern about a syndrome will mandate consideration of a karyotype and/or skeletal radiologic survey; imaging studies to search for anomalies of the brain, heart, and kidneys; and a complex preventive management plan that includes the possibility of mental disability. Even when the family history is unremarkable, malformation syndromes often result from mendelian or chromosomal inheritance that mandates referral for genetic evaluation and counseling.

Isolated congenital anomalies

Every health professional must learn to distinguish anomalies from family or racial characteristics that have no medical significance. *Normal variants*, such as the lumbar Mongolian spot or the aural (Darwinian) tubercle, are sometimes distinguished by their occurrence in more than 4% of the population (Table 1.3; Opitz & Wilson, 1997). *Major anomalies* are those with cosmetic or surgical consequences (e.g., cleft palate, atrial septal defect, malformed pinna). *Minor anomalies*, despite their diagnostic significance, occur in less than 4% of individuals and have little impact on well-being (e.g., epicanthal fold, single palmar crease, fifth finger clinodactyly, shawl scrotum). A scoresheet is available for >90 common minor anomalies that may be recognized during the physical examination (Opitz & Wilson, 1997). The presence of 3 or more minor anomalies should arouse suspicion of a syndrome; multiple minor anomalies also confer increased risk for a major anomaly. In children with Down syndrome, minor anomalies of the face and hands (e.g., epicanthal folds, upslanting palpebral fissures, flattened facial profile, single palmar crease) often alert the physician before signs or symptoms of major anomalies (e.g., cardiac defects) become manifest. The detection of minor anomalies is thus an integral part of the genetic examination, allowing the child with a surgically correctable major anomaly to be distinguished from the child with a complex multiple anomaly syndrome.

Because the developing embryo has a dynamic anatomy, an isolated embryonic anomaly may lead to several abnormalities in the infant. A *sequence* represents a cascade of secondary events that derive from a primary anomaly. Sequences, like isolated anomalies, are usually associated with sporadic occurrence or multifactorial determination. Examples include spina bifida sequence with lower limb hypoplasia and club feet; Pierre Robin sequence with small jaw, protruding tongue, and posterior cleft palate; or Potter sequence with facial changes, limb contractures, lung hypoplasia, and oligohydramnios due to renal agenesis. The key is to recognize that the several consequences of a sequence are related to a single cause; that, like isolated anomalies, they have a lower risk for mental disability or genetic etiology.

Congenital anomaly patterns

When several minor anomalies are recognized, the probability of major defects and of a syndrome is increased. Minor anomalies also help to distinguish syndromes from *associations*, which are groups of major defects thought to derive from a brief period of embryonic injury. Associations, like sequences and isolated anomalies, will generally have lower genetic risks than syndromes.

Syndromes (literally, running together) are patterns of major and minor anomalies that relate to a single cause. In many cases, the cause is unknown. Malformation syndromes are exemplified by disorders such as Goldenhar syndrome, which involves multiple orofacial, cardiac, limb, and vertebral malformations. Note the involvement of several embryologically independent regions in a syndrome (eye, ear, heart, vertebrae, thumb) in contrast to the localized branchial arch error involving ear and jaw in hemifacial microsomia sequence.

Associations consist of major anomalies with similar embryologic timing. The *VATER* association of *V*ertebral, *A*norectal, *T*racheo-*E*sophageal, *R*adial, and *R*enal defects involves mesodermal derivatives that begin differentiation at 20–25 days of embryogenesis (see Chapter 5). Associations usually lack minor anomalies, since there is no persistent influence like an extra chromosome to produce subtle alterations throughout gestation. As a result, individuals with associations do not have a characteristic facial appearance. For associations, identification of a characteristic anomaly stimulates a search for others; for syndromes, facial recognition often prompts evaluation for the characteristic anomaly pattern. In a child with a normal facial appearance, radial aplasia with tracheo-esophageal atresia should prompt concern for associated renal defects that occur in the VATER association. If the craniofacies is abnormal with a prominent occiput and malformed ears, the child should have chromosome studies to evaluate the possibility of trisomy 18 syndrome. Suspicion of the more devastating syndrome requires attention to minor anomalies of the face, ears, chest, hands, and feet; recognition of the trisomy 18 phenotype will then prompt imaging studies to search for major anomalies of the brain, heart, and kidneys.

Diagnostic approach to the child with metabolic disease

Despite the number and variety of metabolic disorders, consideration of the age of onset and the presenting manifestations (Table 1.4) allows a systematic approach to diagnosis. As with other categories of genetic disease, the complexity of laboratory tests and therapies will require the involvement of metabolic disease specialists. However, it is again the primary health care professional that must recognize the initial symptoms. For purposes of recognition, the metabolic disease category

Table 1.4. Presentations of metabolic disease

Presentation	Disease examples	Laboratory abnormalities
Small-molecule diseases		
Lethargy, coma, alkalosis, tachypnea	Urea cycle disorders	Elevated ammonia, abnormal amino acid screen (e.g., elevated glutamine)
Hypoglycemia, lethargy, coma, acidosis	Organic acidemias	Anion gap, low pH, hypoglycemia, abnormal organic acid screen (e.g., methyl malonate)
	Maple syrup urine disease	Abnormal amino acid screen (elevated leucine, isoleucine, valine), abnormal organic acid screen (elevated ketoacids)
Sepsis, hepatic disease, hepatomegaly	Galactosemia	Urine reducing substances
Hypoglycemia, hepatic disease, hepatomegaly	Tyrosinemia	Abnormal amino acid screen (tyrosine), elevated serum succinylacetone
Hypoglycemia ± hepatic disease, hepatomegaly	Fatty acid oxidation disorder	Decreased serum carnitine, abnormal organic acid screen (e.g., dicarboxylic acids), abnormal acylcarnitine profile (e.g., dicarboxoyl carnitine)
Developmental delay, seizures	Phenylketonuria	Abnormal amino acid screen (phenylalanine)
Large-molecule diseases		
Hypoglycemia, hepatic disease, hepatomegaly	Glycogenoses	Hyperuricemia, hyperlipidemia, glycogen on liver biopsy
Developmental regression, seizures ± hepatomegaly	Neurolipidoses	Stored substances in retina, brain, leukocytes, liver biopsy
Developmental regression, dysotosis, hepatomegaly	Mucopolysaccharidoses	Stored substances in brain, leukocytes

can be divided into acute disorders, involving smaller molecules with rapid turnover, and chronic disorders, involving larger molecules with slow turnover (e.g., *storage diseases*). This classification is of course oversimplified, and a more detailed summary of algorithms for metabolic disease can be found in the chapter by Saudubray & Carpentier in Scriver et al. (2001). Since metabolic disorders almost always exhibit autosomal- or X-linked-recessive inheritance, the family history may be helpful in showing consanguinity or siblings with deaths in early childhood. Special laboratory evaluations are also implied for acute versus chronic metabolic diseases, and a definitive diagnosis has the added value of allowing prenatal diagnosis.

Acute metabolic disorders

The metabolic pathways responsible for the interconversion of small molecules are crucial as sources of energy and building blocks for the organism. Amino acids, sugars, fatty acids, and nucleotides are examples of small molecules that are inter-converted by enzyme action to form intracellular networks that are much like a highway interchange; when an enzyme is missing due to a genetic mutation, the proximate molecules (substrates) accumulate and the distal molecules (products) are deficient. Diseases result from these accumulations and/or deficiencies, and from the diversion of substrates into alternative pathways.

Because of rapid interconversion and turnover, small-molecule diseases tend to be acute or episodic in presentation, with hypoglycemia, acidosis, anion gap, or unusual odors, as summarized in Table 1.4. These features contrast with large-molecule diseases, in which protein, carbohydrate, or lipid polymers cannot be catabolized and slowly accumulate in affected tissues. Acute metabolic diseases are not covered in this book because the frequency of specialist involvement and the need for dietary modifications are not easily summarized using the checklist approach. Several of these disorders allow true primary prevention, where disease is eliminated by avoidance of offending metabolites. Large-molecule (storage) dis-orders often have a chronic onset with symptoms such as neurodegeneration and/or hepatosplenomegaly. These more chronic and incurable disorders do require sec-ondary or tertiary preventive management to minimize their complications. Chapter 19 deals with the management of chronic metabolic disorders.

When a child presents with catastrophic illness, the clinician should first con-sider toxic or infectious etiologies. Toxicants such as ethylene glycol or sepsis that causes cardiorespiratory failure can present with severe acidosis and an anion gap. If toxicants are ruled out by history or urine screen, and if the symptoms seem out of proportion to the fever or possible infectious source, then a metabolic etiology should be considered. Routine evaluation of acutely ill children will usually pro-vide a complete blood count together with serum glucose, electrolytes, pH, lactic acid, and hepatic transaminase values. Extending the testing to detect most meta-bolic diseases involving small molecules will require four additional tests: blood ammonia, blood amino acids, urine organic acids, and urine for reducing sub-stances. If a fatty acid oxidation disorder is suspected, then a serum carnitine and acylcarnitine profile should be obtained.

Several categories of acute metabolic diseases will be evident from the initial panel of laboratory tests (Tables 1.2 and 1.4). Marked elevations of blood ammonia in a child with lethargy, coma, and mild alkalosis/tachypnea suggest a urea cycle disorder, although transient hyperammonemia of the newborn can occur. A large anion gap with acidosis is suggestive of an organic acidemia. Examples include methylmalonic or propionic acidemia, which often manifest neutropenia due to bone marrow suppression. Because intermediary metabolism is a network of inter-conversions, urea cycle disorders will have elevations of certain amino acids (e.g., citrulline, ornithine, glutamine, lysine) and certain organic acidemias will have elevated blood ammonia. Hypoglycemia can also occur in methylmalonic or propionic acidemia, but often suggests a disorder of carbohydrate metabolism like galactosemia. Patients with galactosemia will have reducing substances in the urine. Certain disorders with hypoglycemia (e.g., galactosemia), aminoacidemia (e.g., tyrosinemia), or disorders of fatty acid oxidation (e.g., medium chain coenzyme A dehydrogenase deficiency) may present with hepatic disease.

Some children with accumulation of small molecules will not have acute presentations. Classical phenylketonuria is an example where symptoms are minimal until substantial neurologic damage occurs. Organellar diseases involving the peroxisomes or mitochrondria are also intermediate in this classification; they may be associated with lactic acidosis or hepatic disease, but usually have an indolent presentation (see Chapter 19). On the other hand, disorders involving large molecules like the glycogen storage diseases may have an acute presentation because of limited availability of substrate. The inability to degrade glycogen can produce hypoglycemia with seizures and acidosis (Table 1.4). These exceptions emphasize that categorization into small- and large-molecule disorders offers a simplistic approach that must be refined for actual patients.

The clinical goal for children with acute metabolic illness is to stabilize them by treating the acidosis, hypoglycemia, coagulopathies, and/or sepsis until the definitive results of blood amino acids and urine organic acids are available. Children with hyperammonemia or large elevations of organic acids may require peritoneal or hemodialysis for successful therapy, although pharmacologic treatment can reduce milder elevations of ammonia. Once stabilized, the definitive metabolic diagnosis can be made through enzyme assay of leukocytes, cultured fibroblasts, or biopsied liver. A few disorders can be diagnosed specifically by amino acid or organic acid profile (e.g., phenylketonuria), but most require confirmatory demonstration of an enzyme deficiency. Another general characteristic of small-molecule disorders is that they often can be treated by vitamin supplementation or dietary modifications. The diagnosis of disorders such as phenylketonuria or galactosemia not only allows the anticipation and prevention of neurosensory problems, but also dramatically alters the clinical course through dietary therapy.

Disorders involving large molecules

The prototypes for large-molecule disorders are enzyme deficiencies that cause accumulation of polymers in affected tissues. These "storage diseases" are usually more chronic in onset and less susceptible to dietary modification than disorders of small-molecule metabolism. Examples include the glycogen storage diseases, neurolipidoses, and mucopolysaccharidoses (Table 1.4). Instead of acute alterations in amino acid or organic acid profiles, large-molecule disorders are categorized by examination of brain, retina, liver, leukocytes, bone marrow, and/or skeleton for evidence of storage. Recognition of the retinal cherry red spot in Tay–Sachs disease, bone marrow foam cells in Gaucher disease, or leukocyte granules in Hurler disease leads to confirmatory studies such as brain or skeletal imaging. The definitive diagnosis again rests on the demonstration of a specific enzyme deficiency using leukocytes, fibroblasts, or liver. Although dietary therapy is rarely available (continuous starch feedings for glycogenoses being an exception), diagnosis of a storage disease often leads to important preventive measures such as screening for hydrocephalus in the mucopolysaccharidoses (see Chapter 19).

The laboratory diagnosis of genetic/metabolic disease

The direct diagnosis of genetic disease using chromosomal, DNA, or enzyme analysis provides the most reliable information for genetic counseling. In thinking about genetic laboratory diagnosis, it is important to conceive of a typical cell with its large and small molecules in the cytoplasm and chromosomes in the nucleus. Chromosomal analysis (karyotyping) examines the chromosomes for numerical or structural alterations, while DNA analysis examines the structure of a specific gene on one of the 23 chromosome pairs. Metabolic testing examines the protein product of a specific gene by enzyme/antibody assay or, less precisely, by measuring altered metabolite levels that are created by enzyme deficiency. An advantage of DNA diagnosis is the ability to detect mutant alleles in all cell types, while assay of specific tissues may be required for the demonstration of protein or enzyme deficiency. If the diagnostic change in chromosomal, DNA, or enzyme analysis is detectable in amniotic or chorionic villus cells, then prenatal diagnosis can be offered to the at-risk couple.

For couples with multiple miscarriages, or children with a dysmorphic appearance and developmental delay, a chromosomal study or *karyotype* should be considered (Table 1.2). A routine karyotype demonstrates the number of chromosomes in peripheral blood leukocytes, and allows inspection of the paired metaphase chromosomes for rearrangements. Standard *cytogenetic notation* describes the karyotype in terms of total chromosome number (typically 46), the type of sex chromosomes (typically XX or XY), and particular abnormalities relative to landmarks (light and dark *bands*). The chromosomal bands are designated by their location on the short (*p*) or long (*q*) chromosome arms and given consecutive numbers according to their distance from the centromere (e.g., band 15q11 on the chromosome 15 long arm or band 6p21 on the chromosome 6 short arm). Notation such as 47,XX+21 then describes altered chromosome number in a female with Down syndrome, and 46,XY,del(5)(5p14) describes a deletion of chromosome 5 extending to band p14 on the short arm in a male with cri-du-chat syndrome.

Although routine chromosomal analysis is an excellent screening test in children with dysmorphology or developmental delay, fluorescent *in situ* hybridization

(*FISH*) technology allows the search of specific chromosome regions for subtle rearrangements. Small deletions in disorders such as Williams syndrome (chromosome 7q deletion), Prader–Willi syndrome (chromosome 15q deletion), or Shprintzen syndromes (chromosome 22q deletion) are diagnostic if the characteristic alteration is suspected and probed (see Chapter 9). FISH technology has largely replaced prometaphase analysis in which high resolution chromosome banding patterns were produced by arrest in early metaphase.

Because genes are segments of chromosomal DNA analogous to beads on a string, radioactive or fluorescent DNA probes can be designed to distinguish normal from abnormal alleles based on altered *DNA sequences*. DNA diagnostic testing is specific for the disorder in question (e.g., sickle cell anemia), since probes must be targeted to a particular genetic locus (e.g., the A or S β-globin gene alleles). Limitations of DNA diagnosis include disorders where every abnormal allele is different (e.g., Marfan syndrome), single gene disorders where the causative gene has not been identified or isolated (e.g., autosomal recessive Bardet–Biedl syndrome), or polygenic disorders involving environmental and genetic factors (e.g., diabetes mellitus). For many multifactorial diseases (e.g., diabetes mellitus, coronary artery disease, schizophrenia, Alzheimer disease) DNA analysis of family members allows the identification of predisposing alleles with risk modification. The involvement of genetic specialists and DNA diagnostic laboratories is often required in the planning of DNA diagnostic studies, since the selection of at-risk family members and the interpretation of results may be quite complex.

The fragile X syndrome is an example of a disorder where DNA analysis is definitive, but complex to interpret. Like Huntington chorea, Friedreich ataxia, and Steinert myotonic dystrophy, fragile X syndrome is caused by the expansion of DNA regions composed of trinucleotide repeating units. The fragile X syndrome was first correlated with a site on the X chromosome that appeared broken or fragile in affected males, then with DNA instability of gene at that site. Fragile X syndrome is also unusual in that female carriers may have altered behavior and mental disability despite moderate expansion of triplet repeating units on one X chromosome. DNA analysis is thus required for female carriers, since their clinical severity and their risk for severely affected sons can be predicted by documenting the extent of triplet repeat expansion. Fragile X syndrome illustrates the power and complexity of DNA diagnosis, and emphasizes the need for genetic referral when single gene disorders are recognized.

While DNA testing is available for some inborn errors of metabolism, laboratory diagnosis usually involves products of the abnormal allele (e.g., enzyme assay) or metabolites that accumulate as a result of enzyme deficiency. Acute metabolic disorders often present with alterations of blood electrolyte, pH, glucose, ammonia, or lactate levels as listed in Table 1.2, while the more chronic storage diseases present with organ enlargement, progressive brain dysfunction, and the accumulation of polymers in affected tissues. The goal is to characterize the abnormal metabolites in plasma, urine, or affected tissues, which will in turn guide selection of the gene or enzyme to be tested. Participation of a metabolic disease specialist in the initial diagnostic evaluation is strongly recommended for interpretation of complex laboratory results (e.g., urine organic acid profiles). After recognition, referral, and diagnosis, the primary physician assumes an important role by ensuring dietary compliance or coordinating the preventive management program.

2

Providing a primary care medical home for the child with a developmental disability

Health care providers in the primary care medical home are uniquely positioned to identify and initially evaluate developmental differences in young children. They are familiar with aspects of the family history and with psychosocial factors that may place a child at higher risk for developmental delay. Primary health care providers are aware of birth events and usually provide for the care of newborns. For those developmental disabilities that are identifiable prenatally or at birth or that result from perinatal complications, early detection is possible. Finally, and most important, the primary care medical home provides a headquarters for longitudinal anticipatory care during which alterations in developmental course can be recognized, investigated, and managed. For most parents, the primary care physician is the first and most trusted respondent to their worries or concerns about their young child's development. It is important that all primary care physicians feel comfortable with this responsibility, confident in their skills at developmental surveillance and screening, clear about the resources for intervention and further evaluation, and knowledgeable about management, care coordination and advocacy.

This chapter provides an overview of the approach to the child with a developmental delay or disability from the perspective of the primary care medical home. Taking a generic approach that is intended to complement the specific guidelines of other chapters, we review the epidemiology of developmental disabilities. Developmental screening in the medical home is discussed, with guidelines for referral to community-based agencies and for further medical evaluation. The adaptation of families to developmental difference in their children is discussed with reference to the facilitating role that primary health care providers may play in that adjustment. Finally, the concept of *Chronic Condition Management* (CCM) in primary care is introduced to clarify the important but often underemphasized ways in which primary health care providers complement specialists in the long-term co-management of children with developmental disabilities. Further information about the medical home model of care and tools for its implementation are available at: www.medicalhomeimprovement.org

Definitions and epidemiology

Estimates of the incidence of developmental disabilities, like those of chronic illnesses in children, vary depending on the definitions used and the method of ascertainment. Epidemiologic data can be derived from population surveys like the National Health Interview Survey conducted by the National Center for Health Statistics, in which a random selection of households are surveyed, providing information about over 17,000 children (Boyle et al., 1994). Case registries provide more categorical data, but are limited to the range of data sources used by the registry and the timing of registration. Registries that focus on birth and neonatal information may not detect developmental disabilities that become apparent later in the life cycle, and those that focus on identifiable conditions (e.g., birth defects registries) may not include children with developmental delays of unknown cause. Finally, administrative ascertainment data reflect the number of children receiving disability-related services, such as special education, early intervention, or financial benefits (e.g., Supplemental Security Income, SSI). Obviously, such data will include only those children who apply and are then found eligible for the service under study.

Estimates of the incidence of developmental disabilities in children range from 5% to 20%. When higher-prevalence, lower-severity conditions such as speech and language disorders and learning disabilities are included, estimates approach 20%, while a focus on conditions of higher severity shifts the rate toward 3–5%. The World Health Organization estimates the incidence world-wide at around 15–20%, while the National Health Interview Survey data based on parent interviews in the United States suggest a rate of 17% (Lipkin, 1991; Boyle et al., 1994). More recently, the National Survey of Children with Special Health Care Needs identified 12.7% of children in the United States (Strickland et al., 2004). Figures for enrollment in special education services show wide variability from state to state, but provide a national average of about 10% (Ayers, 1994). Most special education services are for learning disabilities, speech, and attentional-behavioral disabilities.

When the focus shifts to specific conditions, each of the identifiable developmental disabilities (except for learning disabilities and attention deficit/hyperactivity disorder) is relatively rare. Though the "bell-shaped curve" for intelligence would predict a 2.5% incidence of mental retardation in the population, actual population data suggest a rate closer to 1% (Munro, 1986). Cerebral palsy occurs in 0.25–0.4% of children, while developmental language disorders affect up to 5%. The incidence of autism spectrum disorders seems to have increased in the past decade with as many as 1 in 200 children affected (Committee on children with disabilities, 2001). Though most developmental disabilities have a similar incidence across ethnic groups and national boundaries, the rates for some vary inversely with income. Males significantly outnumber females for many developmental disabilities, including mental retardation, autism, and attentional disorders. This sex difference suggests sex-linked genetic mechanisms, ascertainment biases, or enhanced vulnerability of males to adverse developmental sequellae when exposed to biological or psychosocial risk factors.

Of major importance is the distinction of developmental disabilities from those that occur in adult life as a result of trauma, stroke, or aging. Developmental disability refers to a long-term impairment in the ability to perform or achieve age-appropriate skills in one or more areas that has its onset prenatally or during the developmental years. By definition, developmental disabilities involve families that require a wide range of supports, services, and professional disciplines, all with varied objectives and definitions of "developmental disability." These variable definitions, services, and outcome goals may cause confusion among families and professionals.

Another distinction in the definition of developmental disabilities has been between a categorical and a functional approach. The former fits within a traditional medical model and, for many years, was used to identify individuals eligible for a variety of services and supports. Categories such as mental retardation, cerebral palsy, sensory impairment, autism, learning disability, and language disorder are familiar chapter or section headings in pediatric textbooks and on benefit application forms. In the early 1980s, the federal government's Administration on Developmental Disabilities adopted a functional definition in which individuals must manifest impairments in at least three of seven functional categories with onset before age 22 years in order to be developmentally disabled. This definition is used in many states to determine eligibility for some non-medical benefits for people with developmental disabilities such as family support services. More recently, new SSI regulations for children require that the determination of eligibility of children for SSI benefits include an individual functional assessment if the child was not found eligible on a categorical basis. These changes reflect the fact that many children who experience obvious developmental disability do not have an identifiable cause or specific diagnosis.

What are the causes of developmental disabilities? Unlike the major chronic illnesses of adult life, the chronic disabling conditions affecting children are often rare. The more severe disorders such as Down syndrome, fragile X syndrome, or cerebral palsy are rare enough that an individual primary care physician may follow only one or two affected children at any time. More common conditions such as borderline cognitive disability or attention deficit disorder will be more familiar to practitioners, but are less likely to be associated with definitive diagnostic tests or etiologies. Given uncertainties of diagnosis and the bias of referral selection, the experience of a tertiary-based developmental evaluation clinic can be summarized as follows (Munro, 1986; Lipkin, 1991; Boyle et al., 1994):

1 Prenatal events are responsible for nearly half of developmental disabilities with genetic and teratogenic factors influencing up to one-third.

2 20% of developmental disabilities were felt to have stemmed from environmental/behavioral influences in which the biologic effect on etiology was absent or of less apparent importance.

3 One-third of children with developmental disability referred for evaluation to a tertiary center remained without a specific diagnosis.

Screening and identification of developmental disorders in the primary care medical home

Responding to the newborn with a condition causing development disability

Some conditions associated with developmental disabilities are recognized at birth based on the presence of birth defects or physical features that characterize a specific syndrome or condition or through routine newborn screening tests. Down syndrome, cleft lip/palate, and spina bifida, which are usually identified in the newborn period, are classic examples. In addition, children with adverse perinatal events (complications of prematurity or low birth weight, asphyxia, or infections) may have obvious early neurologic impairments or may be identified as being at "high risk" for later developmental delays. In these instances of very early identification of developmental concerns, the primary care physician has a series of responsibilities and opportunities to foster optimal outcomes for the child and the family.

Once a disabling condition is recognized (e.g., Down syndrome or evidence of neurologic impairment via seizures, abnormal tone, hydrocephalus), the primary health care provider may be responsible for conveying this news to the parents. Health care providers have learned a great deal in the past decade about how this news should be shared. Though nothing can turn bad news into good, it is possible for the process to help parents to a good start toward adaptation instead of prolonging their recovery from shock or grief. This process of breaking news should be regarded as an active one of empowering parents in the care of their new child in the face of events that have occurred beyond their control. Table 2.1 provides some guidelines about informing parents of diagnoses that were developed from surveys of parents regarding their satisfaction with the process.

In one study, when these simple steps were implemented, parental satisfaction with "how they were told" improved from about 25% to 100% (Cunningham et al., 1984). Informing parents of a diagnosis of disability in their child is not so much a single event as an ongoing process. Initial office visits may need to be more frequent to help support parents through this time and ensure their successful adaptation. They will need access to accurate, comprehensible information that addresses both the challenges ahead and the reasons for hope. The primary physician can aid optimism by listening, emphasizing positive aspects of the child (e.g., the child is

Table 2.1. Recommended techniques for informing parents of the diagnosis of Down syndrome in their child

Parents should be informed:
1 By someone with sufficient knowledge to inspire credibility
2 As soon as possible
3 With both parents together, if possible
4 With the baby present, if possible; refer to the baby by name
5 In a private, comfortable place; away from disturbances; with a minimal audience
6 In a straightforward manner, using understandable language; allow time for questions
7 With a balanced point of view; state something positive instead of a catalogue of problems
8 With follow-up discussion arranged, including a telephone number for more information
9 Followed by uninterrupted time in a private place for parents and child to be alone together

Source: Cunningham et al. (1984).

a child first with assets as well as challenges), and prioritizing supports. Most parents indicate an interest in meeting other parents who have children with the same or similar conditions. These parent-to-parent contacts can be arranged informally with other families in the same primary care practice or through parent advocacy or regional parent-to-parent organizations. Parents might also be encouraged to join regional and national organizations for families who have children with specific conditions. These organizations provide access to information, facilitate contact with other families, and often produce informative newsletters and conferences. Primary care practices should refer parents to appropriate organizations through the annual resource guide of *Exceptional Parent* magazine (www.eparent.com/) or the Alliance of Genetic Support Groups (www.geneticalliance.org/). Many parent support groups now have home pages on the Internet that can be found through standard search engines. Parent support groups provide an enormous, if undistilled, source of information for both parents and professionals.

A recent scenario is the prenatal diagnosis of a birth defect or condition associated with developmental disability. Though the majority of prenatal tests for genetic conditions involve parents who plan to terminate the pregnancy in the event of an abnormal finding, some parents use such tests as information about the status of their child-to-be and plan to continue the pregnancy regardless of the result. When such parents are found to have a fetus affected by Down syndrome or spina bifida, they require the same attentive, careful "news breaking" as the parents of newborns. They may wish to meet other parents who have made the same decision to continue a pregnancy, and they usually will want the same access to information as the parents of an affected newborn. There may be further information about the fetus that will allow the anticipation of additional medical needs or assist planning for the delivery (e.g., looking for congenital heart disease or bowel anomalies in a fetus with Down syndrome or planning a Cesarean delivery for a child with spina bifida). Such parents may be able to prepare family and friends for the arrival of a child with challenges, allowing them to be more supportive and helpful at the time of birth.

All children who have a specific condition that is likely to cause developmental delay or disability (as well as all children simply found to be delayed, but without a diagnosis) should be referred to early intervention services (Majnemer, 1998). All states in the United States currently receive federal funding to provide early intervention services for children with established conditions causing developmental delays or with documented delays, but no specific diagnosis. Some states also provide these services for children who meet "at risk" criteria established by the state, but who are not yet experiencing delays. Many early intervention services are provided through regular home visits by early childhood professionals, though some programs offer "center-based" services in addition to or instead of home visits. Since the passage of the Individuals with Disabilities Education Act (IDEA) in 1986 and several revisions since, early intervention services have been an entitlement for eligible children. Early intervention services have used a family-centered model in which parents are actively involved in the planning and implementation of interventions. Though most early intervention programs include therapeutic services such as physical and speech therapy, they also provide "family support services" such as help with coordinating care, access to information, assistance with applications for benefits, transportation, and respite care. Physicians should not attempt to judge which children with disabling conditions or developmental delays in their practice should be referred, but should simply offer referral to all. The early intervention providers and parents will go through a process of evaluation and develop an Individual Family Service Plan (IFSP) once the referral is made. Involvement of the primary care physician and input into the IFSP process are usually welcome, though busy schedules and lack of reimbursement sometimes make such participation difficult.

In addition to making appropriate referrals, primary care physicians serve two important quality monitoring functions. First, they can make sure that the system is responsive to families with cerebral palsy, Down syndrome, spina bifida, epilepsy, failure to thrive, and technology dependence. Second, they can emphasize that developmental goals must have a whole child perspective with learning through play, exploration, and quality social interaction as the key programmatic components.

Finally, primary health care providers need to be aware of and respond to the condition-specific health care needs associated with specific diagnoses. To a large measure, this book is intended to provide guidelines for the specific primary and specialty care needs of children with genetic and prenatally determined conditions. Generally, it is important for primary care providers to know that many genetic conditions place an affected child at risk for other medical complications, some of which are preventable and some of which will require specific interventions.

Developmental surveillance and screening in the medical home

When prenatal or neonatal diagnosis of a genetic cause of developmental disability is not possible, suspicions usually emerge during the course of well-child care visits or when a change in health suggests an underlying condition that was not previously recognized. Such physical findings as alterations in muscle tone, movement, or reflexes, failure to grow, small or large head circumference, the presence or emergence of skin lesions, impairment of vision, or enlargement of liver and spleen may be clues to an underlying, identifiable syndrome or condition. When such findings are combined with developmental delays, the likelihood of a specific diagnosis increases.

In the majority of children with developmental disabilities, the first clues are delays in expected developmental progress. What constitutes the best approach to developmental screening in primary care is a subject of ongoing debate (Meisels, 1989). Nevertheless, every primary health care provider or agency should have a set of policies and practices aimed at the early identification of developmental delay and the initiation of appropriate interventions. Developmental screening is most effective when it is an ongoing process permeating various aspects of primary care. In this respect, the British experience with "developmental surveillance" is worth reviewing for its success in identifying children and its emphasis that every encounter is an opportunity to consider developmental issues (Dworkin, 1989).

Among the most reliable developmental screening tools is parental concern. When compared with a variety of more formal developmental screening tools, parental opinions or worries have a comparable degree of specificity and sensitivity (Glascoe & Dworkin, 1995). However, there is a temptation for clinicians to dismiss parents' concerns as the products of an anxious imagination or ignorance. Studies suggest that such an attitude is fraught with the risk of future recrimination for postponing the investigation of or intervention for a valid concern. Additional screening information is contained in the child and family's history in the form of "risk factors." Positive family history for developmental disabilities, exposure to risky events or behaviors during pregnancy, very low birth weight, or failure to thrive are all factors that tend to be associated with developmental delays. Furthermore, contributing social factors such as teenage parents, educational underachievement in parent or family members, single parent with decreased social support, and a history of abuse or neglect increase the likelihood of developmental delay or disability.

Many primary care settings undertake periodic formal screening using a variety of standardized instruments. A review of the advantages and disadvantages of such tools is beyond the scope of this chapter, but a number of excellent reviews are available (Glascoe et al., 1990). Some of these tools require direct, hands-on-evaluation of the infant or child, but others are accomplished through information collected from parents. Some can be administered at any time or age, and others are standardized for use at specific ages or in association with specific well-child visits. A new American Academy of Pediatrics statement on developmental screening with an algorithm and specific guidance should be published by Spring 2006.

When clinicians encounter developmental delays in the course of well-child care, they should consider prompt referral for early intervention services. Such a referral provides (usually at no charge) further, more in-depth evaluation of all developmental domains by qualified professionals. If the child is found to be eligible for early intervention services, parents are supported in the feeling that "something is being done" in which they are able to play an important role. In addition, further family needs may be identified and addressed through the IFSP (discussed above). The referral for early intervention need not and should not be postponed until a cause for the developmental delays is identified. As we have seen, at least a third of children may never have a specific diagnosis, and for others, the diagnostic evaluation may take months or even years to complete.

The diagnostic evaluation selected by the primary care physician may vary depending upon the individual case. The primary care provider must constantly question the thoroughness of the undertaking and whether specialists consulted are focusing on narrow issues or broad possibilities. For example, if a child with delays is suspected of having seizures, did the pediatric neurologist simply "rule out" a seizure disorder or did he or she consider other neurologic or genetic conditions affecting development. Some children will benefit from a child development clinic diagnostic team evaluation, including a developmental pediatrician and other allied health professionals (physical therapist, occupational therapist, speech pathologist, psychologist, special educator). As genetic knowledge and technology continues its rapid growth, an increasing number of conditions can be identified through genetic testing and consultation. Most children with developmental delays, physical findings of note (e.g., microcephaly, unusual facial features), or positive family histories should be considered for a genetics or dysmorphology consultation. All older children with significant delays or mental retardation, whether they have other findings or not, should be considered for chromosome analysis and fragile X testing.

In addition to the identification of developmental delays in children, a primary care medical home's collection of developmental information is necessary to recognize those children who are actually losing ground developmentally. Developmental regression as opposed to simple delay raises the more ominous possibilities of an ongoing metabolic disorder. Children showing regression require developmental monitoring and should be considered for prompt metabolic screening. In addition, infants and toddlers with seizures, intractable vomiting, failure to thrive, enlargement of liver and/or spleen, and unusual movements, muscle tone, or reflexes should prompt concerns about a metabolic disorder.

Many conditions causing developmental delays are associated with sensory impairments either on a direct neurologic basis or secondary to problems such as middle ear fluid. All children with significant developmental delays should undergo formal audiologic and, in most cases, pediatric ophthalmologic evaluations. These evaluations can be informative in infants and children of any age. They may provide clues about the diagnosis (e.g., the presence of optic atrophy or "cherry red" spots) as well as important secondary challenges that will need to be addressed to make developmental and educational interventions effective.

Parents of children with developmental disability but no clear diagnosis represent a group of families in need of particularly sensitive consideration. In their efforts to understand their child's challenges and to feel confident that nothing has been overlooked, they may require second opinions. Such parents may have difficulty coming to terms with the absence of a diagnosis and may need to revisit the process at intervals or, in particular, at significant transitions in the child's or family's life (e.g., a new pregnancy, transition into special education, the emergence of a new medical problem). Such reconsideration or reassessment may also be warranted from time to time on the grounds that new information and technology is constantly emerging and providing new approaches to diagnosis. Primary care providers should include questions about this issue at each health maintenance encounter.

CCM in the medical home

Pediatric training and primary care practice has traditionally been structured around two basic activities: (1) health promotion and preventive health maintenance ("well-child care") and (2) the diagnosis and treatment of acute pediatric illnesses. Pediatric primary care providers have played less active roles in the long-term management of chronic conditions in children (Young et al., 1994). Primary care providers have been clear about the reasons for their lack of involvement in long-term care of chronic conditions. These reasons usually are related to issues of training and preparation, time and reimbursement, and poor communication about the roles and responsibilities of specialists and specialty clinics. Pediatric primary care providers have usually trained in settings where the model for care involves specialists. For example, the trainee is expected to learn about juvenile rheumatoid arthritis (JRA) from the rheumatologist and to experience long-term management of JRA in the rheumatology clinic. Seldom is a role for the primary care provider articulated or modeled. Needless to say, specialists play a crucial role in the diagnosis and management of chronic conditions in children, but primary care physicians should play an important and explicit co-management role. Primary care providers are well positioned for a coordinating role with schools and to help monitor such generic issues regarding chronic conditions as access to information, care coordination, instructions about self-care, and advocacy for needed services (Briskin & Liptak, 1995; Cooley, 2004).

A further need is for the explicit definition of roles and services. Parents, school personnel, and health care providers are all subject to confusion about responsibility for various aspects of care (Liptak & Revell, 1989). Rarely do primary care physicians specify in their referral to a specialist the exact level of involvement that they would like the specialist to provide. Such involvement might range from a one-time opinion about a specific management issue to assuming complete responsibility for issues related to a child's chronic illness. Parents are usually left in the dark about whom to call when their child develops a symptom or problem that may be related to a chronic illness. School nurses or educators in need of information about the school implications of a chronic condition or wishing to report on a child's progress may be uncertain about whom to contact.

Unfortunately, most primary pediatric care offices and clinics are structured to provide acute and well-child care through a busy schedule of brief office encounters. The extra time needed by children with chronic conditions and their families is not easily incorporated into a typical office day. To be responsive to children with chronic conditions, primary care offices should consider offering a program of CCM to children with developmental disabilities, in which the entire office system (appointments, record keeping, office visit, billing) and all personnel are geared to respond. Models for such CCM are being developed as generic primary care guidelines as the emergence of managed care places increased responsibilities in the hands of primary care providers (Cooley, 1994b; Cooley & McAllister, 2004). Formalizing such care may allow for the identification of children in need of broader primary care services and in turn allow for enhanced capitated or fee-for-service reimbursement to providers who offer CCM.

Supporting the families of children with disabilities

We have seen the importance of supportive informing about the diagnosis of a genetic or disabling condition to assist parents to the best possible adaptation to their child's needs. To continue to support this adaptation, primary care providers must view families in the light of recent research about coping strategies and resilience. Older theories and assumptions were based on models of either pathology (e.g., chronic sorrow) or grief resolution rather than efforts to evaluate family strengths and resilience (Summers et al., 1989; Singer, 1991). It is now clear from many studies that even when children are affected by the most severe handicaps, at least two-thirds of families cope well. Such families experience stress and periods of great difficulty, but do not have increased rates of divorce, serious mental illness, or other long-term dysfunction (Gath & Gumley, 1984). In fact, many such families frame their overall experience in terms of enrichment, empowerment, and spiritual growth. Much depends on the coping skills and strengths that families possessed prior to the identification of illness or disability in their child. However, it is also clear that families that cope well benefit from the presence of traditional social supports (extended family, friends, and community). Coping families also appear to develop a network of "reliable allies" among those supports. Primary care providers should strive to become and consider it a privilege to be one of those reliable allies (Cooley, 1994c).

Parents of children with disabilities and chronic conditions may be exquisitely sensitive to the words professionals use in characterizing their child. The use of dated or obsolete language not only damages the precarious hopes and self-esteem of parents but also may label the well-meaning professional as backward and out of date. Primary care providers should use care in their prognostic formulations, ensuring that they are speaking from knowledge and experience, not making baseless assumptions. Individuals with disabilities have shown a preference for "people first" language. This means referring to the child before the condition (e.g., the "child with Down syndrome," not the "Down syndrome child") and avoiding global references such as "the mentally retarded" instead of saying "people with mental retardation."

It is important for primary care providers to recognize the importance of the natural supports upon which all families depend, as described above. However, many families need additional formal supports, and these are available through state and community agencies (Cooley, 1994a). Such family support services often include assistance with access to information, contact with other families, and respite care. Some states provide family support in the form of a cash stipend to families to use at their own discretion, while others have discretionary funds for which families in need can apply. Family support services have been shown to make important contributions to the successful adjustment of families to the challenges of raising a child with a disability or other chronic condition. Primary care providers need to know how such services are organized in their communities, and need to consider referring all families of children who might benefit from family supports.

Parents of children with disabilities or other chronic conditions, like other parents, are experts about their child. Their expertise needs to be respected in the process of providing health care services at all levels. The development of a health care partnership between parents and professionals has been articulated as national public health policy. The Surgeon General of the United States has issued a directive that services for children with special health care needs be "family-centered, coordinated, community-based, and culturally competent" (US Department of Health and Human Services, 1987). From this beginning, the characteristics of family-centered care have been further refined as standards against which health

Table 2.2. Key elements of family-centered care

1 Recognizing that the family is the constant in a child's life, while the service systems and personnel within those systems fluctuate
2 Facilitating family/professional collaboration at all levels of health care
3 Honoring the racial, ethnic, cultural, and socioeconomic diversity of families
4 Recognizing family strengths and individuality and respecting different methods of coping
5 Sharing with parents, on a continuing basis and in a supportive manner, complete and unbiased information
6 Encouraging and facilitating family-to-family support and networking
7 Understanding and incorporating the developmental needs of infants, children, and adolescents and their families into health care systems
8 Implementing comprehensive policies and programs that provide emotional and financial support to meet the needs of families
9 Designing accessible health care systems that are flexible, culturally competent, and responsive to family-identified needs

care settings, including clinics and physician offices, can measure their success or toward which they can aspire (Table 2.2).

In conclusion, developmental disabilities and chronic conditions affecting development are common in primary pediatric health care settings. This chapter provided an approach to the primary care of children with such conditions that promotes the best outcomes for health and independence as well as supporting family strengths in the process. When it is linked to the care guidelines for specific conditions described in the remainder of this book, sound and reliable primary health care may be achieved. The combination of the generic aspects of CCM in primary care, the elements of family-centered care, and the specific preventive health care needs of individual children provides a powerful enhancement of the role of pediatric primary care providers in community settings.

3

Approach to preventive management

This book promotes preventive management for children with genetic and developmental disorders as an extension of general preventive care. The central rationale is that accessible reminders of disease complications will facilitate preventive care for affected children, empowering the general physician to give usual and unusual children the benefits of their expertise. In Chapter 2, necessary accommodation to the extra time and planning required by children with disabilities is summarized under the term "Chronic Condition Management (CCM)." In this chapter, CCM is facilitated by presenting two types of preventive medical checklists: a *general checklist* for children with disabilities and, for more common disorders, *disease-specific checklists* based on well-defined natural histories and complications.

The extension of regular pediatric care to the special-needs child is first discussed, with formulation of a general preventive medical checklist for children with disabilities (see checklist at end of Preface). This general checklist can be used for rarer causes of disabilities by transferring their tabulated complications to the appropriate spaces on the checklist form. Specific preventive checklists for more common disorders are then discussed, with their standard format of a summary page, two-page checklist for age-specific measures, and parent information page. An overview of preventive measures used for special conditions is presented, providing a summary that ratifies recommendations on the general preventive checklist.

The remaining portions of this chapter provide background on the formulation of preventive guidelines. They discuss general goals of preventive medicine, challenges in providing and assessing preventive care, and an approach for justifying preventive guidelines for rare diseases with little outcome data. The increased compliance achieved by checklists is reviewed, as is the arbitrary nature of many guidelines herein for which no consensus has been achieved. For this reason, as emphasized on each checklist, clinical judgment and individual circumstance are essential elements of the preventive management program.

Preventive care for children with disabilities

The over-riding rationale for preventive care as presented in this book is improvement in quality of life. Although later discussion emphasizes that more research is needed to prove the value and/or cost-effectiveness of many preventive measures, the prime determinants here are the frequency of a potential complication, its impact on quality of life, and the effectiveness of an intervention in avoiding the complication. Our concept of using a table of complications to design a preventive management checklist is drawn from the idea of a "burden of suffering" inflicted by an illness or medical complication. The "burden of suffering" combines the prevalence with the severity of illness, and has been used frequently in justifying prevention programs (US Public Health Service, 1994). For a child with a congenital anomaly or syndrome, the frequency of a complication combined with its impact on quality of life would constitute the "burden of suffering" that justifies prevention.

Preventive measures for all children

At the core of preventive management for children with disabilities are the principles of anticipatory guidance and preventive care for all children. A first step for all families is access to medical care, enhancing prevention from the "gleam in father's eye" through cradle and grave. The couple planning their first pregnancy would ideally consult their regular gynecologist or family practitioner so that family or prenatal risk factors can be defined. Though general health education is helpful, insurance coverage resulted in a two-fold increase in preventive measures (breast examination, digital rectal examination) from survey of 102,263 Americans (Centers for Disease Control, 1995). Regular pediatric health care is crucial for anticipatory guidance of children, and a major goal of this book is to give primary physicians confidence in providing their extensive expertise to children with developmental and genetic disorders.

Pediatric preventive care should begin with pregnancy planning in concert with parental medical and family histories. In 2004, the US Department of Health and Human Services issued a special initiative on family history, emphasizing its importance for medical care. Although hype about genetic testing for predispositions and susceptibilities has perhaps over-reached its actual application, insights into developmental disorders, heart disease, diabetes, hypertension, and cancers will undoubtedly expand the scope of genetic screening in the near future (ACOG Committee on Genetics, 2004). DNA panels are likely to complement risk factors such as serum lipid profiles in determining risks for sudden cardiac death, and cystic fibrosis DNA screening is already offered to many pregnant couples. Forms for parent and physician documentation of family histories are provided in Chapter 1 (Fig. 1.1), allowing family risk factors to be documented for preventive care of average and special-needs children. Some general preventive measures and those based on specific family risk factors are summarized in Table 3.1. The general and specific preventive checklists provided in this book include spaces for listing individual risk factors as defined by family and socio-environmental histories (Table 3.2).

After the genetic endowment is set at fertilization, there are additional risk factors of pregnancy that include particularly the embryonic period where maternal and fetal susceptibilities may interact to produce disease. Preconceptional counseling for provision of folic acid, for control of maternal disease, and for avoidance of teratogens (see Chapter 6) offers general measures for preventing fetal disease. Once pregnancy is undertaken, good prenatal care minimizes risks for labor and delivery based on knowledge of maternal complications, fetal anomalies, fetal

Table 3.1. Preventive strategies for all children

Category	Key concerns	Management considerations
Preconceptional/prenatal period		
Genetic disorders	Over 4000 single gene and 150 chromosomal disorders; maternal age over 35 years	Planned pregnancy, documentation of family history (see Fig. 1.1)
Birth defects	Risk 1–4 per 1000 for individual defects	Planned pregnancy; folic acid supplementation
	Risk 2–3% for any birth defect/disability	Maternofetal monitoring, ultrasound
Maternal medications	Teratogenic drugs, exposures	Planned pregnancy, counsel for drugs, infections
Newborn period		
Common blood, endocrine disorders	Newborn screen for sickle cell disease, thyroid or adrenal dysfunction	Follow-up of screen and false positive results; hormone, blood treatments
Selected treatable metabolic disorders	Newborn screen for phenylketonuria, galactosemia, biotinidase	Follow-up of screen/false positive results Confirmatory testing, dietary changes
Potentially asymptomatic metabolic disorders	Organic or fatty acid metabolic defects	Expanded neonatal screen,* follow-up results Confirmatory testing, dietary changes as needed
Hearing loss	Neonatal illness, hyperbilirubinemia	Neonatal auditory brainstem evoked response (ABR) screening; parental histories
	Craniofacial, ear anomalies, Congenital infections	Examination of ears, jaw and neck Antibody titers
Vision loss	Eyelid, iris, papillary anomalies	Neonatal examination, ophthalmology consultation

(*cont.*)

Table 3.1. (*cont.*)

Category	Key concerns	Management considerations
Early childhood		
Growth, developmental, common illnesses	Growth, developmental, lead, sickle cell, tuberculosis, urinalysis screening	Early and periodic screening diagnosis and treatment, related programs
Common childhood infections	Immunocompetence	Immunization schedule
Hearing, vision loss	Subtle hearing loss, speech deficits	Routine audiometry; speech therapy
	Amblyopia, ocular alignment	Fix and follow examinations, vision charts
Ethnic background	African-American: rickets, obesity	Vitamin D 200 IU/day, dietary counsel
	Caucasian: skin cancer	Skin protection from infancy
	Hispanic: male obesity	Nutrition counsel
	Native American: male suicide	Behavior checklists; social issues
Socio-economic factors	Health insurance, Medicaid eligibility	Encourage preventive care, regular visits
	Parental smoking, tobacco exposure	Minimize respiratory illnesses, sudden infant death syndrome, otitis
Later childhood/teenage periods		
Nutrition	Obesity, eating disorders, diet, exercise	Dietary counsel, monitor growth
Injury prevention	Motor vehicle accidents, sports injuries	Safety belts, helmets, driver education, drug/alcohol education
School and behavior	Learning disabilities, chemical dependency, depression/ suicide, dysfunctional family	Psychosocial history, monitor school performance Alert for diet, sleep, peer, school problems
Puberty and bone growth	Precocious or delayed puberty, scoliosis	Monitor pubertal development, vertebral curve Dietary counsel for dairy, calcium
	Adult osteoporosis	Exercise
Cancer	Breast and testicular cancers	Breast, testicular self-examination
	Skin cancers	Sun protection
Sexuality	Sexual abuse; gender identity	Psychosocial history, sexual history
	Unwanted pregnancy; STD/HIV	Sexual/HIV education, routine examinations
Cardiovascular	Arrythmias, cardiomyopathies	If chest pain, syncope; consider ECG
	Later coronary artery disease	Cholesterol, dietary, exercise counsel

Note:
*Acylcarnitine profile.

Table 3.2. Preventive strategies based on family or social/environmental risk factors

Family risk factors	Key concerns	Management considerations
Preconceptional/prenatal period		
Specific genetic diseases	Genetic counseling, recurrence risks	Preimplantation diagnosis; prenatal diagnosis
	Genetic testing to define specific diagnosis	Fetal treatment, monitoring, delivery strategies
Neural tube defects	Risk 3–5% if affected primary relative	Planned pregnancy; folic acid supplementation; Prenatal
Cardiac defects	Folate/nutritional deficiencies	α-fetoprotein (AFP), ultrasound, neonatal exam
Maternal diabetes	Fetal cardiac, craniospinal, CNS anomalies	Planned pregnancy, stringent diabetic control, prenatal care, fetal monitoring
	Fetal stillbirth, maternal complications	Neonatal examination, complete cell count, glucose, calcium
Maternal epilepsy	Maternal hydantoin or trimethadione therapy	Taper medicines, switch to phenobarbitol
	Fetal cardiac and developmental defects	Prenatal care, maternofetal monitoring
		Neonatal examination, developmental monitoring
Maternal alcoholism	Fetal alcohol syndrome	Maternal intervention; fetal ultrasound
	Fetal growth	Neonatal exam; monitor growth and development
Maternal acne	Maternal Accutane, retinoic acid therapy	Education, avoid retinoic acid preparations
	Fetal brain, craniofacial, limb defects	Prenatal AFP, ultrasound, neonatal studies
Maternal Rh⁻/O blood types	Prenatal Rhogam, fetal monitoring	Neonatal blood type; antibody testing
Infertility, miscarriages	Artificial reproductive technologies	Monitoring for multiple births, pregnancy loss
	Fetal chromosome anomalies	Prenatal diagnosis; newborn examination
Newborn period		
Birth defects	Associations of anomalies	Physical examination, imaging studies
Hearing loss	Hearing loss	Newborn ABR, later hearing assessments
Prematurity	Respiratory syncytial virus,	Add respiratory syncytial virus and influenza prophylaxis, audiology and
	respiratory illnesses, vision/hearing loss	ophthalmology screening to regular schedule
Prior sudden death	Organic or fatty acid metabolic defects	Expanded neonatal screen, follow-up results; Confirmatory testing, dietary changes as needed
Childhood/teenage periods		
Allergies, respiratory illnesses	Immune deficiencies, allergies	Alert for symptoms, allergic cleanliness, nasal saline, monitoring of pulmonary function
Behavior problems	Attention deficit and hyperactivity disorder, obsessive compulsive patient, suicide/depression	Family/social histories, monitor school performance

(cont.)

Table 3.2. (cont.)

Family risk factors	Key concerns	Management considerations
Cancer-breast	Breast cancer risk	Genetic counseling; BRCA gene testing for parent
Cancer-melanoma	Melanoma	Sun protection; regular exams
Chemical dependency	Parental addictions; dysfunctional family	Social and sexual history; drug/alcohol education
	Changes in lifestyle, performance, friends	Sex education; screening for STD/HIV if needed
Coronary artery disease	Hyperlipidemia, coronary artery disease	Serum cholesterol, dietary and exercise counsel
	Other cardiac risk factors	Lipid panel, homocysteine, etc.
Cardiomyopathy, arrythmias	Expanded neonatal screen*	Cardiology evaluation
Depression	Bipolar, manic-depressive illness	Alert for diet, sleep, peer, school problems
	Suicide	
Developmental disabilities	Inherited disorders, autism, mental disability	Developmental monitoring, neurogenetic testing
Diabetes	Maternal diabetes in pregnancy	Pregnancy planning, monitoring
	Juvenile diabetes in child	Regular urinalyses, alert for symptoms
School problems	Dyslexias, inherited mental disability	Monitor school performance, educational testing
Hypertension	Pregnancy monitoring	Routine blood pressures, dietary counsel
Kidney disease	Urinary tract anomalies (6–10% risk if primary relative affected)	Urinalysis, alert for infections, sonogram and voiding cystourethrogram if infection
Lax joints, joint injuries	Lax joints, connective tissue disease	Examine joints, mobility; consider echocardiogram
		Avoid collision or competitive sports if necessary
Multiple miscarriages, infertility	Parental chromosome translocation	Parental chromosomes, prenatal diagnosis options
	Newborn chromosome disorder	Dysmorphology exam
Obesity	Morbid obesity, decreased mobility	Dietary, exercise counsel; monitor growth
Osteoporosis	Fractures at young age, early osteoporosis	Alert for bone pain, symptoms
Respiratory illnesses	Immune deficiencies, allergies	Alert for symptoms, allergic cleanliness, nasal saline, monitoring of pulmonary function
Scoliosis	Progression, disfigurement	Regular examinations
Sudden death as child	Cardiomyopathy, arrythmias	Expanded neonatal screen*
	Fatty acid oxidation defects	Cardiology evaluation

Note:

*Acylcarnitine profile.

positioning, and fetal heart rate changes. Screening for maternal obstetric complications is a preventive intermediary between family history/preconceptional planning and newborn screening for infections, blood group incompatibilities, and common metabolic disorders.

At birth, a variety of screening procedures have been instituted for metabolic, endocrine, or hearing disorders. All states screen newborns for phenylketonuria, galactosemia, sickle cell anemia and thyroid dysfunction, while some screen additionally for biotinidase deficiency, congenital adrenal hyperplasia, or cystic fibrosis. A supplemental or expanded newborn screen employs the same blood spot technology to perform an acylcarnitine profile, thereby detecting as many as 35 disorders of organic or fatty acid metabolism. Disorders such as medium chain coenzyme A dehydrogenase (MCAD) deficiency cause an undegraded organic acid (e.g., 10–12 carbons in this case) to be attached to carnitine, allowing sensitive detection of the abnormal acylcarnitine by gas chromatography/mass spectrometry.

These limited newborn screens will likely be greatly amplified in the future as DNA chip technology allows screening for thousands of mutant alleles using the white blood cell DNA on neonatal blood spots. Such "gene screens" will include alleles conferring susceptibility to common diseases like diabetes or hemochromatosis (Merikangas & Risch, 2003), emphasizing the importance of family histories to define risk factors as shown in Fig. 1.1. Given the estimated 30,000 human genes and over 4000 genetically influenced diseases, it is likely that newborn genetic screens will be tailored to individual ethnicity (e.g., Caucasions for cystic fibrosis) and family afflictions. Genetic risk factors will complement the detection of rare metabolic diseases by predicting susceptibilities or reactivities that impact subsequent medical care. Detection of the cytochrome p450 gene variants that predict toxicity to 6-mercaptopurine would influence chemotherapy for that patient, and the development of DNA testing panels for the long QT, sodium channel, and cardiomyopathy genes will predict teenagers at risk for sudden cardiac death (Rubinstein & Lopez-Soler, 2001).

Following the neonatal physical examination and screening tests, a standardized approach to well-child care is accepted that embodies the pediatric principle of anticipatory guidance. Important sources of recommendations for preventive well-child care include the books Bright Futures (Greene, 1994) and The Canadian Guide to Clinical Preventive Health Care (Canadian Task Force on the Periodic Health Examination, 1994), and recommendations for adolescent care (Jenkins & Saxena, 1995). Early and Periodic Screening Diagnosis and Treatment (EPSDT) formalized entitled younger children to these measures as part of Medicaid managed care programs (Bauchner et al., 1996).

Primary among these strategies is an immunization schedule that is demonstrably effective for prevention and cost. The resulting schedule of well-child visits includes monitoring for growth, developmental, hearing, or vision problems as well as guidance to minimize child injuries from toxins or accidents. Every pediatric chart documents a sequence of visits at prescribed intervals, accompanied by immunizations, screening, and growth data. Socioeconomic factors like passive exposure to tobacco smoke should not be neglected in preventive care, since risks for respiratory illnesses, middle ear effusions, and sudden infant death syndrome can be lowered by simply asking parents to smoke outside. These general preventive measures should of course be followed for children with disabilities, and the checklists in this book are essentially add-ons to this standard pediatric care.

During later childhood and adolescence, there is general agreement (Elster, 1998; Halpern-Felsher et al., 2000) on specific preventive strategies. Monitoring of growth, development/school progress, hearing, vision, and school/family issues continues as at younger ages. Health promotion includes screening for obesity, eating disorders, tobacco or alcohol/substance abuse, and recommendation of helmets and seat belts to prevent injury. Education is provided regarding sexual dangers, contraception, nutrition, dental care, skin protection, and breast or testicular self-examination. Clinical and laboratory measures (Papanicolau smear, blood pressure, human immunodeficiency/sexually transmitted diseases, tuberculosis, cholesterol, urinalysis, blood counts) reflect the transition to adult medical care. A ceremony of adult passage is the pre-college physical, a "last chance" for the pediatrician to ascertain risks in a young adult who may wait a decade or longer to return to primary care (McMillan, 2002).

Adolescent prevention is the foundation for adult health, and areas deserving particular emphasis are those of behavior, sexuality, and nutrition. Behavior checklists are available to investigate concerns about mental illnesses including depression and suicide, and some organizations have recommended that well-child visits for adolescents should be replaced with discussion and counseling sessions.

Some 15–28% of American girls are sexually abused or exploited by the time they reach their 20s, exacting a considerable economic burden through reactive eating disorders, unwanted pregnancies, and sexually transmitted diseases (including costs of 4 billion dollars for treatment of pelvic inflammatory disease alone – Joffe, 2004). Some 10% of American females aged 15–19 years will become pregnant (higher than in most other industrialized countries, causing almost one million births with substandard preconceptional planning and prenatal care (Kirby, 1999). Sex and HIV education programs as well as physician counseling have been shown to reduce adolescent sexual activity, pregnancy, and venerealdisease – regular preventive visits are at least as important as regular contraception and emergency contraception for adolescents since compliance in taking daily pills or seeking help after intercourse is poor (Gold, 1999; Kirby, 1999).

Native American males and homosexuals are at most risk for suicide, and it accounts for twice as many adolescent deaths as natural causes. Ninety percent of suicide victims have a diagnosable psychiatric disorder, including 40% with an affective disorder, and 8–10% of all children have made at least one suicide attempt (Fleischman & Barondess, 2004). The 30% of victims who have made a prior attempt and the 50–100 suicide attempts for every one that is successful make psychosocial assessment, school and behavioral screening, and firearm prevention important parts of every adolescent visit.

Dietary counsel is important because good eating and exercise habits are under assault by cultural attitudes, mass media advertising, dietary fads, and alternative medicines. Osteoporosis affects over 25 million American adults, with a cost of 14 billion dollars per year in 1998 (Golden, 2000). A major contribution to bone mass is made during adolescence, and emphasis on dairy/calcium intake with exercise can produce a higher peak that lessens the risks of post-menopausal bone mass decline. Adolescent bone mass can be optimized by favoring early breast feeding and later milk over carbonated beverage intake, simple strategies also effective for obesity prevention.

One-third of those destined for obesity as adults become so in childhood, and pediatric obesity-related health costs have increased three-fold in the past two decades (Chakravarthy, 2003). As many as 15% of adolescents and 60% of adults are overweight, at least a third with a metabolic syndrome of serum lipid alterations (high triglycerides, low high-density lipoprotein-cholesterol), increased abdominal girth, high fasting glucose level, and high blood pressure (Cook et al., 2003). The metabolic syndrome has high risks for type II diabetes and premature coronary artery disease, and is estimated to affect 22% of the US adult population. Sedentary behavior is a major contributor to obesity and its resulting morbidity, giving rise to the term "sedentary death syndrome" (Chakravarthy, 2003).

Prevention is needed to alter the pathway from early obesity to metabolic syndrome and cardiac death. There are strong genetic factors, illustrated by the higher prevalence of obesity in Hispanic males and African-American females (both around 25%) and by genetic syndromes such as Prader–Willi, Bardet–Biedl, or Cohen syndromes. A family history of obesity or correlated diseases (type II diabetes, hypertension, dyslipidemias, gall bladder disease) mandates early dietary counseling and careful monitoring of weight, exercise, and eating habits.

Endocrine or genetic causes must be excluded in the child with uncontrolled eating, but most cases will be multifactorial, combining genetic background and family/social problems with diet, exercise, and nutritional knowledge. Special health risks that warrant attention in the obese patient (Eissa, 2003) including headaches or blurred vision (hypertension), sleep problems or day-time sleepiness (sleep apnea), abdominal pain or nausea/vomiting (gall bladder disease), hip or knee pain (joint fatigue or slipped capital femoral epiphysis), menstrual irregularities (hypothyroidism, polycystic ovary syndrome), constipation and fatigue (hypothyroidism), and polyuria or polyphagia (diabetes). Attention to at-risk or obese children is an obvious priority for pediatrics, particularly since simple behavioral interventions (limiting television and soft drinks, encouraging breastfeeding and outdoor play) can improve outcomes (Whitaker, 2003).

General preventive guidelines for teenagers and young adults, and especially those for obesity, are important to bear in mind for individuals with disabilities. These children are more likely to be sedentary due to physical or mental disabilities, more susceptible to infections due to altered homeostasis or genetic factors, and more vulnerable in transition to adult care since fewer family practitioners and internists are comfortable with their health care needs. As emphasized in the next section, many children with special health care needs can be sexually active or at least are at risk of being sexually abused, and recommendations for cholesterol, blood pressure, behavioral, and obesity screening apply even more forcefully to individuals with mental and physical limitations. A willingness on the part of pediatricians to extend their preventive expertise to young adults with disabilities (recognizing their appropriate mental age) can mitigate co-morbidities and optimize adult outcomes.

Preventive measures for children with disabilities: The general preventive checklist

The first consideration for children with disabilities may be a decision of whether treatment is justified at all. The Baby Doe infant with Down syndrome and duodenal atresia prompted much discussion of treatment options and was a factor in the development of hospital ethics committees (Bucciarelli & Eitzman, 1988). It is now accepted that all infants should receive basic life support including feeding and fluids. Extraordinary surgical or resuscitative measures may be withheld after discussion with the parents and ethics committee (Raffin, 1991), but it is essential that accurate prognostic information be available. Parent group information can be helpful in such decisions, and survey of parental experiences may give a very different profile of disease as illustrated by the study of Barr & Cohen (2000) on children with holoprosencephaly. Where available, parent group information is included with the parent information pages of specific checklists or with sections discussing less common disorders.

On the opposite side of congenital disorders and disabilities are those that are not obvious during infancy. As discussed in Chapter 2, every infant has a 5–20% risk for psychosocial, growth, or developmental problems and measured at 27.3% of children in one survey of average pediatric practices (Horwitz et al., 1992). Perinatal problems like prematurity or intrauterine growth retardation are associated with even higher risks. This frequency demands that every pediatric practitioner be alert for the child with disabilities so that developmental monitoring and preventive management can begin.

Chapter 2 suggests that children with disabilities require special considerations for scheduling, billing, and frequency of visits that are summarized by the concept of CCM. This concept is expressed here as a general preventive checklist for children with congenital disorders and their accompanying developmental disabilities. This general preventive checklist can be used for children without a specific diagnosis or for those with rare diagnoses, based on the fact that children with different developmental disorders have many problems in common. Common complications of developmental disabilities can be appreciated by their compilation from the 29 disease-specific checklists in this book (see below).

Every new pediatric patient should have a family history, and the child with risks for disability is often identified before birth based on high-risk pregnancy or fetal ultrasound. Family histories can be efficiently documented (see Fig. 1.1), and risk factors transferred to the appropriate spaces on the general checklist. Consideration of genetic counseling by the primary physician or genetic specialist is indicated on the checklist, and this can be taken to include the family history with consequent risk factors.

Also listed early are neonatal problems that complicate parental adjustment and developmental progress if unrecognized. Feeding problems due to neurologic changes often accompany congenital disorders, including a weak suck, dysphagia, chronic aspiration, and/or gastroesophageal reflux. Assessment needs may go beyond a breast-feeding consultant; a speech therapist (with possible video swallow), neonatologist (to evaluate underlying illness), gastroenterologist (with possible gastrointestinal series), and surgical specialties may be needed. Such team approaches have proven effective (Couriel et al., 1993).

Feeding problems may also reflect internal anomalies, and the child with one birth defect or substantial neurologic alteration should receive ultrasound studies for cerebral, cardiac, and renal anomalies as symptoms dictate. Early growth delays may signal internal anomalies, chronic infections, or subtle feeding problems, necessitating dietary consultation, supplemental feedings, and/or high-calorie formulas. Poor growth is frequent in children with genetic abnormalities (e.g., trisomy 13/18), mandating consideration of genetic testing in children with failure to thrive.

Infancy is also a time that metabolic errors can present with subtle or flagrant symptoms, and consideration of blood counts and chemistries (electrolytes, pH, lactate, ammonia) with acylcarnitine profiles (expanded newborn screening) should be considered where appropriate. Many genetic disorders have increased susceptibility to infection, and sepsis must be suspected in infants with syndromes and neurologic manifestations. Hearing and vision loss should be evaluated by examination and auditory evoked response screening that is available in most nurseries.

Along with alertness and evaluation for neonatal diseases, early management should include consideration of specialty referrals to developmental pediatrics, pediatric neurology, and pediatric genetics. Although local availability and patient symptoms will determine the order of these specialty visits, their primary goal is a specific diagnosis that can anchor subsequent medical management. Children with combinations of problems will usually benefit by seeing all three specialties.

The different perspectives of neurology and genetics will guide imaging and laboratory evaluations, while the developmental pediatrician will identify associated behavioral patterns like autism and assess functional strengths and weaknesses that guide therapy. Although as many as 30% of children with disabilities elude a specific medical diagnosis, their neurosensory, cognitive, behavioral, and motor needs can be defined. Genetic counseling cannot provide precise recurrence risks without a diagnosis, but parents can be informed that most disabilities are inborn and sporadic (new mutations) so as to allay guilt about their genes, lifestyle, or pregnancy. Evaluation by a clinical geneticist is mandatory for dysmorphic children and is often helpful in deciphering prenatal influences such as maternal diabetes or substance abuse. Neurology is obviously needed when seizures, tics, or palsies are prominent but also expands the differential for children with odd behaviors or motor delays. Disorders such as cerebral palsy or spina bifida are traditionally managed by developmental pediatricians, and they usually are more experienced with cognitive/neuropsychologic testing and learning disorders.

As the tumult of neonatal treatment and referral subsides, initiation of therapy programs should begin. Early childhood intervention (ECI) programs (ages 0–3 years) and later preschool (4–6 years) are emphasized on the checklists, and these recommendations should be extended to include the appropriate preschool or special education programs when a disability is recognized after infancy. The primary physician has a pivotal role in guiding therapy and education through their certification of special needs to the appropriate agencies.

Parents of school age children should be informed of their rights for education under the Individuals with Disabilities Education Act (IDEA). This act mandates that an individualized educational plan (IEP) be established for each child with disabilities, gives rights for parents to participate in their child's IEP, and provides due process as recourse if the parents are unhappy with the plan for their child. In other words, the IDEA provides ammunition for inclusion of the child in at least some regular classrooms. Attention to school issues is indicated on all the checklists. Children require specific attention during transitions between school levels, particularly if they are required to change agencies as in the transition between early intervention and preschool programs.

Parents should also begin to learn about insurance and financial issues as soon as a disability is suspected in their child. In 1935, Title V of the Social Security Act provided federal funds for care of "crippled" children, later designated as children with special health care needs (Biehl, 1996). In 1965, the medicaid program was created in Title XIX of the Social Security Act, and eligibility will provide coverage for many costs of outpatient preventive care.

Financial counselors or social workers are available at most hospitals for consultation on these issues. Parents should also recognize that their child will become independent at age 18 and, together with exposure to possible abuse or fraud, will lose medicaid benefits if he or she has assets above certain limits. There are tax considerations in establishing guardianship to safeguard the child, and special needs trusts are available to avert loss of federal benefits after the parent is deceased. Most health care professionals are not expert in these issues, but should become familiar with community resources such as the Association for Retarded Citizens (ARC) and specialized legal services. Financial and insurance issues are included in the "family support" reminder on the checklists.

Because many genetic and developmental disorders have increased risk for behavioral problems, screening for abnormalities in the child or family is an important aspect of health assessment. Behavioral screening instruments are available (Herman-Staab, 1994), and referral to psychology or psychiatric specialists should be made early rather than later when adverse consequences have occurred. Counseling strategies can be effective, as shown by the 44% reduction in drug use achieved by annual workshops in a high-school setting (Botvin et al., 1995). Group settings are extremely powerful in dealing with individual and family behavior problems.

Common considerations on the general preventive checklist should be supplemented with disease-specific information when it is available. Many rarer disorders are summarized briefly in this book as listed in the index. Each has a succinct listing of complications in a standard organ system format. These complications and their accompanying preventive management considerations can be entered in appropriate spaces on the general checklist.

Of major importance on the general and specific checklists, and in particular disease discussions, are sources of parent support and information. For the more common disorders, national and international parent group organizations are available, illustrated by the Little People of America group for skeletal dysplasias or the several parent associations for Down Syndrome. These groups and their associated websites are extremely helpful in providing updated information on the disorder(s) and their management. For example, updated results on clinical trials like growth hormone or special growth factor therapies may be available. For less common disorders, a growing number of general medical websites for parents and professionals can be accessed by searching on the disease name. These websites enlist medical professionals as consultants and writers, and generally have review policies that ensure quality information. Some of them provide links to affected families for guidance and sharing of resources.

Specific medical guidelines for congenital malformations and syndromes

The rationales for improved quality of life (realization of functional potential) and for screening a high-risk population (defined by the anomaly or syndrome) provide a solid foundation for using preventive medical checklists in children with genetic and/or developmental disorders. Our disorder-specific checklist begins with a summary listing definitions, resources and complications. A two-page checklist then lists evaluations and key concerns in a first column followed by management considerations in the second column. Space is left in a third column for progress notes. Key concerns usually guide the history or physical (e.g., constipation, hypotonia), while management options include laboratory testing (e.g., thyroid, cervical spine X-rays) or referrals based on these findings. Beneath each checklist is a summary of important complications (left) and spaces for indicating family risk factors (right). Routine pediatric care including immunizations and anticipatory guidance is expected but not specifically indicated on the checklists – most practices have their own forms and schedules for this data.

Checklists have been developed for two anomalies (cerebral palsy, spina bifida), two associations, and 25 syndromes or syndrome groups, and 3 broader categories like partial aneuploidy, skeletal dysplasias, or arthrogryposes (Table 3.3). Disorders with a combined incidence above 1 in 25,000 were selected for consideration based on the likelihood that an average pediatric practice would include at least one affected individual. Less extensive discussion of preventive management recommendations is provided for an additional 120 disorders.

The preventive guidelines used here for Down syndrome, fragile X syndrome, achondroplasia, neurofibromatosis type 1, and Marfan syndrome are essentially those of the American Academy of Pediatrics, Committee on Genetics (1995a, b, 1996a, b, 2001a, b). Even for these consensus recommendations, justification by outcomes analysis or cost-effectiveness has not been performed (see above discussion). In many cases, complications encountered in other disorders could be related to the consensus guidelines from the American Academy of Pediatrics. For example, the incidence of chronic otitis in Williams syndrome (43%) is comparable to that in Down syndrome (40–60%), allowing consensus recommendations for audiology screening in Down syndrome to be extrapolated to patients with Williams syndrome. Particular caution was exerted in recommending imaging studies or other interventions that would require anesthesia in young children; these recommendations are usually qualified by a footnote that emphasizes the need for clinical judgment.

An overview of the resulting guidelines for 32 disorders or categories (assuming diagnosis in the neonatal period) shows that a total of 3200 preventive considerations were listed for 12 age ranges plus early and later adult (~100 recommendations per disorder). Nine types of preventive measures were specified including imaging studies (3% of recommendations), laboratory tests (7%), functional screening (3%),

Table 3.3. The more common pediatric syndromes and metabolic dysplasias

Syndrome (incidence*)	Impairment or disability (chapter number)
Down syndrome (1 in 600–1000)	Mental, heart, thyroid, hearing, vision, spine (7)
VATER association (1 in 620)	Heart, kidney, lumbar spine (5)
Fetal alcohol syndrome (1 in 670)	Mental, heart, hearing, vision, skeleton (6)
Fragile X syndrome (1 in 800)	Mental, vision (8)
47,XXY (Klinefelter) syndrome (1 in 1000)	Hearing, vision (8)
Fetal hydantoin syndrome (1 in 2000)	Feeding, hearing, vision (6)
Noonan syndrome (1 in 1000–2500)	Mental, heart, hearing, vision (10)
Diabetic embryopathy (1 in 3000)	Heart, vision, spine (6)
Neurofibromatosis type 1 (1 in 3000)	Mental, brain, nerves, spine, skeleton (13)
Shprintzen/DiGeorge spectrum (1 in 2–10,000)	Mental, heart, hearing, vision (9)
Turner syndrome (1 in 5000)	Heart, hearing, kidney (8)
Goldenhar syndrome (1 in 5600)	Mental, heart, hearing, vision, kidney, lungs (15)
Trisomy 13/18 (1 in 8000)	Mental, hearing, vision, heart, kidney, skeleton (7)
Skeletal dysplasias (1 in 10,000)	Mental hearing, vision, skeleton, spine, limbs (11)
Marfan syndrome (1 in 10,000)	Heart, vision, skeleton, joints (16)
Arthrogryposis, amyoplasia (1 in 10,000)	Feeding, lungs, joints, muscles (18)
Cornelia de Lange (1 in 10,000)	Mental, feeding, heart, hearing, vision (10)
Ehlers–Danlos syndromes (1 in 10–20,000)	Heart, vision, skin, joints (16)
Beckwith–Wiedemann (1 in 17,000)	Abdomen, liver, kidney, tumors (12)
Osteogenesis imperfectas (1 in 20,000)	Hearing, skeleton, joints (11)
Prader–Willi syndrome (1 in 16–25,000)	Mental, feeding, vision, skin (9)
Achondroplasia (1 in 16–25,000)	Skeletal, spine, foramen magnum, joints (11)
Glycogen storage diseases (1 in 20–25,000)	Liver, kidney, skeleton (20)
Craniosynotosis syndromes (1 in 25,000)	Cranial, spine, vision, hearing (14)
Tuberous sclerosis (1 in 25,000)	Mental, heart, kidney, skeleton (13)
Sotos/Weaver syndrome (1 in 25,000)	Mental, cranial, brain, skeleton (12)
CHARGE association (1 in 20–50,000)	Mental, heart, hearing, vision, skeleton (6)
Williams syndrome (1 in 20–50,000)	Mental, heart, hearing, vision (9)
Mucopolysaccharidoses (1 in 25,000)	Mental, brain, vision, hearing, skeleton (19)
Partial trisomies/monosomies	Mental, brain, hearing, vision, heart, kidney, thyroid, hearing, vision, spine (7)

Note:
*Per number of live births.

screening by examination (20%), screening by history (30%), examination for key findings (11%), specialty referral (15%), referral for special services (7%), and counseling (4%). Timing of the preventive measures includes 35% for 7 visits during infancy, 33% for 6 visits between ages 15 months and 6 years, and 32% for 7 visits between ages 8 and 18 years.

The additional costs of these guidelines can be estimated relative to the baseline cost of routine pediatric care. These cost estimates are very general, since the costs of a well-child visit ($36.19–49.94) or standard immunizations ($9.95 to $25.51 for diptheria–tetanus–pertussis and $11.25–28.00 for hemophilus influenza) are quite variable (Freed et al., 1996). The baseline cost for routine pediatric care was estimated to be $1500 (1995 dollars) with a range from $1320 to $1670 per healthy individual. Additional costs imposed by the preventive care recommendations (estimated from birth to age 18 years) was highest for children with Down syndrome or CHARGE association (3.2 times baseline) and lowest for children with Saethre–Chotzen syndrome (1.8 times baseline). Costs are heavily dependent on the need for specialty referral, reaching 5.5 times baseline in children with CHARGE or VATER association with long-term survival and multiple anomalies. Costs would also be higher if additional physician time (mean of three extra history/physical items per visit) is considered.

Because of the increased costs and time demanded by preventive care, physicians must decide about the utility of individual recommendations based on clinical experience and patient circumstance. A general discussion of prevention and management guidelines follows, showing that theoretical and practical difficulties attend any generalization of guidelines. These difficulties are particularly evident for groups like children with disabilities where outcomes can be subjective. It is clear that use of a preventive checklist improves compliance (Cheney & Ramsdel, 1987; Maiman et al., 1988; Johns et al., 1992), and that the development of clinical practice guidelines has been endorsed by the Agency for Health Care Policy and Research (1993) and by the Division of Health Care Services at the Institute of Medicine. Such trends, together with extrapolation from consensus guidelines (American Academy of Pediatrics, Committee on Genetics, 1995a, b, 1996a, b, 2001a, b), endorse the use of our checklists as prototypes that will need further validation by outcome studies.

General considerations in preventive medicine

Preventive health care has received much attention in the past few decades, emphasized in the United States by a series of targeted health goals culminating in *Healthy People 2000* (US Public Health Service, 1991). *Healthy People 2000* set forth three goals for American health care: (1) to increase the span of healthy life, (2) to reduce health disparities among individuals, and (3) to improve access to preventive services (McGinnis & Lee, 1995). Among the priority areas were family planning, mental health and mental disorders, maternal and infant health, and clinical preventive services, areas relevant to the care of children with congenital anomalies and syndromes. In their mid-decade assessment of progress toward the goals of *Healthy People 2000*, McGinnis & Lee (1995) cited reductions in childhood lead poisoning and accidents, with increases in childhood immunization rates. These results provide optimism that targeted health care goals can improve preventive care in the general pediatric population. This section will consider the rationale, justification, and practical approach to preventive care, focusing first on general well-child care and then on the child with developmental disabilities. A major advantage of the preventive management approach to genetic disease is that it balances some of the negative consequences that may arise from genetic diagnosis (Holtzman, 1988, 1989).

Types of prevention

Rose (1992) emphasized that few diseases are the inescapable lot of humanity, citing that 10% of eastern Indian children die before age 1 year while only 1% do here. This variability of disease offers opportunities for prevention if the causes and natural history of complications can be defined. Prevention is possible even for genetic diseases, where complications can be forestalled even if the disease cannot be treated. Phenylketonuria, sickle cell anemia, and cystic fibrosis are examples of genetic disorders where preventive management can greatly alter the natural history of disease.

Marge (1984), in the context of communication disorders, has discussed prevention as a primary, secondary, or tertiary process. Primary prevention would involve eliminating the onset of the disorder, as in the removal of an individual from a noisy workplace to prevent hearing loss. Secondary prevention would involve early detection of a problem that already has occurred, as in auditory screening of children at school. Tertiary prevention is reduction of the detected problem through rehabilitation, as in use of hearing aids for individuals with hearing loss (Marge, 1984).

For specific genetic and developmental diseases, primary prevention consists of preconceptional and genetic counseling to prevent the occurrence of a disorder (e.g., avoidance of alcohol during pregnancy, folic acid supplementation to lower the incidence of neural tube defects). As discussed in Chapter 1, documentation of a family history allows more general primary prevention for such problems as sudden cardiac death, obesity, renal failure, or hypertension. The propensity for disease is recognized by its presence in the family, and monitoring for early manifestations allows prevention through early treatment or lifestyle changes. This book is mostly concerned with secondary and tertiary prevention, exemplified by recognizing strabismus in a child with fetal alcohol syndrome and by providing optical or surgical treatment. However, the emphasis on family history and documentation of health risk factors on the general preventive medical checklist (see below) can be added to pediatric anticipatory guidance as primary prevention for all children.

Justification of preventive strategies

Although the rationale for prevention as improving health is sound, the justification of particular preventive measures is often difficult. Table 3.1 lists several rationales for preventive strategies and juxtaposes them with conflicts that may arise. Health is a basic human right, but health, like beauty, is often in the eyes of the beholder. Doctors may define it as the absence of serious illness while the individual defines it as a sense of "well-being." The very definition of "health" is complex, since diseases are often extremes along a continuum of measurement (e.g., hypertension, hypoglycemia) rather than binary well/ill states (Rose, 1992). Lead poisoning is an example where the threshold of "disease" has dramatic implications for the efforts made in primary prevention (Schaffer & Campbell, 1994). Progressive lowering of the tolerable childhood lead level to 10 μg/dl of blood dramatically affects the costs and implications of intervention.

The process of diagnosis itself may lead to a loss of well-being because the person is now aware of his or her differences and potential morbidity. Diagnoses may also become labels that cause family, employment, or insurance consequences (Holtzman, 1989). These problems emphasize that diagnostic screening for the purpose of prevention must lead to clear-cut medical benefits for the patient. Individual benefits may also conflict with societal benefits. A dramatic example is when maternal screening must be considered for the infant's health, as when routine HIV testing of pregnant women can lead to beneficial therapy for their infant (Stiehm, 1995).

In estimating the medical benefits of early detection and screening, it is also a complex task to define the appropriate outcome measures (Wilkin et al., 1993). Justification of preventive measures for children with genetic disorders and/or disabilities may require degrees of functional and/or quality of life as outcomes, since overall morbidity or mortality may not be avoided (see below). Quality of life is often a difficult outcome measure (Hennessy et al., 1994).

Disease incidence is another general issue in prevention (Table 3.4). How many people are affected by a particular preventive strategy? Rose (1992) described a "prevention paradox" in which measures bringing large benefits to a community may offer little to each individual. People may avoid seat belts or helmets because the probability of self-injury is low, despite indisputable evidence of benefit to the general population. It is necessary to immunize several hundred children to prevent one death, and some parents seize on this fact to avoid the pain for their child.

These considerations point out the differences between general versus high-risk prevention strategies (Rose, 1992). In general or population strategies, all individuals undergo the intervention. General screening goes to the root of the problem and seeks to eliminate it from the entire population. All people undergo the same screening procedure, and there is no singling out of one group for specialized management until the screening results are obtained. From the viewpoint of genetic disease, diagnostic activities such as newborn screening would qualify as general population screening that leads to disease elimination by dietary therapy. False positive values can be a significant problem in general population screening, since

Table 3.4. Justifications for prevention

Rationale	Conflict
Ethics	
Health is a universal human right	Is health defined as the absence of disease or a feeling of well-being?
	Personal "well-being" versus personal knowledge of impending complications and labeling as "diseased"
Elimination of disease and disability from society	Individual freedom of choice versus benefits for society
	Is health defined as the absence of disease or a feeling of well-being?
Outcomes	
Preventive measure should improve patient outcomes	Mortality versus quality of life as outcomes
Epidemiologic:	
Target diseases are sufficiently common to have important consequences for society	Large benefits to a community may offer little to each individual
	Screening general population versus high-risk population
Cost-effectiveness	
Early detection of illness	Postponement rather than elimination of disease
	Screening general population versus high-risk population
Disease should be prevented or modified by early detection	Must be resources for counseling and follow-up care to realize benefits

large numbers of individuals may be identified as "abnormal" and require additional intervention.

The alternative strategy of focusing on a high-risk population allows the intervention to be more closely matched to needs of the individual (Rose, 1992). Furthermore, the screening can be more selective and cost-effective than mass screening (Table 3.4). A disadvantage of high-risk screening is that it labels the individual rather than initiating general measures for the entire population (e.g., cholesterol screening). This concern reiterates the need to have effective treatment as part of the rationale for preventive screening. A higher frequency of false positive values can be tolerated in high-risk screening, since fewer individuals will be affected. This rationale underlies the application of maternal serum α-fetoprotein (AFP) screening to women over 35 rather than the entire population. However, as evidenced by the anxiety and additional testing that followed the adoption of maternal serum AFP screening, any medical screening for complications must be weighed against the possibility of false positive or ambiguous results. High-risk screening is the major focus of this book, following the rationale that genetic or developmental diagnoses imply specific interventions and preventive measures.

Cost-effectiveness is a strong justification for prevention, and this has been accomplished effectively for measures such as the measles–mumps–rubella vaccine (White et al., 1985). However, prevention of heart attacks by decreasing cigarette smoking may be socially desirable but not cost-effective if the heart attacks are merely postponed to older ages (Rose, 1992). The eventual toll of age often requires humanitarian rather than strict economic arguments, returning again to quality of life outcomes rather than longevity. Cost and cost-effectiveness obviously depend on other characteristics of screening, such as incidence and severity of the target disease and its predictability in a selected population (Table 3.4).

In summary, the underlying themes of beneficence and health optimization offer powerful rationales for preventive medicine. Justification of specific preventive measures is difficult because of ambiguities in defining health, outcomes, and cost-effectiveness. The justification of any given preventive measure will usually involve several considerations (ethics, outcomes, costs) that may be difficult to assess in children with disabilities.

Problems with physician compliance and the value of preventive checklists

Despite their acceptance of preventive guidelines, physicians often are slow to implement them (Lewis, 1988; Scott et al., 1992). Several barriers for implementation have been cited, including (Thompson et al., 1995):

1 organizational rigidity of the health care system which can squelch new initiatives;
2 lack of compelling evidence for improved outcomes or lack of knowledge of these improvements;
3 a disease-oriented tradition that makes physicians reactive to symptoms rather than proactive towards prevention;
4 constraints that eliminate time required for additional history, examination and counseling;
5 lack of resources.

The rigidity of health care systems may reflect the growing input of non-physicians or a lack of education of older physician-managers. Chi-Lum (1995) commented on the inadequacy of education regarding preventive measures in medical school curricula. The difficulty of selecting and measuring outcomes has already been alluded to. Unfortunately, as cited in the foreword to *Bright Futures* (Greene, 1994), there are few studies demonstrating efficacy of biomedical preventive measures and virtually none demonstrating efficacy of psychosocial measures (Wilson, 1995). Funding is one of the most severe problems in implementing preventive care. Kottke et al. (1993) points out that funding and resources correlate well with the willingness of physicians to devote the extra time needed for preventive practices.

On the positive side, Thompson et al. (1995) reported the successes of a preventive care program operated within the Group Health Program of Puget Sound, a health maintenance organization. This program achieved an 89% completion rate for childhood immunizations, a change in bicycle helmet use from 4% to 48%, and a 67% decrease in bicycle head injuries. Thompson et al. (1995) concluded that several factors were responsible for these and other accomplishments:

1 a population-wide viewpoint to prioritize prevention objectives;
2 evidence-based criteria to demonstrate benefits of preventive measures;
3 involvement of practitioners in the formulation of the preventive guidelines;
4 provision of reminders and checklists to patients and physicians;
5 feedback to practitioners on positive population trends.

To focus on a major strategy employed in this book, there have been several studies demonstrating benefits of checklists on the delivery of preventive care (Cheney & Ramsdel, 1987; Maiman et al., 1988; Johns et al., 1992; Jackson, 1996). Regarding the use of a checklist for behavioral problems in pediatric practice, over half of the 556 pediatricians who responded to the survey felt that checklists were valuable but about 30% felt that they were overly time consuming (Cheng et al., 1996). Availability and ease of use are clearly important if the value of checklists is to be realized.

Defining the effectiveness of preventive measures

Types of outcomes in people with disabilities

A health outcome is a result or visible effect that occurs after a health care intervention. The circumstances of the intervention, such as the type of personnel, the dose of medication, the duration of therapy, are often called *inputs*. It is clear that health care objectives influence selection of outcome criteria (Wilkin et al., 1993), and that these objectives in turn reflect perceptions of health care needs. To speak of a need, such as inadequate immunization rates, is to imply a goal of health care; needs are subject to value judgments about what should be appropriate goals and what constitutes deficiency from these goals (Wilkin et al., 1993).

It follows that the outcomes selected for assessing the health care of children with congenital anomalies and syndromes are highly dependent on attitudes toward the disabled. When the goals of society were oriented towards primary prevention of mental retardation, as in the eugenics movement, then the outcome measure was existence and the ideal outcome elimination (Gould, 1981). When the purported benefits of natural settings led to enthusiasm for institutions, then the outcomes were proportions of individuals receiving these benefits. Now, when inclusive schooling and job training are encouraged to allow integration with society at large, degrees of independent function are more pertinent outcomes in assessing health care of persons with disabilities.

The shift from binary outcomes such as life or death to graded outcomes such as function has also occurred for chronic disease in general. Mortality outcomes can be useful endpoints, as shown by Blair et al. (1995) in demonstrating reduced mortality for males with greater physical fitness. However, in chronic diseases such as asthma, functional indicators such as school attendance, sports participation, etc., will be more appropriate for the endpoints of current interest: household smoking, newer bronchodilator medications, home nebulizers, etc. For chronic diseases, natural history becomes an important baseline against which outcomes can be measures (Wilkin et al., 1993). Because of the rarity of disorders and an emphasis on diagnosis, natural history is poorly defined for many genetic syndromes. Natural history comparisons also require long-term studies, while changes in levels of function can be measure year by year.

Functional outcomes in children with disabilities

In order to appreciate functional status as an endpoint of health care, definitions offered by the World Health Organization are helpful (Wilkin et al., 1993). As mentioned previously, health can be defined as a state of complete physical, mental, and social well-being rather than merely the absence of disease or infirmity. In addition, the functional status of individuals can be categorized by the following definitions:

Impairment: Loss or abnormality of psychiatric, physiologic or anatomic structure and function (e.g., loss of limb).
Disability: Restriction of ability to perform an activity in manner or range considered normal for age.
Handicap: Disadvantage to a person resulting from impairment or disability.

As a parallel to the usual sequence of disease leading to pathogenesis leading to manifestations, the following functional sequence can then be imagined: disease (intrinsic situation) leads to an impairment (experience exteriorized), which leads to a disability (experience objectified), which leads to a handicap (experience socialized). Outcomes can be drawn from each level, with disease or impairment being measures of individual biology and disability or handicap being measures of individual and society. The modern perspective on children with special needs shifts emphasis from disease diagnosis and impairment to the ability of the child to lead a normal life (Wilkin et al., 1993).

The first instrument for measurement of functional status was the activities of daily living (ADL) scale developed by the staff at Benjamin Rose Hospital, Cleveland, in 1959. Their underlying concept was that disease caused loss of functional capacities in a particular order, and that rehabilitation restored these capacities in reverse order. Interventions could thus be evaluated by the level of function restored. While the ADL scale focuses on basic ADL (mobility, dressing, toileting) appropriate for the severely disabled, other scales have evolved to evaluate more complex functions (such as laundry, housework, managing money, or employment). Measures have thus become more inclusive, evaluating not only disease or impairment, but also disability and handicap as discussed above.

Despite the potential utility of functional scales in assessing preventive management interventions, there are virtually no studies combining such assessments with the natural history of particular genetic syndromes. Surprisingly, reliability and validity have not been well demonstrated even for the Cleveland ADL scale (Wilkin et al., 1993), which is not very sensitive to small changes in the patient's condition. Strict functional assessment is also rather limited, since mental health or social support will obviously influence function. Any overall quality of life measurement should also include some estimate of patient satisfaction or well-being. A positive sense of well-being correlates strongly with an individual's motivation for preventive health practices (Gill & Feinstein, 1994; Hennessy et al., 1994). Such estimates have obvious difficulties when applied to people with disabilities, but more emphasis on assessment of personal well-being would parallel the emphasis on self-advocacy in the disability movement.

Several types of measures will be needed for a meaningful assessment of quality of life for people with disabilities. Examples include nominal outcomes (e.g., male/female), ordinal outcomes (e.g., severe, moderate, mild), interval outcomes (e.g., temperature), or ratio outcomes (e.g., developmental quotients). Some of these measures are part of functional scales such as the Guttman (ordinal measure of ability to walk 5, 10 or 50 m) and Likert scale (ordinal measures of "strongly agree" to "strongly disagree," "most important" to "least important"; Wilkin et al., 1993). The numerical approach facilitates statistical analysis for correlations with preventive measures and for inter-test reliability (i.e., Kappa analysis). Issues in the measurement of quality of life for individuals with disabilities include the definition of disease-specific norms against which the disabilities are measured and timing and validity of individual functional assessments.

Msall et al. (1994a, b) provided an instrument that assesses functional independence in children and correlates with their stage of development. The WeeFIM scale includes a broad range of activities plus some psychosocial factors such as parental circumstances (Msall, 1996). If combined with measures of self-satisfaction, the WeeFIM scale should be useful for assessing changes in outcome as a result of preventive interventions. Although there few studies linking preventive measures with functional outcome in children with disabilities, some simple theoretical examples can illustrate the importance of anticipatory health care in improving quality of life. These examples provide rationales for the preventive checklists in this book, and are obvious avenues for future research.

Consider a child with Down syndrome who might be scored as full function (3 points), mildly impaired (2 points), moderately impaired (1 point), or severely impaired (0 points) for a variety of skills and activities enjoyed by the typical young adult (e.g., reading, sports, church attendance, cooking, biking, driving). For 50 activities evaluated on a typical daily living scale, an average adult would score 150 points, while an optimally functioning person with Down syndrome would score about 120 points (80%). The young adult with Down syndrome would have mild dysfunction in activities such as reading or writing, and severe dysfunction in activities such as driving a car or managing money.

If, on the other hand, the person with Down syndrome had unrecognized hypothyroidism or pulmonary hypertension due to inoperable cardiac disease, their estimated score would drop to 90 points (60%) or 70 points (46%), respectively. Prevention of these complications by early thyroid or cardiac screening as recommended on the Down syndrome checklist thus would have a dramatic improvement of the child's eventual quality of daily living. Outcome studies that build on this simple analysis should one day provide compelling justification for preventive measures in children with congenital anomalies and syndromes. These outcome analyses must take in account the average disability/handicap expected for a particular disorder, assess a full range of activities, avoid prejudice about capabilities, and include measures of self-satisfaction and well-being.

Cost and health efficiency issues: Influence of health care reform

Cost-effectiveness is also a complex issue when used to judge preventive management interventions for patients with disabilities. It is ideal when an intervention is cost-effective, as for measles–mumps–rubella immunization programs that save $14 for each dollar invested (White et al., 1985). Increased hospitalization or chronic care expenses will be substantial for disorders such as undetected pulmonary hypertension, but less dramatic for a child with undetected hypothyroidism. In fact, the costs of endocrinology referral and treatment/follow-up may increase costs compared to the individual that is never screened for hypothyroidism. In order to demonstrate cost-effectiveness for measures such as thyroid or audiology screening, the lost income and increased living costs resulting from the cognitive or hearing impairments must be calculated. These will obviously depend on the social context (handicap), since an adult living on the family farm may experience fewer economic consequences than an adult seeking employment and independent living in an urban setting.

While health care professionals must balance the importance of a preventive care measure against its cost, there is no simple formula that can take in account both cost and quality of life issues. The philosophy of this book is to include all preventive measures that can significantly impact the quality of life, consistent with the principles of screening mentioned above (e.g., screening where symptoms cannot be relied upon and where an abnormal result implies some type of beneficial intervention). An example would be the consideration of cranial MR imaging for infants with craniosynostosis (Chapter 14) or mucopolysaccharidosis (Chapter 19) but not for children with neurofibromatosis (Chapter 13); the high frequency of asymptomatic hydrocephalus in the first two disorders, together with a discrete intervention (shunt surgery), provides the rationale. For interventions like MRI scanning, where children are subjected to inconvenience or risk (anesthesia), a footnote is always added to emphasize that clinical judgment is needed.

In the future, preventive care for children with disabilities is likely to be challenged by managed care and federal providers. Children with disabilities are part of a large fraction of children with chronic diseases – 25.2% between ages 6 and 11 years, 35.3% between ages 12 and 17 years (Jessop & Stein, 1995). Children with chronic disease are more costly for healthcare, and special "carve-outs" may be needed to protect families from loss of health insurance or exclusion from managed care organizations (Neff & Anderson, 1995). These considerations dramatize the need for outcomes analysis of preventive measures, but should not deter health care professionals from their responsibilities for good medical care.

Part II

The management of selected single congenital anomalies and associations

The average newborn has a 2–3% chance to have a major congenital anomaly, two-thirds with isolated defects like cleft palate and one-third with patterns of defects (sequences, associations, or syndromes). Paralleling this frequency of structural defects, and exaggerated when they are present, are risks for abnormal brain development that manifest as behavior differences and/or cognitive disability. These children, defined by an IQ two standard deviations below normal or less than 70, will also constitute 2–3% of the population. The result is a 5% chance for physical and/or mental disability in children old enough for assessment, and their increased clinical care ensures that every health care professional will devote much time to children with special needs. This section begins translation of principles from Chapters 1 to 3 into management strategies for specific disabling conditions.

Chapters 4 and 5 will discuss congenital disorders that have no associated birth defects (like some cases of cerebral palsy) or lack the stereotypical and recognizable patterns of anomalies that characterize genetic syndromes. Cerebral palsy encompasses a large group of disorders defined by a typical pattern of neurologic dysfunction; it is a category like autism spectrum disorders where DNA technology is demonstrating an increasing etiologic role for genes as compared to perinatal or environmental influences. Hydrocephalus and spina bifida also have genetic predisposition, but are like cerebral palsy in forcing attention to neuromotor function rather than internal defects or genetic testing. Cerebral palsy, single anomalies, and associations do not have the inexorable risks for mental disability brought by many genetic syndromes, and surgical or developmental specialists are often sufficient for assisting the primary physician.

Chapter 6 will review the abnormalities caused by teratogens, acting through maternal exposure or maternal disease. Many require dysmorphology expertise for recognition and, like genetic syndromes, will often have risks for mental disability. Teratogenic conditions remind all pediatric caregivers of their responsibility for the family's next pregnancy, for they demonstrate the power of prevention through preconceptional counseling (Schrander-Stumpel, 1999).

4

Congenital anomalies associated with developmental disability

Cerebral palsy and congenital brain defects

Terminology

Cerebral palsy embraces a range of conditions characterized by disordered movement or posture resulting from a non-progressive brain lesion or injury occurring prenatally or in early childhood (Palmer & Hoon, 1995). Cerebral palsy may be further defined by its topography (quadraplegia, hemiplegia, diplegia) or by its pathophysiology (pyramidal or extrapyramidal). Pyramidal lesions are associated with spastic types of cerebral palsy, while extrapyramidal insults are associated with hypotonic, choreoathetoid, and ataxic cerebral palsy. Overlap among the forms of cerebral palsy is common.

Cerebral dysgenesis refers to alterations in the formation of the central nervous system (CNS) (e.g., abnormal cellular migration or proliferation) resulting in congenital defects in the size, structure, and function of the brain. Most of these defects result in significant neurologic impairment, including cerebral palsy and mental retardation (Gabriel & McComb, 1985; Rosenbloom, 1995). For example, lissencephaly (smooth brain) or agyria is a disorder of neuronal migration associated with severe developmental consequences (Dobyns, 1987). Absence of the corpus callosum includes a spectrum of alterations in the formation of midline cortical structures with diverse etiologies and a wide range of developmental outcomes (Jeret et al., 1987). Porencephalic cysts result from a specific, destructive event such as a vascular accident *in utero*.

Historical diagnosis and management

Taxonomy and classification were of great interest to early clinicians resulting in much of the terminology still in use (Ingram, 1984). William Little, an orthopedic surgeon, is often credited with the earliest efforts at classification (Little, 1862) and cerebral palsy was once called Little's disease. Sigmund Freud advanced the notion of predisposing factors to expand upon the more narrow assumptions of Little that

Table 4.1. Distribution of types of cerebral palsy

Diagnosis	Number	Percent of total number	Percent of those of known type
Dyskinetic	52	9.8	12.5
Spastic	270	51.2	64.7
Ataxic	39	7.4	9.4
Dyskinetic spastic	40	7.6	9.6
Dyskinetic ataxic	3	0.5	0.7
Ataxic spastic	13	2.5	3.1
Other types/type not known*	110	21.0	
Total	527	100	100

Notes:
*The dyskinetic group includes choreoathetosis and dystonia: six cases were described only as hypotonic, but these are included under other types as it was not clear how many had true hypotonic cerebral palsy (Kuban & Levitan, 1994).
Source: Kuban & Levitan (1994); Pharoah et al. (1998).

cerebral palsy resulted from obstetric trauma and anoxia. Freud was also critical of early efforts to classify cerebral palsy on the basis of etiology or pathology rather than clinical findings until direct causal relationships could be established. With notable exceptions, such as the relationship between kernicterus and choreoathetoid cerebral palsy, the issue of causality remains unresolved 100 years later (Freud, 1897).

Interventions for cerebral palsy have mostly been grounded in notions of massage, bracing, and orthopedic surgery (Cruickshank, 1976; Carlson et al., 1997; Scrutton & Baird, 1997); they have also aimed at the limitation of disability and enhancement of function. Neurosurgical and orthopedic surgical techniques attempted in the early 1900s provided the basis for the use of tendon release and relocation and dorsal rhizotomy in the present. Following the establishment of federal funding for "crippled children's services" in the United States in 1935, multidisciplinary clinics have emerged as the state-of-the-art approach to cerebral palsy.

Incidence, etiology, and differential diagnosis

As discussed in Chapter 2, incidence figures are subject to variability as the result of methodologic factors including definitions of cerebral palsy, exclusions by severity or other criteria, and ascertainment. The overall prevalence of significant cerebral palsy ranges from 1.5 to 2.5 per 1000 live births (Kuban & Leviton, 1994; Pharoah et al., 1998). Tables 4.1 and 4.2 portray the distribution of cerebral palsy according to various subtypes.

Table 4.2. Distribution of subgroups described as spastic

	Number	Percentage
Hemiplegia	97	36
Diplegia	74	28
Quadriplegia	71	26
Monoplegia	6	2
Paraplegia	5	2
Other	17	6
Total	270	100

The largest prospective samplings of prevalence, causal associations, and risk factors for cerebral palsy have used data from the Collaborative Perinatal Study of the National Institute of Neurological and Communicative Disorders and Stroke. The outcomes for 43,437 *full-term* children were reviewed by Naeye et al. (1989). Among the 150 children with cerebral palsy in this population, only nine cases (6%) appeared attributable to birth asphyxia. Of the 34 children with quadriplegic cerebral palsy, possible causes were apparent in 71% with 53% appearing attributable to congenital disorders, 14% to birth asphyxia, and 8% to CNS infections. Among the children with non-quadriplegic cerebral palsy, congenital disorders appeared to account for about one-third of the cases and congenital infections for about 5%. Birth asphyxia was not significantly associated with non-quadraplegic cerebral palsy, and no cause could be identified in 60% of these patients. In another analysis of the Collaborative Perinatal Project data for both term and preterm births, Nelson & Ellenberg (1986) found a "defect" (congenital malformation, low birth weight, microcephaly) in 91% of the children who developed cerebral palsy.

Table 4.3 summarizes data from many studies of risk factors associated with cerebral palsy according to the timing with respect to gestation and birth. Additional risk factors of interest include maternal use of thyroid or estrogen hormones during pregnancy, non-vertex and face presentations at birth, and family history of cerebral palsy. Birth asphyxia or related factors have proven to be weak predictors of later cerebral palsy. Newborn encephalopathy and recurrent neonatal seizures are more strongly linked with cerebral palsy, though this may be an associative rather than causal relationship (Kuban & Leviton, 1994).

In contrast to the weak associations of prenatal and birth events in term infants, a birth weight below 1500 g confers a 25–30 times increased risk of cerebral palsy (Kuban & Leviton, 1994). One-third of all babies who later develop cerebral palsy weighed less than 2500 g at birth: by far the strongest factors associated with low birth weight and the later development of cerebral palsy are the presence of periventricular leukomalacia or other parenchymal brain injury. Whether periventricular

Table 4.3. Factors identified in epidemiologic studies as associated with cerebral palsy

---

Before pregnancy
History of fetal wastage
Long menstrual cycles
During pregnancy
Low social class
Congenital malformation
Fetal growth retardation
Twin gestation
Abnormal fetal presentation
During labor and delivery
Premature separation of the placenta
During the early postnatal period
Newborn encephalopathy

---

leukomalacia causes cerebral palsy or simply shares a common origin remains uncertain. These factors provide strong justification for brain imaging in children at risk.

Though the differential diagnosis of cerebral palsy is rarely complicated, other causes for delayed motor development, altered movement and reflexes, and altered muscle tone deserve consideration. Spinal cord tumors or other lesions are usually notable for sparing involvement of muscle groups above the lesion, while even spastic diplegia may show some upper-extremity involvement. Spina bifida is not likely to be mistaken for cerebral palsy, but consideration of a tethered cord in a child with apparent diplegia or monoplegia is important. Lower motor neuron and myopathic conditions also deserve consideration in a child with hypotonia and motor delays.

Diagnostic evaluation and medical counseling

The diagnosis of cerebral palsy is made through neurologic and developmental observation. The process is complicated by its pattern of emergence and change over time. Spasticity is nearly always preceded by hypotonia, which, while delaying motor milestones, may be less obvious to parents and clinicians. On the other hand, early alterations in movement and tone may subsequently attenuate or disappear. Efforts to standardize or formalize such observations are helpful in infants at high risk or who have suspicious findings from developmental screening during well-child care. Clues during well-child visits include the persistence of infantile reflexes, delayed appearance of postural and protective reflexes, asymmetrical movements or reflexes, variations in muscle tone, and delays in the sequence of motor milestones. Primary care physicians can enhance their assessment through the use of a more rigorous neuromotor examination, such as that of Milani-Comparetti & Gidoni (1976).

Standardized instruments such as the Bayley Scales of Infant Development or the Movement Assessment of Infants (MAI) provide scores that may be predictive of long-term motor impairment (Harris, 1984). The average child with cerebral palsy is not diagnosed until about 12 months of age (Palfrey et al., 1987), and some have suggested that a definitive diagnosis should be deferred until 2 years of age (Kuban & Leviton, 1994). Referral to a pediatric neurologist, developmental pediatrics (child development) clinic, or neuromotor disorders clinic may be helpful in establishing the diagnosis, and are essential in long-term preventive management. Such specialists will assist the primary care physician and family in the development of an initial treatment and care plan.

The consideration of specific underlying causes for the motor delays and impairments found on neurologic examination may be important. Conditions for which an intervention might prove crucial, such as a treatable metabolic disorder or findings that suggest child abuse ("shaken baby syndrome"), must not be overlooked. Other identifiable syndromes and conditions may have prognostic significance, associated complications, or recurrence risks (e.g., Aicardi syndrome or familial forms of cerebral palsy). A dysmorphology or genetics consultation may be useful to rule out specific conditions in which cerebral palsy is one of the characteristics. Brain imaging, usually by MRI, should be carried out in nearly all cases.

When the primary care physician becomes suspicious of cerebral palsy, it is important that he or she share those concerns with the parents. Parents will be more able to understand and cope with the eventual diagnosis of cerebral palsy if they have been partners in the diagnostic process. Furthermore, the symptoms and signs themselves, before they are sufficient for a diagnosis, may already be worrisome to parents and may justify a referral for early intervention services. These delays alone may also make some children eligible for Supplemental Security Income (SSI), which may in turn (in most states) provide eligibility for Medicaid.

When it becomes clear that a fixed pattern of altered movement, muscle tone, and reflexes is associated with delayed motor milestones, then a diagnosis of cerebral palsy is warranted. As with other developmental disabilities, care should be taken in the process of informing parents (see Chapter 2 and the section on Down syndrome in Chapter 7). The diagnosis might be framed in provisional terms for a mildly involved child less than 2 years of age because of the possibility of improvement. The term "cerebral palsy" must be presented and discussed carefully with parents to avoid misunderstandings. The prognosis is uncertain in nearly all children at the time of diagnosis, particularly with respect to specific characteristics such as independent ambulation, language, and cognitive ability. Children with the most severe motor involvement (not rolling over or persistent infantile reflexes at 12 months or not sitting by 24 months) are less likely to be walk independently though this may vary with the type of cerebral palsy (Molnar, 1979; Lepage et al., 1998). Plans need to be made with the family for a definitive diagnostic evaluation. Most children and families will benefit from a referral to a multidisciplinary neuromotor clinic or team. This team usually includes a pediatric orthopedist, developmental pediatrician or neurologist, nurse coordinator, pediatric physical therapist, and orthoticist.

Family and psychosocial counseling

Cerebral palsy usually occurs episodically. However, it is important to inquire about any family history of cerebral palsy, motor disability, other developmental disability (e.g., mental retardation), seizures, or known genetic conditions. Such information may provide clues to diagnoses other than or in addition to cerebral palsy. Furthermore, there are a number of uncommon, but well-described forms of familial cerebral palsy (Cooley et al., 1990).

Parents should be referred to a local or state parent-to-parent organization (a parent support group), which will facilitate specific, one-to-one connections with an experienced parent who has been trained to be a resource to parents of newly diagnosed children. Most parents would benefit from contact with national, state, or local organizations such as United Cerebral Palsy Association Inc. (www.ucpa.org): Ontario Federation for Cerebral Palsy (www.ofcp.on.ca); or Scope-About Cerebral Palsy, UK (www.scope.org.uk). Generic support groups for families of children with various disabilities are available, or they may be specific for cerebral palsy as listed (see checklist). Reading materials for parents are also helpful (Geralis, 1991; Miller & Bachrach, 1995).

The diagnosis of cerebral palsy may be the first of a series of "bad news" experiences for parents. Later conclusions that a child will not walk, will need orthopedic surgery, will require augmentative help with communication, or will have cognitive limitations constitute diagnostic events for which parents may need extra support. Many parents and, later, children with cerebral palsy are led to a perspective of "fixing" the cerebral palsy rather than coping, preventing secondary disability, and accommodating. Sometimes this leads children to the impression that they are "broken," that therapy is aimed at "fixing" them, and, to the degree that a "fix" does not occur, they (parents or child) have failed. This is damaging to self-esteem, morale, and family strengths. Clinicians should use care in how they frame the goals of intervention and ensure that parents and, eventually, the child have clear roles in articulating those goals. Siblings and other family members may require attention and support as well.

Most children with cerebral palsy will be eligible for early intervention services (from birth to age 3 years) and special education services (after age 3 years). The goals of these services are optimal functioning, safety, inclusion in school and community, and self-determination to the degree possible. It should be assumed that most children with cerebral palsy can receive and will benefit from school services

Table 4.4. Ambulatory status and onset of walking in prenatal and perinatal cerebral palsy

Clinical type	Number	Age at onset of walking (years)				Never	Ambulatory	
		1–2	2–3	4–5	5–8		Yes (%)	No (%)
Hemiplegia	107	98	9				100	0
Diplegia	81	31	20	5	5	12	85	15
Quadriparesis	144	12	14	22	19	46	68	32
Athetosis	96	20	19	14	12	23	77	23
Spastic–athetoid	38	3	5	2	2	20	47	53
Ataxic	12	0	2	4	2	0	100	0
Rigid	21					21	0	100
Atonic	14					14	0	100
Total	513	164	69	47	40	136	73	27

provided in regular settings. Often the classroom or curriculum will require modifications to include the student with cerebral palsy. Some school districts have maintained that children with cerebral palsy who appear to have no cognitive impairment do not experience an educational handicap and are, therefore, not eligible for a special education program. While some parents and children may prefer this, primary care physicians should be prepared to advocate for children who have been inappropriately denied school services.

Older children and adolescents with cerebral palsy who do not have mental retardation remain at risk for specific learning disabilities and attention deficits that may not become apparent until elementary school begins. More significant issues of self-esteem and anger may emerge during these years. Innovative efforts including peer-to-peer supports and active programs promoting self-determination should be implemented by the middle school years (Olson & Cooley, 1996). Concerns about dating, sexuality, and other social relationships need to be addressed openly and thoughtfully.

Natural history and complications

Outcomes of cerebral palsy vary from profound, multi-domain disability to mild, almost inapparent involvement. By definition it is assumed that all individuals have a permanent, non-progressive motor impairment. The nature of this impairment (spastic or athetoid, diplegia or quadriplegia) may emerge gradually in the early months and years. All children pass through an initial hypotonic phase, so if spasticity is present at birth, then the initial insult followed by hypotonicity occurred during intrauterine life (Capute & Accardo, 1996). Twenty-five percent of people with cerebral palsy are non-ambulatory, though there is considerable variation among types of cerebral palsy (Table 4.4; Molnar, 1979).

Table 4.5. Neurodegenerative disorders that
may be mistaken for cerebral palsy

Disorder	Inheritance
Spasticity	
Leukodystrophy	
Krabbe	AR
Metachromatic	AR
Adrenoleukodystrophy	XLR
Syndromes	
Zellweger	AR
Cockayne	AR
Small molecule disorders	
Arginase deficiency	AR
Abetalipoproteinemia	AR
Movement disorders	
Wilson's disease	AR
Ataxia–telangiectasia	AR
Lesch–Nyhan syndrome	XLR

Note:
AR, autosomal recessive; XLR, X-linked recessive.

Cerebral palsy can "worsen" through failure to address the orthopedic complications. All children with cerebral palsy should be evaluated and followed, if necessary, by a pediatric orthopedist. This is often best accomplished through a neuromotor team. This approach allows the institution of a comprehensive plan of physical therapy, non-invasive orthopedic techniques (e.g., serial casting), and orthotics to maintain the flexibility and mobility of joints. Therapy may also reduce wasting and weakness as a consequence of disuse. Secondary complications such as scoliosis and hip subluxation can be identified, monitored, and treated. Orthopedic surgery, stereotactic spinal cord surgery (dorsal rhizotomy), and medications affecting movement and tone may be considered for selected individuals.

Cerebral palsy may also "worsen" or appear to progress when there is a failure to address nutritional issues, seizures, or an additional medical illness. In addition, on occasion cerebral palsy is not the correct diagnosis but is temporarily mimicked by another, possibly progressive neurologic condition (Table 4.5).

Epilepsy occurs in about one-third of people with cerebral palsy, with a prevalence of 50% in those with hemiplegia (see checklist). At least 30% have mental retardation, with a greater percentage among those with spastic quadriplegia (Kuban & Leviton, 1994). On the other hand, cognition may be underestimated in individuals with choreoathetoid cerebral palsy due to the severity of the expressive language disorder (Palmer & Hoon, 1995). Even those without mental retardation may have learning disabilities. People with cerebral palsy are at increased risk for impairment of vision or hearing. Oral motor involvement is common in most forms of cerebral palsy, and this may complicate feeding. Some individuals have significant problems with drooling. Alterations in esophageal motility may result in reflux and aspiration hazards. In severe cases, feeding or gastrostomy tubes may be necessary. Inadequate caloric intake may be complicated by increased caloric consumption by spastic muscles and excess movements contributing to failure to thrive. Delays in the acquisition of bowel and bladder control are common. Urologic evaluation may be helpful to determine the nature of the bladder dysfunction and the best treatment (McNeal et al., 1983). Constipation may result from decreased overall mobility and spastic involvement of the anal sphincter (see checklist).

Cerebral palsy preventive medical checklist

Because children with cerebral palsy have such diverse manifestations, the preventive medical checklist is an outline that must be modified according to individual needs. The American Academy of Pediatrics' clinical report titled: *Providing a Medical Home for Children and Youth with Cerebral Palsy* provides management guidance for the primary care provider (Cooley and the Committe on Children with Disabilities, 2004). Timely, comprehensive care in early childhood can prevent chronic secondary disability, emphasizing the importance of obtaining early consultation from a neuromotor multidisciplinary team. Early assessment of feeding (Reilly et al., 1996), neuromotor (Capute & Accardo, 1996; DeLuca, 1996), and orthopedic (Ebara et al., 1996; Wilmshurst et al., 1996; Carlson et al., 1997; Scrutton & Baird, 1997) problems is particularly important, with consideration of new therapies such as intrathecal baclofen (Gerszten et al., 1998), botulinum toxin (Gooch & Sandell, 1996), or glycopyrrolate (Blasco & Stansbury, 1996; Bachrach et al., 1998). It is also essential to involve all children with early intervention or preschool special education. The careful evaluation and monitoring of hearing and vision by qualified specialists should become a regular aspect of preventive care for the child with cerebral palsy. Thorough initial consideration of possible neuropathologic, metabolic, genetic, or familial diagnoses should always be undertaken. The issue of causation and specific diagnosis should be revisited periodically as new knowledge and developments in fields such as genetics or brain imaging may offer fresh diagnostic opportunities.

Though the majority of families of children with moderate to severe cerebral palsy are not permanently disrupted by this challenge, about one-third of such families sustain serious consequences (e.g., divorce, abuse, mental health problems; Singer & Irvin, 1991). The families who cope successfully are more likely to have social and other supports and to have regained a sense of mastery of their situation. Primary care physicians can contribute to positive coping by families by facilitating connections with formal (programs, entitlements, information) and natural sources of support (friends, neighbors, churches, etc.). Even such minor actions as asking about and advocating for a "handicap" license plate may significantly relieve daily stresses for some families. Primary care physicians should strive toward a collaborative partnership with family caregivers rather than a prescriptive, paternalistic approach to care.

Hydrocephalus

Terminology

Hydrocephalus is a condition with diverse etiologies characterized by unbalanced formation and absorption of cerebrospinal fluid (CSF) resulting usually in the enlargement of the cerebral ventricles and often in increased CSF pressure (Gabriel & McComb, 1985). Non-communicating hydrocephalus involves obstruction of the flow of CSF at or before the outlet of the fourth ventricle, while communicating hydrocephalus refers to a more distal obstruction that may also interfere with the reabsorption of CSF (Kinsman, 1996). Arrested and compensated hydrocephalus are terms implying a balance between production and the reabsorption of CSF. There is disagreement among experts regarding the usefulness and validity of this notion. A distinction is sometimes made between congenital and acquired hydrocephalus, depending on the timing of the etiologic event with respect to birth.

Arnold–Chiari malformations, which are regarded as neural tube defects account for 40% of cases of hydrocephalus (Gabriel & McComb, 1985). Hydrocephalus results from the herniation of abnormal cerebellar or brainstem structures through the foramen magnum. In the Dandy Walker syndrome, which accounts for 5% of cases, the fourth ventricle dilates and herniates caudally due to the lack of an opening in its roof (Table 4.6).

Incidence, etiology, and differential diagnosis

Congenital hydrocephalus occurs in 2 per 1000 live births, with 25–50% of these cases associated with spina bifida (Jackson, 1990). "Acquired" hydrocephalus usually occurs as the result of infection, neoplasm, abnormal vascularity, or trauma that results in bleeding. Kinsman (1996) suggested classifying hydrocephalus according to etiology as follows: malformation (e.g., Arnold–Chiari), genetic process (e.g., X-linked or autosomal recessive), inflammation (e.g., meningitis), chemical irritation (e.g., bleeding), and neoplasm.

In newborns and infants, an enlarging head circumference is often accompanied by a bulging fontanel and splitting of sutures. Downward deviation of the eyes ("sunset sign") may occur. Symptoms such as irritability, vomiting, lethargy, poor feeding, apnea, and changes in respiratory pattern may also ensue (Marcus, 1996; Nitahara et al., 1996; Taylor & Madsen, 1996). In older children (after age 3 years),

Table 4.6. Potential complications and consequences of hydrocephalus

General	
Life cycle	Increased mortality associated with cause[a]
	Increased mortality (50%), if untreated
	20% of untreated children reach adulthood
Learning	Cognitive disability (verbal IQ scores exceed performance IQ scores)[b]
	Impaired "executive functions," learning differences
	Hyperverbal syndrome, handwriting and reading problems
	Problems with mathematics, problems with visual scanning
Facial	
Face	Altered cranial growth, prominent forehead, broad nasal root
Eyes	Strabismus, "sun-setting"
Skeletal	
Cranial	Macrocephaly, bulging fontanel, split sutures
Limbs	"Cortical" thumbs
Internal	
Digestive	Vomiting as symptom
Neural	
CNS	Accumulation of CSF, elevated intracranial pressure
Sensory	Vision deficits, visuomotor, visuospatial problems

Notes:
[a]For example, neoplasm, CNS infection; [b]Frequent shunt infections lower IQ scores.

head enlargement is unlikely and symptoms will depend on the rapidity of onset of the hydrocephalus and associated changes in CSF pressure. Headaches are usually present, particularly in the morning, along with vomiting, abnormal eye movements, and altered level of consciousness. Papilledema may be evident.

The differential diagnosis includes conditions that either cause head enlargement or the symptoms associated with increased intracranial pressure. The former include subdural hematoma due to trauma, familial or genetic forms of macrocephaly (e.g., Sotos syndrome), certain metabolic storage diseases, and brain tumors. The latter include CNS infections, pseudotumor cerebri with its variety of causes, and ingestions such as lead poisoning. When imaging studies demonstrate enlarged ventricles, conditions in which this has resulted from cerebral atrophy rather than the accumulation of CSF under excess pressure must be considered.

Diagnostic evaluation and medical counseling

The diagnosis of hydrocephalus depends on some form of brain imaging to identify the presence of ventriculomegaly (Kinsman, 1996). Ultrasonography may be performed in infants with patent fontanels, providing a quick, often crib-side assessment without sedation. In most instances, more complete imaging will be necessary using CT or MRI scans. Since sedation or anesthesia will be necessary in infants and young children for either study, the more informative MRI scan is usually preferable. This provides better detail of some structures and regions (James, 1992). In some individuals, serial studies will be necessary to differentiate static ventriculomegaly from true hydrocephalus.

When a clinician strongly suspects hydrocephalus, confirmation and treatment are urgent matters. Referral to an experienced pediatric neurosurgeon for further evaluation and surgical management is mandatory. However, it is also important to consider a variety of underlying etiologies which might be facilitated through consultations from a geneticist or a pediatric neurologist. Treatment is first directed at the underlying cause (e.g., removal of a tumor). In some cases, particularly in neonates, decompression is accomplished through intermittent lumbar or ventricular punctures or through an external drainage system. When long-term decompression is needed, the installation of a ventriculoperitoneal (VP) shunt is the treatment of choice in most situations. The child with hydrocephalus is at high risk for both obvious and subtle developmental disabilities which may warrant monitoring through a developmental pediatrics consultation and referral to early intervention or special education programs. The nature and severity of the disability will depend in part on the etiology of the hydrocephalus and any associated alterations in CNS structures. However, there are a number of learning disabilities associated specifically with hydrocephalus (Wills, 1993; Fletcher et al., 1996).

Family and psychosocial counseling

As with other serious chronic conditions in children, clinician should convey the news of the diagnosis of hydrocephalus with warmth, empathy, and clarity in the manner described in Chapter 2 and in section Down syndrome in Chapter 7. If trauma is a possible etiology, consideration of child abuse is important. A number of familial forms of hydrocephalus exist, so a careful family history should be elicited.

While parents need reassurance about the prognosis of this condition, they will want to understand the developmental consequences that may occur. Hydrocephalus may have a direct impact on development or may be associated with other brain anomalies (e.g., absence of the corpus callosum) that affect brain function (Fletcher et al., 1992). While all families benefit from accurate, understandable information, the families of children who have severe impairments may require access to family support services, financing sources, and parent-to-parent linkages. Education about the monitoring of intracranial shunt functioning must be balanced with encouragement of normal childhood activities to avoid an overly protective "vulnerable child" scenario. National organizations may provide helpful information and support: ASBAH, the Association for Spina Bifida and Hydrocephalus (www.asbah.org/); the

Hydrocephalus Association (www.hydroassoc.org), HyFI Hydrocephalus Foundation (www.hydrocephalus.org/), and a patient center devoted to those with hydrocephalus (www.patientcenters.com/hydrocephalus/).

Natural history and complications

In the past, untreated hydrocephalus was associated with a mortality of 50%, with severe mental retardation and disability occurring in 50% of survivors (Gabriel & McComb, 1985). Two-thirds of patients with untreated "spontaneously arrested" hydrocephalus experience disabling neurologic impairments. Assuming that hydrocephalus is promptly diagnosed and treated, the complications involve those associated with malfunction or infection of the intracranial shunt, those of the conditions causing or associated with the hydrocephalus, and the specific neuropsychologic consequences that have been associated with hydrocephalus (Table 4.6).

Hydrocephalus preventive medical needs

A number of articles, aimed at primary and allied health care professionals, describe principles of management in narrative form (Jackson, 1990; James, 1992). Special preventive medical measures for children with hydrocephalus relate primarily to the monitoring of shunt status (Iskander et al., 1998), of developmental/educational progress and programming, and of family support needs. In other respects, their preventive health care is similar to that of other children. Children in whom hydrocephalus is associated with spina bifida are discussed in the next section of this chapter.

Linear growth of children with hydrocephalus may be delayed during childhood followed by acceleration during precocious puberty (Lopponen et al., 1995). Head circumference monitoring is important, particularly in the first 3 years, and the measurements should be plotted on head circumference charts extending from birth to age 18 years (Nellhaus, 1986). Such charts also allow plotting the head sizes of parents and other family members to rule out familial macrocephaly. Regular vision assessment (Gaston, 1996) and monitoring for signs of early puberty (Lopponen et al., 1996) should also be considered.

Spina bifida

Terminology

Spina bifida or rachischisis refers to a bony defect of the spine in which enclosure of the spinal cord is incomplete. This defect may be covered by normal skin (spina bifida occulta) or there may be a protruding sac (spina bifida cystica). When such a sac contains only meninges and CSF, it is called a meningocele. The combination of spina bifida and meningomyelocele is sometimes referred to as myelodysplasia (Golden, 1979; Shurtleff et al., 1986).

Neural tube defects include CNS malformations that arise during the first 28–30 days of gestation as the result of incomplete formation, folding, or closure of the neural tube. Neural tube defects range from the most severe with holoanencephaly (complete absence of the brain) and craniorachischisis (absence of the covering skull) to the most distal sacral meningomyelocele in which spinal cord disruption may be minimal. Encephalocele and skin covered spinal cord lesions are sometimes included as neural tube defects though they occur after formation of the neural tube and neuronal disruption may be minimal or absent.

Historical diagnosis and management

Skeletal remains dating back over 10,000 years have revealed evidence of spina bifida (Feremback, 1963). Medical descriptions of spina bifida did not occur until the seventeenth century, and the association with hydrocephalus was first reported in 1769. Efforts to remove, close, or protect the herniated sac began in the nineteenth century with recognition by the early twentieth century that infection and hydrocephalus were the two most common lethal complications (Shurtleff, 1986). By the 1930s, early closure of the sac to prevent infection was advised, but debate remained about whether sac excision exacerbated hydrocephalus. Gradually the contemporary practice of skin closure over the sac and prompt shunting has emerged as the standard of care. The issue of "selection" of infants for aggressive management based on the severity of the lesion remains a topic of controversy. Few, if any, centers impose rigid selection criteria; most favor initial closure followed by a process of empowering parents as decision-making partners.

Incidence, etiology, and differential diagnosis

The prevalence at birth of neural tube defects has a distinct variability with geography and ethnicity as well as over time. For example, prior to 1980, the eastern United States experienced a rate of 3–3.5 per 1000 births while in the West the rate was 1–1.5 per 1000 births (Seller, 1994). However, over time this geographic distinction in the United States has been lost with a general decline in prevalence while in the United Kingdom, the birth prevalence has fallen from 4.5 per 1000 births in 1970 to 0.18 per 1000 in 1991. In the United States, the rate of neural tube defects has declined from 1.3 per 1000 births in 1970 to 0.6 per 1000 in 1989 (Yen et al., 1992).

Most reviews of causative factors for neural tube defects support etiologic heterogeneity. Neural tube defects are associated with chromosomal alterations (e.g., trisomies 13 and 18), prenatal exposures such as alcohol, rubella, or valproic acid, maternal diabetes, prenatal folic acid deficiency, and, rarely, Mendelian inheritance patterns (Shurtleff et al., 1986). Clear ethnic differences have been noted with increased prevalence among those of Celtic, Hispanic, and northern Native American origins and lower prevalence among Blacks, Asians, and Pacific Islanders (Centers for Disease Control, 1992). The recurrence risk in siblings which historically approached 5% in the United Kingdom, is now around 2% (Shurtleff et al., 1986).

Neural tube defects are usually readily suspected at birth based on the visible sac. However, care and expertise are required to determine the severity of the lesion and to identify associated complications or malformations. Careful tertiary level, multi-disciplinary evaluation is essential to this process which is likely to involve intensive neonatal care with neurosurgical, pediatric neurologic, genetics, pediatric urologic, and pediatric orthopedics consultations as well as brain and spinal cord imaging. Rarely, apparent neural tube defects will prove to be more simple meningoceles with minimal neurologic impairment or involve lipomas of the spinal cord. Lipomas of the cord may occur in association with meningomyelocele, duplication of the spinal cord (diplomyelia), or tethering of the cord (Shurtleff et al., 1986).

Diagnostic evaluation and medical counseling

All women having relatives with neural tube defects should receive preconceptional supplementation of folic acid in amounts similar to those in standard multivita-mins (Mulinare et al., 1988). Prenatal screening and diagnostic techniques have increased the frequency with which neural tube defects are identified during preg-nancy. Maternal serum alpha-fetoprotein (MSAFP) levels are used for general population screening with an accuracy of 75–80% in detecting an affected fetus (Johnson et al., 1990). The measurement of AFP in amniotic fluid has an accuracy of close to 95%, but fails to identify 5% of the defects in which there is a covering of epithelial tissue. AFP levels are also elevated in other malformations that disrupt the integrity of the fetal epithelium or that result in the loss of fetal (or placental) blood into the amniotic fluid. Ultrasonography can identify all but the smallest lesions including those with coverings of skin (Nadel et al., 1990).

Prenatal diagnosis allows for the provision of counseling, information, and sup-port to parents. When the diagnosis is made within allowable legal gestational limits for abortion, some parents may elect to terminate the pregnancy. However, all parents should be provided access to balanced information about outcomes including the same information provided to parents of newborns with spina bifida and, upon request, contact with parents of older affected children. Prenatal diagnosis permits planning for the safest delivery (often by Cesarean) in a medical center that can provide an immediate response to the newborn's medical needs. In some instances, prenatal diagnosis may also allow ameliorative prenatal surgery (e.g., to remove CSF).

Whether the diagnosis has occurred prenatally or following birth, early, thorough evaluation of the newborn and implementation of appropriate care may substantially improve the outcome. To prevent the occurrence of infection, the meningomyelocele

Table 4.7. Degree of paralysis and functional implications

Paralysis	Hydrocephalus (%)	Ambulation	Bowel/bladder incontinence (%)
Thoracic or high lumbar (L1, L2)	90	May walk with extensive braces and crutches	>90
Mid-lumbar (L3)	85	Can walk with either extensive, moderate, or minimal braces, and usually with crutches	>90
Low lumbar (L4, L5)	70	Will walk with moderate, minimal, or no bracing with or without crutches	>90
Sacral (S1–S4)	60	Will walk with minimal or no braces and usually without crutches	>90

Source: Charney (1990).

defect is usually closed in the first few days after birth. At this time, the level of the lesion may be clarified (Table 4.7). Lesions in the thoracic or high lumbar areas (L1 or L2) are regarded as "high level" and likely to result in complete paralysis of the lower extremities. Mid-level lesions around L3 may allow hip flexion and knee extension, while low lumber lesions at L4 or L5 allow flexion at hips, knees, and ankles with extension at knees and ankles. Hip extension and ankle flexion may remain weak. Sacral lesions result in mild weakness at the ankles, and toes. The higher the lesion the greater the ambulatory limitation and the need for assistive devices and equipment. Lesions at all levels are likely to affect bowel and bladder function (see checklist).

All newborns with spina bifida require brain imaging for the associated presence of CNS malformations, especially Arnold–Chiari malformation type II in which the brainstem and portions of the cerebellum are herniated downward into the foramen magnum. This malformation occurs in the majority of children with spina bifida, resulting in obstruction of CSF movement and hydrocephalus (Griebel et al., 1991). In most cases, hydrocephalus will require surgical treatment as early as possible. This usually involves the placement of a VP shunt to drain CSF from the enlarged cerebral ventricles to the peritoneal cavity (see section on hydrocephalus of this chapter for additional information).

Family and psychosocial counseling

When a neural tube defect is not suspected prenatally and is diagnosed at birth, care, and attention is needed to counsel and inform parents. Immediate information about severity and complications may not be readily available. However, it is crucial that the informant be knowledgeable about the range of prognoses for newborns with spina bifida as well as appropriate interventions. Principles used to inform parents of a diagnosis like Down syndrome (see Chapter 7) apply in this instance as well. The informing interview should begin an active process of re-empowerment and support as parents cope with and adapt to the news. Parents should be supported by being together in the case of two parents or by the presence of another family member or close friend in the case of a single parent. The baby should be present, if possible, referred to by name, and held or otherwise acknowledged as a baby first and affected by a diagnosis second. Ample time for questions according to the parents' agenda of needs and concerns should be provided with frequent follow-up and ready access for parents to sources of information. Some parents may welcome contact with an experienced family of a child with spina bifida (Cerniglia, 1997). Rarely, parents may be interested in the availability of specialized foster care or adoption for babies with spina bifida.

A history of the pregnancy including prenatal care and nutrition, ultrasound and other tests, and exposure to potential teratogens should be reviewed. This may not only identify etiologic factors, but more likely eliminate sources of parental fear or guilt about unrelated occurrences. The family history should be reviewed for other cases of neural tube and related defects as well as notation of the family's ethnic and geographic background.

As with other developmental disabilities, parents of children with spina bifida require ongoing information, advocacy, and support from primary care providers as well as members of a multidisciplinary specialty team (Liptak et al., 1988; Sarwark, 1996). Early referral to such a team located at the nearest tertiary care medical center, at an outreach location for such a medical center, or through the state's program for children with special health care needs is very important. Ideally, this referral connection will be made during the initial hospitalization as a newborn. In addition to the needed medical and surgical specialists working collaboratively, most spina bifida teams have a specialty nurse coordinator who provides the family with an accessible source of information, support, parent-to-parent contact, and care coordination. Such nurse coordinators can often provide community-based professionals (primary care physicians, early intervention professionals, teachers, etc.) with consultation, technical assistance, in-service training, and reading about spina bifida.

Depending on factors such as family income, many children with spina bifida are eligible for benefits such as Medicaid insurance, Supplemental Security Income from the Social Security Administration, and possible financial and other supports from the state's program for children with special health care needs. Some states provide special "family support services" for families of children with developmental disabilities that may include respite care, discretionary funds, stipends or loan programs, advocacy and care coordination, and parent-to-parent contacts. Primary care physicians should ask about and confirm that families have access to these programs. Nearly all young children with spina bifida are eligible for state early intervention services from birth to age 3 years and preschool special education services from age 3 to 5 or 6 years. Prompt connection with these services will benefit most families.

Parents will require specific information to help them maintain and monitor their child's status and well-being. Spina bifida team nurse coordinators often provide parents with training and information about clean intermittent catheterization techniques (Bomalaski et al., 1995; Johnston & Borzyskowski, 1998) and about the signs of VP shunt malfunction or infection. Additional information about home physical therapy and the encouragement of ambulation and other developmental tasks will come both from the nurse coordinator and from community-based therapists and early interventionists. The encouragement of parents to provide their children a normal range of regular experiences with siblings and other children their age will help to avoid creating a "vulnerable child" situation.

The specific issue of mobility will be an important one for parents and for the child. Depending on the level of the lesion, a goal of independent bipedal ambulation may require a range of training, therapy, orthotics, orthopedic interventions, and assistive devices. However, this goal should be supported in most individuals with spina bifida even in situations where the eventual primary mode of community mobility is likely to be a wheelchair. Restricted mobility may be associated with skin lesions and slow healing (Srivastava, 1995).

Older children should be gradually incorporated into discussions and treatment planning activities while they are given increasing responsibility for their own self-care. Information about spina bifida and its specific manifestations in the individual child should be provided in age appropriate language as early as possible. Children should be taught to perform their own self-catheterization during the early school age years according to the child's readiness and interest. Careful counseling about sexuality and reproductive health is important beginning in the grade school years. The spina bifida team coordinator should have helpful information in this regard. Many children might benefit from periodic meetings with an older peer mentor who has spina bifida (Olson & Cooley, 1996).

Additional information of benefit to individuals with spina bifida, their families, and their caregivers can be obtained from the Spina Bifida Association of America-SBAA (www.sbaa.org/). The SBAA publishes a well-written newsletter entitled *Spina Bifida Spotlight*, as well as an e-newsletter on advocacy. Other parent-oriented organizations include the International Federation for Spina Bifida and Hydrocephalus (www.ifglobal.org/home.asp?lang=1&main=1).

Natural history and complications

The natural history and complications of neural tube defects are highly dependent on the severity of the primary defect and on the nature of any associated birth defects (see checklist). Neural tube defects may be uniformly lethal (anencephaly) or associated with lethal combinations of other defects (e.g., trisomy 13). On the other hand, they may be so mild as to have limited impact. Assuming the presence of a spinal cord lesion (as opposed to a cranial lesion), over 90% of babies who receive early surgical treatment survive into adulthood (Shurtleff, 1986). Early handling and management is aimed at avoiding infection of the CSF, spinal cord, or brain before, during, and after closure of the back. As soon as surgical closure is achieved, plans for installation of a VP shunt under uninfected conditions should be carried out since the majority (up to 90%) of babies will have hydrocephalus. There is growing evidence that shunting should be considered in nearly all neonates with spina bifida even in the absence of an enlarging head circumference. Intellectual outcomes seemed improved by such an aggressive approach. Shunt malfunction or infection-remain complications for the child with spina bifida which require prompt diagnosis and management.

Nearly all children will have bowel and bladder incontinence (Bomalaski et al., 1995; Johnston & Borzyskowski, 1998). While bowel function can usually be managed with a combination of behavioral and dietary plans, urinary retention can lead to a series of complications including urinary tract infection, reflux, and hydronephrosis. Depending on the initial cystometric evaluation, a child's program may involve anticholinergic medication, clean intermittent catheterization, and antibiotics. Urinary diversions such as vesicostomy are rarely indicated. Some children (about 10–20%) who have repeated infections despite adequate bladder regimens and prophylaxis may require anti-reflux surgery (Bauer, 1994).

A tethered cord may develop in up to 10% of individuals as the result of scarring and adhesions at the surgical site or due to small cysts or lipomas of the cord. Newer surgical methods have been aimed at reducing the incidence of tethered cord. Unfortunately, the highest risk occurs among children with the lowest lesions who may experience the most relative loss of function due to tethered cord (Humphreys, 1986). Early diagnosis is important. Back and radiating leg pain, worsening of gait, scoliosis, bladder or bowel control, or long-track neurologic findings are important signs and symptoms that suggest a tethered cord.

The presence of partial or complete lower-extremity paralysis results in an increased risk for secondary orthopedic deformity. Many infants have clubfoot deformities when the lesion is at the L3 level or higher. Milder ankle and foot deformities may also require orthopedic attention. The hips are vulnerable to imbalanced musculature which may lead to contractures or hip dislocation (Frawley et al., 1996). Scoliosis occurs in a large number of children particularly those with thoracic or high lumber levels of involvement in whom the incidence of scoliosis approaches 90% (Mayfield, 1991).

An increased risk of allergic hypersensitivity to latex-containing products is now well-recognized in people with spina bifida (Leger & Meeropol, 1992; Kwittken et al., 1995). Prevention from exposure is not only crucial for those with established sensitivity in whom severe reactions can occur, but also among all others beginning as newborns to reduce the likelihood of acquiring sensitivity. Many products used by infants contain latex (e.g., bottle nipples, pacifiers, teething toys, changing pads and mattress covers, and some diapers). Medical equipment must also be checked (bandages, tape, catheters, gloves, crutch arm pads, brace linings). Common childhood toys such as balloons, balls, racquet handles, water toys must be carefully evaluated. Household products such as rubber cement, erasers, sneakers, spandex products, condoms, and diaphragms (for birth control) contain latex. There may be some cross-reactivity with certain foods (bananas, kiwi, avocados).

Cognitive functioning and school performance is affected in the majority of children with spina bifida though usually in the context of a pattern of strengths and challenges (Wills et al., 1990; Dise & Lohr, 1998). It has become increasingly apparent that spina bifida is not associated with a universal reduction in overall intelligence, but some variation occurs depending on the level of the lesion and the priority given to careful management of hydrocephalus and shunt care. Shurtleff found that lesions below L3 were associated on the whole with average performance on IQ tests, while higher-lesions tended to result in lower scores (Shurtleff, 1986). Children with VP shunts that have been carefully managed (prompt recognition and treatment of malfunction and infection) show verbal intelligence scores in the same range as controls without spina bifida (McClone et al., 1982).

More detailed profiling of cognitive abilities often reveals strengths in the verbal areas with better performance in reading and spelling compared to math. Visual perceptual skills affecting eye–hand coordination may also be impaired causing difficulty with handwriting and other fine motor tasks. There may also be an increased risk for more subtle neuropsychologic challenges affecting attention, memory, sequencing, or reasoning (Cull & Wyke, 1984).

Spina bifida preventive medical checklist

Health promotion and preventive care for the child with spina bifida involves the coordination of important services from several medical and surgical subspecialties with attentive and accessible primary health care services. Children with spina bifida require all of the usual immunizations, health supervision, anticipatory guidance, and treatment of common acute health problems as their brothers and sisters (see checklist). In addition, primary care providers must be attentive to the extra child and family needs that may accompany a chronic condition. These needs include condition specific areas of health supervision (e.g., avoidance of latex exposure in spina bifida) as well as generic issues such as the need for information, contact with other similar families, access to family support services and financial assistance, and school issues. Usually these needs are best addressed in an atmosphere of collaborative partnership between primary care providers and parents.

Growth with respect to weight and length/height requires monitoring in spina bifida. Obviously, careful attention to head circumference measurements is important prior to closure of cranial sutures. In some individuals, the measurement of arm span may be used as a substitute for height. Short stature and obesity have been reported with increased frequency in individuals with spina bifida. Careful evaluation for underlying contributing causes and, in the case of obesity, helpful life style guidance is important.

All children with spina bifida require the services of multiple medical and therapeutic specialists. These services are best provided through a multidisciplinary team which will develop and implement a care plan aimed at coordinating needed treatment and follow-up and communicating with community-based caregivers. The spina bifida medical checklists identify regular contact with the spina bifida team, but they do not attempt to specify the precise nature and timing of specific subspecialty interventions that will vary from team to team and from child to child.

As with cerebral palsy, the spina bifida checklist presented here incorporates guidelines from a number of state programs or tertiary care centers that provide multidisciplinary services for children with spina bifida (Sarwark, 1996). Other authorities recognized by the checklist include the single page "Healthwatch for the person with myelodysplasia" (Crocker, 1989). The Spina Bifida Association of America's Professional Advisory Council has also published a well-referenced outline organized by age groups and by specialty areas including primary care roles (Rauen, 1990).

Preventive management of cerebral palsy

Definition: A clinical pattern with variations in muscle tone, often including spasticity, with an incidence of 1.5–2.5 per 1000 births.

Clinical diagnosis: Clues during well child visits include the persistence of infantile reflexes, delayed appearance of reflexes, asymmetrical movements or reflexes, variations in muscle tone, and delays in the sequence of motor milestones. Early alterations in movement and tone may subsequently attenuate or disappear. Often not diagnosed until age 1–2 years.

Diagnostic aids: Standardized instruments such as the Bayley Scales of Infant Development or the Movement Assessment of Infants (MAI) provide scores that may be predictive of long-term/motor impairment (Harris, 1984).

Genetics: Broad category of disease with most cases having a low recurrence risk. Many genetic disorders can be associated with spasticity, producing a 25% recurrence risk in some cases.

Key management issues: Early consultation from a neuromotor multidisciplinary team, spasticity management, involvement in early intervention and preschool special education, monitoring of hearing and vision, connections with formal (programs, entitlements, information) and natural sources of support (friends, neighbors, churches, etc.).

Growth charts: Arm/leg length or other segmental measurements may be substituted for height as a method of following long bone growth over time (Stevenson, 1995).

Parent groups: United Cerebral Palsy Association Inc. (www.ucpa.org); Ontario Federation for Cerebral Palsy (www.ofcp.on.ca); Scope-About Cerebral Palsy UK (www.scope.org.uk).

Basis for management recommendations: American Academy of Pediatrics Clinical Report (Cooley et al., 2004).

Summary of clinical concerns

General	Learning	**Cognitive disability** (30%), **learning differences** (40%), delayed motor skills, athetoid speech
	Behavior	Attention deficit hyperactivity disorder, autism
	Growth	Prematurity, low birth weight, dysphagia, failure to thrive, muscle wasting or muscle overactivity with increased caloric consumption
Facial	Eyes	Oculomotor dysfunction, **refractive errors** (50%), amblyopia (14%)
	Mouth	Oromotor dysfunction, dysphagia, feeding problems
Surface	Skin	Rashes from drooling or allergies, sores in dependent patients
Skeletal	Cranial	Decreased brain growth, later microcephaly
	Axial	Upper motor dysfunction, abnormal tone, scoliosis
	Limbs	Lower motor dysfunction, hip subluxation, contractures, deformities
Internal	Digestive	Oral hypotonia, autonomic dysfunction, vomiting, GE reflux, drooling, decreased bowel motility, altered sphincter tone, constipation, fecal incontinence
	Pulmonary	Aspiration, bacterial pneumonia
	Circulatory	Restrictive cardiomyopathy due to scoliosis
	Endocrine	Delayed growth, puberty
	Excretory	Altered sphincter tone, urinary incontinence
Neural	Central	**Spasticity** (65%), **hemiplegia** (50%), **seizures** (30%), hypotonia, ataxia (10%), dyskinesis (19%), choreoathetosis
	Motor	Hypotonia, oromotor dysfunction, motor delays
	Sensory	Optic nerve injury, **vision deficits** (50%) hemianopsia that is more frequent with with hemiplegia, acoustic nerve injury, hearing deficits that are increased in kernicterus or with infectious etiologies, altered somatosensation, **abnormal stereognosis** (50%)

Concerns of frequency >20% are **highlighted**

Key references

Cooley, W. C. and the Committee on Children with Disabilities (2004). Providing a primary care medical home for children and youth with cerebral palsy. *Pediatrics* 114:1106–13. (aappolicy.aappublications.org/cgi/content/full/pediatrics;114/4/1106)

Rubin, I. L. & Crocker. A. C., eds (1989). *Developmental Disabilities: Delivery of Medical Care for Children and Adults.* Philadelphia: Lea and Febiger.

Stevenson, R. D. (1995). Use of segmental measures to estimate stature in children with cerebral palsy. *Archives of Pediatrics & Adolescent Medicine* 149:658–62.

Cerebral palsy

Preventive medical checklist (0–3 years)

Name _____ Birth date __/__/__ Number _____

Age	Evaluations: key concerns	Management considerations		Notes
New-born ↓ 1 month	Neuromotor:[2] muscle tone, movement Dysmorphology examination:[2] anomalies Neurology: brain anomalies Hearing, vision:[2] sensory deficits Feeding: reflux, poor intake Parental adjustment Other:	❑ Neurology, developmental pediatrics[1] ❑ Pediatric genetics[3] ❑ Cranial sonogram; head MRI scan[3] ❑ ABR; ophthalmology ❑ Feeding specialist; video swallow[3] ❑ Family support[4] ❑	❑ ❑ ❑ ❑ ❑ ❑ ❑	
2 months ↓ 4 months	Growth and development[5] Neuromotor:[2] tone, movement Hearing, vision:[2] sensory deficits Feeding: dysphagia Stooling: anal tone, poor motility Other:	❑ ECI;[6] family support[4] ❑ Developmental clinic[1,5] ❑ ABR;[3] ophthalmology[3] ❑ Feeding specialist;[3] gastroenterology[3] ❑ Gastroenterology[3] ❑	❑ ❑ ❑ ❑ ❑ ❑	
6 months ↓ 9 months	Growth and development[5] Neuromotor:[2] posture, drooling Hearing, vision:[2] amblyopia GI:[2] feeding, stooling Sleep: sleep apnea[7]	❑ ECI;[6] family support[4] ❑ Developmental clinic[1,5] ❑ ABR;[3] ophthalmology[3] ❑ Supplements;[3] laxatives;[3] oromotor therapy[3] ❑ ENT;[3] sleep study[3]	❑ ❑ ❑ ❑ ❑	
1 year	Growth and development[5] Neuromotor:[2] posture, drooling Hearing, vision:[2] amblyopia[2] Eyes; oculomotor function GI:[2] feeding, stooling Other:	❑ ECI;[6] family support[4] ❑ Developmental clinic[1,5] ❑ ABR; ENT[3] ❑ Ophthalmology ❑ Supplements;[3] laxatives[3] ❑	❑ ❑ ❑ ❑ ❑	
15 months ▼ 18 months	Growth and development[5] Neuromotor:[2] posture, drooling Hearing, vision:[2] amblyopia GI:[2] feeding, stooling	❑ ECI;[6] family support[4] ❑ Developmental clinic[1,5] ❑ ABR; ENT;[3] ophthalmology ❑ Supplements;[3] laxatives[3]	❑ ❑ ❑ ❑	
2 years	Growth and development[5] Neuromotor:[2] posture, drooling Hearing, vision:[2] sensory deficits Eyes; oculomotor, amblyopia Sleep: sleep apnea[7] Other:	❑ ECI;[6] family support[4] ❑ Developmental clinic;[1,5] assistive technology[8] ❑ Audiology ❑ Ophthalmology ❑ Sleep study[3] ❑	❑ ❑ ❑ ❑ ❑ ❑	
3 years	Growth, development, communication[5] Neuromotor:[2] posture, drooling Hearing, vision:[2] sensory deficits Eyes; oculomotor, amblyopia Sleep: sleep apnea[7] Other:	❑ ECI;[6] family support[4] ❑ Developmental clinic;[1,5] assistive technology[8] ❑ Audiology ❑ Ophthalmology ❑ Sleep study[3] ❑	❑ ❑ ❑ ❑ ❑ ❑	

Cerebral palsy concerns		Other concerns from history	
Feeding problems Nutrition, failure to thrive Hearing, vision loss Amblyopia, refractive errors Gastroesophageal reflux Urinary, fecal incontinence Aspiration pneumonia	Orthopedic complications Osteoporosis Microcephaly, seizures Spasticity, muscle wasting Developmental delay Cognitive disability Sleep apnea	**Family history/prenatal** _____ _____ _____ _____ _____	**Social/environmental** _____ _____ _____ _____ _____

Guidelines for the neonatal period should be undertaken at *whatever age* the diagnosis is made; ABR, auditory brainstem evoked response; GI, gastrointestinal; [1]infants with suggestive abnormalities in tone, posture, or reflexes should have developmental and neurologic assessments by pediatric specialists; [2]by practitioner; [3]as dictated by clinical findings; [4]parent group, family/sib, financial, and behavioral issues; [5]consider specialty clinic for cerebral palsy including neuromotor therapy if team available; [6]early childhood intervention including developmental monitoring and motor/speech therapy; [7]snoring, pause in breathing, daytime sleepiness, unusual sleep positioning; [8]position, ambulation, communication.

Cerebral palsy

Preventive medical checklist (4–18 years)

Name _____ Birth date __ / __ / __ Number _____

Age	Evaluations: key concerns	Management considerations	Notes
4 years ↓ 6 years	Growth, nutrition Development:[2] preschool transition Hearing, vision:[2] refractive errors Neuromotor:[2] continence, drooling Sleep: sleep apnea[7] Renal: urinary infection, hypertension Other:	☐ Developmental clinic[1] ☐ Family support;[4] preschool program[5] ☐ Audiology;[3] ophthalmology[3] ☐ Assistive technology;[8] neurobehavioral[9] ☐ ENT;[3] sleep study[3] ☐ Urinalysis; BP; urology[3] ☐	☐ ☐ ☐ ☐ ☐ ☐ ☐
7 years ↓ 9 years	Growth, nutrition: obesity Development:[1] school transition[5] Hearing, vision:[2] refractive errors Neuromotor:[2] continence, drooling Sleep: sleep apnea[7] Other:	☐ Developmental clinic[1] ☐ Family support;[4] school progress[6] ☐ Audiology;[3] ophthalmology[3] ☐ Assistive technology;[8] neurobehavioral[9] ☐ ENT;[3] sleep study[3] ☐	☐ ☐ ☐ ☐ ☐ ☐
10 years ↓ 12 years	Growth, development, communication Hearing, vision:[2] refractive errors Neuromotor:[2] continence, drooling Renal: urinary infection, hypertension Other:	☐ Developmental clinic;[1] school progress[6] ☐ Audiology;[3] ophthalmology[3] ☐ Assistive technology;[8] neurobehavioral[9] ☐ Urinalysis; BP; urology[3] ☐	☐ ☐ ☐ ☐ ☐
13 years ↓ 15 years	Growth, development, communication Hearing, vision:[2] refractive errors Neuromotor:[2] continence, drooling Obesity, precocious puberty Sleep: sleep apnea[7] Other:	☐ Developmental clinic;[1] school progress[6] ☐ Audiology;[3] ophthalmology[3] ☐ Assistive technology;[8] neurobehavioral[9] ☐ Dietician; activities; exercise; endocrinology[3] ☐ ENT;[3] sleep study[3] ☐	☐ ☐ ☐ ☐ ☐ ☐
16 years ↓ 18 years	Growth, development, communication Hearing, vision:[2] refractive errors Neuromotor:[2] continence, drooling Renal: urinary infection, hypertension Other:	☐ Developmental clinic;[1] school progress[6] ☐ Audiology;[3] ophthalmology[3] ☐ Assistive technology;[8] neurobehavioral[9] ☐ Urinalysis; BP; urology[3] ☐	☐ ☐ ☐ ☐ ☐
19 years ↓ 23 years	Adult care transition[4] Hearing, vision:[2] refractive errors Neuromotor:[2] continence, drooling Nutrition: obesity Sleep: sleep apnea[7]	☐ Family support;[4] school progress[6] ☐ Audiology;[3] ophthalmology[3] ☐ Assistive technology;[8] neurobehavioral[9] ☐ Dietary counsel; activities; exercise ☐ ENT;[3] sleep study[3]	☐ ☐ ☐ ☐ ☐
Adult	Adult care transition[4] Hearing, vision:[2] refractive errors Neuromotor:[2] continence, drooling Sleep: sleep apnea[7] Renal: urinary infection, hypertension Nutrition: obesity Other:	☐ Family support[4] ☐ Audiology;[3] ophthalmology[3] ☐ Assistive technology;[8] neurobehavioral[9] ☐ ENT;[3] sleep study[3] ☐ Urinalysis; BP; urology[3] ☐ Dietary counsel; activities; exercise ☐	☐ ☐ ☐ ☐ ☐ ☐ ☐

Cerebral palsy concerns		Other concerns from history	
Growth failure, obesity Hearing, vision deficits Amblyopia, refractive errors Gastroesophageal reflux Urinary, fecal incontinence Spasticity, muscle wasting	Orthopedic complications Osteoporosis Microcephaly, seizures Sleep apnea Cognitive disability Employment, independent living	**Family history/prenatal** _____ _____ _____ _____	**Social/environmental** _____ _____ _____ _____

Guidelines for the neonatal period should be undertaken *at whatever age* the diagnosis is made; BP, blood pressure; [1]consider specialty clinic for cerebral palsy including neuromotor and neurobehavioral therapy if team available; [2]by practitioner; [3]as dictated by clinical findings; [4]parent group, family/sib, financial, and behavioral issues with later focus on independent living and employment; [5]preschool program including developmental monitoring and motor/speech therapy; [6]monitor individual education plan, educational testing, balance of special education and inclusion, academic progress, behavioral differences, vocational planning; [7]snoring, pause in breathing, daytime sleepiness, unusual sleep positioning; [8]position, ambulation, communication; [9]cognition, communication, psychosocial.

Parent guide to cerebral palsy

Cerebral palsy embraces a range of conditions that involve abnormal movement or posture; the cause is a brain injury that occurs before birth or during early childhood. Cerebral palsy does not progress (i.e., it does not become worse as the child ages). Cerebral palsy may be further defined by its distribution – all four limbs (quadriplegia) or one side of the body (hemiplegia diplegia) involved; it can also be defined by manifestations such as spasticity (rigid muscles with toe-walking and increased reflexes), hypotonia (muscle weakness) choreoathetosis (sudden movements and posturing), or ataxia (unsteady walking, balance, and trembling). Overlap among the forms of cerebral palsy is common.

Incidence, causation, and diagnosis

The overall prevalence of significant cerebral palsy ranges from 1.5 to 2.5 per 1000 live births. Many different causes can produce the symptoms that are collectively grouped under the term "cerebral palsy." These include newborn breathing problems (6–14% of cases), abnormal brain development (50–60% of cases), brain infections such as meningitis (8–10% of cases), and prematurity (25–30% of cases). Most children with cerebral palsy (90–95%) have a genetic or congenital disorder rather than injury during labor or delivery. Recent evidence suggests that intrauterine infection may be associated with 12% of cases or more. Diagnosis of cerebral palsy must exclude other disorders such as spinal cord tumors or clefts (spina bifida) and diseases of muscles or nerves (e.g., spinal muscular atrophy). The diagnosis of cerebral palsy requires observation of the child over time because symptoms emerge and change. Spasticity is nearly always preceded by less obvious hypotonia, and the average child with cerebral palsy is not definitively diagnosed until age 1–2 years. Several genetic disorders present as cerebral palsy, so family histories and genetic counseling are important. Brain imaging, usually by MRI, should be carried out in nearly all cases.

Natural history and complications

Outcomes of cerebral palsy vary from profound disability in most areas of brain and motor function to minimal dysfunction. Cerebral palsy may "worsen" or appear to progress when there is a failure to address recognize underlying medical illnesses. Epilepsy occurs in 33% of patients and in 50% of those with hemiplegia. At least 30% have cognitive disability that is more common in those with spastic quadriplegia. Cognition may be underestimated in individuals with choreoathetosis due to speech incoordination, and there is increased risk for learning disability, vision, or hearing loss. Feeding problems include reflux (spitting up), aspiration (swallowing fluid into the lungs with choking), and drooling. Nasogastric or gastrostomy tube feeding may be necessary because caloric intake, coupled with higher energy demands from spastic muscles, may be inadequate for growth. Delays in the acquisition of bowel and bladder control are common. Urologic evaluation for urinary bladder dysfunction may be necessary, and chronic constipation due to altered intestinal mobility may require referral to gastroenterology.

Preventive medical needs

Timely, comprehensive care in early childhood is best coordinated by a neuromotor multidisciplinary team. This team may include a pediatric physiatrist, developmental pediatrician or neurologist, nurse coordinator, pediatric physical therapist, and orthoticist. Early assessment of feeding, neuromotor, and orthopedic problems is particularly important, with consideration of new therapies such as intrathecal baclofen, botulinum toxin, or glycopyrrolate. Also necessary is a comprehensive plan of physical therapy, orthopedic treatments such as serial casting of limbs, and orthotics to maintain the flexibility and mobility of joints. Physical/orthopedic therapy may also reduce muscle wasting and weakness that occur as a consequence of disuse. Surveillance for secondary complications such as scoliosis (curved spine) and hip problems is important. Orthopedic surgery, spinal cord surgery (dorsal rhizotomy), and medications affecting movement/tone may be considered for selected individuals. The issue of causation and specific diagnosis should be revisited periodically as new knowledge about genetics or improvements in brain imaging define new congenital causes of cerebral palsy.

Family counseling

Parents should work to establish realistic goals with the multidisciplinary care team and ensure that other family members and siblings share in their information and support. Connection with formal (programs, entitlements, information, parent groups, see p.1) and natural sources of support (friends, neighbors, churches, etc.) is very useful. Genetic causes of cerebral palsy should be evaluated when planning future pregnancies.

Preventive management of spina bifida

Description: A congenital anomaly caused by failure of neural tube closure to produce a bony defect of the spine with incomplete enclosure of the spinal cord. The incidence is 0.6–1.8 per 1000 births with variation according to ethnic background (higher in the United Kingdom, certain Hispanic groups).

Clinical diagnosis: Although usually evident at birth, the level/severity of spina bifida and the presence of additional malformations must be determined. Rarely, apparent neural tube defects will prove to be more simple meningoceles with minimal neurologic impairment or involve lipomas of the spinal cord.

Genetics: Multifactorial determination with a 2–3% recurrence risk after one affected child. Preconceptional supplementation of folic acid in amounts similar to those in standard multivitamins significantly lowers the recurrence risk.

Key management issues: Intermittent catheterization techniques, signs of ventriculoperitoneal shunt malfunction or infection, control of bowel function, urologic complications (urinary retention, urinary tract infection, reflux, and hydronephrosis), tethered cord (back or leg pain, worsening of gait, scoliosis, long-track neurologic findings), avoidance of latex-containing products, and early intervention/school monitoring for learning differences (Liptak et al., 1988).

Parent groups: Spina Bifida Association of America (www.sbaa.org); Spina Bifida and Hydrocephalus Association of Canada (www.sbhac.ca).

Growth charts: No specific charts are available.

Basis for management recommendations: Healthwatch for the person with myelodysplasia (Rubin & Crocker, 1989); Rauen (1990); Sarwark (1996).

Summary of clinical concerns

General	Learning	Cognitive disabilities (attention, memory, sequencing, reasoning); learning differences (perceptual–motor problems, eye–hand coordination, language skills exceed math skills) Conversational ability may conceal problems with comprehension
	Behavior	School and behavioral problems; learning difficulties may compound adolescent adjustment to disability
	Growth	Feeding problems (hospitalization may delay feeding routines), dysphagia, early short stature, later obesity
Facial	Eyes	Oculomotor dysfunction, **Strabismus** (20%)
	Mouth	Oromotor dysfunction, dysphagia
Surface	Neck/trunk	Altered posture, torticollis
	Epidermal	Open skin wound, decreased mobility, decubital ulcers
Skeletal	Cranial	Altered head shape due to hydrocephalus
	Axial	Abnormal posture, **scoliosis** (up to 90%), orthotic and bracing needs
	Limbs	**Orthopedic problems** (hip dislocation, club foot deformity, osteoporosis), muscle wasting (if non-ambulatory or following immobilization for orthopedic surgery), ambulation problems, appliance needs
Internal	Digestive	Bowel dysfunction, constipation, gastrointestinal and toileting problems
	RES	**Latex sensitivity** (20%)
	Excretory	**Bladder dysfunction** (100%), urinary incontinence, urologic problems (infection, urinary retention, reflux, hydronephrosis)
Neural	Central	**Hydrocephalus** (90%), seizures (10%), anticonvulsant needs
	Motor	**Delayed motor skills**, lower extremity paralysis, impaired mobility, ambulation problems, appliance needs
	Sensory	Loss of sensation, impaired coordination

RES, reticuloendothelial system; **concerns** of frequency >20% are **highlighted**

Key references

Rubin, I. L. & Crocker, A. C., eds (1989). *Developmental Disabilities: Delivery of Medical Care for Children and Adults.* Philadelphia: Lea and Febiger.

Liptak, et al. (1988). The management of children with spinal dysraphism. *Journal of Child Neurology* 3:3–20.

Rauen, K., ed. (1990). *Guidelines for Spina Bifida Health Care Services Throughout Life.* Washington DC: Spina Bifida Association of America.

Sarwark, J. F. (1996). Spina bifida. *Pediatric Clinics of North America* 43:1151–8.

Spina bifida

Preventive medical checklist (0–3 years)

Name _____ Birth date __ / __ / ____ Number _____

Age	Evaluations: key concerns	Management considerations		Notes
New-born ↓ 1 month	Neuromotor:[2] muscle tone, movement Skeletal: bony deformities Neurology: hydrocephalus, level of NTD Hearing, vision:[2] sensory deficits Neonatal: feeding, avoid latex exposure Parental adjustment Other:	☐ Spina bifida team[1] ☐ Radiology; orthopedics[3] ☐ Cranial sonogram; head, spinal MRI scan3[3] ☐ ABR; ophthalmology ☐ Feeding specialist, video swallow[3] ☐ Family support;[4] spina bifida counsel[5] ☐	☐ ☐ ☐ ☐ ☐ ☐ ☐	
2 months ↓ 4 months	Growth and development: hips dislocation Neuromotor:[2] shunt Hearing, vision:[2] strabismus Feeding, nutrition: dysphagia Bowel, bladder: incontinence Parental adjustment Other:	☐ Spina bifida team;[1] ECI[6] ☐ Neurology; caudal sonogram[3] neurosurgery ☐ ABR;[3] ophthalmology[3] ☐ Feeding specialist[3] ☐ Gastroenterology;[3] urology[3] ☐ Family support;[4] spina bifida counsel[5] ☐	☐ ☐ ☐ ☐ ☐ ☐ ☐	
6 months ↓ 9 months	Growth and development: hips dislocation Neuromotor:[2] tethered cord Hearing, vision:[2] sensory deficits Bowel, bladder function: incontinence Parental adjustment	☐ Spina bifida team;[1] ECI[6] ☐ Neurology;[3] caudal sonogram[3] neurosurgery ☐ ABR;[3] ophthalmology[3] ☐ Gastroenterology;[3] urology[3] ☐ Family support;[4] spina bifida counsel[3]	☐ ☐ ☐ ☐ ☐	
1 years	Growth and development: hips dislocation Neural:[2] prelanguage, shunt function Hearing, vision:[2] strabismus Bowel, bladder: incontinence Parental adjustment Other:	☐ Spina bifida team;[1] ECI[6] ☐ Neurology;[3] neurosurgery[3] ☐ ABR;[3] ophthalmology ☐ Gastroenterology;[3] urology[3] ☐ Family support;[4] spina bifida counsel[5] ☐	☐ ☐ ☐ ☐ ☐ ☐	
15 months ↓ 18 months	Growth and development Neural:[2] prelanguage, shunt function Hearing, vision:[2] sensory deficits Bowel, bladder: incontinence	☐ Spina bifida team;[1] spina bifida counsel;[5] ECI[6] ☐ Neurology; neurosurgery[3] ☐ Audiology;[3] ophthalmology[3] ☐ Gastroenterology;[3] urology[3]	☐ ☐ ☐ ☐	
2 years	Growth and development Neural:[2] shunt function, muscle strength Hearing, vision:[2] strabismus Bowel, bladder: incontinence Ambulation plans, seating Other:	☐ Spina bifida team;[1] ECI[6] ☐ Neurology;[3] assistive technology[7] ☐ Audiology;[3] ophthalmology ☐ Gastroenterology;[3] urology[3] ☐ Spina bifida counsel[5] ☐	☐ ☐ ☐ ☐ ☐ ☐	
3 years	Growth and development Neural:[2] shunt function, muscle strength Hearing, vision:[2] sensory deficits Bowel, bladder: incontinence Ambulation plans, seating Other:	☐ Spina bifida team;[1] ECI[6] ☐ Neurology;[3] assistive technology[7] ☐ Audiology;[3] ophthalmology ☐ Gastroenterology;[3] urology[3] ☐ Spina bifida counsel[5] ☐	☐ ☐ ☐ ☐ ☐ ☐	

Spina bifida concerns		Other concerns from history	
Strabismus Incontinence Urinary infections Renal failure Hypertension Latex allergy	Hip dislocation Scoliosis Hydrocephalus Shunt infections Tethered cord Learning differences	Family history/prenatal _____ _____ _____ _____	Social/environmental _____ _____ _____ _____

Guidelines for the neonatal period should be undertaken *at whatever age* the diagnosis is made; [1] including a nurse coordinator with pediatric specialists in development, neurosurgery, urology, orthopedics and, if multiple anomalies, genetics – the timing of follow-up visits may vary from team to team and from patient to patient; [2] by practitioner; [3] as dictated by clinical findings; [4] parent group, family/sib, financial, and behavioral issues; [5] teach avoidance of latex products, bowel management, signs of shunt malfunction with later planning of ambulation, seating, positioning' [6] early childhood intervention including developmental monitoring and motor/speech therapy; [7] position, ambulation, communication.

Spina bifida

Preventive medical checklist (4–18 years)

Name _____ **Birth date** __ / __ / __ **Number** _____

Age	Evaluations: key concerns	Management considerations		Notes
4 years ↓ **6 years**	Growth and development Development:[2] preschool transition Hearing, vision:[2] sensory deficits Neural:[2] shunt function, cognition Bowel, bladder: incontinence Renal: infection, hypertension Other:	❑ Spina bifida team;[1] spina bifida counsel[5] ❑ Preschool program[6] ❑ Audiology;[3] ophthalmology ❑ Assistive technology;[7] neurobehavioral[8] ❑ Gastroenterology;[3] urology[3] ❑ Urinalysis; BP; urology[3]	❑ ❑ ❑ ❑ ❑ ❑	
7 years ↓ **9 years**	Growth: obesity, scoliosis Development:[2] school transition Hearing, vision:[2] refractive errors Neural:[2] shunt function, cognition Renal: infection, hypertension Other:	❑ Spina bifida team;[1] spina bifida counsel[5] ❑ Family support;[4] school progress[6] ❑ Audiology;[3] ophthalmology[3] ❑ Assistive technology;[7] neurobehavioral[8] ❑ Urinalysis; BP; urology[3] ❑	❑ ❑ ❑ ❑ ❑ ❑	
10 years ↓ **12 years**	Growth: obesity, scoliosis Development[2] Hearing, vision:[2] sensory deficits Neural:[2] shunt function, cognition Other:	❑ Spina bifida team;[1] spina bifida counsel[5] ❑ Family support;[4] school progress[6] ❑ Audiology;[3] ophthalmology[3] ❑ Assistive technology;[7] neurobehavioral[8] ❑	❑ ❑ ❑ ❑ ❑	
13 years ↓ **15 years**	Growth and development: puberty Hearing, vision:[2] refractive errors Neural:[2] shunt function, cognition Ambulation, self-care Excretory: infection, high BP Other:	❑ Spina bifida team; [1]school progress[6] ❑ Audiology;[3] ophthal mology[3] ❑ Assistive technology;[7] neurobehavioral[8] ❑ Self-care planning ❑ Urinalysis; BP; urology[3]	❑ ❑ ❑ ❑ ❑	
16 years ↓ **18 years**	Growth and development: scoliosis Hearing, vision:[2] sensory deficits Neural:[2] shunt function, behavior Ambulation, self-care Other:	❑ Spina bifida team;[1] school progress[6] ❑ Audiology;[3] ophthalmology[3] ❑ Assistive technology;[7] neurobehavioral[8] ❑ Self-care promotion	❑ ❑ ❑ ❑	
19 years ↓ **23 years**	Adult care transition[4] Hearing, vision:[2] refractive errors Neural:[2] shunt function, behavior Ambulation, self-care Excretory: infection, high BP Other:	❑ Spina bifida team;[1] school progress[6] ❑ Audiology;[3] ophthalmology[3] ❑ Assistive technology;[7] neurobehavioral[8] ❑ Self-care promotion ❑ Urinalysis; BP; urology[3]	❑ ❑ ❑ ❑ ❑ ❑	
Adult	Adult care transition[4] Hearing, vision:[2] sensory deficits Neural:[2] shunt function, behavior Ambulation, self-care Excretory: infection, high BP Nutrition: obesity Other:	❑ Spina bifida team; [1]family support[4] ❑ Audiology;[3] ophthalmology[3] ❑ Assistive technology;[7] neurobehavioral[8] ❑ Self-care promotion ❑ Urinalysis; BP; urology[3] ❑ Dietary counsel; activities; exercise	❑ ❑ ❑ ❑ ❑ ❑	

Spina bifida concerns		Other concerns from history	
Latex allergy Strabismus Incontinence Urinary infections Renal failure Hypertension	Hip dislocation Scoliosis Learning differences Hydrocephalus Shunt, urinary infections Tethered cord	**Family history/prenatal** _____ _____ _____ _____	**Social/environment** _____ _____ _____ _____

Guidelines for the neonatal period should be undertaken *at whatever age* the diagnosis is made; BP, blood pressure; [1]including a nurse coordinator with pediatric specialists in development, neurosurgery, urology, orthopedics and, if multiple anomalies, genetics – the timing of follow-up visits may vary from team to team and from patient to patient; [2]by practitioner; [3]as dictated by clinical findings; [4]parent group, family/sib, financial, and behavioral issues; [5]teach avoidance of latex products, bowel management, signs of shunt malfunction with later planning of ambulation, seating, positioning; [6]preschool program including developmental monitoring and motor/speech therapy followed by school support for individual education plan, educational testing, balance of special education and inclusion, academic progress, behavioral differences, vocational planning; [7]position, ambulation, communication; [8]including self-care planning with psycho-educational, emotional, cognition, and self-esteem support.

Parent Guide to spina bifida

Spina bifida or rachischisis refers to a bony defect of the spine (backbone) that exposes the spinal cord. This defect may be covered by skin (spina bifida occulta) or protrude as a sac (spina bifida cystica). The sac may contain only spinal cord lining (meninges) and fluid (meningocele) or the cord itself (meningomyelocele). The combination of spina bifida and meningomyelocele is sometimes referred to as myelodysplasia. Spina bifida occurs when the embryonic spinal canal (neural tube) fails to close at 28–30 days after conception. Such neural tube defects result from both genetic and environmental factors, and their incidence is diminished if folic acid is taken before and during early pregnancy.

Incidence, causation, and diagnosis

The prevalence of spina bifida and related neural tube defects has declined from 2 to 4 per 1000 births to less than 0.4 per 1000 because of maternal folic acid supplementation. Genetic and environmental factors associated with spina bifida include chromosome changes or drugs like alcohol and valproic acid. Prenatal screening for spina bifida can be performed by measuring increased alpha-fetoprotein (AFP) in maternal blood or amniotic fluid, followed by fetal ultrasound. Spina bifida is usually obvious after birth because of the visible sac, but several medical specialties are required to determine severity and exclude associated anomalies.

Natural history and complications

The level of the spina bifida (higher on the back means more nerves damaged) and associated birth defects determine its severity, ranging from early death to 90% survival into adulthood for babies with early surgery and prevention of brain/spinal cord infections. Hydrocephalus (water accumulation in the brain), bowel and bladder incontinence, repeated urinary infections, kidney damage, compression of the lower spinal cord (tethered cord), spinal curvature (scoliosis), and allergic hypersensitivity to latex-containing products are frequent problems. Cognitive functioning and school performance are often affected, particularly if hydrocephalus is not aggressively treated. Subtle neuropsychologic defects may alter eye–hand coordination, attention, memory, sequencing, or reasoning.

Preventive medical needs

All children with spina bifida require the services of multiple medical and therapeutic specialists. These services are best provided through a multidisciplinary team that will develop and implement a care plan aimed at coordinating needed treatment and follow-up and communicating with community-based care givers. Spina bifida team nurse coordinators can provide parents with training and information about home physical therapy, encouragement of ambulation, clean intermittent catheterization techniques, and signs of ventriculo peritoneal shunt malfunction or infection. A major goal is to provide affected children with a normal range of peer and sibling experiences so as not to create a "vulnerable child" situation. Attainment of mobility is a key goal that may require a range of training, therapy, orthotics, orthopedic interventions, and assistive devices. Restricted mobility may be associated with skin lesions and slow healing, and obesity has increased frequency in individuals with spina bifida. Older children should be given increasing responsibility for their self-care and taught to perform their own self-catheterization during the early school age years. Many children benefit from periodic meetings with an older peer mentor who has spina bifida.

Family counseling

All women are advised to take folic acid in amounts similar to those in standard multivitamin preparations when they are planning a pregnancy. This precaution applies particularly to those women who already have a child with neural tube defects, or to those with risk factors such as diabetes mellitus, valproic acid therapy, or other affected relatives. With the advent of folic acid therapy, the recurrence risk for couples having a child with isolated spina bifida has declined from 4–5% to 2%. Prenatal diagnosis is accurate, and prospective parents should receive balanced information about spina bifida. Contact with older patients is a helpful adjunct to education about spina bifida during the pre- or postnatal period. Besides the benefits of early education and counseling, prenatal diagnosis allows the parents to choose the safest delivery (often by Cesarean) and a medical center that can provide the important immediate response to their child's medical needs. In some instances, prenatal diagnosis may also allow ameliorative prenatal surgery (e.g., to remove cerebrospinal fluid in the fetus with spina bifida and hydrocephalus). As with other developmental disabilities, parents of children with spina bifida should have access to ongoing information, advocacy, and support from primary care providers as well as from members of a multidisciplinary specialty team. Many children with spina bifida are eligible for benefits such as Medicaid insurance, Supplemental Security Income (SSI) from the Social Security Administration, and possible "family support services" that may include respite care, discretionary funds, stipends or loan programs, advocacy and care coordination, and parent-to-parent contacts. Additional information can be obtained from the Spina Bifida Association of America (SBAA), see front page.

5

Single anomalies, sequences, and associations

Single anomalies are confined to one body region or organ system, while sequences and associations disrupt several systems. Isolated anomalies and sequences that spare the brain usually have good outcomes with proper medical and surgical management.

Because the embryo is a dynamic structure, anomalies occurring at one stage in development may lead to consequences in later stages (see Chapter 1). Renal agenesis (an isolated anomaly) initiates a cascade of consequences including oligohydramnios, facial deformations, and club feet (Potter sequence). This cascade or "sequence" of events has the low recurrence risk expected of isolated anomalies rather than the likelihood of genetic or chromosomal etiology implied by syndromes. Associations are clusters of major anomalies envisioned as parallel responses to early embryonic injury: they lack the minor anomalies of syndromes. Single anomalies, sequences, and associations usually have a low genetic recurrence risk in contrast to syndromes with likelihood of chromosomal or Mendelian inheritance. The single anomalies, sequences, and associations discussed in this chapter are listed in Table 5.1.

Preventive management can be lifesaving for disorders such as Pierre Robin sequence, or facilitate palliative care and postmortem counseling for disorders such as Potter sequence. In anomalies such as cleft palate, informed management prevents complications such as hearing loss and speech delay. One page summaries are presented for common anomalies, followed by short paragraphs on rarer defects and more extensive checklists for the VATER and CHARGE associations.

Amniotic band disruption sequence

Breakdown of the amnion produces tissue remnants (bands) that encircle fetal parts and cause anomalies. Mechanical or physiologic lesions exemplified by amniotic bands are often called disruptions to separate them from true malformations with higher genetic risks. Postulated mechanisms include amnion hypoplasia, inappropriate cell death, and altered vascular supply. Amniotic bands have an

Table 5.1. Single anomalies, sequences, and associations

Anomaly, sequence, or association	Incidence*	Preventive measures
Isolated anomalies and sequences		
Amniotic disruption sequence	1 in 10,000	Orthopedic and/or craniofacial evaluation; hearing, vision, developmental assessment if craniofacial
Cleft lip/cleft palate	1 in 1000	Plastic surgery and craniofacial evaluation; hearing assessment, evaluation for chronic otitis
Cleft palate	1 in 2500	
Craniofacial deformations: plagiocephaly	~1 in 100	Evaluation for craniosynostosis, monitoring of head shape and growth, helmeting
Craniofacial deformations: torticollis	~1 in 500	Monitoring of head shape, neck extension
DiGeorge anomaly	~1 in 10,000	Cardiac, thymus, serum calcium evaluation; cellular immunity, hearing, ECI
Frontonasal malformation	~1 in 50,000	Craniofacial surgery, examination for frontal encephalocele, vision, and hearing testing
Klippel–Feil anomaly, type I (severe)	1 in 6000–10,000	Cervical spine flexion–extension radiographs, ophthalmology, audiology
Klippel–Feil anomaly, type II (mild)	1 in 100	None
Pierre Robin sequence	1 in 8500	Prone positioning, monitoring of growth, nasopharyngeal airway if obstruction
Associations		
VATER association	1 in 6000	See VATER checklist
CHARGE association	1 in 20,000	See CHARGE checklist

Note:
ECI, early childhood intervention.
*Per number of live births.

incidence of 1 per 2000–4000 live births, with a much higher incidence in abortuses (Jones, 1997, pp. 636–9; Gorlin et al., 2001, pp. 10–13).

Modern ultrasonography (Simpson, 2005) allows assessment of amniotic bands to begin before birth. The distribution of bands and the types of associated anomalies will guide diagnosis and management. Anomalies produced by bands can be confused with other birth defects (e.g., anencephaly, cleft palate), and complex band disruptions can be confused with malformation syndromes. Early embryonic disruptions can produce lethal defects of the body wall with complex deformations and organ adhesions – careful inspection for band remnants and necropsy may be needed to distinguish banding complexes from syndromes with potentially higher recurrence risks. Facial amniotic bands may be confused with cleft lip/palate, but have a geographic distribution that reflects adhesion and tearing rather than persistence of an embryonic cleavage plane.

Preventive management begins with assessment of the distribution of anomalies and involvement of the appropriate surgical specialties. Depending on their embryonic timing and distribution, amnion disruption sequence can include limb, craniofacial, and/or lateral body wall defects. Porencephaly (cystic lesion in the brain) or hemifacial microsomia (small ear and jaw on one side) are other disruptions that can be seen with amniotic bands. Mono-chorionic twins have high rates of disruption due to vascular connections and twin-to-twin shunting. Patients with craniofacial involvement require more attention to growth and development while the more common patient with limb anomalies needs only orthopedic care.

Summary of clinical concerns: Amniotic disruption management considerations

General: Evaluate the spectrum of anomalies, particularly looking for craniofacial clefts or asymmetries.

Growth: Monitor growth, feeding, and nutrition if there are orofacial clefts (as for cleft lip/palate below).

Developmental: Follow developmental milestones as indicators of brain abnormalities; orthopedic defects may help qualify complex patients for neurology and developmental pediatric assessment.

Facial-eye: Clefts of the eye adnexa may expose the corneal and require ophthalmology referral and lubricants to prevent keratitis.

Facial-ENT: Bands may cause choanal atresia or Robin sequence with small jaw that necessitate prone positioning and/or respiratory monitoring; ear anomalies and orofacial clefts may require cosmetic surgery, hearing tests, or feeding/growth monitoring.

Skeletal-cranial: Cranial clefts can produce asymmetries or craniosynostoses that need craniofacial team assessment, head imaging, and prostheses, helmets/cranial bands, or surgery.

Skeletal-limbs: Limb amputations and deformations (particularly club feet) may necessitate orthopedic, orthotic, and physical therapy evaluations.

Neural-CNS: Porencephaly and other brain disruptions may mimic neural tube defects and require neonatal ultrasound or head MRI studies.

Neural-sensory: Eye or ear anomalies should initiate hearing/vision monitoring.

Parent information: Disruptions like amniotic bands are usually sporadic with recurrence risks of less than 1% for parents and affected individuals. Physicians must beware of genetic syndromes with open skin lesions that adhere to the amnion and generate bands, illustrated by the scalp defect of trisomy 13 or epidermolysis bullosa. A parent of a child with hand involvement and club feet provides information (www.amnioticbandsyndrome.com/) with links to organizations for children with arm or hand deficiency (www.reach.org.uk/) or limb differences (www.limbdifferences.org).

Cleft lip/cleft palate

True cleft lip/palate reflects failure of the primary palate to close (cleft lip/cleft palate) or failure of the lateral palatine processes to fuse (cleft palate alone). The incidence of cleft lip with or without cleft palate is 1–2 per 1000 live births, that of cleft palate alone is 1 in 2500 live births (Jones, 1997, pp. 236–7; Gorlin et al., 2001, pp. 850–60; Mulliken, 2004). Neonatal examination for associated anomalies discriminates between isolated cleft lip/palate and over 300 syndromes with these defects (this distinction is crucial for genetic/prognostic counseling and management). Non-embryonic clefts due to amniotic bands, midline clefts (with associated brain anomalies), submucous clefts (with velopalatine incompetence), and Robin sequence with small jaw and posterior U-shaped cleft (see below) are important to distinguish from true cleft lip/cleft palate. Bilateral clefts have slightly higher recurrence risks and greater likelihood of syndrome association than unilateral clefts.

Preventive management begins with fetal ultrasound/neonatal examination to exclude associated anomalies of nearby structures (eyes, ears, nose, teeth, jaw) or cleft palate syndromes (brain, choanae, heart, skeletal defects, ectodermal dysplasia). An average 10% of patients with cleft lip, 30–40% with cleft lip/cleft palate, and 35% for isolated cleft palate. Isolated clefts have an excellent prognosis, especially when management is coordinated by specialized cleft palate teams. Earlier surgery for cleft lip aids parental acceptance, and is often guided by the "rule of tens" – age 10 weeks-weight 10 lb-hemoglobin 10 g/dl. Successful repair of cleft lip/palate is important for mid-facial and nasal growth.

Summary of clinical concerns: Cleft lip/palate management considerations

Growth: Higher risks for growth delay in children with cleft lip/cleft palate require monitoring of growth, feeding, and nutrition. Specialized nipples and oral prostheses may be helpful.

Development: Monitor development for speech and hearing problems and consider early childhood intervention for children with severe clefts and/or associated anomalies.

Facial-ENT: Associated chronic otitis, hearing loss, and respiratory obstruction mandate regular otoscopic examination, audiometry, and vigilance for sleep apnea.

Facial-mouth: Examine for submucous clefts and post-repair defects (including velopalatine incompetence) that can cause swallowing and speech problems; follow tooth development, especially in the presence of severe clefts and jaw hypoplasia that increase the chances for missing or malpositioned teeth (Evans, 2004).

Neural-CNS: Evaluate for sleep apnea or nocturnal enuresis due to airway obstruction that can occur with severe clefts or after surgery.

Neural-sensory: Neonatal hearing screens and regular hearing/vision assessment with appropriate ENT referral are critical for the chronic otitis and hearing loss that accompany oral clefting.

Parent information: Isolated cleft lip/palate exhibits multifactorial determination with a 2–3% recurrence risk for future pregnancies of parents or affected patients (increased somewhat if there are other affected relatives). Exclusion of a syndrome allows emphasis on this low risk and the alleviation of guilt. Teratogens (e.g., hydantoin) and folic acid/nutritional deficiencies that predispose to oral clefts should be addressed during pregnancy planning, including the possibility of ultrasound studies for reassurance. Many websites are available by searching on "cleft palate," including those of the Cleft Palate Foundation (www.cleftline. org) or Cleft Lip and Palate Association (CLAPA-UK-www.clapa.com/).

Torticollis

Torticollis is usually a deformation that has an excellent prognosis once birth frees the baby from uterine constraint. Congenital torticollis or wryneck is often accompanied by a mass (fibromatosis) of the sternocleidomastoid muscle, producing decreased extension and tilting of the head toward the affected side. Breech presentation increases the chance for torticollis and other deformations like scoliosis or talipes, and neonatal examiners should be alert for concurrent deformities that suggest severe constraint *in utero* or global neuromuscular disease that rendered the fetus more susceptible to normal uterine pressures (e.g., arthrogryposis, myopathies, neuropathies). Gastroesophageal reflux (Sandifer syndrome) or ocular problems can cause secondary torticollis during later infancy or childhood, necessitating treatment of the underlying process. Congenital torticollis may resolve but sometimes requires bracing, range of motion exercises, botulinum toxin, or minimal intervention surgery (Rahlin, 2005).

Summary of clinical concerns: Torticollis management considerations

General: Examine for associated anomalies of the ears and neck and additional deformities or contractures that may indicate an arthrogryposis syndrome or neuromuscular disease.

Growth: Monitor head shape and head circumference; watch for associated feeding problems.

Development: Provide physical/occupational therapy, head propping, proper sleep positioning for persisting should be recommended; monitor motor milestones and watch for deficits or asymmetries as indicators of additional neurologic problems or congenital anomalies.

Facial: Monitor facial asymmetry with craniofacial surgery evaluation as needed; watch for accompanying ear or neck anomalies that signal hemifacial microsomia or syndromes rather than simple torticollis.

Facial-eye: Monitor for strabismus or visual problems in acquired torticollis.

Internal-gastrointestinal: Consider video swallow and gastrointestinal (GI) referral if torticollis seems reflexive (Sandifer syndrome).

Neural-sensory: Ear and neck are branchial derivatives, mandating neonatal hearing screens, regular hearing/vision assessment, and appropriate specialty referral if sensory deficits accompany torticollis.

Parent information: Isolated torticollis is sporadic or multifactorial, implying a low (<1%) recurrence risk for future pregnancies of parents or affected patients. Some lay websites are available by searching on "torticollis" including www.pedisurg.com and www.torticolliskids.org.

Plagiocephaly

Plagiocephaly (cranial asymmetry) can occur because of uterine constraint, abnormal fetal presentation, or craniosynostosis (Hutchison et al., 2004). Breech presentation is a common cause of plagiocephaly and other deformities such as congenital hip dislocation, scoliosis, torticollis, and talipes equinovarus. Recent recommendations for "baby on back" sleeping during infancy have increased the frequency of occipital plagiocephaly due to postnatal positioning. The prognosis is usually excellent if associated anomalies and underlying neural problems are excluded. The key to management is early monitoring and referral at an age when the cranium is flexible and can be remolded with bands or helmets.

Summary of clinical concerns: Plagiocephaly management considerations

General: Assess degree of asymmetry and examine for other deformities: torticollis, scoliosis, club feet; examine for underlying cranial anomalies: craniosynostosis, macrocephaly, hydrocephalus.

Growth: Follow head circumference and growth to exclude macrocephaly, brain anomalies.

Development: Recommend physical/occupational therapy, floor time, corrective sleep positioning; monitor for delayed motor milestones that may indicate coincident neurologic problems or congenital anomalies.

Facial: Examine for facial and ear anomalies, web neck, cleft tongue.

Skeletal-cranial: Monitor head shape, especially during the first month of life; refer to craniofacial team before age 6 months if necessary since banding/helmeting can prevent surgery.

Skeletal-axial/limbs: Examine for vertebral, rib, or limb anomalies.

Neural-CNS: Consider head MRI scan and/or skull films with severe deformity or developmental delay.

Neural-sensory: Monitor hearing and vision, particularly with ear asymmetry or anomaly.

Parent information: Isolated plagiocephaly is sporadic, implying a low (<1%) recurrence risk for future pregnancies of parents or affected patients. Many websites are available by searching on "plagiocephaly," including www.plagio-cephaly.org/and kidshealth.org.

DiGeorge anomaly

The DiGeorge anomaly involves malformation of the thymus, parathyroid, heart, and craniofacies, producing hypocalcemia, cardiac disease, and cellular immune deficiency (Jones, 1997, pp. 616–17; Gorlin et al., 2001, pp. 820–22; Baldini, 2004). The craniofacial changes are suggestive of a branchial arch abnormality with micrognathia, middle ear anomalies, and down-turned corners of the mouth. The condition is most characteristically associated with a microdeletion of chromosome 22, and it overlaps with other chromosome 22 deletion phenotypes such as Cayler syndrome (asymmetric crying facies), Shprintzen syndrome, and isolated conotruncal heart defects. Patients with DiGeorge anomaly and choanal atresia, laryngomalacia, or palatal defects have similarities to the CHARGE association. The DiGeorge anomaly is a component of many other chromosomal or teratogenic syndromes (including fetal alcohol syndrome) and has an incidence of about 1 in 10,000 births.

Preventive management is complex and best coordinated by using the deletion 22/Shprintzen checklist presented in Chapter 9. Concerns include correction of hypocalcemia to prevent seizures, echocardiography for possible cardiac defects, evaluation for associated anomalies of the palate (including subtle velopalatine incompetence), choanae, thyroid, GI, and immune system. Precautions include avoidance of live viral vaccines until adequate immunity is demonstrated. Growth and developmental delays are frequent due to feeding problems and intercurrent illnesses, particularly if a chromosome 22 deletion or other anomaly is found. The finding of chromosome deletion mandates testing of the parents, but recurrence risk are low if the karyotype is normal. Parent information is listed with the deletion 22/Shprintzen entry in Chapter 9, and search on DiGeorge yields many websites including a parent-oriented site (www.familyvillage.wisc.edu/lib_dig.htm).

Frontonasal malformation

This anomaly has been termed "frontonasal dysplasia" even though there is no evidence that tissue dysplasia is involved. There is striking hypertelorism with a broad nasal root, and associated malformations include midline encephalocele and other brain anomalies, eye, ear, and limb defects (Jones, 1997, pp. 240–41; Lopes et al., 2004).

Summary of clinical concerns: Frontonasal malformation management considerations

General: Examine for associated anomalies, including those of the ears or limbs.

Development: Monitor for developmental delay due to associated brain anomalies including hydrocephalus, and speech delay due to conductive hearing loss.

Facial-eyes: Examine for associated epibulbar dermoids or colobomas of the eyes, optic disc anomalies.

Skeletal-cranial: Monitor head growth and shape, consider cranial imaging to evaluate the presence of frontal encephalocele.

Neural-sensory: Monitor hearing and vision, particularly with ear anomalies.

Parent information: Frontonasal malformation is sporadic, implying a low (<1%) recurrence risk for future pregnancies of parents or affected patients. Useful website include those devoted to craniofacial surgery and cleft palate repair including www.craniofacial.net/.

Klippel–Feil anomaly

Klippel–Feil anomaly involves fusion of the cervical vertebrae (Jones, 1997, pp. 618–19; Gorlin et al., 2001, pp. 1142–5). The fusion may be occult or, in more severe cases, associated with shortening of the neck, limitation of head movement, and pterygium colli (webbed neck). A low hairline, short neck, and pterygium colli should alert the physician to obtain spinal radiographs to document the degree of fusion. The more obvious anomaly has been called type I Klippel–Feil anomaly with an incidence of about 1 in 100 live births, and the milder form type II with an incidence of 1 in 6000–10,000 live births. The anomaly does occur as a component of several syndromes, including the Noonan, Wildervanck, and Goldenhar syndromes. Associated abnormalities include those of the eye (strabismus, nystagmus), hearing (25–50%), mouth (cleft palate in 17%), and heart (septal defects).

Neurologic complications, dysraphic lesions of the spinal cord and even brain anomalies may be associated with severe type I anomalies. Milder type II fusions will usually be detected on routine radiographs taken later in life; they require few precautions and do not pose exercise risks. Effects on cervical spine mobility depend on the site of fusion – some have increased motion of the upper cervical segments with risk for neurologic injury, while others have increased movement of the lower cervical segments with risk for degenerative arthritis.

Summary of clinical concerns: Klippel–Feil management considerations

General: Examine for associated anomalies of the face and heart.

Development: Monitor for delayed motor milestones or motor asymmetries that may indicate coincident craniospinal problems.

Facial: Examine for eye anomalies and oral clefts, consider ophthalmology and craniofacial referrals.

Skeletal-axial/limbs: Examine for vertebral, rib, or limb anomalies.

Neural-CNS: Consider head MRI scan, cervical spine MRI/radiographs, and cervical spine flexion–extension films with more severe defects; warn of dangers during intubation or anesthesia (Nargozian, 2004).

Neural-sensory: Monitor hearing and vision, particularly with eye or ear anomalies.

Parent information: Isolated cases of Klippel–Feil anomaly are sporadic, implying a low (<1%) recurrence risk for future pregnancies of parents or affected patients. Professional and lay information is available by searching on "Klippel–Feil," including a site from the National Institutes of Health (www.ninds.nih.gov/) and a Klippel–Feil Circle of Friends site that has many other links (www.fortunecity.com/millenium/bigears/99/kfs.html).

Pierre Robin sequence

The variable definition of Pierre Robin sequence may account for incidence estimates that range from 1 in 2000 to 1 in 30,000 live births (Gorlin et al., 2001, pp. 860–65). The classic description was by Pierre Robin in 1923, and the anomaly is a component of more than 20 syndromes – a reason not to use the confusing term "Pierre Robin syndrome." The primary defect is thought to be mandibular hypoplasia, which interferes with tongue descent and produces a U-shaped cleft palate (some have commented that a V-shaped cleft can be seen as well). Tongue shape, motility, and coordination are usually quite abnormal, adding to respiratory problems by its posterior position and contributing to dysphagia and speech apraxia. All patients should be screened for associated anomalies, particularly the retinal detachment that may occur with Robin sequence in the Stickler syndrome (see Chapter 16). Isolated Robin sequence has an excellent prognosis, with most studies documenting catch-up growth of the mandible with normal appearance and function in later childhood. Preventive management therefore centers on the high-risk period of infancy, seeking to minimize cardiopulmonary and neurologic damage from feeding and respiratory problems.

Summary of clinical concerns: Pierre Robin management considerations

General: Examine for associated anomalies of the eyes, ears, tongue, and heart. Employ prone positioning to bring the tongue forward and facilitate breathing. Most patients should have craniofacial surgery evaluation to considerable resorbable aids to mandibular growth (Burstein & Williams, 2005).

Growth: Monitor growth and feeding that may be affected by palatal immotility, dysphagia, respiratory obstruction, and sleep apnea (remember that growth hormone is secreted during sleep).

Development: Monitor for delayed motor milestones that may indicate coincident anomalies and for speech problems that may indicate velopharyngeal immotility.

Facial-eyes: Ophthalmology referral should be considered for retinal changes that may precede retinal detachment.

Facial-ENT: Monitor for chronic otitis and respiratory problems due to palate and tongue malfunction.

Internal-pulmonary: Evaluate neonates for signs of respiratory obstruction (stertorous breathing, sternal retractions, apnea) and monitor pulmonary functions and blood gases if present. Consider a nasopharyngeal airway and tube feeding in patients with respiratory problems and dysphagia/aspiration.

Neural-sensory: Monitor for hearing or vision loss due to retinal changes or chronic otitis.

Parent information: Isolated cases of Pierre Robin sequence are sporadic, implying a low (<1%) recurrence risk for future pregnancies of parents or affected patients. Higher recurrence risks may apply if the patient has inherited a chromosomal or Mendelian syndrome such as autosomal dominant Stickler syndrome (parents may be mildly affected). Many professional and lay websites are available by searching on "Pierre Robin" including www.pierrerobin.org/ and the Contact a Family website that joins families with similar disorders (http://www.cafamily.org.uk/Direct/p24.html).

ASSOCIATIONS

Associations have long been emphasized in the surgical literature, where discovery was critical for operative outcome. Associations describe anomalies that occur together more often than would be expected by chance and are like syndromes in defining a pattern of anomalies (Jones, 1997, pp. 664–70). Unlike syndromes, associations do not have an implied unique cause (Opitz & Wilson, 1997). A brief period of embryonic injury is hypothesized for associations, contrasting with the prolonged developmental impact of syndromes. In syndromes, the persistence of abnormal chromosomes or genes throughout the embryonic and fetal periods produces not only major malformations but also minor anomalies that reflect altered "fine-tuning" of structure (Opitz & Wilson, 1997). Minor anomalies often produce a distinctive facial appearance in syndromes that is lacking in associations. In practice, the predominance of major anomalies and sporadic occurrence are the most important aspects of associations, for these guide the approach to diagnosis, management, and counseling.

PHACES association

PHACES is an acronym for a highly variable spectrum of the following: brain malformations of the *P*osterior fossa, *H*emangiomata of the face, *A*rterial dissections or disruptions, *C*ardiac anomalies, *E*ye defects, and thoracic defects such as *S*ternal clefting or *S*upraumbilical raphe (Metry et al., 2001). Most patients have the hemangiomata with only one internal complication. Several have been confused with Sturge–Weber syndrome, emphasizing the need to distinguish hemangiomata that often regress from true malformations that will persist such as the flat port-wine stains of Sturge–Weber syndrome.

Summary of clinical concerns: PHACES management considerations

General: Examine for associated anomalies of the eyes, heart, and central nervous system in patients with large facial and/or sternal hemangiomata (Metry et al., 2001).

Growth: Monitor growth and feeding that may be affected by cleft uvula or palatal immotility, especially with obvious facial clefts.

Development: Monitor for delayed motor milestones that may indicate brain anomalies or arterial disruptions of the carotid arteries that affect brain function.

Facial-eyes: Ophthalmology referral should be considered to evaluate glaucoma or strabismus from central problems.

Facial-ENT: Monitor for chronic otitis and respiratory problems if there are palatal defects.

Internal-cardiac: Consider cardiology referral and echocardiogram in the presence of sternal clefts and hemangiomata. Consider arteriography or sonography if examination suggests possibility of aortic dissection.

Neural-central: Consider head MRI and neurovascular studies since atresia of the carotid artery and calcified cerebral aneurysms have been described.

Parent information: PHACES association is a sporadic disorder, implying a low (<1%) recurrence risk for future pregnancies of parents or affected patients. Definitions can be accessed by searching on the inaccurate term "PHACE syndrome," including a parent-oriented website on Microsoft Network (MSN): groups.msn.com/PHACESyndromeCommunity.

VATER association

Terminology

VATER association is an acronym that represents *V*ertebral defects, *A*nal atresia, *T*racheo*E*sophageal fistula, *R*adial limb and *R*enal defects. Synonyms include VACTERL association, where the "C" and "L" are added to emphasize cardiac and limb defects (Jones, 1997, pp. 664–5).

Historical diagnosis and management

Among many well-known associations of midline anomalies was the frequent concurrence of polydactyly, imperforate anus, and vertebral anomalies. This grouping of anomalies was expanded and popularized by Quan & Smith in 1973 as the VATER association. Surgical advances have greatly improved the management of patients with VATER association, which even in recent studies has an infant mortality rate of close to 50%.

Incidence, etiology, and differential diagnosis

More than 500 individuals with VATER association have been reported in the literature, and the birth incidence for VATER association is estimated at 1.6 per 1000. The etiology of VATER association is unknown, although infants of diabetic mothers show an increased incidence. As currently defined, the diagnosis is excluded if a recognizable chromosomal or genetic syndrome is found. Risks for the full association to recur are minimal, but relatives with component defects of the association have been described in VATER families. The pathogenesis involves injury to developing mesoderm at 20–25 days postconception, resulting in abnormal development of vertebral, anorectal, cardiac, tracheoesophageal, radial, and renal derivatives. As discussed in the overview, dysmorphogenesis seems limited to major organ systems, with few minor anomalies of face, palate, or limbs (single umbilical artery is an exception, being present in 35% of cases).

Differential diagnosis is large because many genetic and chromosomal syndromes include one or more components of the VATER association. Most dangerous is the misdiagnosis of patients with trisomy 18 as VATER association, since the management of their cardiac, radial ray, and renal defects may be inappropriately aggressive and fraught with the operative instability manifested by patients with chromosomal disease. Appreciation of minor anomalies such as malformed ears, aberrant palmar creases, prominent heels, or rocker-bottom feet allows suspicion of trisomy 18, with use of fluorescent *in situ* hybridization (FISH) karyotype techniques to confirm the diagnosis within 3–4 h. Mendelian syndromes such as Holt–Oram (heart, limb defects), Fanconi anemia (heart, limb, vertebral defects), or Townes–Brock (heart, anal defects) may be also resemble VATER association and lead to inappropriate genetic counseling. Radial ray defects can occur in VATER association as well as in many genetic syndromes.

Considerable overlap of the VATER spectrum of anomalies with those of the caudal regression and Goldenhar syndrome/hemifacial microsomia complexes is indicated by the terms "axial mesodermal dysplasia spectrum" and "sacrococcygeal dysgenesis association." Cardiac, tracheoesophageal, renal, upper limb, and genital anomalies are common in VATER association, but overlap with other associations is illustrated by anorectal, lower limb, eye, ear, palatal, and central nervous system anomalies. Vertebral anomalies are more caudal in VATER and sacral dysgenesis association as opposed to cervical bias in Goldenhar syndrome. While different anomaly patterns are certainly evident in VATER association, the manifestations of sacral dysgenesis and Goldenhar/hemifacial microsomia complex must be considered in the management of VATER patients (Kallen et al., 2004).

Diagnostic evaluation and medical counseling

Since there is no biologic marker for VATER association, the diagnosis is made by documenting component anomalies. Severe anorectal, cardiac, tracheoesophageal, and limb defects will present with obvious signs or symptoms, but milder anomalies of these systems plus vertebral or renal defects may require laboratory and imaging studies for diagnosis. VATER association should be considered after one cognate defect is recognized, but the degree of suspicion will depend on the presenting anomaly. For example, children with tracheoesophageal fistula have a 37% frequency of cardiac defects, while those with cardiac defects have less than a 2% chance to have tracheoesophageal fistula. It is thus more important to investigate cardiac status in children with tracheoesophageal fistula than vice versa.

A reasonable approach to the diagnostic evaluation is to screen for all of the cognate VATER anomalies once two of them have been documented. For example, in the absence of identified syndromes, children with limb and cardiac defects should have spinal X-rays, renal sonogram, and surveillance for feeding/respiratory problems. Finding of a third cognate anomaly makes the diagnosis secure. Patients with tracheoesophageal fistula certainly deserve echocardiography and renal sonography, as do patients with imperforate anus (30% likelihood of renal defects once imperforate anus is documented). Patients with renal defects or vertebral defects also deserve echocardiography since 25% of patients with either anomaly have cardiac defects. Patients with initial ascertainment of cardiac or limb anomalies have low risks for associated anomalies.

Family and psychosocial counseling

Patients having three or more of the cognate VATER association defects and no obvious pattern of minor anomalies can be given a firm diagnosis with low recurrence risk (<1%). Although patients with tracheoesophageal fistula and/or severe cardiac defects have considerable mortality (as high as 48% in some studies), the good chance for normal mental development warrants health professionals taking an optimistic attitude toward these children. Psychosocial counseling, as for any child with a serious medical illness, may be useful for emotional and social stresses associated with prolonged and difficult hospitalization. Parent support groups for VATER association are available (see the VATER checklist).

Natural history and complications

Most complications of VATER association are direct consequences of congenital anomalies (see VATER checklist). Occasional patients will have growth failure during infancy or more subtle abnormalities like strabismus, myopia, torticollis, scoliosis, hip dislocation, urinary tract infections (with urolithiasis), neurogenic bladder, or altered gait. These potential complications require surveillance in early childhood. Major roles of the primary physician are to ensure thorough evaluation, to coordinate surgical care, and to provide optimistic case management with the realization that most patients have normal neurologic outcomes. While infancy and early childhood may be turbulent periods for patients with VATER association, specialized adolescent and adult care is required only for residual problems from infantile anomalies.

A documented complication of VATER association is spinal dysraphism with intraspinal lipomas or dermoids, tethering of the distal conus by a thickened filum terminale, diastematomyelia, etc. In 50% of patients, the dysraphism may be heralded by cutaneous surface markers such as lipomas, hemangiomas, sacral sinuses, sacral dimples, or asymmetric gluteal folds. If not detected in infancy, compression or traction of the spinal cord may lead to deterioration of walking, asymmetric leg musculature and strength, enuresis and poor bladder control. Myelomeningocele is a well-documented complication of VATER association, and spinal dysraphism represents the milder side of this spectrum. Although the frequency of spinal dysraphism in VATER association is probably low, spinal ultrasound in infants or spinal MRI in older children should be considered.

VATER association preventive management checklist

The most critical period of management for children with VATER association is in the nursery, where documentation of the component anomalies has immediate medical and surgical consequences (see VATER checklist). Patients with tracheoesophageal fistula or anorectal anomalies certainly warrant echocardiographic investigation as discussed above. Renal anomalies are sufficiently frequent in all VATER association groups that ultrasound study is also justified. Even without surface markers in the sacral area, ultrasound of the lower spine to evaluate spinal dysraphism is justified based on later consequences in several VATER patients. Once the patient is past the early childhood period, care is similar to that for the general population unless residual problems from congenital anomalies are present (see VATER checklist).

CHARGE association

Terminology

CHARGE is an acronym for the Association of *C*oloboma, *H*eart disease, *A*tresia choanae, *R*etarded growth and development, *G*enital anomalies, and *E*ar anomalies.

Patients with facial similarities to those with CHARGE syndrome may have Mendelian conditions such as the Hall–Hittner or Abruzzo–Erickson syndromes, so screening of the family history to exclude familial occurrence is requisite to a diagnosis of CHARGE association (Jones, 1997, pp. 668–70; Gorlin et al., 2001, pp. 1135–7).

Historical diagnosis and management

Multiple congenital anomalies associated with coloboma and choanal atresia were recognized for at least 20 years before their designation as CHARGE association. As with VATER association, surgical improvements have lengthened survival for CHARGE association patients. Since the characterization of CHARGE association, there have been occasional familial occurrences and overlapping anomalies that have raised suspicions of underlying syndromes. Gorlin et al. (2001, pp. 1135–7) discuss the Hall–Hittner syndrome as a recognizable subgroup of CHARGE association, and the X-linked Abruzzo–Erickson syndrome as a condition that must be excluded.

Incidence, etiology, and differential diagnosis

CHARGE association is sufficiently frequent that more than 250 cases have been reported. Based on the incidence of bilateral choanal atresia (1 in 8000 live births) and its 50% risk for associated anomalies, an incidence of 1 in 20,000 live births for CHARGE association seems reasonable (Blake et al., 1990, 1998; Issekutz et al., 2005). Its prevalence in older children will be diminished by significant infant mortality. The choanae are formed between days 35 and 38 of gestation; cardiac septation begins on day 38 of gestation, and closure of the fetal choroid fissure (that fails in colobomata) occurs from 28 to 35 days of gestation, establishing a critical period for causation of CHARGE association.

Differential diagnosis includes consideration of VATER association, where heart defects and esophageal atresia may occur. Craniofacial disorders such as the Crouzon or Treacher–Collins syndrome may include choanal atresia, while Kallman syndrome includes central nervous system and genital defects. The occurrence of colobomata and cardiac disease in patients with trisomy 13, dup(22q), or del(4p) syndromes mandates a normal karyotype before rendering a diagnosis of CHARGE association. An interesting exception to this rule may be the finding of deletions of the proximal long arm of chromosome 22–del(22q11); these deletions are very common in patients with DiGeorge anomaly or Shprintzen syndrome (see above and Chapter 9). Since DiGeorge anomaly occurs in both CHARGE association and Shprintzen syndrome (face and palatal anomalies with conotruncal heart defects), and since the three disorders have similar types of cardiac anomalies, the "CATCH 22" spectrum of disorders may yield insight into the etiology of CHARGE association.

Table 5.2. Comparison of anomalies in CHARGE association, DiGeorge anomaly, and Shprintzen syndrome

| Anomaly | CHARGE association | | | | | DiGeorge | Shprintzen |
	A	B	C	D	(Total) %	E, F	G (%)
Colobomata	16/19	17/20	43/47	15/16	(91/102) <u>89</u>	7	3
Heart defect	12/21	16/20	42/50	14/17	(84/108) 84	95	82
Atresia choanae	13/21	13/20	28/50	6/17	(69/108) <u>64</u>	– (low)	– (low)
Retarded growth	20/21	17/20	39/43	7/7	(83/91) 92	– (high)	33
Developmental delay	20/21	12/20	26/34	2/7	(60/82) 73	– (low)	40
Genital defect (M)	11/15	14/14	28/29	–	(53/58) <u>92</u>	3	10
Ear anomaly	17/21	20/20	50/50	17/17	(104/108) 97	46	70
Renal anomaly	–	6/20	12/50	6/11	(24/81) 30	11	– (low)
Death by 1 year	6/21	1/20	10/50	9/17	(26/108) 24	54	– (low)
Cleft lip/palate	5/21	–	–	6/17	(11/38) 29	6	98
Deafness	–	19/20	34/50	8/9	(61/79) <u>77</u>	2	– (low)
Facial palsy	11/18	12/20	16/50	9/9	(48/97) 50	7	– (low)

Notes:
M, male; percentages that distinguish the disorders are underlined.
Source: Blake et al. (1990, 1993, 1998); Baldini (2004); Issekutz et al. (2005).

Diagnostic evaluation and medical counseling

Diagnosis of CHARGE association is based purely on the pattern of anomalies, since no diagnostic test is yet available (Issekutz et al., 2005). Comparison of anomalies in CHARGE association to those of the DiGeorge anomaly and Shprintzen syndrome is made in Table 5.2. CHARGE association frequencies are totaled from the patients of Blake et al. (1990)–each requiring that four of the cognate anomalies be present. Table 5.2 illustrates that high frequencies of coloboma, choanal atresia, male genital defects, deafness, and facial palsy distinguishes CHARGE association from DiGeorge or Shprintzen syndrome. High frequencies of cleft lip/palate including velopalatine incompetence are characteristic of Shprintzen syndrome, while patients with isolated DiGeorge anomaly will lack cleft lip/palate and the coloboma/choanal atresia/facial palsy characteristic of CHARGE association. Despite these differences, patients with CHARGE association who also have DiGeorge anomaly and/or the prominent nose and palatal defects suggestive of Shprintzen syndrome deserve FISH studies for del(22)(q11) as part of their chromosome study (see Chapter 9). The presence of laryngeal anomalies and/or severe swallowing problems in CHARGE patients may also warrant evaluation of del(22)(q11), since the Opitz syndrome of dysphagia, reflux, and genital anomalies also has been related to this deletion (see Chapter 9).

Family and psychosocial counseling

Most cases are sporadic and predict a low recurrence risk for parents. Reports of familial CHARGE association including concordance in identical twins and higher paternal age, may represent cases of Hall–Hittner syndrome or further heterogeneity within the CHARGE group (Gorlin et al., 2001, pp. 1135–7). Many patients with CHARGE association have a better prognosis for growth and development than would be predicted based on their early feeding problems and developmental delay (Blake et al., 1998). Cautious optimism is thus warranted, particularly for those patients with normal neuroimaging and chromosome studies who survive infancy. Most families will require supportive counseling and services appropriate for raising a child with cognitive and physical disabilities. Parent groups are available (see CHARGE checklist).

Natural history and complications

The spectrum of complications in CHARGE association is derived from the studies cited in Table 5.2. Intrauterine growth retardation occurs in 16% of patients with 92% showing growth delay during infancy. Mortality is high (28%) with about half dying in the neonatal period and half during infancy. Most exhibited developmental delay (73%), with 8 of 47 patients (17%) described as severe (Blake et al., 1998). Cardiac anomalies tend to be severe, with tetralogy of Fallot, atrioventricular septal defect, ventricular septal defects, and patent ductus arteriosus being common in CHARGE association, as opposed to the interrupted aortic arch that is common in patients with DiGeorge anomaly. Pulmonary anomalies are also common. Colobomata are often found in the fundus only (59%), emphasizing the importance of an ophthalmologic evaluation. Deafness may occur because of central nervous system or middle ear anomalies, and 77% of patients will have hearing deficits (Blake et al., 1998). Other anomalies include tracheoesophageal fistula/esophageal atresia, omphalocele, facial palsy, cleft lip/palate, renal anomalies, and genital defects in males (see checklist).

CHARGE association preventive management checklist

Frequent central nervous system, airway, and neurosensory complications in CHARGE association require more comprehensive preventive care than in VATER association. Blake et al. (1990, 1998) emphasize the importance of multidisciplinary management that can reduce exposures to general anesthesia by 25%. The pediatrician's role as case manager is thus very beneficial.

Neonatal evaluation of eyes, nose (airway), palate, heart, brain, kidney, and genitalia are indicated in CHARGE patients, along with early functional assessment of hearing and vision. The frequency of aspiration mandates monitoring of patients after operations and thorough review of feeding/swallowing histories. Most patients will require extensive follow-up by ophthalmology and ENT specialists, and the high rate of growth/developmental problems mandates attention to nutrition, growth, early intervention, and school programs. Because the DiGeorge anomaly may occur, early chest X-ray to look for the presence of a thymus as well as calcium and white blood cell count measurements are indicated. The chest X-ray also is useful to screen for vertebral anomalies, and subsequent examinations for scoliosis should be performed. Significant risks for urinary tract anomalies warrant early sonographic screening and monitoring of urinalysis and blood pressure.

Preventive management of VATER association

Description: VATER association is an acronym that represents *V*ertebral defects, *A*nal atresia, *T*racheo *E*sophageal fistula, and *R*enal defects, sometimes expanded to VACTERL to denote *C*ardiac and *L*imb defects. The incidence is 1.6 per 1000 births.

Clinical diagnosis: Recognition of the characteristic anomalies usually requiring three defects for secure diagnosis. Patients with unusual facial appearance and/or minor anomalies such as single palmar creases should have chromosome studies to exclude other possibilities. Imaging studies are often needed to demonstrate the internal defects.

Laboratory diagnosis: None available.

Genetics: Sporadic with less than 1% recurrence risk unless underlying syndromes like trisomy 18 or X-linked VACTERL with hydrocephalus are present.

Key management issues: Detection and surgical treatment of cardiac, renal, or tracheoesophageal anomalies; monitoring of growth; alertness for complications such as hydrocephalus, choanal atresia, strabismus, myopia, torticollis with cervical spine anomalies, lower spine anomalies with scoliosis, hip dislocation, urinary tract infections, urolithiasis, tethered cord with neurogenic bladder or altered gait.

Growth charts: Mapstone et al. (1986) distinguished two patient groups with VATER association, one with low normal and one with delayed growth; many but not all of the delayed group had cardiac disease.

Parent groups: Searching on the term VATER association yields several websites, including the parent-oriented sites VATER connection (www.vaterconnection.org/) and Contact a Family (www.cafamily.org.uk/Direct/v12.html); searches on cognate anomalies are also useful.

Basis for management recommendations: Complications noted below as documented by, Rittler et al. (1996), Kallen et al. (2004). It should be noted that spinal dysraphism is a recently recognized complication, and that the sensitivity of spinal sonography in detecting this anomaly is not known.

Summary of clinical concerns

General	Life span	Stillbirth (12%), **increased infant mortality** (48%)
	Growth	Low birth weight, dysphagia, **failure to thrive**
Facial	Eyes	Microphthalmia, strabismus, myopia
	Ears	Chronic otitis, preauricular tags, malformed pinna (10–39%)
	Nose	Choanal atresia, respiratory obstruction
	Mouth	Cleft lip/palate, oromotor dysfunction
Surface	Neck/trunk	Klippel–Feil anomaly, torticollis, **inguinal hernia** (23%), hernia incarceration
Skeletal	Cranial	Large fontanels, plagiocephaly
	Axial	**Vertebral anomaly** (80%), **rib anomaly** (23%), **scoliosis** (32%)
	Limbs	**Upper limb defect** (35% – radial aplasia, preaxial polydactyly); **lower limb defect** (36% – clubfoot, dislocated hip, flexion contractures)
Internal	Digestive	**Anorectal anomaly** (70%), gastroesophageal reflux, intestinal obstruction, vomiting, constipation
	Pulmonary	**Tracheoesophageal fistula** (28–60%), horseshoe lung
	Circulatory	**Cardiac anomaly** (50% – VSD, ASD, PDA, tetralogy of Fallot, coarctation)
	Excretory	**Renal anomaly** (24–85% – renal agenesis, renal cysts, small or horseshoe kidney); **Urinary tract anomaly** (48% – patent urachus, hydronephrosis, hydroureter); obstructive uropathy, urinary tract infections
	Genital	**Genital anomaly** (44–55% – cryptorchidism, hypospadias, micropenis, vaginal atresia)
Neural	Central	Spina bifida, hydrocephalus, spinal dysraphism (tethered cord), enuresis
	Motor	Ambulation problems
	Sensory	Vision and hearing deficits

Concerns of frequency >20% are **highlighted**

Key references

Kallen, et al. (2004). Relation between oculo-auriculo-vertebral (OAV) dysplasia and three other non-random associations of malformations (VATER, CHARGE, and OEIS). *American Journal of Medical Genetics* 127A:26–34.

Mapstone, et al. (1986). Analysis of growth in the VATER association. *American Journal Disease of Children* 140:386–90.

Rittler, et al. (1996). VACTERL association, epidemiologic definition and delineation. *American Journal of Medical Genetics* 63A:529–36.

VATER association

Preventive medical checklist (0–3 years)

Name _____		Birth date __/__/___	Number _____	
Age	**Evaluations: key concerns**	**Management considerations**		**Notes**
New-born ↓ 1 month	Dysmorphology examination: anomalies Respiratory function: TE fistula Feeding, stooling: GI, anal anomalies Urinary function: renal anomalies Spine, back: bony defects, tethered cord Heart: murmur, tachycardia Parental adjustment	❑ Evaluate associated anomalies, syndrome[1] ❑ Chest X-rays; upper GI studies ❑ Rectal examination; video swallow[3] ❑ Renal sonogram; urinary tract studies ❑ Spinal X-rays; caudal MRI studies[3] ❑ Echocardiogram; cardiology ❑ Family support[4]	❑ ❑ ❑ ❑ ❑ ❑ ❑	
2 months ↓ 4 months	Growth and head size:[5] hydrocephalus Hearing and vision[2] Feeding, stooling: GI, anal anomalies Urinary function: infection Urinary stream, cryptorchidism, hip click Neck length, mobility: Klippel–Feil Parental adjustment Other:	❑ Head MRI;[3] ECI[3,6] ❑ Craniofacial surgery if ear anomalies ❑ Feeding specialist;[3] GI referral[3] ❑ Urinalysis ❑ Urology;[3] orthopedics[3] ❑ Anesthesia precautions; C-spine films[3] ❑ Family support[4] ❑	❑ ❑ ❑ ❑ ❑ ❑ ❑ ❑	
6 months ↓ 9 months	Growth and head size:[5] hydrocephalus Hearing and vision:[2] strabismus Feeding, stooling: GI, anal anomalies Urinary stream, inguinal hernia, hip click Neck length, mobility: Klippel–Feil Other:	❑ Head MRI;[3] ECI[3,6] ❑ ABR;[3] ENT;[3] ophthalmology[3] ❑ Feeding specialist;[3] nutrition;[3] GI referral[3] ❑ Urology;[3] orthopedics[3] ❑ Anesthesia precautions; C-spine films[3] ❑	❑ ❑ ❑ ❑ ❑ ❑	
1 year	Growth and head size:[5] hydrocephalus Hearing and vision:[2] strabismus Feeding, stooling: GI, anal anomalies Urinary stream, cryptorchidism Neck length, mobility: torticollis Sacral dimples, enuresis: tethered cord Other:	❑ Head MRI;[3] ECI[3,6] ❑ ABR;[3] ENT;[3] ophthalmology[3] ❑ Feeding specialist;[3] nutrition;[3] GI referral[3] ❑ Urinalysis; BP; urology[3] ❑ Anesthesia precautions C-spine films[3] ❑ Spinal X-rays;[3] caudal MRI studies[3] ❑	❑ ❑ ❑ ❑ ❑ ❑ ❑	
15 months ↓ 18 months	Growth and head size:[5] hydrocephalus Urinary stream, inguinal hernia Neck length, mobility: Klippel–Feil Other anomalies: spine, heart, GI	❑ Head MRI;[3] ECI[3,6] ❑ Urinalysis, BP; urology[3] ❑ Anesthesia precautions; C-spine films[3] ❑ Cardiology;[3] neurosurgery;[3] pediatric surgery[3] ❑	❑ ❑ ❑	
2 years	Growth and development[5] Hearing and vision:[2] strabismus Urinary stream, inguinal hernia Neck length, mobility: torticollis	❑ ECI;[3,6] nutrition;[3] family support[3,4] ❑ Audiology[3] ENT[3] ophthalmology[3] ❑ Urinalysis; BP; urology[3] ❑ Anesthesia precautions; C-spine films[3]	❑ ❑ ❑ ❑	
3 years	Growth and development[5] Hearing and vision:[2] strabismus Urinary stream, cryptorchidism Neck length, mobility: Klippel–Feil Gait, enuresis: tethered cord Other anomalies: spine, heart, GI Other:	❑ ECI;[3,6] nutrition;[3] family support[3,4] ❑ Audiology;[3] ENT;[3] ophthalmology[3] ❑ Urinalysis; BP; urology[3] ❑ Anesthesia precautions; C-spine films[3] ❑ Spinal X-rays;[3] caudal MRI studies[3] ❑ Cardiology;[3] neurosurgery;[3] pediatric surgery[3] ❑ ❑	❑ ❑ ❑ ❑ ❑ ❑	

VATER association concerns		**Other concerns from history**	
Growth deficiency TE fistula Choanal atresia Cleft lip/palate Torticollis Urinary tract anomaly	Cryptorchidism Clubfoot Cardiac anomaly Vertebral anomaly Hydrocephalus Spinal dysraphism	**Genetic/prenatal** _____ _____ _____ _____	**Social/environmental** _____ _____ _____ _____

Guidelines for the neonatal period should be undertaken *at whatever age* the diagnosis is made; TE, tracheoesophageal; GI, gastrointestinal; C-spine, cervical spine; ABR, auditory brainstem evoked response; BP, blood pressure; [1] consider chromosomes if multiple minor anomalies, unusual facial appearance; [2] by practitioner; [3] as dictated by clinical findings; [4] parent group, family/sib, financial, and behavioral issues; [5] consider developmental pediatrician/neurologist/geneticist if cranial anomalies, developmental concerns; [6] early childhood intervention including developmental monitoring and motor/speech therapy.

VATER association

Preventive medical checklist (4–18 years)

Name _____ Birth date __/__/__ Number _____

Age	Evaluations: key concerns	Management considerations	Notes
4 years ↓ **6 years**	Growth and head size:[5] hydrocephalus Development:[2] preschool transition Hearing and vision[2] Urinary stream, urinary infections Neck length, mobility Gait, enuresis: tethered cord Other anomalies: spine, heart, GI Other:	❑ Revisit possibility of syndrome[1] ❑ Family support;[4] preschool program[5] ❑ Audiology;[3] ENT;[3] ophthalmology[3] ❑ Urinalysis; BP; urology[3] ❑ Anesthesia precautions; C-spine films[3] ❑ Spinal X-rays;[3] caudal MRI studies[3] ❑ Cardiology;[3] neurosurgery;[3] pediatric surgery[3] ❑ ❑ ❑ ❑ ❑ ❑ ❑ ❑	
7 years ↓ **9 years**	Growth and head size:[5] hydrocephalus Development:[1] school transition[5] Hearing and vision[2] Urinary stream, urinary infections Neck length, mobility: Klippel–Feil Other:	❑ Family support;[4] school progress[6] ❑ Audiology;[3] ENT;[3] ophthalmology[3] ❑ Urinalysis; BP; urology[3] ❑ Anesthesia precautions; C-spine films[3] ❑ ❑ ❑ ❑ ❑ ❑	
10 years ↓ **12 years**	Growth and development[5] Hearing and vision[2] Urinary stream, urinary infections Gait, enuresis: tethered cord Genitalia: cryptorchidism, micropenis Other:	❑ Family support;[4] school progress;[6] puberty ❑ Audiology;[3] ENT;[3] ophthalmology[3] ❑ Urinalysis; BP; urology[3] ❑ Spinal X-rays;[3] caudal MRI studies[3] ❑ Urology[3] ❑ ❑ ❑ ❑ ❑ ❑	
13 years ↓ **15 years**	Growth and development[5] Hearing and vision[2] Urinary stream, urinary infections Neck length, mobility: Klippel–Feil Genitalia: micropenis	❑ Family support;[4] school progress;[6] puberty ❑ Audiology;[3] ENT;[3] ophthalmology[3] ❑ Urinalysis; BP; urology[3] ❑ Anesthesia precautions; C-spine films[3] ❑ Urology[3] ❑ ❑ ❑ ❑ ❑	
16 years ↓ **18 years**	Growth and development[5] Urinary stream, urinary infections Gait, enuresis: tethered cord Other anomalies: spine, heart, GI Other:	❑ Family support;[4] school progress;[6] puberty ❑ Urinalysis; BP; urology;[3] ❑ Spinal X-rays;[3] caudal MRI studies[3] ❑ Cardiology;[3] neurosurgery;[3] pediatric surgery[3] ❑ ❑ ❑ ❑ ❑ ❑	
19 years ↓ **23 years**	Adult care transition[5] Hearing and vision[2] Urinary stream, urinary infections Gait, enuresis: tethered cord	❑ Family support[4] ❑ Audiology;[3] ENT;[3] ophthalmology[3] ❑ Urinalysis; BP; urology[3] ❑ Spinal X-rays;[3] caudal MRI studies[3] ❑ ❑ ❑ ❑	
Adult	Adult care transition[5] Hearing and vision[2] Urinary stream, urinary infections Gait, enuresis: tethered cord Other anomalies: spine, heart, GI Other:	❑ Family support[4] ❑ Audiology;[3] ENT;[3] ophthalmology[3] ❑ Urinalysis; BP; urology[3] ❑ Spinal X-rays;[3] caudal MRI studies[3] ❑ Cardiology;[3] neurosurgery;[3] pediatric surgery[3] ❑ ❑ ❑ ❑ ❑ ❑ ❑	

VATER association concerns		Other concerns from history	
Growth deficiency Cleft lip/palate Torticollis Klippel–Feil anomaly	Cervical spine anomalies Cardiac anomaly Urinary tract anomaly Cryptorchidism, micropenis Spinal dysraphism	**Genetic/prenatal** _____ _____ _____ _____	**Social/environmental** _____ _____ _____ _____

Guidelines for the neonatal period should be undertaken *at whatever age* the diagnosis is made; BP, blood pressure; GI, gastrointestinal; C-spine, cervical spine; [1] consider chromosomes if growth failure, multiple minor anomalies, unusual facial appearance; [2] by practitioner; [3] as dictated by clinical findings; [4] parent group, family/sib, financial, and behavioral issues with later focus on independent living and employment; [5] consider developmental pediatrician/neurologist/geneticist if developmental concerns, learning disabilities; [6] monitor individual education plan, educational testing, balance of special education and inclusion, academic progress, behavioral differences, later vocational planning.

Parent guide to VATER association

VATER association is an acronym where the *V* is for Vertebral (spinal) defects, the *A* for Anal anomalies (narrowing or absence of the anus and rectum), the *TE* for TracheoEsophageal fistula (connection between the trachea or windpipe and the esophagus), the *R* for both Radial (hand defects on the thumb side) and Renal (kidney) defects. Synonyms include VACTERL association, where the "*C*" and "*L*" are added to emphasize the cardiac (heart) and limb defects that occur in this condition. Children without neurologic complications have potential for normal mental development, emphasizing the importance of preventive management during the turbulent neonatal period

Incidence, causation, and diagnosis

VATER association has an incidence estimated at 1.6 per 1000 live births. The term "association" indicates that the children have several co-existing anomalies without the recognizable facial appearance and subtle anomalies that characterize a syndrome. A diagnosis of VATER association should be considered after one cognate defect is recognized and considered likely with three or more typical anomalies. Other anomaly constellations such as trisomy 18, Holt-Oram, or Goldenhar syndromes may be confused. A reasonable approach to the diagnostic evaluation is to screen for all of the cognate VATER anomalies once two of them have been documented. For example, in the absence of identified syndromes, children with limb and cardiac defects should have spinal X-rays, renal sonogram, and surveillance for feeding/respiratory problems. Patients with tracheoesophageal fistula certainly deserve echocardiography and renal sonography, as do patients with imperforate anus (31% likelihood of renal defects once imperforate anus is documented). Patients with renal defects or vertebral defects also deserve echocardiography (26% and 25% respective risks for cardiac defects). Patients with initial ascertainment of cardiac or limb anomalies have low risks for associated anomalies.

Natural history and complications

Most complications of VATER association are direct consequences of congenital anomalies. Occasional patients will have growth failure during infancy or more subtle abnormalities like a wandering eye (strabismus), myopia, wryneck (torticollis), curved spine (scoliosis), hip dislocation, kidney or urinary tract infections, dysfunctional (neurogenic) bladder, or altered gait. Urinary tract problems may lead to kidney stones. These potential complications require surveillance in early childhood. Spinal cord abnormalities include fatty tumors, tethered cord (fixation of the spinal cord to surrounding tissues in the lower back region), or cysts within the cord (diastematomyelia). In 50% of affected children, the spinal cord anomaly may be heralded by surface markers on the skin of the lower back such as fatty tumors, birthmarks, or small indentations (sacral sinuses or dimples). The folds of the buttocks (gluteal folds) may be asymmetric, appearing different on the two sides. If not detected in infancy, these spinal cord anomalies may lead to deterioration of walking, asymmetric leg musculature and strength, bed-wetting, and poor bladder control.

Preventive medical needs

The most critical period of management for children with VATER association is in the nursery, where documentation of the component anomalies has immediate medical and surgical consequences (see the preventive medical checklist for VATER association). Patients with tracheoesophageal fistula or anorectal anomalies certainly warrant echocardiographic investigation of the heart. Renal anomalies are sufficiently frequent in all VATER association groups that ultrasound study of the abdomen and kidneys is also justified. Even without surface markers in the sacral area, ultrasound of the lower spine to evaluate spinal cord anomalies is justified based on later consequences in several VATER patients. Families of severely affected children should work with their health care providers to arrange financial and developmental services. Social services may be very helpful for those families undergoing prolonged and difficult hospitalizations. Early intervention services may be indicated for children with delayed development due to prolonged hospitalization, visual difficulties, or physical handicaps from limb or spinal abnormalities. Once the patient is past the early childhood period, care is similar to that for the general population unless residual problems from congenital anomalies are present.

Family counseling

Patients having three or more of the cognate VATER association defects and a normal facial appearance can be given a firm diagnosis. Once genetic or chromosomal syndromes have been excluded, the recurrence risk for parents having a child with VATER association is less than 1%. Although patients with tracheoesophageal fistula and/or severe cardiac defects have considerable mortality, the normal potential for mental development warrants an optimistic attitude toward these children.

Preventive management of CHARGE association

Description: CHARGE is an acronym that denotes the association of *Coloboma*, *Heart* disease, *Atresia* choanae, *Retarded* growth and development, *Genital* anomalies, and *Ear* anomalies. The nasal changes with clefts and ear anomalies may produce a similar facial appearance among affected patients, and some Mendelian syndromes are difficult to distinguish. The incidence is about 1 in 10,000 live births.

Clinical diagnosis: CHARGE association must be diagnosed by recognizing the characteristic anomalies, with most observers requiring that four of the cognate defects be present. High frequencies of coloboma, choanal atresia, male genital defects, deafness, and facial palsy distinguish CHARGE association from DiGeorge or Shprintzen syndrome, but chromosome studies should probably be performed for exclusion.

Laboratory diagnosis: None.

Genetics: Once a normal karyotype is documented, most cases of CHARGE association will be sporadic with a low recurrence risk. Overlap of manifestations with Mendelian conditions like Hall–Hitter or Abruzzo–Erickson syndromes may produce higher recurrence risks in some families (Issekutz et al., 2005).

Key management issues: Neonatal evaluation for choanal atresia, feeding problems, and cardiac defects; ophthalmology evaluation for colobomata or strabismus, audiology for hearing deficits due to CNS or middle ear anomalies, monitoring of feeding with alertness for tracheoesophageal fistula/esophageal atresia, omphalocele, facial palsy, cleft lip/palate, and urogenital anomalies.

Growth Charts: Blake et al. (1990) summarize growth data from 44 affected children.

Parent groups: CHARGE Syndrome Foundation (www.chargesyndrome.org), charge syndrome Canada (www.chargesyndrome.ca/).

Basis for management recommendations: Blake et al. (1998) published recommendations for the multidisciplinary management of CHARGE association.

Summary of clinical concerns

General	Lifespan	**Increased infant mortality** (35% die within first 3 months of life)
	Learning	**Cognitive and learning differences** (73%); severe delay (17%), speech problems
	Growth	Low birth weight (16%); **failure to thrive** (77%); **short stature** (92%)
Facial	Eyes	Oculomotor dysfunction, **eye anomalies** (colobomata, 89%; iris defects, 30%, fundus defects, 59%); **nystagmus** (26%), **strabismus** (32%)
	Ears	**External ear anomaly** (97%), **middle ear anomaly** (38%)
	Nose	**Choanal atresia** (64%), respiratory obstruction
	Mouth	**Feeding problems** (75%), **cleft lip/palate** (29%), dysphagia, small mouth
Surface	Neck/trunk	**Short neck** (20%)
Skeletal	Cranial	**Microcephaly** (25%), micrognathia
	Axial	Hemivertebrae, scoliosis (16%)
	Limbs	Clinodactyly, syndactyly
Internal	Digestive	**Gastroesophageal reflux** (37%), gastrointestinal obstruction, tracheoesophageal fistula/atresia (10%), omphalocele, anal atresia
	Pulmonary	Respiratory problems, **laryngeal anomaly** (20%)
	Circulatory	**Cardiac anomalies** (84%) – septal defects, endocardial cushion defects, aortic defects, tetralogy of Fallot, vascular rings
	Endocrine	Hormonal deficiencies (hypothyroidism; growth hormone deficiency, flat luteinizing hormone releasing hormone response, low testosterone)
	RES	DiGeorge anomaly (14%), immune deficiency (14%), frequent infections
	Urogenital	**Renal anomaly** (30%), hydronephrosis, microphallus, cryptorchidism
Neural	Central	**Brain anomalies** (50% – arrhinencephaly, cerebellar Dysplasia); seizures.
	Motor	**Facial palsy** (50%), facial asymmetry
	Sensory	Acoustic nerve dysfunction, **nerve deafness** (38%), **mixed hearing loss** (30%), **hearing deficits** (60–77%)

RES, reticuloendothelial system; **concerns** of frequency >20% are **highlighted**

Key references

Blake, et al. (1990). Growth in CHARGE association. *Archives of Disease in Childhood* 68:508–9.

Blake, et al. (1998). CHARGE association: an update and review for the primary pediatrician. *Clinical Pediatrics* 37:159–73.

Issekutz, et al. (2005). An epidemiological analysis of CHARGE syndrome: Preliminary results from a Canadian study. *American Journal of Medical Genetics* 133A:1–7.

CHARGE association

Preventive medical checklist (0–3 years)

Name _____ Birth date __/__/__ Number _____

Age	Evaluations: key concerns	Management considerations		Notes
New-born ↓ 1 month	Dysmorphology examination: anomalies Eyes, nose, hearing, breathing Feeding: facial palsy, oral clefts Heart: murmur, tachycardia Urinary function: renal anomalies DiGeorge anomaly Parental adjustment	❑ Evaluate associated anomalies[1] ❑ Colobomata; choanal atresia; ABR ❑ Video swallow;[3] pulmonology[3] ❑ Echocardiogram, cardiology ❑ Renal sonogram, urinary tract studies ❑ Chest X-ray for thymus, calcium, WBC ❑ Family support[4]	❑ ❑ ❑ ❑ ❑ ❑ ❑	
2 months ↓ 4 months	Growth and head size:[5] brain anomalies Hearing and vision[2] Feeding: facial palsy, oral clefts GI: GE reflux, intestinal anomalies Urinary function: renal anomaly Short neck, vertebral anomalies Parental adjustment Other:	❑ Head MRI;[3] ECI[3,6] ❑ Ophthalmology;[3] ENT[3] ❑ Feeding specialist;[3] nutrition;[3] pulmonology[3] ❑ GI specialist[3] ❑ Urinalysis; BP; urology[3] ❑ Anesthesia precautions;[3] spine films[3] ❑ Family support[4] ❑	❑ ❑ ❑ ❑ ❑ ❑ ❑ ❑	
6 months ↓ 9 months	Growth and head size:[5] brain anomalies Hearing and vision:[2] strabismus Feeding: dysphasia, aspiration, reflux Genitourinary anomalies: cryptorchidism Short neck, vertebral anomalies Other:	❑ Head MRI;[3] ECI[3,6] ❑ ABR;[3] ENT;[3] ophthalmology[3] ❑ Nutrition;[3] GI specialist;[3] pulmonology[3] ❑ Urinalysis; BP; urology[3] ❑ Anesthesia precautions;[3] spine films[3] ❑	❑ ❑ ❑ ❑ ❑ ❑	
1 year	Growth and head size:[5] brain anomalies Hearing and vision:[2] strabismus Feeding: dysphasia, aspiration, reflux Genitourinary anomalies: cryptorchidism Other anomalies: facial, heart, GI Other:	❑ ECI[3,6] ❑ ABR;[3] ENT; ophthalmology ❑ Nutrition;[3] GI specialist;[3] pulmonology[3] ❑ Urinalysis; BP; urology[3] ❑ Cardiology;[3] neurosurgery;[3] pediatric surgery[3] ❑	❑ ❑ ❑ ❑ ❑	
15 months ↓ 18 months	Growth and head size:[5] brain anomalies Hearing and vision:[2] sensory deficits Feeding: dysphasia, aspiration, reflux Other anomalies: facial, heart, GI	❑ ECI[3,6] ❑ ENT;[3] ophthalmology[3] ❑ Nutrition;[3] GI specialist;[3] pulmonology[3] ❑ Cardiology;[3] neurosurgery;[3] pediatric surgery[3]	❑ ❑ ❑ ❑	
2 years	Growth and development[5] Hearing and vision:[2] strabismus Feeding: dysphasia, aspiration, reflux Genitourinary anomalies, scoliosis	❑ ECI;[3,6] nutrition;[3] family support[3,4] ❑ Audiology; ENT; ophthalmology ❑ Nutrition;[3] GI referral[3] ❑ Urinalysis; BP; urology;[3] orthopedics[3]	❑ ❑ ❑ ❑	
3 years	Growth and development[5] Hearing and vision:[2] sensory deficits Feeding: dysphasia, aspiration, reflux Genitourinary anomalies, scoliosis Other anomalies: facial, heart, GI Other:	❑ ECI;[3,6] nutrition;[3] family support[3,4] ❑ Audiology; ENT; ophthalmology ❑ Nutrition;[3] GI specialist;3 pulmonology3 ❑ Urinalysis; BP; urology;[3] orthopedics[3] ❑ Cardiology;[3] neurosurgery;[3] pediatric surgery[3] ❑	❑ ❑ ❑ ❑ ❑ ❑	

CHARGE association concerns		Other concerns from history	
Choanal atresia Facial palsies DiGeorge anomaly Iris or fundus coloboma Ear anomalies, hearing loss Cleft lip/palate	TE fistula, omphalocele Laryngeal anomaly Cardiac anomaly Urogenital anomalies Developmental disability Brain anomalies, seizures	**Genetic/prenatal** _____ _____ _____ _____ _____	**Social/environmental** _____ _____ _____ _____ _____

Guidelines for the neonatal period should be undertaken *at whatever age* the diagnosis is made; WBC, white blood cell count; GE, gastroesophageal: GI, gastrointestinal; ABR, auditory brainstem evoked response; TE, tracheoesophageal; [1]consider chromosomes if multiple minor anomalies, unusual facial appearance; [2]by practitioner; [3]as dictated by clinical findings; [4]parent group, family/sib, financial, and behavioral issues; [5]consider developmental pediatrician/neurologist/geneticist if cranial or multiple anomalies, developmental concerns; [6]early childhood intervention including developmental monitoring and motor/speech therapy.

CHARGE association

Preventive medical checklist (4–18 years)

Name _____ **Birth date** __/__/__ **Number** _____

Age	Evaluations: key concerns	Management considerations	Notes
4 years ↓ **6 years**	Growth and head size:[5] brain anomalies Development:[2] preschool transition Hearing and vision[2] Feeding: dysphasia, aspiration, reflux Thyroid, growth problems, obesity Genitourinary anomalies, scoliosis Other anomalies: facial, heart, GI Other:	❏ Head MRI;[3] revisit possibility of syndrome[1] ❏ ❏ Family support;[4] preschool program[5] ❏ ❏ Audiology; ENT; ophthalmology ❏ ❏ Nutrition;[3] GI specialist;[3] pulmonology[3] ❏ ❏ T4, TSH; endocrinology[3] ❏ ❏ Urinalysis; BP; urology;[3] orthopedics[3] ❏ ❏ Cardiology;[3] neurosurgery;[3] pediatric surgery[3] ❏ ❏ ❏	
7 years ↓ **9 years**	Growth and head size:[5] Development:[1] school transition[5] Hearing and vision[2] Feeding: dysphasia, aspiration, reflux Thyroid, growth problems, obesity Other:	❏ Head MRI;[3] revisit possibility of syndrome[1] ❏ ❏ Family support;[4] school progress[6] ❏ ❏ Audiology; ENT; ophthalmology ❏ ❏ Nutrition;[3] GI specialist;[3] pulmonology[3] ❏ ❏ T4, TSH; endocrinology[3] ❏ ❏ ❏	
10 years ↓ **12 years**	Growth and development[5] Hearing and vision[2] Feeding: dysphasia, aspiration, reflux Thyroid, growth problems, obesity Genitourinary anomalies, scoliosis Other:	❏ Family support;[4] school progress;[6] puberty ❏ ❏ Audiology;[3] ENT;[3] ophthalmology[3] ❏ ❏ Nutrition;[3] GI specialist;[3] pulmonology[3] ❏ ❏ T4, TSH; endocrinology;[3] ❏ ❏ Urinalysis; BP; urology;[3] orthopedics[3] ❏ ❏ ❏	
13 years ↓ **15 years**	Growth and development[5] Hearing and vision[2] Feeding: dysphasia, aspiration, reflux Renal anomalies, scoliosis Puberty: micropenis, obesity	❏ Family support;[4] school progress[6] ❏ ❏ Audiology;[3] ENT;[3] ophthalmology[3] ❏ ❏ Nutrition;[3] GI specialist;[3] pulmonology[3] ❏ ❏ Urinalysis; BP; urology;[3] orthopedics[3] ❏ ❏ Urology;[3] endocrinology[3] ❏	
16 years ↓ **18 years**	Growth and development[5] Renal anomalies, scoliosis Puberty: micropenis, obesity Other anomalies: facial, heart, GI Other:	❏ Family support;[4] school progress;[6] puberty ❏ ❏ Urinalysis; BP; urology;[3] orthopedics[3] ❏ ❏ Urology;[3] endocrinology[3] ❏ ❏ Cardiology;[3] neurosurgery;[3] pediatric surgery[3] ❏ ❏ ❏	
19 years ↓ **23 years**	Adult care transition[5] Hearing and vision[2] Renal anomalies, scoliosis Puberty: micropenis, obesity	❏ Family support[4] ❏ ❏ Audiology;[3] ENT;[3] ophthalmology[3] ❏ ❏ Urinalysis; BP; urology;[3] orthopedics[3] ❏ ❏ Urology;[3] endocrinology[3] ❏	
Adult	Adult care transition[5] Hearing and vision[2] Feeding: dysphasia, aspiration, reflux Renal anomalies, scoliosis Other anomalies: facial, heart, GI Other:	❏ Family support[4] ❏ ❏ Audiology;[3] ENT;[3] ophthalmology[3] ❏ ❏ Nutrition;[3] GI specialist;[3] pulmonology[3] ❏ ❏ Urinalysis; BP; urology;[3] orthopedics[3] ❏ ❏ Cardiology;[3] neurosurgery;[3] pediatric surgery[3] ❏ ❏ ❏	

CHARGE association concerns		Other concerns from history	
Short stature Failure to thrive Strabismus, nystagmus Middle ear anomalies Hearing loss Hypothyroidism	Cardiac anomalies Urogenital anomalies Scoliosis Immune deficiency Growth hormone deficiency Cognitive disability	**Genetic/prenatal** _____ _____ _____ _____	**Social/environmental** _____ _____ _____ _____

Guidelines for the neonatal period should be undertaken *at whatever age* the diagnosis is made; TSH, thyroid stimulating hormone; BP, blood pressure; GI, gastrointestinal; [1] consider chromosomes if growth failure, multiple minor anomalies, unusual facial appearance; [2] by practitioner; [3] as dictated by clinical findings; [4] parent group, family/sib, financial, and behavioral issues with later focus on independent living and employment; [5] consider developmental pediatrician/neurologist/geneticist if developmental concerns, learning disabilities; [6] monitor individual education plan, educational testing, balance of special education and inclusion, academic progress, behavioral differences, later vocational planning.

Parent guide to CHARGE association

CHARGE is an acronym in which each letter refers to a characteristic problem in affected children. *C* refers to Coloboma, a cleft in the pupil and/or retina of the eye; *H* to Heart disease that includes holes in the atrial or ventricular septum; *A* to Atresia choanae, a narrowing or occlusion of the nasal passages in the skull; *R* to Retarded growth and development, *G* to Genital anomalies that are particularly obvious in males with small penis and undescended testicles; *E* to Ear anomalies. The term "association" indicates that these characteristics cluster together in certain individuals without having the typical facial appearance and more extensive pattern of anomalies that is termed a "syndrome."

Incidence, causation, and diagnosis

CHARGE association has an incidence of about 1 in 10,000–20,000 live births. Its prevalence in older children will be diminished by significant infant mortality. The critical period for the causation of CHARGE association is at 4–6 weeks after fertilization. The cause or causes of the defects in CHARGE association are not defined, and there is no specific genetic or chromosomal test for the pure condition. Some patients with CHARGE association have signs of DiGeorge anomaly or other genetic conditions and need chromosome studies.

Natural history and complications

Intrauterine growth retardation resulting in low birth weight occurs in 16% of patients; 92% have growth delay during the first year of life. Infant mortality is high (25–40%) because of facial and respiratory anomalies, and most survivors exhibit developmental delay (73%). Heart, lung, and gastrointestinal defects are common; these plus associated aspiration or immune defects often cause chronic respiratory infections. The clefts in the eye (coloboma) may be found only in the back of the eye (retina), emphasizing the importance of an ophthalmologic evaluation. Deafness may occur because of central nervous system or middle ear anomalies, and 77% of patients will have hearing deficits. Other anomalies include connections between the trachea and esophagus (tracheo esophageal fistula), protrusion of the abdominal organs (omphalocele), weaknesses in facial muscles (facial palsies), cleft lip/palate, and kidney anomalies.

Preventive medical needs

The high rate of brain, airway, and hearing/vision complications in CHARGE association requires multidisciplinary management, and integrated care can reduce the number of anesthesia exposures by 25%. One particular risk is that of aspiration (swallowing liquid into the lungs); monitoring of children after operations and thorough review of feeding/swallowing histories are thus important. Neonatal evaluation of eyes, nose (airway), palate, heart, brain, kidney, and genitalia are indicated in CHARGE patients, along with early functional assessment of hearing and vision. Most patients will require extensive follow-up by ophthalmology and ENT specialists, and the high rate of growth/developmental problems mandates attention to nutrition, growth, early intervention, and school programs. Because the DiGeorge anomaly may occur, early chest X-ray to look for the presence of a thymus as well as calcium and white blood cell count measurements are indicated. The chest X-ray also is useful to screen for spinal anomalies, and subsequent examinations for spinal curvature (scoliosis) should be performed. Significant risks for anomalies of the kidney and urinary tract warrant abdominal sonograms and monitoring for urinary infections or high blood pressure.

Family counseling

Most cases of CHARGE association are sporadic (i.e., occur with no family history). The recurrence risk is thus less than 1% for parents of an affected child unless a specific syndrome or chromosomal disorder is found. In patients with DiGeorge anomaly who have chromosome 22 deletions, parental chromosomes should be performed. If the child has a syndrome rather than CHARGE association, then parental recurrence risks can be as high as 25% for an autosomal or X-linked recessive disorder – parents may wish to have level II ultrasound studies in their next pregnancy because there is no definitive laboratory diagnosis (or prenatal diagnosis) for CHARGE association. Many patients with CHARGE association have a better prognosis for growth and development than would be predicted based on their early feeding problems and developmental delay. Cautious optimism is thus warranted, particularly for those children who have normal brain imaging and chromosome studies. As with other conditions causing mental disability, early intervention and preschool services with hearing and vision screening are appropriate.

6

Teratogenic syndromes

It is quite remarkable that only about 20 of the more than 50,000 drugs and chemicals in common use are proven human teratogens (Jones, 1997, pp. 555–79; Schardein, 2000; Gorlin et al., 2001, pp. 14–34). Considerably more – about 180 of 2800 tested – are teratogenic in two or more animal species (Schardein, 2000). The example of Dr. Lenz, the pediatrician who identified thalidomide babies in 1961, emphasizes the need for physicians to be alert and knowledgeable about potential teratogens. The reference of Schardein (2000) and telephone hotlines and websites offer guides to specific teratogens, including ReproTox (www.reprotox.org); TERIS plus Shephard's Catalogue of Teratogenic Agents (http://depts.washington.edu/~terisweb/index.html), International Toxicity Estimates for Risk Database (www.tera.org/iter/), and parent-oriented literature from the Organization of Teratology Information Services (www.otispregnancy.org). Although teratology is a general term for the study of developmental anomalies, it is used here in the more limited sense to describe anomalies caused by environmental agents (physical, chemical, or infectious).

Parents are frequently concerned about environmental exposures to substances such as pesticides or industrial agents when their child has a congenital anomaly. It is again reassuring that only one environmental chemical, methyl mercury, is a proven human teratogen. The many lawsuits concerning agents such as dioxin or Bendectin are truly an American tragedy (Brent, 2004). These unscrupulous awards provide sad testimony to our inadequate science of congenital anomalies.

Brent (2004) has reviewed the criteria required to prove that an agent is a human teratogen:

1 Human population studies associate an agent with a syndrome or specific type of congenital anomaly.

2 Human population studies demonstrate a correlation between the frequency of the anomaly and exposure to the agent.

3 Animal models yield the same types of anomalies at equivalent dosage/exposure ranges of the agent.

Table 6.1. Human teratogenic syndromes

Causal agent	Complications	Preventive measures, evaluations*
Ethanol	IUGR, DD, growth, brain, eye, heart, joints	Ophthalmology, ENT cardiology
Hydantoin	IUGR, DD, growth	Limb X-rays
Maternal diabetes	IUGR or macrosomia, brain, heart, skeleton	Cardiology, head imaging, vertebral X-rays
Maternal hyperthermia	DD, brain, limbs, eye, craniofacies, genitalia	Ophthalmology, ENT, orthopedics, urology
Maternal PKU	IUGR, DD, brain, heart, joints	Head imaging, cardiology
Methyl mercury	IUGR, DD, brain, vision, hearing	Head imaging, ENT, ophthalmology
Retinoic acid	DD, craniofacies, brain, heart	Head imaging, ENT, ophthalmology, cardiology
TORCH	IUGR, DD, brain, eye, hearing, liver, spleen, blood	Head imaging, ENT, ophthalmology, GI, hematology
Trimethadione	IUGR, heart	Cardiology
Valproic acid	Neural tube, DD, heart	Cardiology
Varicella	IUGR, DD, eye, limbs, skin	Ophthalmology, dermatology
Warfarin	IUGR, craniofacies, nose	Head imaging

Notes:

IUGR, intrauterine growth retardation; DD, developmental disability; PKU, phenylketonuria.

*Early childhood intervention screening should be done for all exposed infants.

4 The frequency and/or severity of anomalies show correlation with dosage of the agent.

5 A mechanism for teratogenesis is understood and/or the results make biologic sense.

All of these criteria are fulfilled for agents such as thalidomide or alcohol, while none is fulfilled for Bendectin. Claims that an agent increases the frequency of all types of congenital anomalies, rather than a pattern of specific malformations, are particularly suspect. It is important for physicians to emphasize the 2–3% risk of congenital anomalies in an average pregnancy, to allay parental guilt about exposures when appropriate, and to avoid naive or deliberate support for unscientific claims.

Table 6.1 lists many of the agents that fulfill the criteria for human teratogenesis, including major complications and preventive measures. Important among these are congenital infectious agents, some remembered by the TORCH acronym: *Toxo-plasmosis*, *Other* (syphilis, maternal viral infections), *Rubella*, *Cytomegalovirus*, *Herpes*. Less common conditions that affect the embryo (embryopathy) or fetus (fetal syndrome) are then summarized, followed by detailed recommendations for the management of children with fetal alcohol syndrome (FAS), fetal anticonvulsant exposure (FAE), and diabetic embryopathy.

A fetal cocaine syndrome?

The 30% of adults in the United States who admit to at least one use of cocaine, coupled with the 9–30% rates of positive cocaine testing at delivery indicate a potentially common neonatal disorder. Detection of cocaine may reach 70–80% when meconium or hair is screened after delivery of women who have had no prenatal care. Although severe effects of fetal cocaine exposure have been reported by specialists seeing referral populations, blinded examination of exposed newborns has failed to demonstrate a characteristic appearance (Little et al., 1996). The study of Chiriboga et al. (1999) is most definitive, comparing 104 cocaine-exposed and 136 cocaine-unexposed maternal–child pairs to document complications as cited below. Based on the mechanism of drug action in adults, fetal vascular disruptions might be anticipated as supported by pregnancy complications and disruption defects cited below.

Summary of clinical concerns: Cocaine exposure management considerations

General: Higher rates of intrauterine growth retardation (24% versus 8% as per the observation of Chiriboga et al., 1999) and higher frequencies of abortion, placental abruption, and prematurity require monitoring of fetal growth and perinatal status for those mothers receiving prenatal care.

Growth: Head circumference was below the 10th percentile (20% versus 5% as per the observation of Chiriboga et al., 1999; 30% in Gorlin et al., 2001, p. 17), and birth parameters are generally below the 25th centile in cocaine-exposed infants. Monitoring of head size and growth is needed, particularly in small-for-gestational age infants.

Developmental: Higher frequencies of neurologic problems, developmental delays, and behavior problems emphasize the need for early intervention assessment and regular developmental monitoring.

Craniofacial: Large fontanel, low hairline, short palpebral fissures, short nose, and shallow nasal bridge have been observed.

Facial-eye: Microphthalmia and retinal dysplasias or clefts can occur, requiring careful neonatal examination and regular vision testing with ophthalmology referral for concerns.

Internal: Some studies have indicated higher frequencies of cardiac defects and urogenital anomalies, so these systems should be evaluated carefully by neonatal examination, urinalyses, and, if suspected, by ultrasonography.

Neural-CNS: Chiriboga et al. (1999) documented global hypertonia (32% versus 11%), coarse tremor (40% versus 15%), and extensor leg posture (20% versus 4%) in cocaine-exposed versus non-exposed infants. Brain anomalies can include porencephaly, agenesis of the corpus callosum, septo-optic dysplasia, and schizencephaly (Gorlin et al., 2001, p. 17), and infants with microcephaly or severe neurologic problems should have a head MRI scan. Other neurologic complications such as sleep disorders, autism, learning problems, and attention deficit–hyperactivity disorders have been observed, emphasizing the need for annual behavioral assessments.

Neural-sensory: Eye changes and possible optic nerve damage mandate regular hearing and vision checks.

Parent information: The Organization of Teratology Information Services (OTIS) provides parent information about cocaine and pregnancy in Adobe Acrobat format (www.otispregnancy.org/pdf/cocaine.pdf).

Congenital cytomegalovirus infection

Congenital infection with cytomegalovirus (CMV) is estimated to be present in 0.5–2% of newborns, producing variable consequences that range from no symptoms (80%) to mild or disseminated neonatal disease with hepatosplenomegaly, coagulopathy, jaundice, and anemia (Schleiss & McVoy, 2004; Naessens et al., 2005). Maternal infection occurs in 0.7–4.0% of pregnancies with transmission rates to the fetus averaging about 40% (www.otispregnancy.org). About 10% of infected fetuses show symptoms of congenital CMV infection, and 5–15% of asymptomatic neonates may demonstrate long-term neurologic effects (www. otispregnancy.org).

Serologic screening of pregnant women is effective in detecting infants with CMV infection as demonstrated by Naessens et al. (2005). Screening of 7140 unselected mother–infant pairs showed evidence of past CMV infection in 3850 women (~54%), with 192 (2.7%) having IgG and IgM CMV antibodies when first tested and another 44 (1.4%) developing CMV antibodies during pregnancy. Infants of these 236 mothers were cultured, yielding 44 (0.62%) with CMV infection and detection of an estimated 82% of all CMV-infected infants.

Fetal infection may produce intrauterine growth retardation, microcephaly, and optic atrophy in addition to the complications of acute neonatal disease. As with rubella or toxoplasmosis, continuing infection in the infant may cause chorioretinitis, hematologic abnormalities, obstructive hydrocephalus, and intracranial calcifications. Inguinal hernias also occur.

Recent data suggests that ganciclovir therapy is effective in ameliorating hearing loss from CMV infection, and other antiviral drugs are being tested (Schleiss & McVoy, 2004). Early pregnancy screening is important for detecting mildly affected infants, and seronegative mothers should be counseled for good hygiene around young children and avoidance of cat-litter boxes and sandlots. Infants of mothers with early positive CMV antibodies or seroconversion should have urine CMV culture and leukocyte CMV DNA studies to document infection. Those with positive cultures should be considered for antiviral treatment after evaluation of the extent and severity of infection. CMV vaccines are under development and should be considered for mothers since recurrent infections are milder.

Clinical trials of antiviral therapy and recommendations for the diagnosis and management of congenital CMV infection are available on several websites (http://home.coqui.net/myrna/cmv.htm; http://cancer.gov/clinicaltrials/FHCRC-1577.00; http://www.clinicaltrials.gov/ct/show/NCT00016068; Collaborative Antiviral Study Group – http://www.niaid.nih.gov/daids/PDATguide/casg.htm).

Summary of clinical concerns: Congenital cytomegalovirus management considerations

General: Fetal infection may produce intrauterine growth retardation and/or microcephaly, providing indicators for team management by neonatal follow-up, general pediatrics, ophthalmology, and neurology specialists.

Growth: Monitor growth, feeding, and head size, especially in infants with low birth weight or small birth head circumference.

Developmental: Monitor developmental milestones and be alert for behavior differences since autism spectrum disorders have been reported.

Facial-eye: A retinal examination is necessary at birth, and annual ophthalmology evaluations are needed in all infected neonates since retinitis can occur later in childhood.

Internal-reticuloendothelial: Neonatal examination of liver/spleen size with blood count, peripheral smear, platelet count, liver transaminase, and bilirubin levels are indicated, with appropriate monitoring of symptomatic infants.

Neural-CNS: The severe side of CMV infection is shown by survivors of disseminated neonatal disease, with high frequencies of developmental disability (60%), hyperactivity with seizures or spasticity (35%), and hearing loss (30%). Head circumference should be documented at birth and monitored for evidence of obstructive hydrocephalus. Infected infants should have cerebrospinal fluid cell counts, protein, and glucose levels with CT scans for intracranial calcifications (cranial ultrasound is not sufficiently sensitive). Those with positive findings deserve early childhood intervention and more careful developmental/behavioral monitoring.

Neural-sensory: Sensorineural deafness should be evaluated by auditory brainstem-evoked response (ABR) in the nursery and followed by annual vision and hearing checks.

Congenital and neonatal herpes infection

Neonatal infection with herpes virus occurs in 1500–2000 infants each year in the United States (0.5–0.75 per 1000 births), usually transmitted from mothers with primary genital infection (Bale & Miner, 2005). Ninety percent of these infections are due to herpes simplex virus-2, and only 4% of herpes infections are truly congenital (acquired prenatally) as compared to 86% acquired natally and 10% postnatally. Preventive management of neonatal herpes infection mainly concerns Cesarean delivery to avoid exposure to genital lesions and subsequent treatment of exposed infants with vidarabine and acyclovir to lower mortality and neurologic sequellae. The diagnosis of neonatal infection is best made by viral culture from maternal genital lesions or fluids (establishing exposure) or from neonatal vesicles, eye swabs, mouth swabs, buffy coat, or cerebrospinal fluid. It is important to suspect the diagnosis in infants with pustular lesions.

Summary of clinical concerns: Congenital herpes management considerations

General: Infants who survive congenital or neonatally acquired herpes infection have significant frequencies of neurologic sequellae. Joint care with neonatal follow-up, ophthalmology, and neurology specialists would provide an ideal management team, with the pediatrician coordinating specialty and support services.

Growth: Monitor growth, feeding, and head size, especially in the 85% with low birth weight due to prematurity or intrauterine growth retardation.

Developmental: Follow developmental milestones as indicators of brain abnormalities; orthopedic defects may help qualify complex patients for neurology and developmental pediatric assessment.

Facial-eye: 57% have microphthalmia and chorioretinitis, requiring early and annual ophthalmology evaluation.

Neural-CNS: Developmental monitoring and early childhood intervention are often needed for microcephaly (67%) that may be accompanied by seizures and intracranial calcifications.

Neural-sensory: Eye changes and possible optic nerve damage mandate regular hearing and vision checks.

Parent information: Parental education and planning of future pregnancies with neonatal and obstetric specialists is also essential, since 5–7% of neonatal infections occur in offspring of women with recurrent or asymptomatic herpes virus shedding. The website www.herpes.com/pregnancy.shtml provides parent-oriented information and discussion of pregnancy risks. Searching on herpes simplex viruses 1 and 2 yields abundant information about these viruses and their human diseases.

Congenital human immunodeficiency virus infection

Over 1 million children worldwide have acquired infection with human immunodeficiency virus-1 (HIV-1), most due to congenital infection. Prior studies showed vertical transmission rates of 15–40%, equally divided between transplacental or perinatal infection (including breast-feeding) from HIV-positive mothers. Prenatal treatment with antiviral agents is now very effective in preventing HIV-1 transmission (Semprini & Fiore, 2004). Nevertheless, the severity and frequency (~0.3–0.5 per 1000 births in the United States) of symptomatic congenital/neonatal HIV-1 infection remains a considerable public health problem.

The most effective means of preventive management would be preconceptional screening to identify women with HIV infection – recent analyses suggest that screening high-risk populations every 3 years would cost 85,000 dollars per quality-adjusted life-year gained, and one-time screening of the entire United States population would cost 113,000 dollars per quality-adjusted life-year gained (Paltiel et al., 2005). Such screening is cost-effective based on enhanced survival alone, and would be even more effective if the advantages of early detection and antiviral treatment to prevent congenital infections were considered (Paltiel et al., 2005).

Summary of clinical concerns: Congenital HIV management considerations

General: Although characteristic facial features such as frontal bossing, prominent eyes, hypertelorism, and thick lips have been described in infants with congenital HIV-1 infection, most complications seem due to postnatal rather than fetal alterations. A multidisciplinary team devoted to HIV-positive children is needed for optimal management of complex nutritional, immune, and infectious problems (Semprini & Fiore, 2004).

Growth: Monitor head size, growth, and nutrition.

Developmental: Follow developmental milestones as indicators of brain abnormalities.

Facial: Minor features such as frontal bossing, prominent eyes, hypertelorism, and thick lips have been described in some infants, but clefts are rare.

Reticuloendothelial: Susceptibility to frequent infections may require prophylaxis (e.g., trimethoprim sulfamethoxazole against *Pneumocystis*, rifabutin against atypical mycobacteria); anemia may require iron supplementation.

Skin: Dermatitis is common in immunosuppressed children.

Neural-CNS: Microcephaly and developmental delays can occur, requiring monitoring with hearing/vision checks and early childhood intervention.

Parent information: Social and family supports are needed for ill children, particularly in families where a parent is incapacitated or absent. Several organizations are available for parental support and information, including the Children with AIDS Project (www.aidskids.org/), the Children with AIDS Charity (www.cwac.org/), and the Children with AIDS Foundation (www.caaf4kids.org/).

Retinoic acid embryopathy

The ingestion of large amounts of vitamin A (retinol) or smaller amounts of its potent derivatives (isotretinoin, retinoic acid) during pregnancy may be associated with a severe malformation syndrome (Coberly et al., 1996). It is estimated that 25% of fetuses exposed to isotretinoin (Accutane) in the first trimester, during treatment for acne, will have major malformations (Gorlin et al., 2001, p. 24). Though isotretinoin is cleared rapidly form the body, other retinoids such as etretinate that are used for psoriasis may require 2 years before elimination from fat stores is adequate for safe conception.

Summary of clinical concerns: Retinoic acid embryopathy management considerations

Growth: Growth deficiencies may attend neurologic, cardiac, or craniofacial defects and require involvement of feeding specialists, dieticians, and gastroenterology.

Developmental: Cognitive defects occur in at least 50%, justifying early childhood intervention and regular developmental assessments. Mental deficiency is often severe, necessitating early intervention and parental counseling appropriate for children with severe mental disability.

Facial-eye: Retinal dysplasias, strabismus, and myopias occur in 20%, mandating early and annual ophthalmology assessments.

Facial-ENT: Cleft palate and micrognathia with associated ear anomalies may occur, requiring team management of surgeries, feeding, and hearing problems due to serous otitis.

Internal-cardiac: Transposition of the great vessels, septal defects, and tetralogy of Fallot with DiGeorge anomaly may occur, justifying neonatal echocardiograms and chest X-rays for thymus visualization in exposed infants. Screening for neonatal hypocalcemia and later immune deficiencies should be considered.

Internal-immunology: Immune assessment should precede the administration of live viral vaccines, since DiGeorge anomaly can occur.

Neural-CNS: Brain anomalies occur in 70% including microcephaly, hydrocephalus, cerebellar anomalies, and cranial nerve deficits such as Moebius sequence. Head MRI scan and alertness for seizures or dystonias are indicated.

Neural-sensory: Eye and ear anomalies require annual vision and hearing assessment including annual ophthalmology and ENT referrals.

Parent information: A fact sheet on Accutane and other retinoids is available from the Organization of Teratology Information Services (OTIS – www.otispregnancy.org).

Rubella embryopathy

Congenital rubella infection is now rare due to universal immunization programs. It was one of the first teratogenic syndromes to be detected, by the Australian ophthalmologist Gregg in 1941 (Gorlin et al., 2001, p. 25), and a recent report from that country indicates the occasional cases encountered due to local outbreaks of rubella. Such outbreaks are most common among immigrants from countries without routine immunization. Women at risk to deliver infants with congenital rubella are those less likely to have prenatal care – younger or minority women, with 40% of cases following a previous live birth. Routine rubella immunization after pregnancy is recommended, and is likely responsible for the decrease in congenital rubella from 0.45 per 100,000 births in 1990 to 0.1 per 100,000 in 1999 observed in the United States (American College of Obstetrics & Gynecology, 2002). As with other congenital infections, the best prevention of congenital rubella is good prenatal care and widespread immunization, since maternal antibodies to rubella virus prevent damage to the fetus. The need for continued surveillance and immunization (despite shortages of vaccine – American College of Obstetrics & Gynecology, 2002) is indicated by the estimated 25,000 babies damaged by the 1964 United States epidemic of 2 million cases (Gorlin et al., 2001, p. 25).

The timing of maternal rubella infection is critical for the congenital syndrome, in that virtually 100% of gestational infections occurring before 11 weeks, 35% of those occurring between 13 and 16 weeks, and less than 1% of those occurring after 16 weeks produce fetal birth defects (Gorlin et al., 2001, p. 25).

Summary of clinical concerns: Congenital rubella management considerations

General: Major anomalies affecting the eye, ear, and heart are correlated with the degree of intrauterine growth retardation, making ultrasound screening a useful strategy for women with negative rubella titers. There is a 5–10% incidence of abortion or stillbirth.

Growth: Growth and head circumference should be monitored, especially in infants with neonatal thrombocytopenia or intrauterine growth retardation, and supplemental or high-calorie feedings may be necessary.

Developmental: Cognitive defects occur in over half of symptomatic infants, mandating early childhood intervention with particular alertness for hearing loss.

Facial-eye: Retinopathy, strabismus, glaucoma, cataract, and myopia, are common, requiring early and annual ophthalmology assessments.

Facial-mouth: Enamel hypoplasia occurs in 20%, emphasizing the need for regular dental care (Gorlin et al., 2001, p. 26).

Skeletal: Enlarged anterior fontanel and microcephaly may signal underlying neurologic problems; growth plate abnormalities may add to growth delays.

Internal-cardiac: Septal defects and pulmonary artery stenosis are common in infants exposed early in gestation, so cardiology and echocardiographic assessment is important for symptomatic infants.

Internal-reticuloendothelial system: Hepatosplenomegaly, thrombocytopenia with purpura, interstitial pneumonia, and immune deficiencies may require evaluation during infancy and early childhood.

Internal-endocrine: Diabetes mellitus occurs in 30% of adults with rubella embryology, so urinalysis screening is important for survivors of the 1964 epidemic.

Neural-CNS: Mental deficiency is likely in cases with microcephaly and may be exacerbated by ongoing encephalitis.

Neural-sensory: Hearing loss is well-known and underlines the need for neonatal ABR screening. Frequent eye anomalies mandate regular hearing and vision screening, with more intensive rehabilitation programs for infants with growth delay that correlates with neurodevelopmental problems.

Congenital syphilis

Presentations of congenital syphilis range include early abortion, symptomatic infants with Hutchinson triad (keratitis, sensorineural deafness, dental anomalies), or asymptomatic infants with positive serology (Peeling & Ye, 2004). For less severely affected neonates, early diagnosis through antibody testing allows treatment with penicillin or comparable antibiotics and produces an excellent prognosis. Women who have or acquire syphilis during early pregnancy will usually have an infected, symptomatic child with secondary syphilis; antibiotic therapy can prevent maternal disease, maternal transmission, and markedly improve outcomes for congenitally infected infants.

Congenital syphilis, like other consequences of sexually transmitted diseases, has exhibited recent increases in frequency. Although effective prevention and therapy are available, lack of prenatal care and the predominance of asymptomatic maternal infection perpetuate the congenital syndrome (Peeling & Ye, 2004). Diagnosis is made by detecting *Treponema pallidum* IgM antibodies in mother or infant.

Summary of clinical concerns: Congenital syphilis management considerations

General: Placental hyperplasia and fetal hydrops are common, as is spontaneous abortion or stillbirth yielding a macerated fetus. Serologic studies are important in such cases when prenatal care was lacking, since treatment of the mother prevents subsequent congenital disease. Antibiotic therapy should be initiated as soon as the diagnosis is made, as ongoing spirochetemia can cause gummatous necrosis and later complications.

Growth and development: Monitoring of development, growth, hearing, and vision is important, particularly for neonates exhibiting intrauterine growth retardation.

Facial-eye: Chorioretinitis may result from intrauterine or neonatal infection, requiring early and annual ophthalmology assessments.

Facial-mouth: Notched teeth and tapering of the incisors can require early dental care.

Skeletal: Osteochondritis can cause subperiosteal elevations and saber shins, leading to severe limb pain, persistent crying, and pseudoparalysis. Skeletal X-rays are important to document infection and resolution after treatment.

Internal-various: Gummatous necrosis can affect the liver, lung (pneumonia alba), thymus, and kidney. Extramedullary hematopoesis, hepatosplenomegaly, nephrotic syndrome, intestinal atresias, hypoalbuminemia, coagulopathies, and cardiopulmonary failure must be suspected even after neonatal treatment.

Neural-CNS: Gummas may cause cysts, microcephaly, and mental deficiency with neurosensory deficits.

Toluene embryopathy

Toluene sniffing during pregnancy may produce a fetal syndrome of microcephaly, micrognathia, renal anomalies, and growth failure (Hersch, 1989). The facies is subtle, so a maternal history is usually necessary to consider the diagnosis. Preventive management should consist of monitoring growth and development, with consideration of an abdominal ultrasound if renal anomalies are suspected through growth failure or urinary tract infection. Early childhood intervention is needed because of developmental delay.

Congenital toxoplasmosis infection

Congenital toxoplasmosis infection occurs at a rate of 0.1–2 per 1000 births in the United States, with the overall rate of vertical transmission being 30–40% (Lopez et al., 2000). Maternal infection during the first trimester is associated with more severe neonatal symptoms, with a transmission rate estimated at 15%. Maternal infection later in gestation is associated with higher transmission rates (~60%) but mild or asymptomatic neonatal disease. Prevention is best accomplished by maternal education to avoid contact with cat litter, undercooked meat, or soil through gardening or poorly washed vegetables. In France, where the incidence of toxoplasmosis and congenital infection is 2–3-fold higher than in the United States, spiramycin treatment of pregnant women with acute toxoplasmosis infection has been shown to lower fetal transmission and the severity of neonatal disease.

Congenital toxoplasmosis infection may be asymptomatic or manifest during the neonatal or later infantile period. The acute presentation may include fever, respiratory illness, hepatosplenomegaly, anemia, and jaundice that mimics other congenital infections. Diagnosis by the detection of specific IgM antibody allows effective treatment using pyrimethamine, sulfadiazine, and folinic acid to ablate pyrimethamine toxicity. Neonatal screening programs allowing early treatment have demonstrated effectiveness by lowering the frequency of subsequent neurologic and ophthalmologic complications.

Summary of clinical concerns: Congenital toxoplasmosis management considerations

General: The placenta may be large and hydropic, with villitis and spontaneous abortion or stillbirth (Lopez et al., 2000). A specific preventive management program is recommended for surviving infants to evaluate complications during and after pyrimethamine therapy.

Growth and development: Monthly pediatric and neurodevelopmental assessment is recommended with monitoring of head circumference, hearing, and vision. After treatment, less than 4% of infants had motor deficits, none had cognitive or hearing deficits, and 8% acquired new retinal lesions with some visual impairment.

Facial-eye: Retinal lesions (18–60%) and visual impairment (15–43%) require initial ophthalmology evaluation with assessments every 3 months until age 18 months and annually thereafter.

Internal-various: Hepatosplenomegaly, jaundice, extramedullary hematopoesis, hepatitis, cholestasis, and immune glomerulonephritis may occur, mandating alertness for these complications during infancy. Blood IgG/IgM antitoxoplasmosis antibody measurements, blood counts, liver function tests, and urine culture for toxoplasmosis should be performed every 3 months until age 18 months. Biweekly blood counts are recommended during pyrimethamine therapy.

Neural-CNS: Intracranial calcifications (25–71%), hydrocephalus (7–17%), seizures (6%), and microcephaly (4–14%) mandate initial cranial CT scan, lumbar puncture, and complete neurologic evaluation. Severe cases may develop hydrocephalus *in utero* and present with hydranencephaly.

Warfarin embryopathy

Exposure of the fetus to coumarin anticoagulants during pregnancy may produce a syndrome of nasal hypoplasia and stippling of the epiphyses that must be distinguished from genetic forms of chondrodysplasia punctata (Gorlin et al., 2001, pp. 31–2). The most characteristic anomaly is the "fleur-de-lys" nose with its shallow bridge and hypoplastic tip. Additional abnormalities include prenatal growth deficiency, failure to thrive, microcephaly, hydrocephaly, seizures, hearing loss, ocular anomalies (cataracts, strabismus), and choanal atresia. Preventive management should include an initial skeletal radiographic survey to assess the extent of skeletal involvement, monitoring of feeding and growth, monitoring of head circumference and neurosensory development, initial ophthalmology evaluation and audiologic screening.

Fetal alcohol syndrome

Terminology

FAS denotes a pattern of physical and behavioral anomalies related to exposure to ethanol during pregnancy. Some use the term fetal alcohol effects for alcohol-exposed children with milder abnormalities or characteristic behaviors, but most discourage this term and acknowledge a broad spectrum of findings that depends on the gestational timing and amount of ethanol exposure (Jones, 1997, pp. 555–8; Gorlin et al., 2001, pp. 14–17; Hoyme et al., 2005).

Historical diagnosis and management

Dangers of drinking during pregnancy were mentioned in biblical times and were specifically emphasized during England's Gin Epidemic of 1720–50. Specific patterns of physical anomalies in offspring of alcoholic women were documented by Jones & Smith (see Hoyme, 2005) in 1975.

Incidence, etiology, and differential diagnosis

The incidence of FAS is heavily dependent on socioeconomic status and ethnic background. The overall incidence is now estimated at about 1 per 1000 live births in the United States, reaching as high as 40 per 1000 among "heavy" drinkers. This general incidence is 10–20 times higher than in Europe and other countries (0.08 per 1000), representing higher rates in areas characterized by low socioeconomic status and African American or Native American background (2.29 cases per 1000). Because births with FAE are 3–4 times more common than those with FAS, some authors suggest that 10–20% of all mental retardation may be related to pre-natal exposure to ethanol. Isolated communities with low socioeconomic status and high-risk ethnic backgrounds can have incidences reaching 20%.

Brain anomalies and small eyes have been documented in several animal models of FAS, including rodents and non-human primates. Correlation of alcohol dosage and timing with teratogenesis establishes ethanol as the etiologic agent, but its mode of action has not been defined. Maternal nutrition seems to play a minor role, with acetaldehyde and prostaglandins implicated as mediators of teratogenesis. Ethanol injected into pregnant mice can produce growth retardation, neural anom-alies, and facial changes similar to human FAS, and a strong influence of genetic background explains why certain mothers and fetuses seem susceptible to FAS.

Diagnosis of FAS is based on subjective recognition of minor anomalies com-bined with disproportionate microcephaly and failure to thrive. Facial anomalies include small eyes, shallow nasal bridge, upturned nose, abnormal ears (posteri-orly rotated or low placed), thin upper lip, and absent philtrum; anomalies of the eye, heart, and skeleton are common. Stoler & Holmes (2004) have devised criteria for neonatal diagnosis that requires four of six typical facial anomalies be present.

Some authors argue against the false dichotomy between FAS and FAE on the grounds that all teratogens exhibit a range of effects according to the severity of the exposure. Regardless of the terminology, it is important to realize that ethanol teratogenesis may not produce an obvious phenotype at birth. Several studies suggest that less than half of children with FAS will be identified at birth. Until a biochemical "footprint" of exposure to ethanol is defined that can be used for objective diagnosis, FAS has a very broad differential that includes many children with microcephaly and growth and developmental delay. Offspring of mothers with untreated phenylketonuria resemble those with FAS, as do children with a long list of genetic or chromosomal conditions with microcephaly and growth failure. Severely affected infants may have abnormal brains with heterotopias (abnormal cell migration), prompting consideration of other neurologic disorders. Milder effects of FAS include learning disabilities, poor impulse control, and hyperactivity that can be present in numerous other syndromes. A broad differential diagnosis and high degree of suspicion are essential for FAS, since the definitive maternal history may require skill and experience to elicit.

Diagnostic evaluation and medical counseling

A major aspect of diagnosis is a good parental history. Blunt or judgmental questions often meet with denial or underestimates of drinking that are classic for alcoholic persons. Questioning of both parents (social customs are often congruent), initial focus on non-threatening agents such as carbonated beverages, and specific mention of beer and wine (sometimes not considered "drinks") are important strategies. Smoking histories are important, since cigarette smoking is a common correlate of alcoholism that also contributes to fetal growth restriction.

Because of difficulties in neonatal diagnosis, follow-up is a key tool for diagnosis of FAS. Even with strong evidence of maternal alcoholism, the "hit" rate in offspring varies between 20% and 70%. In the presence of a clear-cut maternal history and the typical FAS appearance discussed above, cardiac, renal, and perhaps even head ultrasound are warranted in the newborn period. Examination for minor anomalies is warranted, with careful documentation of subsequent growth and development. When available, experienced dysmorphologists may assist in recognizing the diagnosis as confirmed by controlled studies. Since no medical test is diagnostic, counseling must emphasize abstinence in future pregnancies, but acknowledge uncertainty in relating specific infant problems to maternal drinking.

Ongoing debate concerns the reliability and specificity of a behavioral phenotype in FAS. Of concern is the use of soft neurologic signs or behavioral symptoms as diagnostic criteria for FAS, particularly when objective changes in growth, craniofacial morphology, and organ development are not present. Heavy drinking does cause IQ deficits in offspring regardless of morphologic findings.

Family and psychosocial counseling

Although most children with recognizable FAS are born to persons with chronic alcoholism, better awareness of the condition may identify moderate drinkers who have children with milder growth and behavioral problems. Intervention can be very successful in more moderate drinkers, and should be attempted with chronic alcoholic persons to prevent alcohol in breast milk or even in formula as an infant tranquilizer. The familial predisposition to chemical dependency and recurrent affliction of siblings predicts that FAS will affect several family members; one study showed that 17% of older sibs and 77% of younger sibs had evidence of FAS after an index case was identified. The first goals of family counseling are to intervene in the cycle of alcohol abuse and to protect the newly diagnosed infant from the hazards of further alcohol exposure or neglect. Since the incidence of FAS is strongly correlated with low socioeconomic status, initial counseling, and intervention will usually require the involvement of protective and social services. Several parent groups and organizations for FAS are available as indicated on the checklist. Public education is important because there seems to be no safe period for alcohol use in pregnancy.

Natural history and complications

Major complications of the FAS include increased pregnancy loss and subsequent low birth weight. Impact of alcohol on the developing brain is evidenced by a high frequency of neurologic problems and learning deficits with a mean IQ of 41–65. Older children often have attention deficits with hyperactive, distractible, and impulsive behavior (Gorlin et al., 2001, pp. 14–16; Hoyme et al., 2005). Children with FAS have different behaviors than controls with similar IQ, and are at risk for mental illness (Famy et al., 1998). Abnormal behaviors include peculiar language, hyperacusis, memory and sleep disturbances, impulsivity and other personality disorders. Neurosensory damage is also common, with abnormal ABR, hearing loss, and diminished vision (due to optic nerve or eye anomalies) are found in a majority of patients. The cognitive and neurosensory problems produce a high incidence of speech delay that needs attention.

FAS commonly affects the digestive, cardiac, immune, and skeletal systems. Cleft palate, delayed dentition, and feeding problems are common. The DiGeorge anomaly with hypoparathyroidism and immune defects has been described, and the incidence of many types of infections, including otitis media, is increased. Cardiac anomalies are found in 40–50% of and include atrial or ventricular septal defects, tetralogy of Fallot, peripheral pulmonary artery stenosis, and dextrocardia.

Upper airway obstruction due to midface hypoplasia has produced apnea or chronic hypoxia in some patients, placing them at risk to develop pulmonary hypertension. Subclinical renal tubular defects with impaired acidification have been documented in FAS, as have frank renal anomalies.

A variety of skeletal and connective tissue defects occur, including Klippel–Feil anomaly, transverse limb defects, limb contractures, hip dislocation, scoliosis, chest deformities, and the radiographic finding of stippled epiphyses. An elevated cancer rate has been suggested for FAS, with examples of neuroblastoma, hepatoblastoma, sacrococcygeal teratoma, medulloblastoma, adrenal carcinoma, and acute lymphocytic leukemia being published. Whether these tumors reflect carcinogenic effects of alcohol that have been documented in adults or increased scrutiny of FAS patients is unknown.

Fetal alcohol syndrome preventive medical checklist

Because of the relatively high incidence and economic impact of FAS and FAE, there is probably no condition in which preventive management can have greater importance. A major goal is family intervention before further damage is inflicted on the developing infant and sibs. Provision of alcohol in breast milk or as an infant sedative is well-recognized, and social/protective service intervention is mandated when the diagnosis of FAS is made. High rates of affected sibs emphasize the need for family evaluation and a thorough parental history for children with suspect FAS or FAE.

In those cases where the diagnosis is recognized during infancy, imaging or X-ray studies for cardiac, vertebral, and renal anomalies are indicated. Physical examination for orthopedic defects, including congenital hip dislocation, is important. Sensorineural or conductive hearing loss and eye anomalies are as common as in Down syndrome, so similar recommendations for vision and hearing assessment are included in the checklist. The high frequency of failure to thrive (50–75%) and microcephaly (disproportionately small in 90%) mandates careful monitoring of growth and nutrition. Growth hormone secretion in children with FAS is lower than normal but comparable to that of other children with intrauterine growth retardation.

Referral to early childhood intervention and assistance with social, school, and financial issues that affect children with special needs are appropriate. Challenging behaviors in most children with FAS or FAE should be emphasized in discussions with foster or adoptive parents, and avenues for behavioral therapy provided. Behavior problems are particularly difficult in the adolescent and adult, including poor judgment, distractibility, and difficulty perceiving social clues. Pregnancy counseling, school/job support, and violence prevention are thus of even greater importance in the care of adolescents with FAS.

Fetal anticonvulsant exposure

Terminology

Anticonvulsant use in pregnancy is associated with a 5–7 increased risk for fetal birth defects and developmental delay (Moore et al., 2000). Because many women with epilepsy use multiple medications, it has been difficult to match particular patterns of anomalies with particular anticonvulsants. Specific abnormalities have been associated with hydantoin (growth deficiency, developmental delay, microcephaly, cardiac defects, genital anomalies, hypoplasia of the terminal digits/nails), primidone (similar to hydantoin without the genital defects), trimethadione (mild developmental/growth delay, cardiac defects, hernias, tracheoesophageal anomalies), and valproic acid (developmental delay, spina bifida, cardiac defects, genital defects, distal phalangeal/nail dysplasia with more severe limb deficiencies). The overlap among anomaly patterns, coupled with claims that epilepsy itself is teratogenic, justifies their grouping under fetal anticonvulsant exposure for the purpose of this discussion.

Historical diagnosis and management

Anticonvulsant therapy was initiated with the use of potassium bromide in 1853, with the first recognition of congenital anomalies in offspring of epileptic women occurring in 1963 (Schardein, 2000). The introduction of hydantoins in the 1930s was followed by a similar delay before Hanson & Smith in 1975 (see Pennell, 2003) described a syndrome of craniofacial anomalies, nail and digital hypoplasia, intrauterine growth retardation, and mental deficiency in offspring of hydantoin-treated women. Similar patterns were then observed in infants exposed to primidone, trimethadione, and valproic acid, and the current view is that these drugs plus the maternal epileptic state are synergistic in producing the various anomalies. Modern management is therefore oriented towards finding minimal dosage and number of anticonvulsants that will control seizures (Pennell, 2003). Planning of pregnancies is particularly important in epileptic women, since drug titration before pregnancy, preconceptional supplementation of folic acid, and minimization of first trimester exposures are key to preventing neural tube defects and other anomalies.

Incidence, etiology, and differential diagnosis

It is estimated that 1% of all individuals have epilepsy, and that anticonvulsants account for about 0.5% of drug sales (Schardein, 2000; Wide et al., 2004). These figures translate to about 30,000 annual United States births to women on anticonvulsants, and a 5–10% risk for exposed infants to have abnormalities (based on hydantoin exposure) translates to 3000 infants with anticonvulsant-associated abnormalities (about 1 in 1000 births).

Moore et al. (2000) illustrate the spectrum of abnormalities in their description of 57 infants exposed to anticonvulsants. These included 60% exposed to valproate alone, 7% to carbamazepine alone, 7% to phenytoin alone, and 26% to more than one anticonvulsant. Behavioral problems were noted in two-thirds, with about half of these having hyperactivity or poor concentration and six (about 10%) having a diagnosis of autism or Asperger syndrome. Learning difficulties, speech delay, gross or fine motor delays, glue ear, joint laxity, and myopia were also common findings.

The pathogenesis of major or minor anomalies caused by anticonvulsants is still unknown. General effects of maternal epilepsy on fetal development, and possible synergies of multiple anticonvulsant medications have not been adequately dissected from the effects individual agents like hydantoin. Animal studies offer the best evidence for primary hydantoin effects, including face/limb and behavioral abnormalities that are comparable to those produced in humans. Differences in response among mouse strains predicted genetic factors in human susceptibility, and there is correlation between maternal arene oxidase levels and fetal abnormalities after hydantoin exposure.

Differential diagnosis includes conditions with hirsutism, nail or digital hypoplasia, and similar facial features. FAS is associated with growth/developmental delays and nail hypoplasia, as are the genetic Coffin–Siris and Coffin–Lowry syndromes. Maternal and family history together with the pattern of anomalies should differentiate these conditions from anticonvulsant associations.

Diagnostic evaluation and medical counseling

When the positive maternal history, various facial anomalies, typical defects, and especially digital/nail hypoplasia are present, few diagnostic tests are needed. Chromosomal and radiographic studies may be indicated when atypical anomalies or severe growth/developmental retardation are present. Counseling should focus on subsequent pregnancies, aiming to minimize anticonvulsant dose and number while avoiding seizures. Lowering of folic acid levels by hydantoin and the association of neural tube defects with valproic acid amplifies the importance of preconceptional folic acid supplementation.

Family and psychosocial counseling

New parents are confronted with risks for developmental and chronic medical problems in their child. Their shock may be heightened by guilt or blame attached to the maternal seizure disorder. Counseling regarding the common occurrence of congenital anomalies regardless of maternal status and an optimistic scheme for management may be helpful. Early childhood intervention should be encouraged and social and/or psychiatric services made available.

Natural history and complications

Common complications in anticonvulsant-exposed infants include pre- or postnatal growth delay, microcephaly with developmental delay, feeding problems due to facial clefts or gastrointestinal anomalies, and anomalies of the eye, heart, skeleton, and urogenital systems (see checklist). The face after hydantoin exposure may be distinctive, with hypertelorism, shallow and broad nasal bridge, short nose, wide mouth, and increased subcutaneous tissue (coarse facies). V-shaped eyebrows and similar facial changes have been associated with trimethadione exposure, and a shallow nasal bridge, ear anomalies, flat philtrum, and small jaw have been associated with valproic acid exposure. The general association includes eye anomalies (ptosis, colobomata, strabismus), oral clefts, cardiac anomalies (septal defects, coarctation of the aorta, tetralogy of Fallot), genitourinary anomalies (urinary tract obstruction, micropenis, cryptorchidism), skeletal defects of the ribs, vertebrae, and limbs (particularly of the terminal digits and nails), and neural tube defects or holoprosencephaly (Gorlin et al., 2001, pp. 21–31). A worrisome finding in mouse or rat models is the prominence of behavioral abnormalities, and autism spectrum disorders have been observed in humans. Tumors of neural crest origin occur at increased frequency in fetal hydantoin syndrome, and phenytoin is carcinogenic in adults.

Fetal anticonvulsant exposure preventive management checklist

Preventive management is directed toward detection of neonatal anomalies and evaluation for abnormal growth, development, feeding, hearing, vision, gastrointestinal, cardiac, skeletal, and urinary tract function. Neonatal evaluation for positional deformities such as club feet or congenital hip dislocation is important, since these have a cumulative frequency of 11% (Schardein, 2000). Although developmental and behavioral problems are not as frequent or severe as with the FAS, the frequency of disabilities in the study of Moore et al. (2000) mandates consideration of early childhood intervention with occupational and speech therapy. Eye problems such as strabismus and urinary tract infections due to anomalies of the outflow tract require appropriate screening and referral. Abdominal examination is important because of early risk for renal anomalies and later risk for neural crest tumors. The low frequency of these complications (less than 1%) probably does not justify routine abdominal ultrasound examinations.

Diabetic embryopathy

Terminology

Infants of diabetic mothers (IDM) have increased risk for congenital malformation that correlates with the degree of metabolic aberration during pregnancy. The malformation process and its resulting pattern of anomalies are referred to as diabetic embryopathy (Nold & Georgieff, 2004).

Historical diagnosis and management

As the complications of stillbirth, neonatal hypoglycemia, and respiratory distress syndrome were ameliorated through better maternal management, a pattern of birth defects and even occasional growth retardation were recognized in IDM. Several typical malformations in IDM (such as anencephaly) occur before 4 weeks of pregnancy, so control of diabetes before conception must be emphasized to safeguard the embryo.

Incidence, etiology, and differential diagnosis

The prevalence of diabetes mellitus during pregnancy is about 3%, with about 0.3% being pre-existing diabetes. Of the 50 to 150,000 IDM that are born each year in the United States, those who experience problems with maternal diabetic control during gestation will have a 6–10% incidence of major congenital anomalies (Schardein, 2000). These anomalies account for 50% of all perinatal deaths.

The etiology of anomalies resulting from maternal diabetes is still unclear. Maternal vasculopathy was first implicated as a predisposing factor, with a 10–11% risk for anomalies in offspring of women with Class D or F diabetes, compared with 3–4.5% in Class B or C diabetes. More recent studies have not confirmed these trends, and experiments with *in vitro* embryo culture have emphasized the teratogenic effects of hypo- and hyperglycemia, ketonemia, and somatomedin inhibitors (Reece et al., 1993). Deficiencies of zinc and arachidonic acid, high levels of free oxygen radicals, and differences in genetic susceptibility have also received experimental support as factors in diabetic embryopathy. Of great interest is a paradoxical growth *retardation* in some severely affected IDM; delayed growth along with delayed maturation of lung and hematologic functions may be a unifying theme in the disorder (Wilson, 1987). The pattern of malformations in diabetic embryopathy and suggest that somite mesoderm and cephalic neural crest cells may be prime targets in the embryo.

Diagnostic evaluation and medical counseling

Unless other disorders are suspected, neonates should be evaluated for major anomalies of the brain, heart, GI tract, urinary tract, and vertebrae (complications are listed in the checklist). Since the frequency of any given anomaly is low, clinical examination rather than routine screening should guide the use of expensive imaging studies. Medical counseling should review the correlation of poor diabetic control with anomaly risk, particularly emphasizing the achievement of good control before attempting another pregnancy. Gestational diabetes is not associated with a higher risk for congenital anomalies, so these mothers can be reassured and their offspring evaluated for other causes of anomalies.

Family and psychosocial counseling

Diabetes mellitus is a multifactorial disorder with significant genetic predisposition. Parents with type I diabetes confer a 5–10% risk to their offspring for developing type I (insulin-dependent) diabetes. These offspring have an even higher risk for developing type II (adult-onset) diabetes. These risks increase slightly if additional family members are affected. As with other teratogens, maternal guilt and blame may be counseling issues that require specialty participation. For women who can achieve and maintain good control of their diabetes, an optimistic outlook for future pregnancies is appropriate. Many anomalies associated with diabetic embryopathy can be detected by prenatal ultrasound at or before 16–18 postmenstrual weeks. Abundant information on IDM can be found by entering those words into a web browser, and information for people with diabetes mellitus can be found on the websites of the American Diabetes Association (www.diabetes.org/home.jsp), Diabetes UK (www.diabetes.org.uk/), and the Canadian Diabetes Association (www.diabetes.ca/).

Natural history and complications

The checklist, part 1 lists major anomalies affecting the eye, jaw, heart, gastrointestinal tract, urinary tract, and central nervous system that occur in IDM whose mothers had pre-existing diabetes mellitus (Gorlin et al., 2001, pp. 18–19; Nold & Georgieff, 2004). All of the anomalies occur at fairly low frequencies (1–3%). Caudal regression, ranging from sirenomelia (mermaid anomaly) to sacral agenesis, is the most characteristic anomaly, being present in about 1% of patients. Some children may require orthopedic, urologic, and neurosurgical follow-up when severe caudal regression produces limb hypoplasia, bladder dysfunction, and/or tethered cord/ diastematomyelia.

Diabetic embryopathy preventive management checklist

Preventive measures in diabetic embryopathy are oriented more toward physical examination than toward routine screening, since all of the characteristic anomalies occur at low frequency (see checklist). Neonatal evaluation for eye, ear, oral, cardiac, skeletal, urinary tract, and neurologic anomalies is important. Management during later childhood is focused on preventing obesity and detecting subtle neurodevelopmental problems. For children with caudal regression, or the full VATER association of anomalies, more aggressive orthopedic, urologic, and neurosurgical management is required. In such children, the VATER association preventive checklist may be more appropriate as a guide for management.

Preventive management of fetal alcohol syndrome

Description: Clinical pattern in infants exposed to alcohol during gestation, with an estimated incidence of 1.5–1.9 births.

Clinical: Variable findings low birth weight, microcephaly, growth failure, small eyes, shallow or absent philtrum, thin upper lip, anomalous ears, ocular, orthopedic, and cardiac problems.

Laboratory: No specific biochemical or genetic tests.

Genetics: Sporadic disorder related to maternal alcohol use during pregnancy.

Key management issues: Monitoring of growth, vision, and hearing; surveillance for ocular, cardiac, and orthopedic problems, early intervention with alertness for behavior problems and school difficulties.

Growth charts: None available; failure to thrive and microcephaly are characteristic.

Parent information: National Organization on Fetal Alcohol Syndrome (www.nofas.org/) and its state affiliates (e.g., www.calfas.org in California). Many links to sites relevant to fetal alcohol syndrome are available at (www.acbr.com/fas/faslink.htm and www.come-over.to/FAS/fasonline.htm). Parents contemplating adoptions from high-risk areas (eastern Europe, Russia) can find relevant information at www.adopting.org/rwfas.html.

Summary of clinical concerns

General	Learning	**Cognitive disability** (60%), **speech delay** (93%), **learning differences** (89% – mean IQ 41–65)
	Behavior	**Behavior problems** (80%), hyperactivity, psychiatric problems
	Growth	**Low birth weight** (57–89%), **short stature** (84%), **failure to thrive** (50–75%)
	Cancer	Increased cancer risk (rhabdomyosarcoma, Wilms tumor, leukemias)
Facial	Eyes	**Small eyes** (92%), **optic nerve defects** (39%), **myopia** (88%), **astigmatism** (50%), **strabismus** (56%)
	Ears	Ear anomalies (22%), **otitis media** (93%), **hearing loss** (38%)
	Nose	**Shallow nasal bridge** (61%), chronic nasal discharge
	Mouth	**Dysphagia** (91%), **high palate** (30%), **cleft palate** (7%), dental anomalies
Surface	Neck/trunk	Pectus excavatum
	Epidermal	Hemangiomata and hirsutism
Skeletal	Cranial	**Microcephaly** (93%)
	Axial	Cervical and thoracic vertebral fusions
	Limbs	Decreased fetal mobility, radioulnar fusion (14%), **hip dislocation** (9–33%), limb contractures
Internal	Digestive	**Dysphagia, feeding problems** (91%)
	Pulmonary	Airway obstruction, apnea
	Circulatory	**Cardiac defects** (40–50% – septal defects, tetralogy of Fallot, transposition of great vessels)
	Endocrine	Hypoparathyroidism and hypocalcemia if DiGeorge anomaly present
	RES	Frequent respiratory infections
	Excretory	**Renal defects** (20–66% – pyelonephritis, hematuria, renal hypoplasia)
	Genital	Genital defects (46% – hypospadias, micropenis, cryptorchidism)
Neural	Central	Brain anomalies, holoprosencephaly, neural tube defects (1–3%), **seizures** (10–50%), irritability
	Motor	Hypertonia, oromotor dysfunction, motor delays
	Sensory	**Vision and hearing deficits** (20–30%)

RES, reticuloendothelial system; **concerns** of frequency >20% are **highlighted**

Key references

Famy, et al. (1998). Mental illness in adults with fetal alcohol syndrome or fetal alcohol effects. *American Journal of Psychology* 155:552–4.

Hoyme, et al. (2005). A practical clinical approach to diagnosis of fetal alcohol spectrum disorders: clarification of the 1996 institute of medicine criteria. *Pediatrics* 115:39–47.

Stoler, et al. (2004). Recognition of facial features of fetal alcohol syndrome in the newborn. *American Journal of Medical Genetics* 127C:21–7.

Fetal alcohol syndrome

Preventive medical checklist (0–3 years)

Name —————————— Birth date —/—/—— Number ——————————

Age	Evaluations: key concerns	Management considerations		Notes
New-born ↓ 1 month	Parental adjustment; family evaluation Dysmorphology examination:[2] anomalies Hearing, vision:[2] deafness, eye anomalies Feeding: dysphagia, cleft palate Heart: murmur, tachycardia Renal: small kidneys, hydronephrosis Skeletal: Klippel–Feil, limb defects	❑ Maternal counsel;[1] family support[4] ❑ Imaging of head; C-spine[3] ❑ ABR; opthalmology[3] ❑ Feeding specialist; video swallow[3] ❑ Echocardiogram; cardiology ❑ Renal sonogram ❑ Orthopedics[3]	❑ ❑ ❑ ❑ ❑ ❑ ❑	
2 months ↓ 4 months	Growth and development:[5] microcephaly Nutrition: feeding, poor suck Hearing and vision:[2] otitis Renal: small kidneys, hydronephrosis Skeletal: hip dislocation, limb defects Neck flexibility: Klippel–Feil, torticollis Parental adjustment Other:	❑ ECI;[6] monitor head circumference ❑ Extra feeding;[3] feeding specialist[3] ❑ Repeat ABR;[3] opthalmology[3] ❑ Urinalyses ❑ Orthopedics[3] ❑ Anesthesia precautions ❑ Family support[4] ❑	❑ ❑ ❑ ❑ ❑ ❑ ❑ ❑	
6 months ↓ 9 months	Growth and development[5] Nutrition: dysphagia, poor suck Hearing and vision:[2] otitis, strabismus Renal: small kidneys, hydronephrosis Skeletal: hip dislocation, limb defects Other:	❑ Family support;[4] ECI[6] ❑ Oromotor therapy[3] ❑ Repeat ABR;[3] opthalmology[3] ❑ Urinalyses ❑ Orthopedics[3] ❑	❑ ❑ ❑ ❑ ❑ ❑	
1 year	Growth and development:[5] microcephaly Nutrition: dysphagia, poor suck Hearing and vision:[2] otitis, strabismus Renal: small kidneys, hydronephrosis Skeletal: hip dislocation, limb defects Neck flexibility: Klippel–Feil, torticollis Other:	❑ Family support;[4] ECI;[6] head circumference ❑ ❑ Oromotor therapy[3] ❑ Repeat ABR;[3] opthalmology[3] ❑ Urinalyses ❑ Orthopedics[3] ❑ Anesthesia precautions ❑	❑ ❑ ❑ ❑ ❑ ❑	
15 months ↓ 18 months	Growth and development[5] Hearing and vision:[2] otitis, strabismus Skeletal: hip dislocation, limb defects Neck flexibility: Klippel–Feil, torticollis	❑ Family support;[4] ECI;[6] head circumference ❑ ❑ Repeat ABR;[3] opthalmology[3] ❑ Orthopedics[3] ❑ Anesthesia precautions	❑ ❑ ❑	
2 years	Growth and development:[5] microcephaly Nutrition: dysphagia Hearing/vision:[2] otitis, strabismus Skeletal: hip dislocation, limb defects Neck flexibility: Klippel–Feil, torticollis	❑ Family support;[4] ECI;[6] head circumference ❑ ❑ Dietician[3] ❑ Audiology; ENT;[3] ophthalmology[3] ❑ Orthopedics[3] ❑ Anesthesia precautions	❑ ❑ ❑ ❑	
3 years	Growth and development:[5] microcephaly Hearing/vision:[2] otitis, strabismus Skeletal: hip dislocation, limb defects Renal: small kidneys, hydronephrosis Neck flexibility: Klippel–Feil, C-spine fusion Increased cancer risk Other:	❑ Family support;[4] ECI;[6] head circumference ❑ ❑ Audiology; ENT;[3] ophthalmology[3] ❑ Orthopedics[3] ❑ Urinalyses; BP ❑ Anesthesia precautions; C-spine X-rays[3] ❑ Alert for Wilms tumor, leukemias ❑	❑ ❑ ❑ ❑ ❑	

Fetal alcohol syndrome concerns		Other concerns from history	

Poor feeding, weight gain
Low birth weight
Thin upper lip,
  absent philtrum
Eye and ear anomalies
Cardiac anomalies
Renal anomalies
	Genital anomalies
	Hip dislocation
	Feeding problems,
	  growth delay
	Microcephaly
	Irritability, seizures
	Motor and speech delay
		Family history/prenatal
		——————————
		——————————
		——————————
		——————————
			Social/environmental
			——————————
			——————————
			——————————
			——————————

Guidelines for the neonatal period should be undertaken *at whatever age* the diagnosis is made; ABR, auditory brainstem evoked response; BP, blood pressure; C-spine, cervical spine; [1]may have to consider foster care and adult intervention/social services; [2]by practitioner; [3]as dictated by clinical findings; [4]parent group, family/sib, financial, and behavioral issues including other at-risk or affected sibs; [5]consider developmental pediatrician/neurologist/behavior therapist according to symptoms and availability; [6]early childhood intervention including developmental monitoring and motor/speech therapy; [7]snoring, pause in breathing, daytime sleepiness, unusual sleep positioning .

Fetal alcohol syndrome

Preventive medical checklist (4–18 years)

Name ——————————————— **Birth date** —/—/—— **Number** ———————————

Age	Evaluations: key concerns	Management considerations		Notes
4 years ↓ 6 years	Growth:[5] microcephaly Development: behavior differences Hearing/vision:[2] otitis, strabismus Dental: small teeth, thin enamel Renal: small kidneys, hydronephrosis Skeletal: cervical, limb defects Other:	❑ Monitor head circumference[1] ❑ Family support;[4] preschool program[5] ❑ Audiology; ENT;[3] ophthalmology[3] ❑ Dentistry ❑ Urinalyses; BP ❑ Orthopedics;[3] anesthesia precautions ❑	❑ ❑ ❑ ❑ ❑ ❑ ❑	
7 years ↓ 9 years	Growth[1] Development:[1] school transition[5] Behavior: impulsivity, hyperactivity Hearing/vision:[2] hearing loss, myopia Renal: small kidneys, hydronephrosis Skeletal: cervical, limb defects Other:	❑ Consider specialists[1] ❑ Family support;[4] school progress[6] ❑ Behavioral therapy[3] ❑ Audiology; ENT;[3] ophthalmology[3] ❑ Urinalyses; BP ❑ Orthopedics;[3] anesthesia precautions ❑	❑ ❑ ❑ ❑ ❑ ❑ ❑	
10 years ↓ 12 years	Growth and development[1] Behavior: impulsivity, hyperactivity Hearing/vision:[2] hearing loss, myopia Dental: small teeth, thin enamel Other:	❑ Family support;[4] school progress[6] ❑ Behavioral therapy[3] ❑ Audiology; ENT;[3] ophthalmology[3] ❑ Dentistry ❑	❑ ❑ ❑ ❑ ❑	
13 years ↓ 15 years	Growth and development[1] Hearing/vision:[2] hearing loss, myopia Renal: small kidneys, hydronephrosis Skeletal: C-spine fusion, scoliosis Puberty: genital hypoplasia Other:	❑ School progress[6] ❑ Audiology; ENT;[3] ophthalmology[3] ❑ Urinalyses; BP ❑ Orthopedics;[3] anesthesia precautions ❑ Endocrinology;[3] urology[3]	❑ ❑ ❑ ❑ ❑	
16 years ↓ 18 years	Growth and development[1] Behavior: impulsivity, hyperactivity Hearing/vision:[2] hearing loss, myopia Puberty: genital hypoplasia Other:	❑ Family support;[4] school progress[6] ❑ Behavioral therapy[3] ❑ Audiology; ENT;[3] ophthalmology[3] ❑ Endocrinology;[3] urology[3] ❑	❑ ❑ ❑ ❑ ❑	
19 years ↓ 23 years	Adult care transition[5] Behavior: impulsivity, hyperactivity Hearing/vision:[2] myopia, astigmatism Renal: small kidneys, hydronephrosis Skeletal: scoliosis, limb defects	❑ Family support;[4] school progress[6] ❑ Behavioral therapy[3] ❑ Audiology; ENT;[3] ophthalmology[3] ❑ Urinalyses; BP ❑ Orthopedics[3]	❑ ❑ ❑ ❑ ❑	
Adult	Adult care transition[5] Hearing/vision:[2] myopia, astigmatism Renal: small kidneys, hydronephrosis Skeletal: C-spine fusion, scoliosis Dental: small teeth, thin enamel Increased cancer risk Other:	❑ Family support;[4] behavior issues[7] ❑ Audiology;[3] ENT; ophthalmology ❑ Urinalyses; BP ❑ Orthopedics;[3] anesthesia precautions ❑ Dentistry ❑ Alert for rhabdosarcoma, leukemias ❑	❑ ❑ ❑ ❑ ❑ ❑ ❑	

Fetal alcohol syndrome concerns		Other concerns from history	
Hearing, vision Dental problems Irritability, seizures Hearing loss Cardiac anomalies Renal anomalies	Scoliosis Learning differences Behavioral problems Increased cancer risk Employment, independent living	**Family history/prenatal** ———————— ———————— ———————— ————————	**Social/environmental** ———————— ———————— ———————— ————————

Guidelines for the neonatal period should be undertaken *at whatever age* the diagnosis is made; BP, blood pressure; C-spine, cervical spine; [1]consider developmental pediatrician/neurologist/behavior therapist according to symptoms and availability; [2]by practitioner; [3]as dictated by clinical findings; [4]parent group, family/sib, financial, behavioral, and psychosocial issues with later focus on independent living and employment; [5]preschool program including developmental monitoring, motor/speech therapy, alertness for psychosocial and behavior problems; [6]monitor individual education plan, educational testing, balance of special education and inclusion, academic progress, behavioral differences, later vocational planning; [7]smonitor for impulsivity, adult hyperactivity, depression with suicidal tendencies.

Parent guide to fetal alcohol syndrome

Fetal alcohol syndrome (FAS) denotes a pattern of physical and behavioral anomalies related to exposure to ethanol during pregnancy. Children with milder abnormalities may be described as having fetal alcohol effects (FAE). Some have argued against the false dichotomy between FAS and FAE on the grounds that all teratogens (chemicals that produce birth defects) exhibit a range of effects according to the severity of the exposure. Although the dangers of drinking during pregnancy had been mentioned since biblical times, specific patterns of physical anomalies in offspring of alcoholic women were not documented until the late 1960s and early 1970s.

Incidence, causation, and diagnosis

The incidence of FAS is heavily dependent on socioeconomic status and ethnic background. The overall incidence is now estimated at 0.97–1.9 cases per 1000 live births in the United States, reaching 43 per 1000 among "heavy" drinkers. The correlation of alcohol dosage and timing with the severity of FAS in these animals clearly establishes ethanol as the causative agent. Genetics factors and maternal nutrition may influence the impact of alcohol ingestion on a particular pregnancy. The diagnosis of FAS is based on subjective recognition of distinctive facial anomalies combined with a small head size and poor growth. Facial anomalies include small eyes, shallow nasal bridge, upturned nose, abnormal ears (posteriorly rotated or low placed), thin upper lip, and absent philtrum (the crease between the nose and upper lip. In the presence of a clear-cut maternal history and typical findings of FAS, cardiac, renal, and perhaps even head ultrasound studies may be considered to document characteristic anomalies that can substantiate the diagnosis. Since no medical test is diagnostic, counseling must emphasize abstinence in future pregnancies, but acknowledge uncertainty in relating specific infant problems to maternal drinking. Heavy drinking does cause IQ deficits in offspring regardless of morphologic findings.

Natural history and complications

Severely affected infants may have brain anomalies with potential for multiple neurologic deficits. Milder effects of FAS include learning disabilities, poor impulse control, and hyperactivity that can be present in numerous other syndromes. Children with FAS have a high frequency of neurologic problems and learning deficits with a mean IQ of 41–65. Older children often have attention deficits with hyperactive, distractible, and impulsive behavior. Neurosensory damage is also common, with abnormal brainstem evoked response or hearing loss in 79–90% of patients and diminished vision in 50%. The cognitive and neurosensory problems produce a high incidence of speech delay that needs attention. The DiGeorge anomaly with hypoparathyroidism and immune defects has been described, and the incidence of many types of infections, including otitis media, is increased. Cardiac anomalies are found in 40–50%, including atrial or ventricular septal defects, tetralogy of Fallot, peripheral pulmonary artery stenosis, and dextrocardia. Upper airway obstruction due to underdevelopment of the midface has produced cessation of breathing (apnea spells) or decreased blood oxygen (hypoxia) in some patients. Subtle abnormalities of kidney function have been documented in FAS, and rare children have kidney malformations that can be identified by ultrasound. Skeletal defects include Klippel–Feil anomaly (cervical spine fusions), dislocated hip, spinal curvature (scoliosis), or chest deformities. An elevated cancer rate has been suggested for FAS, with examples of neuroblastoma, hepatoblastoma, sacrococcygeal teratoma, medulloblastoma, adrenal carcinoma, and acute lymphocytic leukemia being published.

Preventive medical needs

In those cases where the diagnosis is recognized during infancy, imaging or X-ray studies for cardiac, vertebral, and renal anomalies are indicated. Physical examination for orthopedic defects, including congenital hip dislocation, is important. Hearing loss and eye anomalies are common, mandating vision and hearing assessment. The high frequencies of failure to thrive (50–75%) and small head size (disproportionately small in 93%) mandate careful monitoring of growth and nutrition. Referral to early childhood intervention is important, and challenging behaviors with complicating psychosocial factors may require various types of therapists. Behavior problems are particularly difficult in the adolescent and adult, including poor judgment, distractibility, and difficulty perceiving social clues. Pregnancy counseling, school/job support, and violence prevention are thus of even greater importance in the care of adolescents with FAS.

Family counseling

Better awareness of alcohol effects may identify moderate drinkers who have children with milder growth and behavioral problems. Intervention can be very successful in more moderate drinkers, and should be attempted with chronic alcoholic persons to prevent alcohol in breast milk or even in formula as an infant tranquilizer. The familial nature of FAS is emphasized by the 17% of older sibs and 77% of younger sibs who had evidence of FAS after an index case was identified. The first goals of family counseling are to intervene in the cycle of alcohol abuse and to protect the newly diagnosed infant from the hazards of further alcohol exposure or neglect. Initial counseling and intervention will usually require the involvement of protective and social services.

Preventive management of fetal anticonvulsant exposure

Description: Spectrum of abnormalities seen in infants exposed to anticonvulsants such as hydantoin, primadone, trimethadione, and valproic acid. Overlap of anomalies and multiple anticonvulsant exposures often confuse the identification of specific syndromes. There is a 5–7-fold increased risk for birth defects in infants exposed to anticonvulsants with a potential birth incidence of anticonvulsant effects of 1 in 1000.

Clinical diagnosis: Typical minor anomalies include hypertelorism, shallow nasal bridge, upturned nares, ear changes, long or flat philtrum, and wide mouth. Major anomalies of the ocular, gastrointestinal, cardiovascular, skeletal, urogenital, and central nervous systems and not specific, but a compatible pattern with history of maternal exposure makes the diagnosis. Some of the more specific changes include small terminal digits and nails and club feet, dislocated hip, or scoliosis; neural tube defects are associated with valproic acid exposure.

Laboratory diagnosis: None available.

Genetics: Multifactorial, synergistic causation with a role for genetic factors shown by correlation of maternal epoxide hydrolase levels and fetal anomalies.

Key management issues: Thorough neonatal evaluation to determine the extent of anomalies and the potential for developmental disabilities. If a major anomaly like cleft palate or clubfoot is present, then aggressive imaging and radiographic studies to evaluate internal anomalies is justified. Microcephaly, alterations in tone, or craniospinal defects may herald later developmental disabilities including autism spectrum and hyperactivity/attention deficit disorders. Early monitoring of hearing and vision with consideration of early childhood intervention is necessary, along with checks for clefts and dysphagia, club feet, hip dislocations, urinary anomalies, renal function, and abdominal tumors.

Growth Charts: None available but growth delay and microcephaly occur in 25% of patients with hydantoin exposure.

Parent groups: American Epilepsy Society (www.aesnet.org/) Epilepsy Canada (www.epilepsy.ca/); The International League Against Epilepsy (http://www.ilae-epilepsy.org/), and Epilepsy Action (www.epilepsy.org.uk/) provide general information on epilepsy, including pregnancy risks.

Basis for management recommendations: Drawn from the complications below:

Summary of clinical concerns

General	Learning	Mild cognitive disability, **learning differences** (25%)
	Behavior	**Behavior problems** (20–80%) – hyperactivity, attention deficit, autism spectrum disorders including Asperger syndrome
	Growth	**Low birth weight** (36%), **growth delay** (52%), short stature
	Cancer	Cancer diathesis, neural crest tumors, lymphomas
Facial	Eyes	**Hypertelorism** (21%), ptosis (5%), colobomata, strabismus, unusual eyebrows
	Ears	Simplified or posteriorly rotated ears, chronic serous otitis
	Nose	**Shallow nasal bridge** (21%)
	Mouth	Broad alveolar ridges, high palate, cleft palate, cleft lip (3%)
Surface	Neck/trunk	Short neck, cystic hygroma, inguinal hernias (9%)
	Epidermal	Nail hypoplasia (11%), hirsutism (3%)
Skeletal	Cranial	**Microcephaly** (29%), wide anterior fontanel (10%), cranial asymmetry, metopic ridging (8%)
	Axial	Rib and vertebral anomalies (<1%), scoliosis
	Limbs	Hypoplastic distal digits, hip dislocation, club feet
Internal	Digestive	GI anomalies (pyloric stenosis, duodenal atresia, imperforate anus, diaphragmatic hernia)
	Circulatory	Cardiac anomalies (3%), mitral valve prolapse
	RES	Hyposplenism, thrombosis, coagulopathy
	Excretory	Renal hypoplasia, urinary tract anomalies
	Genital	Hypospadias, cryptorchidism, micropenis, shawl (bifid) scrotum
Neural	Central	Holoprosencephaly, seizures, lumbosacral myelomeningocele
	Motor	Motor delays
	Sensory	Vision loss and conductive hearing loss

RES, reticuloendothelial system; **concerns** of frequency >20% are **highlighted**

Key references

Moore, et al. (2000). A clinical study of 57 children with fetal anticonvulsant syndromes. *Journal of Medical Genetics* 37:489–97.

Pennell. (2003). The importance of monotherapy in pregnancy. *Neurology* 60(11 Suppl. 4):S31–8.

Fetal anticonvulsant exposure

Preventive medical checklist (0–3 years)

Name _____ Birth date __/__/__ Number _____

Age	Evaluations: key concerns	Management considerations	Notes
New-born ↓ 1 month	Dysmorphology examination: anomalies Morphologic: internal, skeletal defects Morphologic: external anomalies[2] Hearing, vision:[2] ear, eye anomalies Feeding: clefts, dysphagia Neurologic: CNS anomalies Parental adjustment	☐ Maternal counsel[1] ☐ ☐ Craniospinal, cardiac, GI, renal imaging[3] ☐ ☐ Cranial and skeletal X-rays;[3] urology[3] ☐ ☐ ABR; ENT;[3] ophthalmology[3] ☐ ☐ Feeding specialist; video swallow[3] ☐ ☐ Neurology;[3] neurosurgery;[3] spina bifida team[3] ☐ ☐ Family support[4] ☐	
2 months ↓ 4 months	Growth and development:[5] head size Hearing, vision:[2] strabismus, otitis Feeding: clefts, dysphagia Skeletal: craniospinal, hip, limb defects Urogenital: hypospadias, renal anomalies Neurologic: CNS anomalies Other:	☐ ECI;[3,6] family support[4] ☐ ☐ Repeat ABR;[3] ENT;[3] ophthalmology[3] ☐ ☐ GI;[3] feeding specialist[3] ☐ ☐ Orthopedics;[3] neurosurgery[3] ☐ ☐ Urology;[3] BP; urinalysis ☐ ☐ Neurology;[3] neurosurgery;[3] spina bifida team[3] ☐ ☐ ☐	Predis-posed to epilepsy
6 months ↓ 9 months	Growth and development:[5] head size Hearing, vision:[2] strabismus, otitis Feeding: clefts, dysphagia Skeletal: craniospinal, hip, limb defects Urogenital: hypospadias, renal dysplasia Other:	☐ ECI;[3,6] family support[4] ☐ ☐ Repeat ABR;[3] ENT;[3] ophthalmology[3] ☐ ☐ GI;[3] feeding specialist[3] ☐ ☐ Orthopedics;[3] neurosurgery[3] ☐ ☐ Urology;[3] BP; urinalysis ☐ ☐ ☐	Be alert for abdominal tumors
1 year	Growth and development:[5] head size Hearing, vision:[2] strabismus, otitis Feeding: clefts, dysphagia Skeletal: craniospinal, hip, limb defects Urogenital: hypospadias, renal anomalies Tumors: Wilms, neuroblastoma Other:	☐ ECI;[3,6] family support[4] ☐ ☐ Repeat ABR;[3] ENT;[3] ophthalmology[3] ☐ ☐ GI;[3] feeding specialist[3] ☐ ☐ Orthopedics;[3] neurosurgery[3] ☐ ☐ Urology;[3] BP; urinalysis ☐ ☐ Alert for abdominal masses, asymmetries ☐ ☐ ☐	
15 months ↓ 18 months	Growth and development:[5] head size Hearing, vision:[2] strabismus, otitis Feeding: clefts, dysphagia	☐ ECI;[3,6] family support[4] ☐ ☐ Repeat ABR;[3] ENT;[3] ophthalmology[3] ☐ ☐ GI;[3] feeding specialist[3] ☐	
2 years	Growth and development:[5] head size Hearing, vision:[2] strabismus, otitis Nutrition: feeding Skeletal: craniospinal, hip, limb defects Urogenital: hypospadias, renal anomalies	☐ ECI;[3,6] family support[4] ☐ ☐ Audiology; ENT;[3] ophthalmology[3] ☐ ☐ GI;[3] feeding specialist[3] ☐ ☐ Orthopedics;[3] neurosurgery[3] ☐ ☐ Urology;[3] BP; urinalysis ☐	
3 years	Growth and development:[5] head size Hearing, vision:[2] strabismus, otitis Nutrition: feeding Skeletal: craniospinal, hip, limb defects Urogenital: hypospadias, renal anomalies Tumors: Wilms, neuroblastoma Other:	☐ ECI;[3,6] family support[4] ☐ ☐ Audiology; ENT;[3] ophthalmology[3] ☐ ☐ GI;[3] feeding specialist[3] ☐ ☐ Orthopedics;[3] neurosurgery[3] ☐ ☐ Urology;[3] BP; urinalysis ☐ ☐ Alert for abdominal masses, asymmetries ☐ ☐ ☐	

Anticonvulsant exposure concerns		Other concerns from history	
Poor feeding and nutrition Vision, hearing deficits Strabismus Chronic serous otitis Cleft palate, TE, GI anomalies Embryonal tumors (e.g., Wilms)	Cardiac anomalies Urinary tract anomalies Cryptorchidism, micropenis Club feet, hip dislocation Spina bifida, seizures Microcephaly, motor delays	**Family history/prenatal** _____ _____ _____ _____ _____	**Social/environmental** _____ _____ _____ _____ _____

Guidelines for the neonatal period should be undertaken *at whatever age* the diagnosis is made; BP, blood pressure; GI, gastrointestinal; ABR, auditory brainstem evoked response; TE, tracheoesophageal; [1]document timing and dosage of anticonvulsants, plan future pregnancies; [2]by practitioner; [3]as dictated by clinical findings; [4]if potential disability (family/sib, financial, and behavioral issues); [5]consider developmental pediatrician/neurologist/behavior therapist if neurologic abnormalities; [6]early childhood intervention including developmental monitoring and motor/speech therapy.

Fetal anticonvulsant exposure

Preventive medical checklist (4–18 years)

Name _____ Birth date __ / __ / __ Number _____

Age	Evaluations: key concerns	Management considerations	Notes
4 years ↓ 6 years	Growth:[1] head size Development:[2] preschool transition Hearing, vision:[2] hearing loss Nutrition: feeding, intake Skeletal: scoliosis, limb defects Urogenital: hypospadias, renal anomalies Other:	❑ Family support[4] ❑ Preschool program[5] ❑ Audiology; ENT;[3] ophthalmology[3] ❑ GI;[3] feeding specialist[3] ❑ Orthopedics[3] ❑ Urology;[3] BP; urinalysis ❑	Predisposed to epilepsy
7 years ↓ 9 years	Growth[1] Development:[1] school transition[5] Hearing, vision:[2] hearing loss Nutrition: feeding, intake Skeletal: scoliosis, limb defects Urogenital: hypospadias, renal anomalies Other:	❑ Family support[4] ❑ School progress[6] ❑ Audiology; ENT;[3] ophthalmology[3] ❑ GI;[3] feeding specialist[3] ❑ Orthopedics[3] ❑ Urology;[3] BP; urinalysis ❑	Be alert for abdominal tumors
10 years ↓ 12 years	Growth and development[1] Hearing, vision:[2] hearing loss Nutrition: feeding, intake Urogenital: urinary tract anomalies Other:	❑ School progress[6] ❑ Audiology; ENT;[3] ophthalmology[3] ❑ Dietary counsel; activities; exercise ❑ Urology;[3] BP; urinalysis ❑	
13 years ↓ 15 years	Growth and development[1] Hearing, vision:[2] hearing loss Nutrition: feeding, intake Puberty; urogenital anomalies Skeletal: scoliosis, limb defects Other:	❑ School progress[6] ❑ Audiology; ENT;[3] ophthalmology[3] ❑ Dietary counsel; activities; exercise ❑ Urology;[3] endocrinology;[3] BP; urinalysis ❑ Orthopedics[3] ❑	
16 years ↓ 18 years	Growth and development[1] Nutrition: obesity Puberty, urogenital anomalies Skeletal: scoliosis, limb defects Other:	❑ Family support;[4] school progress;[6] ❑ Dietary counsel; activities; exercise ❑ Urology;[3] endocrinology;[3] BP; urinalysis ❑ Orthopedics[3] ❑	
19 years ↓ 23 years	Adult care transition[5] Hearing, vision:[2] hearing loss Nutrition: obesity Urogenital: urinary tract anomalies Skeletal: scoliosis, limb defects	❑ Family support;[4] school progress[6] ❑ ENT, ophthalmology ❑ Urology;[3] BP; urinalysis ❑ Dietary counsel; activities; exercise ❑ Orthopedics[3]	
Adult	Adult care transition[5] Hearing, vision:[2] hearing loss Nutrition: obesity Heart: mitral valve prolapse Urogenital: urinary tract anomalies Skeletal: scoliosis, limb defects Other:	❑ Family support[4] ❑ Audiology;[3] ENT; ophthalmology ❑ Dietary counsel; activities; exercise ❑ Cardiology[3] ❑ Urology;[3] BP; urinalysis ❑ Orthopedics[3] ❑	Be alert for lymphomas, other tumors

Anticonvulsant exposure concerns		Other concerns from history	
Hearing, vision loss Ptosis, amblyopia Mitral valve prolapse Vertebral fusions Scoliosis Hernias	Urinary tract anomalies Genital hypoplasia Growth delays, later obesity Seizures, developmental disabilities Autism spectrum disorders Embryonal tumors (e.g., Hodgkin)	**Family history/prenatal** _____ _____ _____ _____	**Social/environmental** _____ _____ _____ _____

Guidelines for the neonatal period should be undertaken *at whatever age* the diagnosis is made; BP, blood pressure; GI, gastrointestinal; [1]consider developmental pediatrician/neurologist/behavior therapist if neurologic abnormalities; [2]by practitioner; [3]as dictated by clinical findings; [4]parent group, family/sib, financial, and behavioral issues with later focus on independent living and employment; [5]preschool program including developmental monitoring and motor/speech therapy; [6]monitor individual education plan with regular educational testing, balance of special education/inclusion, behavioral assessment, and later vocational planning.

Parent guide to fetal anticonvulsant exposure

Anticonvulsant use in pregnancy is associated with a 5–7-fold increased risk for fetal birth defects and developmental delay. Congenital anomalies affecting the eye, heart, kidneys, urinary tract, spine, limbs, and nervous system have been noted after exposure to hydantoin, primidone, trimethadione, and valproic acid when prescribed singly or in combination. Specific facial changes and anomaly patterns in some exposed infants have defined fetal hydantion, fetal trimethadione, and fetal valproic acid syndromes, but their overlapping features and combined use justifies their grouping under the general term of fetal anticonvulsant exposure.

Incidence, causation, and diagnosis

The 1% of women who have epilepsy predicts a substantial frequency of anticonvulsant-exposed births. Since fetuses exposed to anticonvulsants like hydantoin (Dilantin) have a 5–10% risk for congenital anomalies, an estimated 1 in 1000 live births will suffer consequences of fetal anticonvulsant exposure. General effects of maternal epilepsy on fetal development, and likely synergies of multiple anticonvulsant medications have not been adequately separated from the effects of individual medicines. Differences in anticonvulsant effects on model organisms predict genetic factors in human susceptibility, and this has been confirmed for hydantoin by relating maternal levels of an enzyme called arene oxidase to risks for fetal abnormalities. The diagnosis of fetal anticonvulsant exposure is highly dependent on the history of maternal therapy; appreciation of a distinctive pattern of anomalies supports the diagnosis during infancy. Other conditions can exhibit the increased facial hair (hirsutism), small nails and digits, and subtle facial features. Fetal alcohol syndrome is associated with growth/developmental delays and nail hypoplasia, as are the genetic Coffin–Siris and Coffin–Lowry syndromes. Maternal and family history together with the pattern of anomalies should distinguish genetic disorders from the consequences of fetal anticonvulsant exposure.

Natural history and complications

Major complications of fetal anticonvulsant exposure include low birth weight or delayed growth after birth, small head circumference with developmental delays, hearing loss due to serous otitis, vision loss due to ptosis (hooding of the upper lids) or strabismus (wandering eyes), feeding problems due to gastrointestinal anomalies, and a variety of internal defects affecting the heart, skeleton, or urinary tract. The face may appear different, with widely spaced eyes, shallow and broad nasal bridge, short nose, and wide mouth. Cleft or high palate with broad ridges near the gums can be noted inside the mouth, and the neck is often short with webbing or redundant skin. Small ends of the digits and small nails are the most distinctive skeletal anomaly, but congenital hip dislocation, club feet, rib anomalies, spinal anomalies, and scoliosis (curved spine) can occur. Significant behavioral abnormalities have been documented in about 10% of infants exposed to anticonvulsants, including hyperactivity and autism spectrum disorders. Tumors of embryonic origin such as neuroblastoma, Wilms tumor, and Hodgkin lymphoma occur at increased frequency after hydantoin exposure.

Preventive medical needs

Preventive management is directed toward the treatment of neonatal anomalies and evaluation for abnormal growth, development, hearing, vision, cardiac, skeletal, and urogenital function. Neonatal evaluation for positional deformities such as club feet or congenital hip dislocation is important, and early childhood intervention with occupational and speech therapy should be considered and definitely initiated in children with small head circumference. Eye problems such as strabismus and urinary tract infections due to anomalies of the outflow tract require appropriate screening and referral. Periodic examination of the abdomen is important because of early risk for renal anomalies and later risk for neural crest tumors. The low frequency of these complications (less than 1%) probably does not justify routine abdominal ultrasound examinations. Also infrequent are cleft palate and dental anomalies due to high-arched palate, but occasional patients may require plastic surgery and/or dentistry referral.

Family counseling

When the positive maternal history, characteristic anomalies, and particularly small fingertips/nails are present, the diagnosis of fetal anticonvulsant exposure is secure. The recurrence risk depends entirely on anticonvulsant management of future pregnancies, so planning of future pregnancies is crucial. Trials to minimize medication dosage and to avoid multiple drugs should be considered, particularly in the preconceptional period. Since Dilantin can interfere with folic acid action, and spina bifida is increased after valproic acid exposure, folic acid supplementation should be begun when planning a pregnancy. In addition to confronting risks for developmental and chronic medical problems in their child, new parents may experience guilt or blame attached to the maternal seizure disorder. It is important to recognize the 2–3% risk for congenital anomalies in every pregnancy, regardless of maternal medications, and to focus on the optimistic outlook for most children with fetal anticonvulsant exposures. Early childhood intervention is appropriate for some children, and parents may find social and/or psychiatric services to be helpful in supporting chronic care needs. Educational information is available from numerous organizations devoted to epilepsy (see part 1 of this checklist).

Preventive management of diabetic embryopathy

Description: A broad pattern of defects in infants of diabetic mothers (IDM) including cranial, cardiac, and caudal anomalies (sacral agenesis, lower limb hypoplasia, urogenital anomalies).

Clinical: Poor diabetic control early in pregnancy can cause abnormal development of the nervous system (anencephaly, holoprosencephaly, eye defects), skeleton (hemifacial microsomia, rib and vertebral defects, caudal dysplasia), gastrointestinal system (intestinal defects, situs abnormalities), heart (transposition of the great vessels, septal defects), and kidneys (renal agenesis, urinary tract anomalies). This pattern of anomalies must be considered in IDM with classic macrosomia and hypoglycemia.

Laboratory: Neonatal hypoglycemia, hypocalcemia, hypomagnesemia, and polycythemia should alert physicians to the pattern of anomalies seen in diabetic embryopathy.

Genetics: Diabetes mellitus is a multifactorial disorder with a 5–10% risk for primary relatives (e.g., offspring of mothers with type I diabetes) to become affected with type I diabetes.

Key management issues: Neonatal metabolic alterations including low glucose, calcium, magnesium and high blood count; neonatal anomalies including facial (eye and ear anomalies, cleft palate), cardiac (transposition, septal defects), vertebral, limb, and urogenital defects; potential developmental problems with later obesity and propensity for diabetes mellitus.

Specific growth charts: None available; there is predisposition to obesity beginning in mid-childhood (Reece et al., 1993).

Parent information: American Diabetes Association (www.diabetes.org/home.jsp), Diabetes UK (www.diabetes.org.uk/), and the Canadian Diabetes Association (www.diabetes.ca/).

Summary of clinical concerns

General	Learning	Developmental delay, learning differences
	Growth	Large birth weight, macrosomia, growth delay with neurologic defects and feeding problems
Facial	Eyes	Anophthalmia, microphthalmia
	Ears	Ear anomaly (2%), ear atresia, hearing loss, chronic otitis media
	Mouth	Oromotor dysfunction, cleft lip/palate (5%)
Skeletal	Cranial	Hemifacial microsomia, cranial asymmetry
	Axial	Rib and vertebral anomalies (<1%), scoliosis, sacral agenesis (1–2%)
	Limbs	Caudal dysplasia with small lower limbs (1%), femoral hypoplasia, hip aplasia
Internal	Digestive	Intestinal malrotation, omphalocele, imperforate anus, heterotaxy with asplenia or polysplenia)
	Pulmonary	Immature lungs, respiratory distress
	Circulatory	Cardiac anomalies (3% – transposition, ventricular septal defect)
	Endocrine	Hypoglycemia, hypocalcemia, hypomagnesemia, cyanosis, irritability, tetany, seizures
	RES	Polycythemia, jaundice, clotting diathesis
	Excretory	Renal agenesis, ureteral duplication, urinary tract anomalies, obstructive uropathy, urinary tract infections
	Genital	Micropenis, hypospadias, cryptorchidism
Neural	Central	Holoprosencephaly, neural tube defects, tethered cord, seizures, developmental disability
	Motor	Motor delays
	Sensory	Vision or hearing deficits due to eye and ear anomalies

RES, reticuloendothelial system; **concerns** of frequency >20% are **highlighted**

Key references

Nold & Georgieff (2004). Infants of diabetic mothers. *Pediatric Clinics of North America* 51:619–37.

Reece, et al. (1993). Metabolic fuel mixtures and diabetic embryopathy. *Clinics in Perinatology* 20:517–32.

Sperling & Menon (1997). Infant of the diabetic mother. *Current Therapy in Endocrinology and Metabolism* 6:405–9.

Diabetic embryopathy

Preventive medical checklist (0–3 years)

Name _____ Birth date __ / __ / ____ Number _____

Age	Evaluations: key concerns	Management considerations	Notes
New-born ↓ 1 month	Metabolic: low glucose, Ca, Mg Morphologic: internal, skeletal defects Morphologic: external anomalies[2] Color: polycythemia, jaundice Hearing, vision:[2] ear, eye anomalies Feeding: clefts, dysphagia Parental adjustment[4]	☐ Glucose, Ca, Mg levels ☐ ☐ Craniospinal, cardiac, GI, renal imaging[3] ☐ ☐ Cranial and skeletal X-rays;[3] urology[3] ☐ ☐ CBC, differential; bilirubin ☐ ☐ ABR; ENT;[3] ophthalmology[3] ☐ ☐ Feeding specialist; video swallow[3] ☐ ☐ Family support[4] ☐	
2 months ↓ 4 months	Growth and development:[5] head size Hearing, vision:[2] ear, eye anomalies Nutrition: feeding, stooling Facial: hemifacial microsomia Morphologic: external anomalies[2] Skeletal: craniospinal, hip, limb defects Parental adjustment[4] Other:	☐ ECI;[3,6] family support[4] ☐ ☐ Repeat ABR;[3] ENT;[3] ophthalmology[3] ☐ ☐ GI;[3] feeding specialist[3] ☐ ☐ Alert for dysphagia, weak pharyngeal muscles ☐ ☐ Cranial and skeletal X-rays;[3] urology[3] ☐ ☐ Orthopedics;[3] neurosurgery[3] ☐ ☐ Family support[4] ☐ ☐ ☐	
6 months ↓ 9 months	Growth and development:[5] head size Hearing, vision:[2] ear, eye anomalies Nutrition: feeding, stooling Facial: hemifacial microsomia Neurologic: neural defects, tethered cord Other:	☐ ECI;[3,6] family support[4] ☐ ☐ ABR;[3] ENT;[3] ophthalmology[3] ☐ ☐ GI;[3] feeding specialist[3] ☐ ☐ Alert for dysphagia, weak pharyngeal muscles ☐ ☐ Orthopedics;[3] neurosurgery;[3] urology[3] ☐ ☐ ☐	
1 year	Growth and development:[5] head size Hearing, vision:[2] ear, eye anomalies Nutrition: feeding, stooling Facial: hemifacial microsomia Skeletal: craniospinal, hip, limb defects Urogenital: hypospadias, renal dysplasia Other:	☐ ECI;[3,6] family support[4] ☐ ☐ Repeat ABR;[3] ENT;[3] ophthalmology[3] ☐ ☐ Dietician;[3] GI[3] ☐ ☐ Alert for dysphagia, weak pharyngeal muscles ☐ ☐ Orthopedics;[3] neurosurgery[3] ☐ ☐ Urology;[3] BP, urinalysis ☐ ☐ ☐	
15 months ↓ 18 months	Growth and development:[5] head size Hearing, vision:[2] ear, eye anomalies Nutrition: intake, dysphagia Skeletal: craniospinal, hip, limb defects	☐ ECI;[3,6] family support[4] ☐ ☐ Repeat ABR;[3] ENT;[3] ophthalmology[3] ☐ ☐ Dietician;[3] GI[3] ☐ ☐ Orthopedics;[3] neurosurgery[3] ☐	
2 years	Growth and development:[5] head size Hearing, vision:[2] ear, eye anomalies Nutrition: intake, dysphagia Skeletal: craniospinal, hip, limb defects Urogenital: hypospadias, renal dysplasia	☐ ECI;[3,6] family support[4] ☐ ☐ Audiology;[3] ENT;[3] ophthalmology[3] ☐ ☐ Dietician;[3] GI[3] ☐ ☐ Orthopedics;[3] neurosurgery[3] ☐ ☐ Urology;[3] BP; urinalysis ☐	
3 years	Growth and development:[5] head size Hearing, vision:[2] ear, eye anomalies Nutrition: intake, dysphagia Skeletal: craniospinal, hip, limb defects Urogenital: hypospadias, renal dysplasia Neurologic: neural defects, tethered cord Other:	☐ ECI;[3,6] family support[4] ☐ ☐ Audiology;[3] ENT;[3] ophthalmology[3] ☐ ☐ Dietician;[3] GI[3] ☐ ☐ Orthopedics;[3] neurosurgery[3] ☐ ☐ Urology;[3] BP, urinalysis ☐ ☐ Orthopedics;[3] neurosurgery;[3] urology[3] ☐ ☐ ☐	

Diabetic embryopathy concerns		Other concerns from history	
Low glucose, Ca, Mg Polycythemia Cleft palate, feeding problems Microphthalmia, vision defects Ear defects, hearing loss VATER association defects	Cardiac anomalies Scoliosis, tethered cord Urogenital anomalies Limb anomalies Brain, neural tube defects Developmental delay	**Family history/prenatal** _____ _____ _____ _____	**Social/environmental** _____ _____ _____ _____

Guidelines for the neonatal period should be undertaken *at whatever age* the diagnosis is made; Ca, calcium; Mg, magnesium; BP, blood pressure; GI, gastrointestinal; ABR, auditory brainstem evoked response; [1]evaluate for polycythemia, metabolic consequences, anomalies; recall that child has increased genetic risk for diabetes; [2]by practitioner; [3]as dictated by clinical findings; [4]emphasize preconceptional diabetic control for next pregnancy, address family/sib, financial, and behavioral issues if brain or neurologic abnormalities; [5]consider developmental pediatrician/neurologist/behavior therapist if neurologic dysfunction – if spina bifida, follow that checklist; [6]early childhood intervention including developmental monitoring and motor – speech therapy.

Diabetic embryopathy

Preventive medical checklist (4–18 years)

Name _____ Birth date __/__/__ Number_____

Age	Evaluations: key concerns		Management considerations		Notes
4 years ↓ 6 years	Growth:[1] obesity Development:[2] preschool transition Hearing, vision:[2] ear, eye anomalies Nutrition: intake, dysphagia Skeletal: scoliosis, caudal dysplasia Urogenital: hypospadias, renal dysplasia Other:	❑ ❑ ❑ ❑ ❑ ❑ ❑	Consider specialists[1] Family support;[4] preschool program[5] Audiology;[3] ENT;[3] ophthalmology[3] Dietician;[3] GI[3] Orthopedics;[3] neurosurgery[3] Urology;[3] BP; urinalysis	❑ ❑ ❑ ❑ ❑ ❑ ❑	
7 years ↓ 9 years	Growth[1] Development:[1] school transition[5] Hearing, vision:[2] hearing or vision loss Nutrition: obesity versus poor intake Skeletal: scoliosis, caudal dysplasia Urogenital: hypospadias, renal dysplasia Other:	❑ ❑ ❑ ❑ ❑ ❑ ❑	Consider specialists[1] Family support;[4] school progress[6] Audiology;[3] ophthalmology Dietician;[3] GI[3] Orthopedics;[3] neurosurgery[3] Urology;[3] BP; urinalysis	❑ ❑ ❑ ❑ ❑ ❑ ❑	
10 years ↓ 12 years	Growth and development[1] Hearing, vision:[2] hearing or vision loss Nutrition: obesity versus poor intake Skeletal: scoliosis, caudal dysplasia Other:	❑ ❑ ❑ ❑ ❑	School progress[6] Audiology;[3] ENT;[3] ophthalmology[3] Dietician;[3] activities; exercise Orthopedics;[3] neurosurgery[3]	❑ ❑ ❑ ❑ ❑	
13 years ↓ 15 years	Growth and development[1] Hearing, vision:[2] hearing or vision loss Puberty; genital hypoplasia Nutrition: obesity versus poor intake Skeletal: scoliosis, caudal dysplasia	❑ ❑ ❑ ❑ ❑	School progress[6] Audiology;[3] ENT;[3] ophthalmology[3] Urology;[3] endocrinology[3] Dietician;[3] activities; exercise Orthopedics;[3] neurosurgery[3]	❑ ❑ ❑ ❑ ❑	
16 years ↓ 18 years	Growth and development[1] Puberty; genital hypoplasia Nutrition: obesity versus poor intake Skeletal: scoliosis, caudal dysplasia Other:	❑ ❑ ❑ ❑ ❑	Family support;[4] school progress;[6] Urology;[3] endocrinology[3] Dietician;[3] activities; exercise Orthopedics;[3] neurosurgery[3]	❑ ❑ ❑ ❑ ❑	
19 years ↓ 23 years	Adult care transition[5] Hearing, vision:[2] hearing or vision loss Nutrition: obesity versus poor intake Skeletal: scoliosis, caudal dysplasia Urogenital: urinary tract anomalies	❑ ❑ ❑ ❑ ❑	Family support;[4] school progress;[6] ENT; ophthalmology Dietician;[3] activities; exercise Orthopedics;[3] neurosurgery[3] Urology;[3] BP; urinalysis	❑ ❑ ❑ ❑ ❑	
Adult	Adult care transition[5] Hearing, vision:[2] hearing or vision loss Nutrition: obesity Heart: valvular defects, post surgery Skeletal: scoliosis, caudal dysplasia Urogenital: urinary tract anomalies Other:	❑ ❑ ❑ ❑ ❑ ❑ ❑	Family support[4] Audiology;[3] ENT; ophthalmology Dietary counsel; activities; exercise Cardiology[3] Orthopedics;[3] neurosurgery[3] Urology;[3] BP; urinalysis	❑ ❑ ❑ ❑ ❑ ❑ ❑	

Diabetic embryopathy concerns		Other concerns from history	
Hearing, vision loss Optic nerve, eye defects Cardiac anomalies Renal hypoplasia Urinary tract anomalies Cryptorchidism, micropenis	Scoliosis, spinal fusions Tethered cord (altered gait, enuresis) Limb fusions, hypoplasias Neural tube defects Developmental disabilities Obesity versus poor intake	**Family history/prenatal** _____ _____ _____ _____	**Social/environmental** _____ _____ _____ _____

Guidelines for the neonatal period should be undertaken *at whatever age* the diagnosis is made; GI, gasterointestinal; BP, blood pressure; [1]consider developmental pediatrician/neurologist/behavior therapist for children with neurologic dysfunction; [2]by practitioner; [3]as dictated by clinical findings; [4]parent group, family/sib, financial, and behavioral issues with later focus on independent living and employment; [5]preschool program including developmental monitoring and motor/speech therapy for those with disabilities; [6]monitor individual education plan – for individuals with disability, include regular educational testing, balance of special education and inclusion, monitor academic progress with screening for behavioral differences and later vocational planning.

Parent guide to diabetic embryopathy

Infants of diabetic mothers (IDM) have increased risk for congenital malformation that correlates with the success of diabetic control during pregnancy. The malformation process and its resulting pattern of anomalies are referred to as diabetic embryopathy. As other complications in offspring of mothers with diabetes (stillbirth, low blood sugar, respiratory problems) were ameliorated by better maternal management, a continuing risk for congenital anomalies gained attention.

Incidence, causation, and diagnosis

The prevalence of diabetes mellitus during pregnancy is about 3%, with about 0.3% being pre-existing diabetes. Of the 50 to 150,000 IDM that are born each year in the United States, those who experience problems with maternal diabetic control during gestation will have a 6–10% incidence of major congenital anomalies. These anomalies account for 50% of all deaths in the delivery and neonatal period. Several malformations in IDM occur before 5 weeks of pregnancy, a time when pregnancy may not be recognized. Diabetic women must therefore establish good control of their diabetes when they begin planning a pregnancy so as to safeguard the embryo. The way that maternal diabetes causes anomalies is still unclear. Maternal blood vessel disease may be one predisposing factor, since women with more longstanding and severe diabetes (Class D or F) have a 10–11% risk for anomalies in their offspring compared to women with Class D or F diabetes (3–4.5%). Chemical changes of diabetes may also contribute, including low or high sugar concentrations, ketones, deficiencies of zinc or certain fatty acids, hyperglycemia, ketonemia, and somatomedin inhibitors. Although the classic IDM has a larger birth weight due to higher insulin levels, fetuses destined to develop congenital anomalies may exhibit a paradoxical growth delay. Delayed growth along with delayed maturation of lung and other organs may be a unifying theme in the causation of anomalies in IDM. The diagnosis of diabetic embryopathy is based on recognition of typical anomalies of the brain, heart, gastrointestinal tract, urinary tract, and spine. Infants with macrosomia, plethora, and metabolic changes should be carefully examined for evidence of internal or external anomalies.

Natural history and complications

Major anomalies affecting the eye, jaw, heart, gastrointestinal tract, urinary tract, and central nervous system can occur in IDM. Underdevelopment of the tail end of the embryo (caudal regression) is the most characteristic anomaly of diabetic embryopathy, ranging from sacral agenesis (small sacral spine in the lower back) to sirenomelia (failure of the lower limbs to separate or "mermaid" anomaly). Caudal regression occurs in about 1% of IDM, necessitating orthopedic, urologic, and neurosurgical follow-up for severely affected children. The caudal underdevelopment may produce lower limb defects, urinary bladder dysfunction, and lower spinal cord anomalies such as tethered cord. Tethered cord involves fixation of the spinal cord to surrounding tissues, causing symptoms such as lower leg asymmetry, altered gait, or bed-wetting.

Preventive medical needs

Preventive measures in diabetic embryopathy should involve regular physical examinations rather than routine imaging studies, since all of the characteristic anomalies occur at low frequency. Neonatal evaluation for eye, ear, oral, cardiac, skeletal, urinary tract, and neurologic anomalies is important. Management during later childhood is focused on preventing obesity and detecting subtle neurodevelopmental problems. In children with caudal regression, more aggressive orthopedic, urologic, and neurosurgical management is required. Some children will have the more extensive vertebral (spinal), anal, tracheoesophageal (windpipe and esophagus), and renal (kidney) anomalies that are known as the VATER association. For these IDM, the preventive checklist and parent guide for VATER association may be more appropriate as a guide for management.

Family counseling

Diabetes mellitus is a multifactorial disorder, meaning that both genes and the environment interact to cause the disease. Parents with type I diabetes confer a 5–10% risk to their offspring for developing type I (insulin-dependent) diabetes. IDM have an even higher risk for developing type II (adult-onset) diabetes when they mature. These risks increase slightly if additional family members are affected. As with other maternal diseases that cause birth defects, families may benefit from counseling to alleviate maternal guilt and blame. For women who can achieve and maintain good control of their diabetes, an optimistic outlook for future pregnancies is appropriate. Many anomalies associated with diabetic embryopathy can be detected by prenatal ultrasound at or before 16–18 postmenstrual weeks. Families should appreciate the correlation of poor diabetic control with anomaly risk, emphasizing the achievement of good control before attempting another pregnancy. Gestational diabetes is not associated with a higher risk for congenital anomalies, so these mothers can be reassured and their offspring evaluated for other causes of anomalies.

Part III

Chromosomal syndromes

Chromosomal disorders are the most common genetic conditions, occurring in 50% of miscarriages, 4% of stillbirths, and 0.5% of newborns. Chromosome aberrations may disrupt any phase of embryonic and fetal development, producing a broad range of congenital anomalies and mental disabilities. Their preventive management will be discussed in three chapters corresponding to autosomal aneuploidy, sex chromosome aneuploidy, and submicroscopic deletions that require diagnosis using fluorescent technology.

7

Autosomal aneuploidy syndromes

Embryonic or fetal death is most likely when chromosomes 1–22 (autosomes) are deficient or duplicated (chromosomal aneuploidy). Fetuses that do survive to be born will usually have multiple medical problems, including growth failure, developmental delay, predisposition to infection, and multiple major or minor anomalies. Sex chromosome aneuploidies (e.g., Turner or Klinefelter syndromes) are discussed in a separate chapter (see Chapter 8) since their milder mental disability, specific behavioral issues, and fewer congenital anomalies are different from the autosomal aneuploidies. The new category of microdeletions revealed by fluorescent *in situ* hybridization (FISH) techniques (e.g., Prader–Willi, Smith–Magenis syndromes) are discussed in Chapter 9.

There are three major categories of chromosome aneuploidy – extra or missing whole chromosomes (trisomy, monosomy), extra or missing parts of a chromosome (partial trisomies or duplications, partial monosomies or deletions), and mixtures of normal and aneuploid cells (mosaicism). Few complete trisomies (except for 8, 9, 13, 18, and 21) and probably no complete monosomies (with possible exceptions for 21 and 22) survive the prenatal period to be born. The majority of live births with trisomies other than 13/18/21 are mosaic, and it is not surprising that prenatal diagnostic studies reveal a significant frequency of mosaicism.

The key to management for individually rare but categorically significant autosomal disorders is to merge common complications shared by these disorders, as outlined in Table 7.1, with risks unique to the particular chromosome aberration (Tables 7.2 and 7.3). Description of specific chromosomal disorders can be found in specialized references (Jones, 1997; Schinzel, 2001; Gorlin et al., 2001) and an increasing number of websites accessed by searching on the appropriate description (e.g., duplication 13p, deletion 8q). Several websites are available that provide details on rare genetic conditions (e.g., the Jablonski database, www.nlm.nih.gov/cgi/jablonski/syndrome; Online Medical Dictionary, cancerweb.ncl.ac.uk/cgi-bin/).

This chapter begins with an autosomal trisomy/monosomy checklist based on common complications of chromosome disorders listed in Table 7.1. This aneuploidy checklist can be augmented with specific manifestations discussed in

Table 7.1. Anomalies characteristic of chromosomal syndromes

Category	Common anomalies	Uncommon anomalies
General		
Gestational	Low birth weight	Conjoint twins
Cancers	Adenocarcinomas, leukemias	Teratomas
Facial		
Eyes	Microphthalmia, iris coloboma, cataracts	Lens dislocations
Mouth	Cleft lip/palate, dental anomalies	
Surface		
Neck/trunk	Short neck, cervical instability, hernias	
Skin	Depigmented spots, atrophic areas	
Skeletal		
Cranial	Microcephaly, metopic synostosis	Exencephaly
Axial	Vertebral anomalies, kyphoscoliosis	Spina bifida
Limbs	Polysyndactyly, hip dislocation, club feet, radial or tibial ray defects	Ulnar or fibular ray defects, amelia, phocomelia, extrodactyly
Internal		
Pulmonary	Tracheoesophageal fistula, diaphragmatic hernia, abnormal lung lobation	
Circulatory	Cardiac and great vessel anomalies	Situs inversus, acardius
Digestive	Omphalocele; esophageal, duodenal, or anal atresias; malrotation, rectal fistulae	Gastroschisis; jejunal, ileal atresias, congenital arthrogryposis
Excretory	Small kidneys, decreased tubule number, urinary tract anomalies	Exstrophy of the bladder or cloaca, sirenomelia
Genital	Cryptorchidism, hypospadias, labial hypoplasia	Ambiguous genitalia
Neural		
Central	Holoprosencephaly, agenesis corpus callosum, microencephaly	Anencephaly, otocephaly

Source: In part from Schinzel (2001).

individual sections for the more common aneuploidies or for rare conditions, in Table 7.2 (partial aneuploidies) or Table 7.3 (mosaic disorders). More detailed discussion and checklists are presented for trisomy 13/18 (Patau/Edwards syndromes, each with an incidence of 1 in 8000), and for trisomy 21 (Down syndrome with

Table 7.2. Unique complications of rare partial trisomy/monosomy syndromes

Disorder	Complications
Del(1p)	Amaurosis (blindness)
Del(1q)	Large anterior fontanel, bifid or broad thumbs, ambiguous genitalia, osteoporosis
Dup(1p)	Iris coloboma, protruding tongue, contractures
Dup(1q)	Omphalocele, malrotation, duodenal atresia, duplicated thumbs, syndactyly, occipital encephalocele, lumbar spina bifida, holoprosencephaly
Ring(1)	Pleasant personality, hypothalamic dysfunction, acute myelogenous leukemia
Del(2p)	Radioulnar synostosis, finger contractures
Del(2q)	Abnormal lung lobation with severe pneumonia, situs inversus with complex cardiac anomalies, anal atresia, radioulnar synostosis, postaxial polydactyly, hydrocephalus, occipital encephalocele
Dup(2p)	Diaphragmatic hernia, intestinal atresia, absence of gall bladder, lumbar spina bifida, ectopic anus, neuroblastoma
Dup(2q)	Glaucoma, iris coloboma, intestinal ectasias, dry skin with depigmentation
Ring(2)	Retinal dysplasia, bifid scrotum, congenital lymphedema of hands and feet
Del(3p)	Optic atrophy, anterior anus, duodenal stenosis, reduced hip mobility
Del(3q)	Camptodactyly, joint contractures
Dup(3p)	Choanal atresia, iris coloboma, cloudy cornea, esophageal atresia, renal cysts, duplication right ureter, bicornuate uterus, syndactyly, joint contractures
Dup(3q)	Microphthalmia, corneal opacities, hernias, Chiari defect, cerebellar hypoplasia
Ring(3)	Anal atresia, absent thumbs, hirsutism
Del(4p)	See text entry for Wolf–Hirschhorn syndrome*
Del(4q)	Rieger anomaly of the iris, microphthalmia, Robin sequence, TE fistula, pulmonary atresia, absent gall bladder, anterior anus, depigmented skin and hair
Ring(4)	Epispadias, hypospadias, seizures
Dup(4p)	Obesity, bilateral anophthalmia, iris coloboma, duplicated thumbs, absence corpus callosum, hydrocephalus
Dup(4q)	Choanal stenosis, omphalocele, TE fistula, seizures
Del(5p)	See text entry for *cri-du-chat* syndrome; ring(5) has similar features
Del(5q)	Optic atrophy, narrow anus, syndactyly toes 3/4
Dup(5p)	Iris coloboma, microphthalmia, corneal opacities, hiatal hernia, anal atresia
Dup(5q)	Microphthalmia, microstomia, micrognathia, diaphragmatic hernia, omphalocele, anal atresia, mesomelic shortening of limbs, cortical atrophy, hydrocephalus
Del(6p)	Renal tubular hypoplasia, seizures
Del(6q)	Tall stature, atresia lacrimal ducts, choanal atresia, diaphragmatic hernia, seizures
Ring(6)	Microphthalmia, iris coloboma, chorioretinitis
Dup(6p)	Microphthalmia, cataract, umbilical hernia, multiple hemangiomata
Dup(6q)	Tower skull, microphthalmia, kyphosis, joint contractures, holoprosencephaly, hydrocephalus, absent corpus callosum, seizures
Del(7p)	Craniosynostosis, skull ossification defect, choanal stenosis, eventration of diaphragm, recto-vaginal fistula, vertebral defects, joint contractures

(cont.)

Table 7.2. (*cont.*)

Disorder	Complications
Del(7q)	Leprechaunism, glaucoma, hypothyroidism, thumb anomaly, synbrachydactyly, holoprosencephaly, seizures (hypsarrhytmia), deafness
Ring(7)	Craniosynostosis, iris coloboma, sacral agenesis
Dup(7p)	Choanal atresia, micrognathia, limb contractures, hydrocephalus, encephalocele
Dup(7q)	Skull ossification defect, iris coloboma, renal tubular acidosis, vertebral anomalies, kyphosis, menstrual irregularity, hydrocephalus
Dup(7q)	FTT, hydrocephalus, coloboma, cleft, cardiac anomaly
Del(8p)	Nystagmus, inguinal hernia, vertebral defects, kyphosis, primary amenorrhea, cerebral atrophy, hydrocephalus
Del(8q)	Microphthalmia, small thumbs, exostoses, sparse hair, hydrocephalus
Ring(8)	Tower skull, pectus excavatum, inguinal hernias
Dup(8p)	Cataract, diaphragmatic hernia, rib and vertebral defects, scoliosis, joint contractures, absent corpus callosum, cerebellar hypoplasia, seizures
Dup(8q)	Choanal atresia, TE fistula, absent gall bladder, camptodactyly, Dandy–Walker malformation
Del(9p)	See text entry on deletion 9p syndrome
Del(9q)	Sclerocornea, duodenal atresia, malrotation, synpolydactyly
Ring(9)	Thumb hypoplasia, ambiguous genitalia, agitated and disruptive behaviors
Dup(9p)	See text entry on duplication 9p syndrome
Dup(9q)	Aortic dilation, mitral valve prolapse, pyloric stenosis, joint contractures, short lower limbs, renal cysts
Del(10p)	Microphthalmia, iris coloboma, hypothyroidism, hypoparathyroidism, syndactyly digits 3/4, seizures
Del(10q)	Web neck, anal atresia, recto-vaginal fistula, syndactyly toes 2/3
Ring(10)	Retinal choroid atrophy, posterior urethral valves, skin depigmentation, thyroid adenocarcinoma
Dup(10p)	Skull ossification defects, iris coloboma, biliary atresia, renal cysts
Dup(10q)	Microphthalmia, cataract, iris coloboma, pectus, kyphoscoliosis, polydactyly
Del(11p)	See text entry on deletion 11p syndrome
Del(11q)	Optic atrophy, iris coloboma, pyloric stenosis, anal stenosis, cystic or duplicated kidneys, polysyndactyly
Ring(11)	
Dup(11p)	Microphthalmia, omphalocele, malrotation, inguinal hernia, absent thumb, seizures
Dup(11q)	Microphthalmia, abnormal lung lobation, bicornuate uterus, radioulnar synostosis, holoprosencephaly, absent corpus callosum, cerebellar hypoplasia, seizures
Del(12p)	Crowded teeth, omphalocele, inguinal hernia, pectus excavatum, seizures; ring(12) is similar
Del(12q)	No distinct features with moderate to severe mental disability
Dup(12p)	Tower skull with brachycephaly, aniridia, anal atresia, duplicated great toes; patients with an extra 12p isochromosome have Pallister–Killian syndrome (see text entry)

Table 7.2. (*cont.*)

Disorder	Complications
Dup(12q)	Macrostomia, hypoplastic lungs, malrotation, anal stenosis, camptodactyly, short limbs, radioulnar synostosis, syndactyly toes 2/3, hydrocephalus
Del(13q)	See text entry on deletion 13q syndrome; ring(13) is similar
Dup(13q)	Cloverleaf skull, microphthalmia, iris coloboma, glaucoma, inguinal hernia, syndactyly toes 3/4, sacral myelomeningocele, cerebellar hypoplasia
Del(14q)	Retinitis pigmentosa, pectus excavatum, cartilage exostoses, skin hypopigmentation, seizures; ring(14) is similar.
Dup(14q)	Sagittal synostosis, microphthalmia, glaucoma, abnormal lung lobation, camptodactyly, syndactyly toes 2/3, absent corpus callosum, deafness
Del(15q)	Microcorneae, scoliosis, joint contractures, absent olfactory nerves, hydrocephalus
Ring(15)	Micrognathia, ectopic anus, radial aplasia, syndactyly toes 2/3
Dup(15q)	Facial asymmetry, cloverleaf skull, nystagmus, diaphragmatic hernia, anal atresia, inguinal hernia, vertebral defects, kyphosis, joint contractures, syndactyly digits 2/3, hirsutism
Del(16q)	Microphthalmia, ectopic anus, malrotation
Ring (16)	Ptosis, hypoparathyroidism, catatonic psychosis
Dup(16q)	Microphthalmia, micrognathia, anal atresia, malrotation, common cloaca, ambiguous genitalia, absent thumbs, joint contractures, ovarian dysgenesis, bicornuate uterus, holoprosencephaly
Ring(17)	Retinitis pigmentosa, multiple café-au-lait spots, seizures
Dup(17p)	Microphthalmia, corneal clouding, microcornea, inguinal hernia
Dup(17q)	Skull ossification defects, microphthalmia, retinitis pigmentosa, iris coloboma, pyloric stenosis, omphalocele, megacolon, kyphoscoliosis, hydrocephalus, seizures, Dandy–Walker anomaly
Del(18p)	See text entry on deletion 18p
Del(18q)	See text entry on deletion 18q; ring(18) has similar features
Dup(18p)	Branchial sinus, hemifacial microsomia, laryngomalacia, kyphoscoliosis, polydactyly, limb contractures, osteoporosis, ataxia, spasticity
Dup(18q)	Duplications encompassing 1/3 to 1/2 of the long arm will have features of trisomy 18
Dup(18q) q21 to qter	Duplications of the distal 1/3 to 1/5 of 18q have a phenotype milder than trisomy 18 with iris coloboma, choanal atresia, malrotation, umbilical hernia, camptodactyly, seizures
Ring(19)	Minimal dysmorphic features, few characteristic anomalies
Dup(19q)	Brachycephaly, ptosis, small gall bladder, renal cysts, kyphosis, thumb duplication, seizures
Del(20p)	Minimal dysmorphology, respiratory infections, seizures; ring(20) is similar
Dup(20p)	Cataract, iris coloboma, umbilical hernia, inguinal hernia, seizures
Del(21q)	Most cases of "monosomy 21;" microphthalmia, corneal clouding, abnormal lung lobation, absent corpus callosum, hydrocephalus
Ring(21)	Craniosynostosis, microphthalmia, glaucoma, corneal clouding, coloboma retina and choroids, choanal stenosis, vertebral defects, syndactyly toes 2/3, myoclonic seizures

(*cont.*)

Table 7.2. (*cont.*)

Disorder	Complications
Dup(21q)	Duplications of 21q below the key band causing Down syndrome (21q22) have minimal dysmorphology with inguinal hernia, umbilical hernia, short digits, attention deficit behaviors
Del(22q)	Microphthalmia, DiGeorge anomaly, polydactyly, ectrodactyly, holoprosencephaly
Ring(22)	Microphthalmia, iris coloboma, inguinal hernia, cyst in septum pellucidum, highly variable pattern
Dup(22q)	Includes "cat-eye" syndrome; microphthalmia, iris coloboma, atresia of ear canals, malrotation, biliary atresia, anal atresia, short limbs, holoprosencephaly, highly variable pattern
Dup(22q)/ Dup(11p)	Hypoplasia of diaphragm, malrotation, anal atresia, rib anomalies, lumbar myelomeningocele, hydrocephalus, other brain anomalies, stereotypic behaviors

Notes:

Listed abnormalities are in addition to those common to all partial aneuploidy syndromes (see partial trisomy/monosomy checklist): pre- and postnatal growth delay with microcephaly, moderate to severe mental disability, feeding problems including cleft palate and dysphagia, cardiac defects, renal and urinary tract anomalies, genital anomalies, skeletal anomalies including hip dislocation, scoliosis, and club feet, neurosensory deficits due to eye, ear, and/or brain anomalies.

Dup, duplication; del, deletion; p, short arm; q, long arm; TE, tracheoesophageal; FTT, failure to thrive.
* These are larger deletions/duplications than those discussed in the text (e.g., larger deletion than the 4p− of Wolf–Hirschhorn syndrome).
Source: Schinzel (2001).

an incidence of 1 in 800). The checklist for Down syndrome was pioneered by the pediatrician Dr. Mary Coleman, and it is the prototype for all checklists in this book.

The general trisomy/monosomy checklist addresses three global features of chromosome disorders – developmental disability with hearing and vision deficits, multiple anomalies often affecting internal organs, and susceptibility to environmental insults due to altered homeostasis (Shapiro, 1983). Patients with autosomal aberrations have frequent or more severe infections, vulnerability to stress (cold–heat–sounds–diet – Cabana et al., 1997), complications from procedures or operations (Roodman et al., 2003), and exaggerated reactions to drugs or stressful social situations. Physicians should be alert for early signs or progression of infections, for instabilities of physiology or metabolism following operations and injuries, and for behavioral changes in response to breaks in routine, school/ employment pressures, and family/social crises.

Table 7.3. Complications of trisomies (mostly mosaic)

Disorder	Complications
Trisomy 1 mosaicism	Mild developmental delay and dysmorphology
Trisomy 2 mosaicism	IUGR, pulmonary aplasia, absent gall bladder, cystic left kidney, extra rib, unilateral clubfoot
Trisomy 3 mosaicism	Decreased lifespan, mild dysmorphology
Trisomy 4 mosaicism	Ranges from normal appearance to prenatal growth retardation, postnatal growth delay, facial asymmetry, high palate, micrognathia, absent thumb, small nails, sacral dimple
Trisomy 5 mosaicism	Developmental and growth delay, eventration of the diaphragm, heart defect
Trisomy 7 mosaicism	Growth delay with Russell–Silver phenotype in some cases, strabismus, enamel dysplasia, cleft lip/palate, bifid tongue, left torticollis, hypoplastic lungs, patient ductus arteriosus, narrow thoracic aorta, renal agenesis, anal atresia, hemivertebrae, radial hypoplasia and absent thumb, inguinal hernia, limb contractures
Trisomy 8 mosaicism	See text entry on trisomy 8 mosaicism
Trisomy 9 mosaicism	Growth and developmental delays, wide sutures and fontanels, microphthalmia, micrognathia, cardiac septal defects, polycystic kidneys, kyphosis, hip dislocation, joint contractures, myelomeningocele, hydrocephalus, Dandy–Walker anomaly
Trisomy 10 mosaicism	Decreased lifespan, hydrops fetalis when diagnosed prenatally, cleft lip, metatarsus adductus, hypopigmented skin
Trisomy 11 mosaicism	Uniparental disomy for chromosome 11 can result from loss of one chromosome 11 in embryos with trisomy 11, with residual mosaicism. Such children have features of Beckwith–Wiedemann syndrome with large size, omphalocele, tumor risks
Trisomy 12 mosaicism	Early death, growth retardation, complex heart defects, polysyndactyly, hypopigmented skin
Trisomy 13 mosaicism	Range from minimal dysmorphology and mild mental disability to multiple anomalies with choroidal and retinal coloboma, cleft lip/palate, scoliosis, brachydactyly, camptodactyly, absence of corpus callosum, hydrocephalus, conductive hearing loss
Trisomy 14 mosaicism	Severe growth and developmental delay, microcephaly, macroglossia, cleft palate, tetralogy of Fallot, renal failure, neonatal hepatitis, cryptorchidism, clubfoot, hip dislocation, hearing loss, absent corpus callosum, holoprosencephaly
Trisomy 15 mosaicism	May correct to cause uniparental disomy 15 with features of Prader–Willi or Angelman syndrome; otherwise mild dysmorphology with growth and developmental delay, progressive right hemihypertrophy
Trisomy 16 mosaicism	Severe IUGR and growth/developmental delay, cardiac septal defects, hypospadias, imperforate anus, inguinal hernia, clubfoot, hydrocephalus

(cont.)

Table 7.3. (*cont.*)

Disorder	Complications
Trisomy 17 mosaicism	Moderate growth and developmental delay, seizures, microcephaly, attention deficit hyperactivity and autistic disorders, hearing loss
Trisomy 18 mosaicism	Higher-degree mosaicism cause Edwards syndrome; lower degrees range from normal intellect to moderate growth and developmental delay with facial asymmetry reminiscent of Russell–Silver syndrome, ventricular septal defect, urinary tract obstruction, infertility, kyphoscoliosis bilateral equinovarus, seizures, structural cerebral malformations, frequent respiratory infections
Trisomy 19 mosaicism	Early death with minor facial anomalies, laryngeal stridor, neutropenia, thrombocytopenia, short chest, short limbs, club feet, spoon-shaped nails, decreased cerebral gyration
Trisomy 20 mosaicism	Usually normal if detected only in amniotic fluid; moderate growth and developmental delay, multiple minor anomalies, delayed closure of fontanel, kyphosis, extensive Mongolian spot, central hypotonia with peripheral hypertonia
Trisomy 21 mosaicism	Usually presents with features of Down syndrome, but patients with low or undetectable mosaicism may present with transient myeloproliferative disorder or leukemia, showing trisomy 21 in the leukemic cells. Children with low degrees of mosaicism have a better prognosis than those with full trisomy 21
Trisomy 22 mosaicism	IUGR with growth and developmental delay, microcephaly, cleft palate, hemifacial microsomia with body asymmetry, webbed neck, transposition of the great vessels, malrotation, anal atresia, ectopic kidney, ovarian dysgenesis, joint laxity, hypoplastic distal digits, thumb anomalies; some patients have Turner syndrome features
Triploidy mosaicism	Early death, IUGR, iris coloboma, TE fistula, diaphragmatic hernia, omphalocele, renal cysts, hypospadias, cryptorchidism, club feet, thumb duplication, syndactyly digits 3/4, holoprosencephaly, cerebellar hypoplasia
Tetraploidy	Severe growth and developmental delay, microcephaly, anophthalmia, cataract, pulmonary and thymic hypoplasia, hydronephrosis, scoliosis, Arnold–Chiari malformation; variable with some patients having Turner syndrome features

Notes:
IUGR, intrauterine growth retardation; TE, tracheoesophageal; defects such as cleft palate, cardiac, and urogenital anomalies are listed for these rare disorders rather than assuming their presence from the list in Table 7.1; all mosaic patients may have areas of skin depigmentation.
Source: Review of the literature by Schinzel (2001) and Gorlin et al. (2001).

Partial aneuploidy

Terminology

Most autosomal aneuploidies are partial, involving extra or missing material from the short (p) or long (q) arm of the chromosome. Short-hand terminology for these partial trisomies and monosomies employs a plus for extra or duplicated (dup) material and a minus for missing or deleted (del) material. Thus 13q−, 13q deletion, or del(13q) syndrome describes individuals who are missing a portion of the long arm of one chromosome 13, while 10p+, 10p duplication, or dup(10p) syndrome describes individuals who have extra material from the short arm of chromosome 10. Sometimes the precise chromosome region is specified by indicating the band numbers that demarcate the duplicated or deleted region: dup(13)(p11→p22) indicates extra chromosome material extending from band 11 to band 22 of the chromosome 13 short arm (see Chapter 1 for more discussion).

Historical diagnosis and management

With availability of accurate chromosome analyses since 1970 or so, duplications and deletions of the long or short arms of all 22 autosomes have been defined. Each chromosomal excess or deficiency is associated with its own particular syndrome. The length of the unbalanced region is one factor, illustrated by the severity of trisomy 13 (2 times longer than chromosome 21) or trisomy 18 (1.5 times longer than chromosome 21) compared to Down syndrome. In addition to length (quantity), the particular genes on a duplicated chromosomal segment (quality) must be important in determining phenotypic severity. Chromosomes 16 and 18 are of about equal length, but trisomy 16 almost always presents as early miscarriage. There is much to learn about the mechanisms by which chromosomal aneuploidy causes an abnormal phenotype. Why, for example, would triploidy (e.g., 69,XXX), with its extra 23 chromosomes in each cell, be more compatible with fetal survival than trisomy 16?

Because most partial trisomies and monosomies are extremely rare, their typical appearance is not encountered frequently enough to be recognized by clinical inspection. Chromosome studies are therefore ordered rather unscientifically in children with multiple anomalies, particularly those with growth and/or developmental problems. Children with isolated malformations are unlikely to have chromosomal disorders unless subtle anomalies have been missed (see Chapter 1).

As patients with particular duplication or deletion were encountered, the particular syndromes and likely complications were compiled from collected cases. Sadly, waning interest in case studies has left this process incomplete, so that the natural history and variability of most partial aneuploidies remain ill-defined. Nevertheless, preventive management can be designed by considering general features of chromosome disorders (Table 7.1), then adding provisions for specific complications on the appropriate sections of the partial trisomy/monosomy checklist. Complications of the rarer aneuploidies are summarized in Table 7.2, and specific recommendations for the more common deletions/duplications (e.g., cri-du-chat syndrome) are listed in the sections following this trisomy/monosomy checklist discussion.

Incidence, etiology, and differential diagnosis

Chromosome disorders have an overall incidence of 1 in 200 live births and 50% of miscarriages, but complete trisomies or monosomies like trisomy 21 (Down syndrome) or monosomy X (Turner syndrome) account for most of these conditions. The rare partial aneuploidies shown in Table 7.2 usually comprise a dozen or so literature cases and an incidence of about 1 in 100,000 births. More common partial aneuploidies like Wolf–Hirschhorn syndrome (4p−) will have incidences from 1 in 25 to 50,000 births with over 100 cases in the literature or known to parent groups.

The etiology of a partial aneuploidy syndrome is defined by chromosome analysis, and the individual syndrome is caused by the specific chromosome segment(s) that are duplicated or deficient. The cytogenetic notation of the laboratory report must therefore be interpreted to define the unbalanced chromosome region that foretells the expected syndrome. For example, the notation 46,XX, −9, +t(9;22) (9pter→9q31::22q21→22qter) indicates a female in which a normal chromosome 9 has been replaced by a translocation between chromosomes 9 and 22. This causes missing material (partial monosomy or deletion 9q) from band 9q31 to the 9q end, replaced by material (yielding partial trisomy 22q or duplication 22q) from chromosome 22, band 22q21 to the 22q end. The clinical pattern would be a combination of that described for patients with del(9q) and dup(22q). While many cytogenetic laboratories now provide interpretation of the extra or missing material, it is usually worthwhile to consult a clinical geneticist so that accurate interpretation and genetic counseling is provided to families with complex chromosome rearrangements.

The differential diagnosis will include many chromosomal, single gene, or multifactorial syndromes that produce multiple anomalies of the type presenting in the individual patient. Rare partial aneuploidies cannot be recognized even by experienced dysmorphologists, so documentation of a karyotype in all neonates with unusual appearance and several minor and/or major anomalies is essential for diagnosis (see Chapter 1).

Diagnostic evaluation and medical counseling

Rapid FISH studies that are available for common aneuploidies (trisomies 13, 18, 21, X, Y or monosomy X) will not be useful for partial aneuploidies unless extra or missing long or short arm happens to correspond with the regions targeted by the mixture of fluorescent DNA probes. A routine banded karyotype is thus essential for diagnosis, and even in emergencies will require 3–4 days to stimulate lympho-cyte cell division, arrest in metaphase, and spread on slides to obtain banded and well-separated chromosomes. Medical counseling will then be guided by the unbalanced chromosome region(s) defined. While waiting for karyotype results, and/or for clarification of the precise partial trisomy/monosomy, the common complications listed in Table 7.1 can be considered. Evaluation of head size and head ultrasound for signs of abnormal brain development; monitoring for conse-quent apnea, seizures, swallowing incoordination, or diabetes insipidus; and alertness for internal anomalies of the pulmonary, cardiac, gastrointestinal, or urogenital systems can be instituted. While partial monosomies or trisomies will almost always cause some degree of developmental disability, they will usually not be suf-ficiently severe to prompt decisions about palliative versus aggressive care.

Family and psychosocial counseling

Partial monosomies and trisomies arise by chromosome rearrangement, meaning that chromosomes have been broken and rejoined rather than segregating abnor-mally by non-disjunction (see Chapter 1). Once the partial aneuploidy is defined, the parents should have chromosome studies to determine if the aneuploidy is spontaneous (deriving from one egg or sperm) or inherited from a parent with a balanced translocation. Rarely, a parent may actually carry the same partial aneu-ploidy, as in patients with ring 22 where deletion of the terminal short- and long-arm regions to form a ring causes mild symptoms.

If the parental chromosomes are normal, they have a very low (<1%) recur-rence risk in future pregnancies (the low but not zero risk is mentioned because rare parents may have germline mosaicism – mixtures of normal and translocation cells in their gonads). If a parent carries a balanced chromosome rearrangement, then there are four possibilities for offspring: liveborn child with partial aneu-ploidy (mental disability, birth defects) due to unbalanced translocation (5–10% risk), miscarriage due to unbalanced translocation (20–30% risk), normal child with the same balanced rearrangement (20–30% risk), or normal child with nor-mal chromosomes (40–50% risk). These numbers will vary slightly for each type of parental translocation, and experience with these rare aneuploidies is usually not sufficient of provide accurate risk data. Parental carriers should be informed about prenatal diagnosis options such as chorionic villus sampling (8–10-week gesta-tion), amniocentesis (13–18-week gestation), and the increasingly affordable and safe option of pre-implantation diagnosis.

There are a growing number of parent support groups for chromosome disorders, and these can be found through the directories of the Genetic Alliance (www.geneticalliance.org). Examples for chromosomal disorders include Chromosome Deletion Outreach, Inc. (www.chromodisorder.org), the Rare Chromosome Disorder

Support Group (www.rarechromo.org), Recombination 8 Syndrome Family Support Group (www.rec8.org), the Chromosome 9p− Network (www.9pminus.org), the Isodicentric 15 Exchange (www.idic15.org), and the Chromosome 18 Registry and Resource Society (www.chromosome18.org).

Natural history and complications

As mentioned above, natural history and even the range of complications are not well-defined for the rarer partial aneuploidies (Table 7.2). More is known about the more common disorders, as summarized under individual headings after this chapter. Even small amounts of extra or missing chromosome material can cause severe anomalies and moderately severe mental disability, so lifespan is often limited and complex needs of patients with disabilities often must be anticipated. Provisions for early childhood intervention, regular developmental assessments, and specialty follow-up should be made in the neonatal period as dictated by the documented or anticipated pattern of congenital anomalies.

Partial trisomy/monosomy preventive management checklist

Once a pattern of altered facial appearance with minor and major anomalies is appreciated, a routine karyotype should be sent to the cytogenetics laboratory with request for rapid reporting. The common complications from Table 7.1 are included on the checklist, and evaluation of the brain, heart, alimentary tract, heart, and urinary tract should be considered while awaiting the karyotype results. Once results are available and interpreted, disorder-specific complications can be entered from Table 7.2 or sections on common partial aneuploidies (see below), and the management plan consolidated. Neonatal and pediatric follow-up, early childhood intervention, and parental supports should be planned during the perinatal period.

SPECIFIC PARTIAL ANEUPLOIDIES

A few of the partial trisomy or monosomy syndromes are sufficiently common to warrant specific discussion.

Deletion 4p (Wolf–Hirschhorn) syndrome

Larger deletions of the distal chromosome 4 short arm (4p−) cause the Wolf–Hirschhorn syndrome, while smaller deletions detected by FISH techniques cause the Pitt–Rogers–Danks syndrome. The face is distinctive in this 4p deletion spectrum, with prominent supraorbital ridges, broad nasal root, and down-turned corners of the mouth. Battaglia & Carey (1999) provide a thorough summary of preventive management.

Summary of clinical concerns: Wolf–Hirschhorn management considerations

General: Infant mortality of 30% due to cardiopulmonary problems.

Growth and development: Low birth weight is followed by microcephaly in 90% with severe growth and developmental delay in 75%, severely delayed or absent speech: Early childhood intervention – developmental pediatrics, genetics, and/or neurology.

Craniofacial: Asymmetry with high forehead, broad nasal root, down-slanting palpebral fissures, short philtrum, down-turned corners of the mouth, micrognathia.

Eye: Colobomata, ptosis, and strabismus: Ophthalmology.

ENT: Cleft lip/palate, dysphagia with feeding problems, simplified ears with narrow canals, chronic otitis, small teeth: Feeding specialist, swallow studies, feeding tubes and nutrition, otolaryngology, dentistry.

Cardiac: Septal defects in 50%: Cardiology, echocardiogram.

Urogenital: Small kidneys with few tubules, cryptorchidism, and hypospadias: Renal ultrasound and functional monitoring, urology, nephrology.

Skeletal: Club feet, dislocated hips, vertebral fusions, kyphoscoliosis, radioulnar synostosis, digital defects: Examination of neck, hips, limbs with selected X-rays; orthopedics, anesthesia precautions.

Neural-CNS: Seizures, hypotonia: Alert for apnea, seizure equivalents; neurology, sleep studies.

Neural-sensory: Sensorineural hearing loss in 25%, conductive hearing loss: auditory brainstem evoked response (ABR), audiology, hearing and vision monitoring.

Parental counseling and support: Most cases are *de novo* deletions with minimal recurrence risks, but parents should have chromosome studies to exclude the 10–15% of cases that arise by translocation. Parent-oriented information can be found at the Family Village (www.familyvillage.wisc) or Contact a Family (www.cafamily.org.uk) websites and includes a specific 4p− Support Group (www.4p-supportgroup.org).

Deletion 5p (cri-du-chat or Lejeune) syndrome

Deleted material from the tip of the chromosome 5 short arm (5p−) produces brain alterations that cause a cat-like cry (*cri-du-chat*) with moderate to severe developmental disability. Severity correlates with the extent of chromosome deletion, being worse in those inheriting parental translocations (Cornish & Bramble, 2002).

Summary of clinical concerns: Cri-du-chat management considerations

General: Reduced lifespan with more severe disability, frequent respiratory infections: Aggressive influenza, pneumovax vaccination, screen for aspiration.

Growth and development: Low birth weight (70%) with postnatal growth delay and microcephaly, moderate to severe disability: Specific growth charts (Marinescu et al., 2000), early childhood intervention – developmental pediatrics, genetics, and/or neurology.

Facial: Hypertelorism, down-slanting palpebral fissures, preauricular tags, and small jaw are common, but the facies may not be distinctive.

Eye: Strabismus, optic atrophy, myopia: Ophthalmology.

ENT: Chronic otitis and early dysphagia with cleft lip/palate, frequent dental malocclusion: Feeding specialists, otolaryngology, dentistry, cleft palate team.

Surface: Inguinal hernias, prematurely gray hair.

Cardiac: Conotruncal and septal defects in 30%: Cardiology, echocardiogram.

Urogenital: Absent kidney, cryptorchidism: Abdominal ultrasound, monitoring of blood pressure and urine cultures, urology.

Skeletal: Club feet, dislocated hips: Examination of hips, limbs with selected X-rays, orthopedics.

Neural-CNS: Infantile hypotonia with later increased reflexes.

Neural-sensory: Sensorineural and conductive hearing loss: ABR, audiology, hearing and vision monitoring.

Parental counseling and support: From 10% to 15% are inherited translocations, mandating parental chromosome studies to differentiate a ≈10–20% recurrence risk in the case of parental balanced translocation versus <1% if parental chromosomes are normal. Parent groups are available in several countries, and include Cri-du-Chat Syndrome Support Group (www.cridchat.u-net.com/), Five P Minus Society (www.fivepminus.org/), and Cri-du-Chat Support Group of Australia (www.criduchat.asn.au/).

Duplication 9p syndrome

Extra material from the chromosome 9 short arm (9p+) produces a recognizable syndrome with large anterior fontanel, high forehead, small eyes, down-slanting palpebral fissures, bulbous tip of the nose, and large mouth with down-turned corners. Tetrasomy 9p with four equivalents of 9p material (extra small chromosome with mirror-image 9p arms) is also fairly common, and produces a similar pattern with more severe disability and higher complication frequencies.

Summary of clinical concerns: Dup(9p) management considerations

Growth and development: Variable growth delay with continued growth in the second and third decades due to delayed puberty, average IQ of 30–65 with more severe language impairment: Early childhood intervention with regular developmental, language, and behavioral assessment.

ENT: Narrow ear canals with chronic otitis, cleft lip/palate: Feeding specialists, otolaryngology, cleft palate team.

Surface: Small nails.

Cardiac: Conotruncal and septal defects in 15–20%: Cardiology, echocardiogram.

Skeletal: Contractures and fusions of the digits, scoliosis, kyphosis: Examination of extremities and spine with selected X-rays, orthopedics, hand surgeons.

Neural-CNS: Hypotonia, hydrocephalus: Monitor head circumference, head MRI scan, neurosurgery.

Parental counseling and support: Parental chromosomes are needed to differentiate a ≈10–20% recurrence risk in the case of parental balanced translocation versus <1% if parental chromosomes are normal. Numerous websites with parent-oriented information can be found by searching on the term "duplication 9p syndrome."

Deletion 9p syndrome

Deleted material encompassing variable extents of the chromosome 9 short arm (9p−) causes a distinct syndrome, usually with severe mental disability.

Summary of clinical concerns: Del(9p) management considerations

Growth and development: Delayed growth with a minority of patients having an IQ above 50: Early childhood intervention – developmental pediatrics, genetics, and/or neurology.

Craniofacial: Prominent metopic suture producing trigonocephaly with up-slanting palpebral fissures, shallow midface, malformed ears, and small jaw: Skull X-rays/MRI, craniofacial surgery to evaluate metopic sutural synostosis.

ENT: Cleft lip/palate: Feeding specialists, otolaryngology, cleft palate team.

Surface: Inguinal hernias, umbilical hernia, diastasis recti.

Cardiopulmonary: Septal defects, patent ductus arteriosis, pulmonic stenosis in 33–50%, diaphragmatic hernia: Cardiology, echocardiogram, chest X-ray.

Urogenital: Hydronephrosis, cryptorchidism, hypoplastic labia: Abdominal ultrasound, monitoring of blood pressure and urine cultures, urology.

Skeletal: Rib and vertebral defects, scoliosis: Skeletal examination, selected X-rays, orthopedics.

Neural-sensory: Vision and hearing deficits: ABR, monitoring, audiology, ophthalmology.

Parental counseling and support: Parental chromosomes are needed to differentiate a ≈10–20% recurrence risk in the case of parental balanced translocation versus <1% if parental chromosomes are normal. Numerous websites with parent-oriented information can be found by searching on the term "deletion 9p syndrome."

Deletion 11p syndrome including WAGR anomalies

Deleted material from the chromosome 11 short arm (11p−) causes a distinct syndrome that includes propensity to Wilms tumor and aniridia if band 11p13 is included in the deletion. Some patients will have the WAGR syndrome that is an acronym for *W*ilms tumor, *A*niridia, *G*enitourinary anomalies, and *R*etardation. Large 11p deletions produce more dramatic facial changes and additional anomalies, while submicroscopic deletions confined to band 11p13 are limited to the cognate abnormalities.

Summary of clinical concerns: WAGR-del(11p) management considerations

General: Wilms tumor occurs in 50% of patients with deleted band 11p13, and is more frequently bilateral (35% versus 1–2%) and of early onset (2–3 versus 4–5 years) than in patients with no chromosome abnormality: Abdominal examinations, serial abdominal ultrasounds in infancy and childhood.

Growth and development: Growth deficiency and microcephaly in 50%, moderate to severe disability: Early childhood intervention – developmental pediatrics, genetics, and/or neurology.

Facial: Ptosis, small palpebral fissures, ear anomalies, prominent lips, micrognathia.

Eye: Aniridia, glaucoma, cataracts, nystagmus: Ophthalmology.

Skeletal: Fifth finger clinodactyly, hemihypertrophy as sign of Wilms tumor.

Urogenital: Hypospadias, cryptorchidism, urinary tract anomalies, inguinal hernia: Urology, nephrology, blood pressure monitoring.

Parental counseling and support: Most cases of deletion 11p are sporadic, but parental chromosome studies should be performed to rule out translocations and 10–20% recurrence risks. Support and information are available at the International WAGR Syndrome Parent Group website (www.wagr.org/pages/432553/index.htm).

Duplication 12p mosaicism: Pallister–Killian syndrome

Pallister–Killian syndrome was delineated before skin fibroblast studies demonstrated mosaicism for an extra chromosome formed by fusion of two chromosome 12 short arms (isochromosome 12p). The syndrome is distinct from that caused by partial duplication of 12p caused by translocation (Table 7.2). Skin biopsy with karyotyping of cultured fibroblasts is most accurate, since the mosaic isochromosome 12p decreases in frequency with age.

Summary of clinical concerns: Pallister–Killian/dup(12p) management considerations

General: Unexplained fevers, pineal tumors, early death.

Growth and development: Early gigantism followed by growth and developmental delay, ranging from severe delay and absent speech in those with

Pallister–Killian phenotype to mild dysmorphology and mental disability with lower degrees of isochromosome 12p mosaicism: Growth and developmental monitoring, early childhood intervention – developmental pediatric, clinical genetic, and neurology specialists depending on symptoms and availability.

Facial: Characteristic coarse facies with sparse frontal hair and hypertelorism.

Eye: Strabismus, ptosis: Ophthalmology.

ENT: Micrognathia, macroglossia, mandibular prognathism, delayed tooth eruption: Dentistry, otolaryngology.

Surface: Webbing of neck, supernumerary nipples.

Cardiopulmonary: Diaphragmatic hernia, heart defects (25%, septal defects most common): Chest X-ray, cardiology, echocardiogram.

Skeletal: Joint laxity or contractures, atlanto-occipital instability, scoliosis, polydactyly, broad hallux, club feet: Skeletal examination with selected X-rays including cervical spine flexion–extension, orthopedics, anesthesia precautions.

Neural: Hyper- or hypotonia, seizures, vision and hearing deficits: ABR, audiology, hearing and vision monitoring, neurology.

Parental counseling and support: Parental chromosome studies are not needed. Parent information is available by searching on Pallister–Killian.

Deletion 13q syndrome, ring 13 syndrome

Most patients with 13q− syndrome are missing two-thirds of the chromosome 13 long arm, and retinoblastoma occurs in patients with deletion of band 13q14. The facial characteristics and degree of disability vary with the extent and location of deletion. Patients with ring(13) have similar patterns to those with small 13q deletions.

Summary of clinical concerns: Del(13q)/ring(13) management considerations

General: Retinoblastoma in 15% of patients with deletions encompassing band 13q14: Serial ophthalmology evaluations.

Growth and development: Low birth weight with postnatal growth delay and moderate to severe disability: Early childhood intervention – developmental pediatrics, genetics, and/or neurology.

Facial: Prominent forehead and metopic suture with trigonocephaly, broad nasal root, large and malformed ears.

Eye: Strabismus, ptosis, colobomata: Evaluate during serial ophthalmology examinations.

ENT: Chronic otitis and early dysphagia with cleft lip/palate, frequent dental malocclusion: Feeding specialists, otolaryngology, dentistry, cleft palate team.

Surface: Short neck with extra skin folds, inguinal hernias, prematurely gray hair.

Cardiac: Conotruncal and septal defects in 35%: Cardiology, echocardiogram.

Gastrointestinal: Anal atresia: Pediatric surgery.

Genital: Hypospadias, cryptorchidism, micropenis, delayed bone age: Urology, endocrinology.

Skeletal: Club feet, dislocated hips, thumb anomalies, osteosarcoma: Examination of hips, limbs with selected X-rays, orthopedics.

Neural-CNS: Brain anomalies including holoprosencephaly and agenesis of the corpus callosum: Head MRI scan, monitoring for absent olfaction, diabetes insipidus.

Neural-sensory: Vision and hearing deficits: ABR, audiology, hearing and vision monitoring.

Parental counseling and support: Parental chromosome studies are needed to differentiate a ≈10–20% recurrence risk for those with translocations from <1% for those with normal chromosomes (Parent groups).

Deletion 18p syndrome

Patients with deletion of material from the short arm of chromosome 18 (18p− syndrome) have extremely variable degrees of mental deficiency, and this does not correlate with the extent of deletion.

Summary of clinical concerns: Del(18p) management considerations

Growth and development: Moderate growth delay with microcephaly and occasional growth hormone deficiency, more severe language than motor delays with broad IQ range from 25 to 75: Growth monitoring with alertness for growth hormone deficiency, regular developmental assessment: Endocrinology if growth hormone deficiency suspected, early childhood intervention – developmental pediatrics, genetics, and/or neurology.

Facial: Round face with hypertelorism, broad nose, large and malformed ears, down-turned corners of the mouth, micrognathia.

Eye: Strabismus, ptosis: Ophthalmology.

ENT: Frequent dental caries: Dentistry.

Surface: Short neck, alopecia.

Cardiac: Septal defects, coarctation of the aorta, patent ductus arteriosus in a minority (5–10%): Cardiac examination, cardiology if symptoms.

Gastrointestinal: Anal atresia: Pediatric surgery.

Reticuloendothelial system (RES): Immunoglobulin A deficiency, usually asymptomatic.

Genital: Hypospadias, cryptorchidism, micropenis, delayed bone age: Urology, endocrinology.

Skeletal: Club feet, dislocated hips, kyphoscoliosis, rheumatoid arthritis symptoms: Examination of spine, hips, limbs with selected X-rays, orthopedics, rheumatology.

Neural-CNS: Brain anomalies including holoprosencephaly in 10%, may present with single central incisor: Head MRI scan if signs and symptoms, monitoring for absent olfaction, diabetes insipidus.

Neural-sensory: Vision and hearing deficits: ABR, audiology, hearing and vision monitoring.

Parental counseling and support: Parental chromosome studies are needed to differentiate a ≈10–20% recurrence risk for those with translocations from <1% for those with normal chromosomes (Parent groups).

Deletion 18q syndrome; ring(18) syndrome

Patients with deletion of material from the long arm of chromosome 18 (18q− syndrome) usually have severe mental deficiency except for the 10% of patients who are mosaic. Ring(18) causes a similar syndrome.

Summary of clinical concerns: Del(18q)/ring(18) management considerations

Growth and development: Short stature, developmental delay with broad IQ range from 40 to 85, and frequent behavior problems: Growth, developmental, and behavioral monitoring, early childhood intervention – developmental pediatrics, genetics, behavioral specialists, and/or neurology.

Facial: Characteristic facies with deep-set eyes, shallow midface, down-turned corners of the mouth.

Eye: Cataract, strabismus, retinal defects, optic disk malformations: Ophthalmology.

ENT: Cleft palate (30%), chronic otitis: Otolaryngology, cleft palate team.

Surface: Widely spaced nipples, eczema, inguinal hernia, acromial dimples.

Cardiac: Septal defects, pulmonic stenosis, patent ductus arteriosus in 35%: Cardiology, echocardiogram.

RES: Immunoglobulin A deficiency contributing to chronic otitis: Immunology with possible immunoglobulin shots.

Genital: Hypospadias, cryptorchidism, micropenis, hypoplasia of labia: Urology.

Skeletal: Rib anomalies, coxa valga, club feet, vertical talus: Skeletal examination with selected X-rays, orthopedics.

Neural-sensory: Vision and hearing deficits: ABR, audiology, hearing and vision monitoring.

Parental counseling and support: Parental chromosome studies are needed to differentiate a ≈10–20% recurrence risk for those with translocations from <1% for those with normal chromosomes (Parent groups).

Full trisomies and monosomies

The majority of complete autosomal trisomies or monosomies are aborted in early embryonic life; surviving patients are almost always mosaics with minority cell lines containing the aneuploidy. Autosomal monosomy syndromes are particularly rare, reflecting the more severe consequences of multiple gene deficiencies compared to the multiple excesses of trisomies. Even Turner syndrome with monosomy X (see next chapter) has a 95% miscarriage rate, and only monosomies for the smallest autosomes (21, 22) are seen as live births. Complete autosomal trisomies of these small chromosomes (Down syndrome, trisomy 22) do survive (although even trisomy 21 has a miscarriage rate of 10%), and complete trisomy 22 is listed in Table 7.3 along with the mosaic aneuploidies. Trisomy 13/18 and Down syndrome are sufficiently common to warrant individual discussion.

Mosaic trisomies and monosomies have the same common abnormalities of chromosomal syndromes listed in Table 7.1. Management guidelines can incorporate recommendations of the general chromosome disorder checklist after adding the unusual complications listed in Table 7.3. While it might be expected that complications of a complete trisomy could be derived from Table 7.2 by adding those of its partial short- and long-arm aneuploidies, these mosaic conditions are often unique. Many will have minor facial alterations, fewer major anomalies, and milder mental disability that depends somewhat on the degree of mosaicism. Many of the mosaic aneuploidies will be difficult to diagnose based on their minimum dysmorphology, and management is often focused on their mild to moderate mental disability rather than on a pattern of congenital anomalies.

Trisomy 8/trisomy 8 mosaicism syndrome

The majority of patients with trisomy 8 are mosaic (85%), but their pattern of malformations is similar to those with full trisomy. The aberration occurs in 10% of abortuses and 1 in 25–50,000 live births with an interesting 5:1 predilection for males (Gorlin et al., 2001, p. 51). Trisomy 8 is usually evident in blood studies of mosaic patients but becomes less frequent with age.

Summary of clinical concerns: Trisomy 8 mosaicism management considerations

Growth and development: Mild growth and developmental delay with IQ range from 40 to 75 with occasional near-normal intelligence: Growth and developmental monitoring with early childhood intervention.

Cancer: Wilms tumor and leukemias have been reported.

Eye: Corneal opacities, strabismus, retinal defects, optic disk malformations: Ophthalmology.

ENT: Small mandible with occasional cleft palate: Otolaryngology, cleft palate team.

Cardiac: Septal defects, pulmonic stenosis, patent ductus arteriosus, coarctation of the aorta in 25%: Cardiology, echocardiogram.

RES: Immunoglobulin A deficiency contributing to chronic otitis: Immunology with possible immunoglobulin shots.

Urogenital: Cryptorchidism in 50%, hydronephrosis and obstructive anomalies in 40%: Monitoring of urinalysis and blood pressure, urology.

Skeletal: Rib anomalies, vertebral defects, scoliosis, absent patellae: Skeletal examination with selected X-rays, orthopedics, anesthesia precautions.

Neural-sensory: Vision and hearing deficits: ABR, audiology, hearing and vision monitoring.

Parental counseling and support: Parental chromosome studies are not necessary; parent information can be found by searching on trisomy 8.

Trisomy 13/18

Terminology

Children with extra chromosomal material representing an entire chromosome 13 or 18 are affected with the trisomy 13/18 syndrome (Jones, 1997, pp. 14–23; Gorlin et al., 2001, pp. 42–8). The extra chromosomal material may arise by trisomy or translocation. Although each syndrome has a distinctive pattern of anomalies, trisomy 13 and 18 are discussed together because they have many overlapping features and a similar natural history. Patients with mosaicism for trisomy 13/18 have variable proportions of normal and trisomic cells among different tissues. Those with low percentages of mosaicism as judged from blood or fibroblast karyotyping will have a much milder phenotype than is typical for trisomy 13/18 syndrome (Slavotinek et al., 2003).

Historical diagnosis and management

The terms "Patau syndrome" and "Edwards syndrome" indicate the respective descriptions of trisomies 13 and 18 in 1960. They have remarkable similarities in their clinical patterns, with trisomy 18 more likely to exhibit intrauterine growth retardation or limb anomalies and trisomy 13 more likely to exhibit scalp defects and forebrain anomalies.

Incidence, etiology, and differential diagnosis

Trisomy 13 due to non-disjunction or translocation occurs in about 1 in 12,000 live births, with a frequency in miscarriages some 100-fold higher (Gorlin et al., 2001, pp. 42–8). Trisomy 18 is slightly more common, with a frequency between 1 in 5000 and 1 in 7000 live births. Aneuploidy leads to the characteristic pattern of malformation, but the pathogenesis is poorly understood. Brain anomalies often bias the facial appearance in trisomy 13, with variable degrees of microphthalmia, nasal hypoplasia, and/or cleft lip caused by underlying holoprosencephaly (Rios et al., 2004). Isolated holoprosencephaly, Meckel syndrome with encephalocele and polydactyly, and the Pallister–Hall syndrome of brain anomalies and polydactyly may be confused with trisomy 13. Patients with trisomy 18 often have a characteristic "clenched fist" with overlapping fingers. Following the general rule that no one anomaly is pathognomonic for a syndrome, the clenched fist may occur in other disorders associated with decreased movement or innervation of the hands. Patients with the Pena–Shokeir syndrome of arthrogryposis and microcephaly, other disorders with decreased fetal movement, and trisomy 13 may resemble patients with trisomy 18.

Diagnostic evaluation and medical counseling

Rapid laboratory confirmation of trisomy 13/18 is available using FISH or bone marrow karyotyping when surgical decisions are pending. Patients with trisomy 13/18 are at risk for a variety of internal malformations that require evaluation in the newborn period. Initial management often will require imaging of the brain, heart, urinary tract, and abdomen along with careful observation of feeding and respiratory status. Hypertonia, seizures, and uncoordinated swallowing place these patients at high risk for aspiration, which may further increase their risks for apnea. Cardiac anomalies in trisomy 13/18 include septal defects, polyvalvular disease, patent ductus arteriosus, coarctation of the aorta, and, in trisomy 13, dextrocardia with or without aberrant venous return and/or aortic positioning (trisomy 13/18 checklist, part 1). Medical counseling should emphasize the risks for internal anomalies and be realistic but not hopeless concerning the developmental potential of patients with trisomies 13 and 18.

Crucial perinatal decisions involve the aggressiveness of medical and surgical management. Trisomy 13 and 18 patients are often recognized prenatally, offering the opportunity to counsel the parents concerning delivery and neonatal resuscitation options. Avoidance of Cesarean delivery or extreme resuscitation measures is often appropriate, especially in infants with major organ anomalies who may not survive the infantile period. Early neonatal diagnosis facilitates medical counseling regarding the management of anomalies such as hydrocephalus, meningomyelocele, cleft palate, tetralogy of Fallot, ventricular septal defect, or cryptorchidism/hypospadias; each of these anomalies, together with requirements for artificial ventilation or gastrostomy feedings, involves different levels of intervention and different consequences from withholding therapy. A reasonable strategy is to recommend simple surgeries and supportive care that alleviate suffering or ease management for parents. However, cardiac surgery has been accomplished with good outcome (Graham et al., 2004) even though there are increased risks from anesthesia. Appropriate fluid and nutritional support are always indicated, and an overly negative and dehumanizing outlook by the health professional may provoke parental resistance and delay agreement on palliative care. It is important to recall that about 10% of patients will survive at least 1 year, and to emphasize the preventive management that can be provided for these children. As with any medical crisis, social and pastoral services should be included in the medical counseling.

Family and psychosocial counseling

For patients with free-standing trisomy of chromosome 13 or 18, the recurrence risk is about 1%, increasing in the usual way with maternal age (2–3% total risk by maternal age of 40 years). Parental karyotyping is required if the infant has translocation 13 or 18, with risks in the 5–10% range if one parent is a balanced translocation carrier. A recent study suggests that most children with apparent Robertsonian translocation (joining of one chromosome 13 to another at its end) actually have an isochromosome 13 (mirror-image duplication of chromosome 13) of paternal origin (Bugge et al., 2005). Although parental chromosome studies are still necessary if the child has apparent translocation, the majority of these will show normal parental chromosomes with low recurrence risk. If genetic counseling is not available during the neonatal period, then referral to a genetics clinic is essential. Prenatal diagnosis is an option for subsequent pregnancies, with chorionic villus biopsy or amniocentesis recommended rather than the less specific lowering of maternal serum α-fetoprotein (MSAFP).

The most crucial counseling issue concerns the high infant mortality and severe developmental disability faced by patients with trisomy 13/18. Survey of more than 100 families with trisomy 18 demonstrated some developmental progress in these children (Baty et al., 1994a, b), so initial counseling should be realistic but not overly bleak (see below). Options for palliative care, including the chance to ameliorate some of the disabilities, should be mentioned when the parents have had a chance to adjust to the diagnosis. Parent support groups are listed on the trisomy 13/18 checklist.

Natural history and complications

Survival rates in trisomy 18 are about 70% to age 1 month and <10% to age 1 year. Patients without cardiac anomalies live longer, with a mean survival of 40 days. Survival in trisomy 13 is somewhat better, with 55% surviving 1 month and 14% surviving 1 year (Jones, 1997, pp. 20–1; Gorlin et al., 2001, pp. 42–8). Mortality figures vary considerably among studies, influenced by occasional long-term survivors. Patients with full trisomy 13/18 have survived into their late teens.

Baty et al. (1994a) documented the natural history of 130 patients with trisomy 13/18 using parental questionnaires and medical record review. Brain anomalies with seizures are common in both syndromes, with holoprosencephaly being prevalent in trisomy 13. Each disorder may include early hypertonia with clenched fists, although this sign is more emphasized in trisomy 18. Eye, external ear, and inner ear anomalies are common, causing visual and/or hearing impairment in most patients who are properly assessed. Severe feeding problems with failure to thrive and multiple internal anomalies can be expected (see checklist). Urinary tract infections occurred in 11–19% of patients with trisomy 13/18 according to the survey of Baty et al. (1994a). Other complications include spinal dysraphism, myeloid malignancy, and pigmentary lesions.

An important addition to the literature is the study of Baty et al. (1994b) that documents some psychomotor development in patients with trisomy 13/18. Developmental quotients (developmental age divided by chronologic age) averaged 0.18 in 50 trisomy 18 individuals (age 1–232 months) and 0.25 in 12 trisomy 13 individuals (age 1–130 months), according to assessments from the medical record (Baty et al., 1994b). Older children responded to words or phrases, communicated with simple words or signs, crawled, used a walker, interacted with others, and achieved some toileting skills.

Trisomy 13/18 preventive management checklist

After initial evaluations for internal anomalies, agreement on the various surgical versus palliative care options should be reached with the parents. Neurologic dysfunction may superimpose poor feeding on underlying pre- and postnatal growth retardation, particularly in patients with trisomy 18. Careful monitoring of growth, feeding, and nutrition is thus necessary throughout life, and feeding specialists may be required to achieve adequate caloric intake in these hypertonic, irritable, and neurologically immature patients. Malformations of the eye, external ear, and inner ear are frequent, emphasizing the need for frequent hearing and vision assessment to ensure maximal function. Urinary tract anomalies are frequent in both trisomies, and hepatoblastoma or Wilms tumor has been encountered in longer survivors with trisomy 18. These risks should be monitored by performing periodic urinalyses and abdominal palpation. The debilitated state of many patients requires vigilance for respiratory infections and attention to social or local services such as social work, clergy, occupational or physical therapy, respite, and hospice care. Medical interventions listed on the trisomy 13/18 checklist should obviously be tailored to prognosis, since palliative care is appropriate for patients with severe anomalies.

Down syndrome

Terminology

Patients with an entire extra copy of chromosome 21 have Down syndrome (Jones, 1997, pp. 8–13; Gorlin et al., 2001, pp. 36–42). The extra chromosome may arise by non-disjunction (trisomy 21) or translocation (translocation Down syndrome). Patients with mixtures of normal and trisomic cells (mosaic Down syndrome) often have milder phenotypes, but it should be realized that percentages of normal cells among peripheral lymphocytes used for karyotyping may differ from percentages in brain.

Historical diagnosis and management

Down syndrome was first described in 1866 by Dr. J. H. Langdon Down, a British physician. Diagnosis was clinical until 1959, when Lejeune reported the extra number 21 chromosome in patients with Down syndrome. Early in this century, patients with Down syndrome and those with congenital hypothyroidism ("cretinism") were mistaken for each other because each displayed mental retardation, hypotonia, thyroid dysfunction, and growth failure. Patients with Down syndrome, like others with moderate mental retardation, were often institutionalized because of overly pessimistic views of their potential. Improvements in cardiac surgery, immunizations, and thyroid treatment have ameliorated the major complications of Down syndrome and provided the modern expectations of family living, inclusive schooling, and prolonged lifespan (Cooley & Graham, 1991).

Incidence, etiology, and differential diagnosis

The incidence of Down syndrome is 1 in 650 to 1 in 1000 live births and shows little variation by ethnic groups (Gorlin et al., 2001, pp. 36–42). Increasing maternal age is a significant risk factor, rising from about 1 in 2000 at age 20 to 1 in 50 at age 40. The disorder is caused by duplicated material from the distal long arm of chromosome 21 through non-disjunction (trisomy 21) or translocation (translocation Down syndrome). Extensive mapping of genes on this "critical region" of chromosome 21 is under way as part of the human genome initiative. The mechanisms by which increased dosage of these genes leads to the Down syndrome phenotype are as yet unknown.

The newborn with Down syndrome is often recognized because of an unusual facies and hypotonia. In some newborns, especially premature infants, facial recognition may be difficult. Characteristic minor anomalies may be needed for diagnosis, including a central hair whorl, brachycephaly, up-slanting palpebral fissures, epicanthal folds, Brushfield spots, anteverted nares, redundant neck skin, single palmar creases, clinodactyly, broad space between the first and second toes, and a deep-plantar crease. The tongue frequently protudes, more because of hypotonia than true enlargement. As with all syndromes, the pattern of minor and major defects in Down syndrome varies from individual to individual. None of the anomalies is pathognomonic.

Diagnostic evaluation and medical counseling

All patients with Down syndrome have duplicated chromosomal 21 material, but the origin of this duplicated material may vary. The most typical finding is trisomy 21 where the extra number 21 chromosome is free-standing. Translocation refers to joining or exchange of chromosome 21 material with another chromosome. Translocation of chromosome 21 usually involves an acrocentric chromosome (chromosomes 13–15, 21, 22) as an end-to-end "Robertsonian" translocation. When a translocation is found, the parents must be karyotyped to determine if they "carry" the translocation in a balanced form. Occasionally, patients with Down syndrome will be mosaic, having a mixture of normal and trisomy 21 cells. Trisomy 21 is the etiology for Down syndrome in 96% of cases, with translocation (3%) and mosaic Down syndrome (1%) being less common.

Initial disclosure that Down syndrome is suspected is best made during the neonatal period when both parents are present or when other family members are available for support (Cooley & Graham, 1991). Avoidance of pejorative terms such as "mongolism" or "simian" crease is desirable, and the use of people-first language (e.g., the infant with Down syndrome rather than the "Down's baby") is encouraged. Counseling should stress the improved prognosis for children with Down syndrome and emphasize the importance of anticipatory guidance. Genetic counseling can begin when the karyotype results are available, usually 1–2 weeks after birth. If counseling must be delayed for 1–2 months, karyotype results should be communicated as soon as possible, to minimize parental anxiety. The recurrence risk for trisomy 21 is 1% if the mother is under age 35 and increases with maternal age thereafter. Depending on the nature of the balanced translocation, carriers can have risks between 5% and 100% to have another child with Down syndrome. Prenatal diagnosis using chorionic villus biopsy or amniocentesis allows detection of fetuses with Down syndrome by documenting the fetal karyotype. Screening for low maternal serum markers during pregnancy is also possible and is recommended as a standard of care for women over age 35 years.

Family and psychosocial counseling

Cooley (1999, see Chapter 2) has emphasized the importance of family support as part of his Chronic Condition Management Program for children with disabilities. Supports include contact with representatives of a Down syndrome parent group who can inform new parents about the many psychosocial issues involved in raising a child with disabilities. Such contacts can be facilitated through one of the national organizations listed below, with most urban areas having active Down syndrome guilds or parent groups. Msall (1996) discussed ways in which a partnership can be forged between families, health care professionals, and early intervention specialists. Natal psychosocial issues include the options for adoption or foster care for parents who cannot accept a child with a handicap or who have insufficient resources. Few parents will opt to place children for adoption if they receive supportive counseling from informed professionals and parent representatives. Institutionalization is no longer a realistic option and should be mentioned only as an example of negative and inaccurate information that may be found in the older literature on Down syndrome. Marital and sibling stress that occurs during the adjustment to a child with disabilities should be discussed and appropriate counseling resources provided. Sibling and parent workshops available through Down syndrome organizations are helpful with these adjustments.

Later issues include the challenges in obtaining educational resources faced by many parents. Local parent groups and chapters of the Association for Retarded Citizens are often helpful in preparing parents as advocates in the educational process. While there is controversy and some resistance surrounding inclusive education of children with moderate disabilities, much anecdotal evidence attests to positive experiences for both "normal" and disabled children. Key indicators will be the child's level of function and the availability of assistance for the teacher. Behavioral and psychiatric disorders are more prevalent in children with Down syndrome, ranging from attention deficit disorders to psychoses. Child psychologists and behavioral therapists may be needed, with the provision that observation for problems triggering the behavior should precede and accompany pharmacologic intervention.

Medical issues include educating the parents about the importance of comprehensive pediatric care using a medical checklist. Care coordinated by a primary care physician in conjunction with specialized Down syndrome clinics is optimal where available, and improved anticipation of complications can be demonstrated even in a semi-rural setting (Lovell & Saul, 1999). Parents should know about symptoms of sleep apnea (excessive sweating, gasping respirations, unusual sleep positioning, daytime somnolence) as well as those of atlantoaxial instability (easy tiring, abnormal gait, neck pain, limited neck mobility, head tilt, clumsiness, spasticity, hyperreflexia, extensor–plantar reflex, other upper motor neuron signs). Simple preventive measures like anal dilation (for infants with stenosis and painful stooling), scrubbing of eyelids during baths (to prevent blepharitis) and nasal saline drops (to prevent mucosal drying and consequent respiratory infections) can be helpful for new parents who are already under stress.

Issues for mid-childhood and adulthood include behavior differences that can interfere with schooling, socialization, and employment readiness. Problems can include attention deficit or conduct disorders with stubborn, impulsive, disobedient, and distracted behaviors (Clark & Wilson, 2003). Older children are more likely to have depression and communication problems, merging with later aggressive and autistic tendencies that may reflect dementia (Van Allen et al., 1999). Pubertal children are very aware of sexuality and require education about appropriate personal boundaries and private behavior. Contraception is an important consideration in females. Job training is important to anticipate, beginning at age 15–16 years to prepare for the end of mandated education after age 21–22 years. Parents must also confront issues of guardianship and financial support of older dependent children. Resources to assist with legal and estate planning issues can be obtained through the Down syndrome organizations and the Association of Retarded Citizens. While parents are usually too overwhelmed to confront these later issues in the first counseling session, they should be addressed in early childhood so that the parents can begin investigation and planning. Parent information and educational resources are listed on the checklist.

Natural history and complications

Cooley & Graham (1991) emphasized the improvements in the length and quality of life enjoyed by individuals with Down syndrome. They cite a 50% mortality by age 5 in 1965, compared with 80% survival to age 30 or beyond in 1991. Much of this improvement reflects advances in pediatric and cardiothoracic surgery, allowing the correction of the gastrointestinal and cardiac anomalies that are prominent among the complications listed on the checklist. If no congenital anomalies are manifested in the newborn period, then more subtle abnormalities of the ocular, otic, dental, immune, urinary, and skeletal systems must be suspected. Transient myeloid proliferation may occur as an asymptomatic presentation with abnormal blood counts or (in 20%) as an acute multisystemic disease with hydrops fetalis, liver failure, and significant mortality (Massey, 2005). Most infants will have a spontaneous remission, but have a 13–35% risk for contracting acute megakaryoblastic leukemia that is fatal without chemotherapy (Massey, 2005). Neonatal jaundice, feeding problems, and anal stenosis are common problems that often respond to parental counseling and resolve spontaneously (Spahis & Wilson, 1999).

Respiratory infections are more frequent and severe in children with Down syndrome, including chronic otitis, sinusitis, and pneumonia. Many children have a stormy course in the first 3 years, with abatement after age 3–4 years. Tonsillectomy and adenoidectomy may be required for children with sleep apnea or frequent upper respiratory infections. Correctable problems such as constipation, strabismus, hypothyroidism, dental anomalies, atlantoaxial instability, and cryptorchidism are important not to miss.

Although 15% of individuals with Down syndrome have radiographic evidence of atlantoaxial instability, few are symptomatic (Committee on Sports Medicine and Fitness, 1995). Precautions are reasonable, however, when children undergo anesthesia (Hata & Todd, 2005). It is symptomatic children who are at highest risk for spinal cord injury, but consensus guidelines still call for cervical radiographic screening (Committee on Genetics, 2001b). Developmental delays, learning differences, and speech problems are universal, and there is a 10% risk for psychiatric problems in older individuals with Down syndrome. Despite neuropathologic changes typical of Alzheimer disease in 100% of individuals over 35, symptomatic dementia is fortunately much less frequent (Cooley & Graham, 1991).

With better survival and more emphasis on adult preventive measures, specific complications for the adult with Down syndrome are being recognized. Van Allen et al. (1999) report complications in middle-aged (age 30–45 years) and elderly (age 46–68 years) adults with Down syndrome. The middle-aged group had onset of cataracts, keratoconus, blindness, recurrent pneumonias, seizures, self-abusive behaviors, vitiligo with alopecia, and hepatitis B antigen positivity while the elderly group had these complications plus osteoporosis with compression fractures of the vertebrae, arthritis, long-bone fractures, bladder infections, and symptoms of Alzheimer disease (15 of 20 patients). Preventive measures tailored for the adult population can be found in Van Allen et al. (1999).

Down syndrome preventive management checklist

An early version of the preventive medical checklist was designed by Dr. Mary Coleman and adapted by authors such as Cooley & Graham (1991), Carey (1992), and the Committee on Genetics, American Academy of Pediatrics (2001b) Cooley & Graham (1991) provide an especially useful discussion of modern preventive management.

Neonatal evaluation of Down syndrome includes attention to feeding and bowel function, since cardiac and gastrointestinal anomalies may occur. All children need an echocardiogram in the first few weeks, since large septal defects may not be audible by auscultation and present later with inoperable pulmonary hypertension. Hypotonia often complicates breastfeeding, so extra support and expertise should be provided to interested mothers. The nasal, otic, and anal canals are narrow in children with Down syndrome, causing anal stenosis in some neonates that can be relieved by gentle dilation or lubrication. Blood for karyotyping should be obtained in all cases, with referral for genetic counseling, early intervention, and parent group support. These services are potentially coordinated by a Down syndrome clinic in areas where one is available. Preventive care in childhood includes annual thyroid testing, monitoring of hearing and vision, and referral to ophthalmology at age 6–8 months to prevent later amblyopia. A "high thyroid-stimulating hormone

(TSH)" form of hypothyroidism is common, requiring repeat thyroid function tests and possible hormone therapy. X-rays of the cervical spine are recommended at age 3 years and at 10-year intervals thereafter. Sleep apnea is common in children with hypotonia, obesity, and respiratory infections; a "GRIMES" acronym may be used as a screening tool. The acronym stands for Gasping respirations, Retractions, Inspiratory stridor, Mouth breathing, and Excessive Sweating in children with Down syndrome (Spahis, 1994), to which one should add abnormal sleep positioning and daytime somnulence. Because of their susceptibility to infection, children and adolescents with Down syndrome should receive all immunizations, including pneumococcal, varicella, and influenza vaccines in children with respiratory difficulties.

Pediatric visits should continue through adolescence with particular attention to moderating obesity, recognizing visual or auditory deficiencies, and early recognition of school and behavior problems. Nutritional monitoring, with encouragement of dieting and exercise, is important, and some children may be more susceptible to vitamin deficiencies (Cabana et al., 1997). There is a higher risk for several autoimmune disorders, including type I diabetes and celiac disease. Pubertal males with micropenis may be subject to ridicule, and early testosterone treatment may be considered. Although males are rarely fertile, adolescents may be sexually active and need protection from sexually transmitted diseases and pregnancy. Many females with Down syndrome can schedule and manage birth control pills with supervision, and Norplant or depot hormone injections may be considered for individuals with lower function.

Simple preventive treatments may include eyewash scrubs for blepharitis and nasal saline drops for sinusitis. Blepharitis is evidenced by erythema and/or swelling of the eyelids and can result in unsightly deformities of the lid or even keratitis. Washing of the eyelids with baby shampoo (or saline, if shampoo is irritating) during baths is helpful. Nasal saline drops (two in each nostril, morning and night) prevent drying of the mucosa and help with the rhinorrhea, nasal obstruction, and sinusitis that is so common in the first 3–4 years.

The adult with Down syndrome should have continued monitoring of vision, hearing, thyroid, heart, gastrointestinal, and genitourinary function with particular attention to exercise and employment activities that will combat depression, withdrawal, and obesity. Nutritional counseling and weight management will in turn lessen joint problems from osteoporosis and arthritis, and the importance of activity in delaying symptoms of dementia is well documented in the literature on Alzheimer disease. A growing number of specialty clinics focus on adults with Down syndrome, and they can be consulted regarding results of clinical trials with anti-Alzheimer medications.

Several unproven therapies have been promoted for Down syndrome, including recent attention to the memory-enhancing drug piracetam. This drug has been tried in European patients with Alzheimer disease, but has a minimal track record and no proven benefit in children with Down syndrome. Vitamin supplements have a long history of use in Down syndrome, despite a lack of scientific evidence for true vitamin deficiencies. Fortunately, neither piracetam nor the common vitamin/nutrient mixtures seem to be harmful. Parents should be warned against costly biochemical analyses, "cellular" treatments by injection of animal cell mixtures, or "patterning" treatments that impose rigid schedules on families already dealing with the added stress of disability (Cooley & Graham, 1991). Plastic surgery to alter tongue size or to correct facial features is also controversial.

Although a consensus approach to preventive management of Down syndrome has been in place for more than 20 years, areas of controversy remain. These include the frequency of thyroid studies, the value of cervical spine films in predicting risk of atlantoaxial instability, and the frequency of referrals to genetic or Down syndrome clinics. While yearly thyroid studies are often recommended, relaxation of this schedule in children with appropriate growth and development should be considered. As mentioned above, counseling for symptoms of atlantoaxial instability is considered more useful than cervical spine radiographs by the Committee on Sports Medicine and Fitness (1995). Pediatricians familiar with Down syndrome and its preventive health care recommendations are certainly capable of managing these families without involvement of a Down syndrome or genetics clinic. However, initial genetic referral for counseling and family support is essential, and referral to a multidisciplinary Down syndrome clinic is useful during transition stages (preschool, school, puberty, adulthood – see Lovell & Saul, 1999).

Description: More than 100 syndromes caused by extra or missing material from chromosomes 1 to 22, some partial and some complete trisomies with mosaicism. They range in incidence from less than 1 in 100,000 to 1 in 50,000 live births.

Clinical: Specific manifestions are predicted by determining the short (p) or long (q) arm material that is deleted (−) or duplicated (+). Problems common to all aneuploidies include pre- and postnatal growth delay; developmental disability ranging from IQ 25 to 75; early feeding problems due to hypotonia, oral clefting, or GI defects; hearing and vision deficits due to eye anomalies and ear dysplasia; cardiac anomalies such as septal defects and arterial stenoses; urogenital anomalies such as dysfunctional kidneys, urinary tract obstruction, and genital hypoplasia; skeletal defects including cervical spine anomalies, scoliosis, hip dislocation, club feet, and limb deficiencies; immune deficiencies with frequent infections, brain anomalies ranging from holoprosencephaly to microencephaly; and altered homeostasis causing exaggerated reactions to stress and procedures; unique or unusual complications can be found in Tables 7.2 and 7.3, and added to the checklist.

Laboratory: The blood chromosome study (karyotype) is definitive, defining partial monosomies such as 5p− (deleted material from the chromosome 5 short arm = cri-du-chat syndrome), partial trisomies such as 13q+ (duplicated material from the chromosome 13 long arm), and mosaics like 46,XX/47,XX+7 (trisomy 7 mosaicism in a female). Complex karyotypes may require interpretation by a clinical geneticist to determine the extra or missing segments and thereby guide management.

Genetics: The majority (85–95%) of partial aneuploidies or mosaics arise spontaneously, giving parents a low recurrence risk. Parental karyotypes are needed for partial trisomies/monosomies to recognize the minority (5–15%) that are inherited from a parent with a balanced translocation, conferring a 5–10% recurrence risk for future pregnancies.

Key management issues: Recognition of major and minor anomalies that mandate a chromosome study, neonatal evaluation for hearing, feeding, heart, urogenital, skeletal, and neurologic defects pending karyotype results, design of early intervention and developmental/behavioral monitoring programs. Mosaic patients may be difficult to recognize.

Specific growth Charts: Available for a few common disorders such as cri-du-chat syndrome.

Parent information: Educational websites and parent support groups can be found by searching on the disorder (e.g., 18p deletion syndrome), and on the Family Village (www.familyvillage.wisc) or Contact a Family (www.cafamily.org.uk) web sites.

Summary of clinical concerns

General	Learning	**Cognitive and learning differences, speech and behavior problems**
	Growth	**Low birth weight, feeding problems, short stature, microcephaly**
Facial	Eyes	**Myopia**, **strabismus**, cataracts
	Ears	Small ear canals, **chronic otitis**
	Mouth	Cleft lip/palate, **dental anomalies**, frequent caries
	Other	
Surface	Neck/trunk	**Short neck**, inguinal hernias
Skeletal	Cranial	Microcephaly, metopic synostosis
	Axial	Vertebral anomalies and fusions, kyphoscoliosis
	Limbs	Reduction defects, **hip dislocation**, **club feet**
	Other	
Internal	Digestive	Neonatal jaundice, gastrointestinal anomalies including anal atresia, gastroesophageal reflux
	Pulmonary	Increased severity and frequency of respiratory infections
	Circulatory	**Cardiac anomalies** (5–50%), cardiac failure, pulmonary hypertension
	RES	**Frequent infections**, immune defects like immunoglobulin A deficiency
	Excretory	Small kidneys, decreased tubule number, urinary tract anomalies
	Genital	**Cryptorchidism**, hypospadias, labial hypoplasia
	Other	
Neural	Central	Holoprosencephaly, agenesis corpus callosum, microencephaly, obstructive and central sleep apnea
	Motor	**Hypotonia**, oromotor dysfunction, motor delays
	Sensory	**Vision and hearing deficits**

RES, reticuloendothelial system; **concerns** of frequency >20% are **highlighted**

Key references

Gorlin, et al. (2001). *Syndromes of the Head and Neck*, 4th edn. Oxford: Oxford University Press.
Jones (1997). *Recognizable Patterns of Human Malformation*. Philadephia, PA: W.B. Saunders.
Schinzel, A. (2001). *Catalogue of Unbalanced Chromosome Aberrations in Man*. Berlin: de Gruyter.

Partial trisomy/monosomy

Preventive medical checklist (0–3 years)

Name _____ Birth date __ / __ / __ Number _____

Age	Evaluations: key concerns	Management considerations		Notes
New-born ↓ 1 month	Dysmorphology examination: anomalies	❑ Karyotype, genetic counseling[1]	❑	
	Hearing, vision:[2] eye, ear anomalies	❑ ABR; ENT;[3] opthalmology[3]	❑	
	Feeding, stooling: dysphagia, anomalies	❑ GI imaging; feeding specialist, GI[3]	❑	
	Heart: murmur, tachycardia	❑ Echocardiogram; cardiology	❑	
	Urogenital: anomalies	❑ Abdominal sonogram;[3] urology[3]	❑	
	Skeletal examination: anomalies	❑ Orthopedics[3]	❑	
	Parental adjustment	❑ Family support[4]	❑	
2 months ↓ 4 months	Growth and development[5]	❑ ECI[6]	❑	
	Hearing, vision:[2] eye, ear anomalies	❑ ABR; ENT;[3] opthalmology[3]	❑	
	Feeding, stooling: dysphagia, anomalies	❑ GI imaging; feeding specialist, GI[3]	❑	
	Heart: murmur, tachycardia	❑ Echocardiogram; cardiology	❑	
	Urogenital: anomalies	❑ Abdominal sonogram;[3] urology[3]	❑	
	Skeletal examination: anomalies	❑ Orthopedics[3]	❑	
	Parental adjustment	❑ Family support[4]	❑	
	Other:	❑	❑	
6 months ↓ 9 months	Growth and development[5]	❑ ECI[6]	❑	
	Hearing and vision[2]	❑ ABR; ENT;[3] opthalmology[3]	❑	
	Nutrition: feeding	❑ Feeding specialist; GI[3]	❑	
	Urogenital: urinary tract anomalies	❑ Urinalysis, BP;[3] urology[3]	❑	
	Skeletal examination: hip dislocation, club feet	❑ Orthopedics[3]	❑	
	Other:	❑	❑	
1 year	Growth and development[5]	❑ ECI[6]	❑	
	Hearing and vision[2]	❑ ABR; ENT;[3] opthalmology[3]	❑	
	Nutrition: feeding	❑ Feeding specialist; GI[3]	❑	
	Urogenital: urinary tract anomalies	❑ Urinalysis, BP;[3] urology[3]	❑	
	Skeletal examination: hip dislocation, club feet	❑ Orthopedics[3]	❑	
	Neck flexibility	❑ Anesthesia precautions	❑	
	Other:	❑	❑	
15 months ↓ 18 months	Growth and development[5]	❑ ECI[3]	❑	
	Hearing and vision[2]	❑ ABR; ENT;[3] opthalmology[3]	❑	
	Nutrition: feeding	❑ Feeding specialist, GI[3]	❑	
	Urogenital: urinary tract anomalies	❑ Urinalysis, BP;[3] urology[3]	❑	
2 years	Growth and development[5]	❑ ECI[6]	❑	
	Hearing and vision[2]	❑ ABR; ENT;[3] opthalmology[3]	❑	
	Nutrition: feeding	❑ Feeding specialist; GI[3]	❑	
	Urogenital: urinary tract anomalies	❑ Urinalysis, BP;[3] urology[3]	❑	
	Sleep: sleep apnea[7]	❑ Sleep study[3]	❑	
3 years	Growth and development[5]	❑ ECI[6]; family support[4]	❑	
	Hearing and vision[2]	❑ ABR; ENT;[3] opthalmology[3]	❑	
	Nutrition: feeding	❑ Feeding specialist; GI[3]	❑	
	Urogenital: urinary tract anomalies	❑ Urinalysis, BP;[3] urology[3]	❑	
	Skeletal examination: hip dislocation, club feet	❑ Orthopedics[3]	❑	
	Neck flexibility	❑ Anesthesia precautions	❑	
	Other:	❑	❑	

Partial aneuploidy concerns		Other concerns from history	
		Family history/prenatal	Social/environmental
Poor feeding, weight gain	Limb, vertebral anomalies		
Vision, hearing deficits	Renal, urinary tract anomalies	_____	_____
Eye (cataracts, strabismus)	Genital anomalies, hypoplasia	_____	_____
Chronic otitis, other infections	Brain anomalies, microcephaly	_____	_____
Jaundice, GI anomalies	Central, obstructive sleep apnea	_____	_____
Cardiac anomalies	Motor and speech delay	_____	_____

Guidelines for the neonatal period should be undertaken *at whatever age* the diagnosis is made; GI, gastrointestinal; BP, blood pressure; ABR, auditory brainstem evoked response; [1]parental chromosomes needed to look for balanced translocation and higher recurrence risk; [2]by practitioner; [3]as dictated by clinical findings; [4]parent group, family/sib, financial, and behavioral issues; [5]consider developmental pediatrician/neurologist/behavior therapist/genetics clinic according to symptoms and availability; [6]early childhood intervention including developmental monitoring and motor/speech therapy; [7]snoring, pause in breathing, daytime sleepiness, unusual sleep positioning.

Partial trisomy/monosomy

Preventive medical checklist (4–18 years)

Name _____ Birth date __ / __ / __ Number _____

Age	Evaluations: key concerns	Management considerations		Notes
4 years ↓ **6 years**	Growth:[1] microcephaly, short stature Development:[2] preschool transition Hearing and vision[2] Nutrition: feeding Urogenital: urinary tract anomalies Skeletal examination: scoliosis, contractures Other:	❑ Special growth charts if available ❑ Family support;[4] preschool program[5] ❑ Audiology; ENT;[3] opthalmology[3] ❑ Feeding specialist; GI[3] ❑ Urinalysis; BP;[3] urology[3] ❑ Orthopedics[3] ❑	❑ ❑ ❑ ❑ ❑ ❑ ❑	
7 years ↓ **9 years**	Growth[1] Development:[1] school transition[5] Hearing, vision:[2] hearing loss, myopia Urogenital: urinary tract anomalies Skeletal examination: scoliosis, contractures Neck flexibility Other:	❑ Special growth charts if available ❑ Family support;[4] school progress[6] ❑ Audiology; ENT;[3] opthalmology[3] ❑ Urinalysis; BP;[3] urology[3] ❑ Orthopedics[3] ❑ Anesthesia precautions ❑	❑ ❑ ❑ ❑ ❑ ❑ ❑	
10 years ↓ **12 years**	Growth and development[1] Hearing, vision:[2] hearing loss, myopia Urogenital: urinary tract anomalies Sleep: sleep apnea[7] Other:	❑ School progress[6] ❑ Audiology; ENT;[3] opthalmology[3] ❑ Urinalysis; BP;[3] urology[3] ❑ ENT;[3] sleep study[3] ❑	❑ ❑ ❑ ❑ ❑	
13 years ↓ **15 years**	Growth and development[1] Hearing, vision:[2] hearing loss, myopia Urogenital: urinary tract anomalies Skeletal examination: scoliosis, contractures Neck flexibility Other:	❑ School progress[6] ❑ Audiology; ENT;[3] opthalmology[3] ❑ Urinalysis; BP;[3] urology[3] ❑ Orthopedics[3] ❑ Anesthesia precautions ❑	❑ ❑ ❑ ❑ ❑ ❑	
16 years ↓ **18 years**	Growth and development[1] Puberty; genital hypoplasia Urogenital: urinary tract anomalies Skeletal examination: scoliosis, contractures Other:	❑ Family support;[4] school progress[6] ❑ Urology;[3] endocrinology[3] ❑ Urinalysis; BP;[3] urology[3] ❑ Orthopedics[3] ❑	❑ ❑ ❑ ❑ ❑	
19 years ↓ **23 years**	Adult care transition[5] Hearing, vision:[2] hearing loss, myopia Urogenital: urinary tract anomalies Skeletal examination: scoliosis, contractures Sleep: sleep apnea[7]	❑ Family support;[4] school progress[6] ❑ Audiology; ENT;[3] opthalmology[3] ❑ Urinalysis; BP;[3] urology[3] ❑ Orthopedics[3] ❑ ENT;[3] sleep study[3]	❑ ❑ ❑ ❑ ❑	
Adult	Adult care transition[5] Hearing, vision:[2] hearing loss, myopia Urogenital: urinary tract anomalies Skeletal examination: scoliosis, contractures Neck flexibility Other:	❑ Family support[4] ❑ Audiology;[3] ENT; ophthalmology ❑ Urinalysis; BP;[3] urology[3] ❑ Orthopedics[3] ❑ Anesthesia precautions ❑	❑ ❑ ❑ ❑ ❑ ❑	

Partial aneuploidy concerns		Other concerns from history	
Vision, hearing deficits Eye (strabismus, myopia) Chronic otitis, infections GI anomalies Cardiac anomalies Limb, vertebral anomalies	Renal, urinary tract anomalies Genital anomalies, hypoplasia Brain anomalies, microcephaly Central, obstructive sleep apnea Learning disabilities Employment, independent living	**Family history/prenatal** _____ _____ _____ _____	**Social/environmental** _____ _____ _____ _____

Guidelines for the neonatal period should be undertaken *at whatever age* the diagnosis is made; GI, gastrointestinal; BP, blood pressure; 1consider developmental pediatrician/neurologist/behavior therapist/genetics clinic according to symptoms and availability;2by practitioner; 3as dictated by clinical findings; 4parent group, family/sib, financial, and behavioral issues with later focus on independent living and employment; 5preschool program including developmental monitoring and motor/speech therapy; 6monitor individual education plan, educational testing, balance of special education and inclusion, academic progress, behavioral differences, later vocational planning; 7snoring, pause in breathing, daytime sleepiness, unusual sleep positioning.

Parent guide to partial trisomy/monosomy syndromes

Patients with extra or missing chromosome material have a pattern of medical and developmental changes that reflect the region of chromosome that is unbalanced. General characteristics of chromosome disorders, together with complications specific to the unbalanced segment, allow formulation of a preventive management program to optimize health and educational potential.

Incidence, causation, and diagnosis

Chromosome analysis (routine karyotype) can identify more than 150 disorders with extra (duplicated) or missing (deleted) chromosome material, including those with an entire extra or missing chromosome (complete aneuploidy) or part of a chromosome (partial trisomy/monosomy). Duplications and deletions of the long or short arms of all 22 autosomes have now been defined, including more common disorders (incidence 1 in 25–50,000 live births) like 5p– syndrome (deletion of the chromosome 5 short arm) or extremely rare disorders (less than 1 in 100,000 live births) like 6q+ syndrome (duplication of the chromosome 6 long arm). Each partial aneuploidy is accompanied by a specific pattern of anomalies (syndrome) which is determined by the specific chromosome segment that is duplicated or deficient.

Natural history and complications

Nearly all patients with chromosome disorders have growth and developmental delays, with resulting short stature and mental disability (IQs in 25–75 range according to the disorder and individual). Congenital anomalies and later abnormalities can affect any organ system including particularly the eye (wandering eyes or strabismus, cataract), ear (external ear anomalies, chronic otitis), mouth (cleft lip/palate, dental abnormalities) gastrointestinal tract (poor swallowing, gastrointestinal reflux, gastrointestinal anomalies causing obstruction), heart, urinary tract (kidney defects and defects obstructing urine flow), genital defects (cleft penis or hypospadias, undescended testicles, hernias, underdeveloped labia), skeletal defects (short neck, spinal fusions, spinal curvature or scoliosis, hip dislocation, club feet, missing fingers or toes), brain abnormalities (absent forebrain, absent corpus callosum, small brain causing microcephaly, seizures, sleep apnea), and neurosensory defects consequent to anomalies (nerve or bone, hearing loss, vision loss). Patients with chromosome abnormalities often exaggerated reactions to infectious agents (frequent or more severe infections), physical agents (cold, heat, noise), medical interventions (procedures, surgeries, drugs, anesthesia), feeding/dietary problems (vitamin deficiencies), or psychosocial changes (breaks in routine, school/employment pressures, family/social crises).

Preventive medical needs

Preventive measures include neonatal evaluation to determine the spectrum and extent of external and internal anomalies. Imaging studies of the heart, gastrointestinal tract, abdomen (kidneys, urinary tract), skeleton (spine, sacrum), and brain should be considered. Monitoring of hearing/vision, feeding, bowel function, and growth (including particularly head circumference) and neurologic function/developmental progress should be initiated in early infancy, and continued jointly with developmental pediatric, genetic, and/or neurology clinics according to symptoms and availability. Preventive management should reflect general risks for chromosome disorders as well as complications specific to the particular chromosome segment that is extra or missing.

Family counseling

Parents should have chromosome studies to see if they carry a balanced translocation that was transmitted in unbalanced form to cause partial aneuploidy in their child. Parental carriers have a 5–10% risk for partial aneuploidy with each future pregnancy, and should be counseled regarding their increased risk for miscarriage and prenatal diagnosis options. Parents with normal chromosomes have minimal risks to have another child with partial aneuploidy. Parent-oriented websites can be accessed by searching on the particular partial aneuploidy (e.g., duplication 18p), particularly within the Family Village (www.familyvillage.wisc) or Contact a Family (www.cafamily.org.uk) websites, and several specific parent support groups are available – for example, Chromosome Deletion Outreach, Inc. (www.chromodisorder.org), the Rare Chromosome Disorder Support Group (www.rarechromo.org), Recombination 8 Syndrome Family Support Group (www.rec8.org), the Chromosome 9p-Network [www.9pminus.org]; the Isodicentric 15 Exchange (www.idic15.org), and the Chromosome 18 Registry and Resource Society (www.chromosome18.org).

Preventive management of trisomy 13/18

Description: Clinical pattern caused by extra chromosome 13 material (trisomy 13 or Patau syndrome) or extra chromosome 18 material (trisomy 18 or Edwards syndrome). Trisomy 13 occurs in 1 in 12,000 and trisomy 18 in 1 in 5000–7000 live births; they have a 50–100-fold higher frequency in miscarriages.

Clinical diagnosis: Variable findings include scalp defect, microphthalmia, cleft lip and palate, polydactyly, facial changes caused by forebrain anomalies with trisomy 13; small face and jaw, abnormal ears, clenched fists, convex soles, more frequent prenatal growth retardation with trisomy 18. Both syndromes have high frequencies of major organ defects.

Laboratory: Karyotype to demonstrate trisomy 13/18 or translocation, with occasional mosaicism.

Genetics: Approximate 1% recurrence for pure trisomy 13/18, 5–10% for translocation if a parent is a carrier.

Key management issues: Neonatal recognition of brain anomalies, seizures, apnea for trisomy 13; gastrointestinal and cardiac anomalies for both trisomies; family support and palliative care options, hearing, vision, genitourinary anomalies.

Growth charts: Baty et al. (1994) reported measurements from 76 individuals with trisomy 18, 17 individuals with trisomy 13.

Parent information: Support Organization for Trisomy 18, 13, and Related Disorders (www.trisomy.org/), Trisomy 18 Support Organization (www.trisomy18support.org/), and Trisomy Online: Support for Families by Families (www.trisomyonline.org/).

Basis for management recommendations: Recommendations of Carey (1992).

Summary of clinical concerns

General	Aging	**Infant mortality** (T13: 45% at 1 month, 70% at 1 year; T18: 50% at 1 month, 90% at 1 year)
	Learning	**Severe disability** (100%)
	Growth	**Failure to thrive** (T13: 87%; T18: 96%)
	Cancer	Leukemia, neuroblastoma, Wilms tumor
Facial	Eyes	**Eye anomalies** (T13: 74% – microphthalmia, iris coloboma; T18: 27% – corneal clouding, cataracts, microphthalmia, glaucoma)
	Ears	**Malformed ears** (T18: 88%; T13: 87%), inner ear defects
	Nose	Malformed nose with underlying holoprosencephaly (T13: 70%)
	Mouth	**Oromotor dysfunction**, feeding problems, cleft lip (T13: 50%; T18: 6%), cleft palate (T13: 55%; T18: 7%)
Surface	Neck/trunk	Short neck (T13: 79%), **inguinal hernia** (T13: 40%; T18: 56%); umbilical hernia
	Epidermal	Scalp defect (T13: 60%); Redundant neck skin
Skeletal	Cranial	**Microcephaly** (T13: 86%; T18: 70%), wide sutures and fontanel (T18)
	Axial	Short neck (T13: 79%), rib anomalies, vertebral anomalies, short sternum (T18)
	Limbs	Polydactyly (T13: 60%), **overlap of fingers** (T13: 68%; T18: 89%), clubfoot (T13: 15%; T18: 89%), radial aplasia
Internal	Digestive	GI anomalies: omphalocele (T13: 11%; T18: 9%), esophageal atresia, anal atresia, Meckel diverticulum, incomplete fixation of colon
	Circulatory	**Cardiac anomalies** (T13: 75% – septal defects, patent ductus arteriosus (PDA), dextrocardia; T18: 85% – valvular disease, patent foramen ovale (PFO), septal defects, PDA, coarctation of aorta)
	Endocrine	T13 – pancreatic dysplasia, exocrine insufficiency; T18 – ectopic pancreas, thyroglossal duct cyst, hypothyroidism
	Excretory	**Renal anomalies** (T13: 70% – polycystic kidneys, urinary tract anomalies; T18: 30% – cystic kidneys, horseshoe kidney, double ureter), urinary tract infections
	Genital	**Cryptorchidism** (T13,T18: 100%), prominent clitoris (T18: 89%), bicornuate uterus
Neural	Central	**Hypertonia** (T13, T18: 60%), **seizures** (T13: 37%; T18: 45%), apnea (T13: 58%), holoprosencephaly (T13: 70%), absent corpus callosum (T18: 20%), spina bifida (T13: 4%; T18: 1%)
	Sensory	Hearing deficits (T13: 50%), sensorineural deafness, blindness

Concerns of frequency >20% are **highlighted**

Key references

Baty, et al. (1994). Natural history of trisomy 18 and trisomy 13: I. Growth, physical assessment, medical histories, survival and recurrence risk; II. Psychomotor development. *American Journal of Medical Genetics* 49A:175–88; 189–94.

Carey (1992). Health supervision and anticipatory guidance for children with genetic disorders (including specific recommendations for trisomy 21, trisomy 18, and neurofibromatosis). *Pediatric Clinics of North America* 39:25–53.

Trisomy 13/18

Preventive medical checklist (0–3 years)

Name _____ Birth date __ / __ / __ Number _____

Age	Evaluations: key concerns		Management considerations		Notes
New-born ↓ 1 month	Dysmorphology examination: anomalies	☐	Karyotype, genetic counseling[1]	☐	
	Hearing, vision:[2] eye, ear anomalies	☐	ABR, ophthalmology[3]	☐	
	Feeding, stooling: dysphagia, anomalies	☐	GI imaging; feeding specialist; GI[3]	☐	
	Heart: murmur, tachycardia	☐	Echocardiogram; cardiology	☐	
	Urogenital: anomalies	☐	Abdominal sonogram;[3] urology[3]	☐	
	Neurologic: seizures, apnea	☐	Head MRI;[3] neurology[3]	☐	
	Parental adjustment	☐	Family support[4]	☐	
2 months ↓ 4 months	Growth and development[5]	☐	ECI;[6] family support[4]	☐	
	Hearing, vision:[2] deafness, cataracts	☐	ABR, ophthalmology[3]	☐	
	Feeding, stooling: dysphagia, anomalies	☐	GI imaging; feeding specialist; GI[3]	☐	
	Heart: murmur, tachycardia	☐	Echocardiogram; cardiology	☐	
	Urogenital: anomalies	☐	Abdominal sonogram;[3] urology[3]	☐	
	Neurologic: seizures, apnea	☐	Head MRI;[3] neurology[3]	☐	
	Parental adjustment	☐	Family support[4]	☐	
	Other:	☐		☐	
6 months ↓ 9 months	Growth and development[5]	☐	ECI;[6] family support[4]	☐	
	Hearing and vision[2]	☐	ABR; ENT;[3] opthalmology[3]	☐	
	Nutrition: feeding	☐	Feeding specialist; GI[3]	☐	
	Urogenital: urinary tract anomalies	☐	Urinalysis; BP;[3] urology[3]	☐	
	Skeletal examination: hip dislocation, club feet	☐	Orthopedics[3]	☐	
	Other:	☐		☐	
1 year	Growth and development[5]	☐	ECI;[6] family support[4]	☐	
	Hearing and vision[2]	☐	ABR; ENT; opthalmology	☐	
	Nutrition: feeding	☐	Feeding specialist, GI[3]	☐	
	Urogenital: urinary tract anomalies	☐	Urinalysis; BP;[3]urology[3]	☐	
	Neurologic: seizures, apnea	☐	Head MRI;[3] neurology[3]	☐	
	Neck flexibility	☐	Anesthesia precautions	☐	
	Other:	☐		☐	
15 months ↡ 18 months	Growth and development[5]	☐	ECI;[6] family support[4]	☐	
	Hearing and vision[2]	☐	ABR; ENT;[3] opthalmology[3]	☐	
	Nutrition: feeding	☐	Feeding specialist; GI[3]	☐	
	Urogenital: urinary tract anomalies	☐	Urinalysis; BP;[3] urology[3]	☐	
2 years	Growth and development[5]	☐	ECI;[6] family support[3]	☐	
	Hearing and vision[2]	☐	ABR; ENT; ophthalmology	☐	
	Nutrition: feeding	☐	Feeding specialist; GI[3]	☐	
	Neurologic: seizures, apnea	☐	Head MRI;[3] neurology[3]	☐	
	Heart: murmur, tachycardia	☐	Sleep study[3]	☐	
3 years	Growth and development[5]	☐	ECI[6]; family support[4]	☐	
	Hearing and vision[2]	☐	ABR; ENT; ophthalmology	☐	
	Nutrition: feeding	☐	Feeding specialist; GI[3]	☐	
	Urogenital: urinary tract anomalies	☐	Urinalysis; BP;[3] urology[3]	☐	
	Neurologic: seizures, apnea	☐	Head MRI;[3] neurology[3]	☐	
	Heart: murmur, tachycardia	☐	Echocardiogram;[3] cardiology[3]	☐	
	Other:	☐		☐	

Trisomy 13/18 concerns		Other concerns from history	
		Family history/prenatal	Social/environmental
Poor feeding, weight gain	Limb, vertebral anomalies		
Vision, hearing deficits	Renal, urinary tract anomalies	_____	_____
Eye (microphthalmia, strabismus)	Genital anomalies	_____	_____
	Brain anomalies, microcephaly	_____	_____
Chronic otitis, other infections	Severe developmental delays	_____	_____
GI anomalies	Infant mortality, palliative care		
Cardiac anomalies			

Guidelines for the neonatal period should be undertaken *at whatever age* the diagnosis is made; ABR, auditory brainstem evoked response; BP, blood pressure; GI, gastrointestinal; [1]parental chromosomes only if child has translocation; [2]by practitioner; [3]as dictated by clinical findings; [4]discuss palliative care options, parent group, family/sib, financial, and behavioral issues; [5]consider developmental pediatrics/genetics clinic/neurology according to symptoms and availability; [6]early childhood intervention including developmental monitoring and motor/speech therapy.

Trisomy 13/18

Preventive medical checklist (4–18 years)

Name _____ Birth date __/__/__ Number _____

Age	Evaluations: key concerns	Management considerations		Notes
4 years ↓ 6 years	Growth:[1] microcephaly, short stature Development:[2] preschool transition Hearing and vision[2] Nutrition: feeding Urogenital: urinary tract anomalies Skeletal examination: osteoporosis, fractures Other:	❑ Trisomy 13/18 growth data ❑ Family support;[4] preschool program[6] ❑ Audiology; ENT;[3] opthalmology[3] ❑ Feeding specialist; GI[3] ❑ Urinalysis; BP;[3] urology[3] ❑ Orthopedics[3] ❑	❑ ❑ ❑ ❑ ❑ ❑ ❑	
7 years ↓ 9 years	Growth[1] Development:[1] school transition[6] Hearing, vision:[2] hearing loss, myopia Urogenital: urinary tract anomalies Abdominal examination: tumors, obstipation Neck flexibility Other:	❑ Down syndrome charts[1] ❑ Family support;[4] school care plan[5] ❑ Audiology; ENT;[3] opthalmology[3] ❑ Urinalysis; BP;[3] urology[3] ❑ GI specialist[3] ❑ Anesthesia precautions ❑	❑ ❑ ❑ ❑ ❑ ❑ ❑	
10 years ↓ 12 years	Growth and development[1] Hearing, vision:[2] hearing loss, myopia Urogenital: urinary tract anomalies Skeletal examination: osteoporosis, fractures Other:	❑ Family support;[4] school care plan[5] ❑ Audiology; ENT;[3] opthalmology[3] ❑ Urinalysis; BP;[3] urology[3] ❑ Orthopedics[3] ❑	❑ ❑ ❑ ❑ ❑	
13 years ↓ 15 years	Growth and development[1] Hearing, vision:2 hearing loss, myopia Urogenital: urinary tract anomalies Abdominal examination: tumors, obstipation Heart: murmurs, valvular disease Other:	❑ Family support;[4] school care plan[5] ❑ Audiology; ENT;[3] opthalmology[3] ❑ Urinalysis; BP;[3] urology[3] ❑ GI specialist[3] ❑ Echocardiogram,[3] cardiology[3] ❑	❑ ❑ ❑ ❑ ❑ ❑	
16 years ↓ 18 years	Growth and development[1] Hearing, vision:2 hearing loss, myopia Urogenital: urinary tract anomalies Skeletal examination: osteoporosis, fractures Other:	❑ Family support;[4] school care plan[5] ❑ Audiology; ENT;[3] opthalmology[3] ❑ Urinalysis; BP;[3] urology[3] ❑ Orthopedics[3] ❑	❑ ❑ ❑ ❑ ❑	
19 years ↓ 23 years	Adult care transition[5] Hearing, vision:[2] hearing loss, myopia Urogenital: urinary tract anomalies Abdominal examination: tumors, obstipation	❑ Family support;[4] school care plan[5] ❑ Audiology; ENT;[3] opthalmology[3] ❑ Urinalysis; BP;[3] urology[3] ❑ GI specialist[3]	❑ ❑ ❑ ❑	
Adult	Adult care transition[5] Hearing, vision:[2] hearing loss, myopia Urogenital: urinary tract anomalies Skeletal examination: osteoporosis, fractures Heart: murmurs, valvular disease Abdominal examination: tumors, obstipation Other:	❑ Family support[4] ❑ Audiology;[3] ENT; ophthalmology ❑ Urinalysis, BP;[3] urology[3] ❑ Orthopedics[3] ❑ Echocardiogram;[3] cardiology[3] ❑ GI specialist[3] ❑	❑ ❑ ❑ ❑ ❑ ❑ ❑	

Trisomy 13/18 concerns		Other concerns from history	
Vision, hearing deficits Eye (strabismus, myopia) Hearing loss GI anomalies Cardiac valve anomalies Limb, vertebral anomalies	Renal, urinary tract anomalies Genital anomalies, hypoplasia Osteoporosis, fractures Leukemias, Wilms tumor Seizures, microcephaly Severe mental disability Chronic care issues	**Family history/prenatal** _____ _____ _____ _____	**Social/environmental** _____ _____ _____ _____

Guidelines for the neonatal period should be undertaken *at whatever age* the diagnosis is made; BP, blood pressure; GI, gastrointestinal; [1]consider developmental pediatrics/genetics clinic/neurology according to symptoms and availability; [2]by practitioner; [3]as dictated by clinical findings; [4]parent group, family/sib, financial, and behavioral issues with focus on respite, hospice, and chronic care issues; [5]school care plan for severe disabilities.

Parent guide to trisomy 13/18

Children with extra chromosomal material representing an entire chromosome 13 or 18 are affected with the trisomy 13/18 syndrome. The terms "Patau syndrome" and "Edwards syndrome" derive, respectively, from the physicians who described trisomy 13 and 18 syndrome in 1960. The extra chromosomal material may be present as a free-standing chromosome (trisomy) or be attached to another chromosome as a translocation. Patients with mosaicism for trisomy 13/18 have variable proportions of normal and trisomic cells a much milder phenotype. Although each syndrome has a distinctive pattern of anomalies, trisomies 13 and 18 are discussed together because they have many overlapping features and a similar natural history.

Incidence, causation, and diagnosis

Trisomy 13 as a free-standing chromosome or translocation occurs in about 1 in 12,000 live births, with a frequency in miscarriages some 100-fold higher. Trisomy 18 is slightly more common, with a frequency between 1 in 5000 and 1 in 7000 live births. Brain anomalies often bias the facial appearance in trisomy 13, with small eyes, underdeveloped nose, and/or cleft lip. Patients with trisomy 18 often have a characteristic "clenched fist" with overlapping fingers. Following the general rule that no one anomaly is characteristic of one syndrome, the clenched fist may occur in other disorders associated with decreased movement or nerve supply to the hands. Patients with the genetic Pena–Shokeir syndrome of fixed joints and small head, disorders with decreased fetal movement, and trisomy 13 may resemble patients with trisomy 18. The karyotype (chromosome study) establishes the diagnosis of trisomy 13/18 when these syndromes are suspected. Fluorescent *in situ* hybridization (FISH) testing can provide a diagnosis in a few hours, but should be followed by routine chromosome testing to determine the presence of trisomy versus translocation.

Natural history and complications

Significant infant mortality occurs in trisomy 13 (55% survive 1 month, 14% survive 1 year) and trisomy 18 (35% survive 1 month, 5% survive year). Mortality figures vary considerably among studies, with some full trisomy 13/18 patients surviving into their late teens. Severe feeding problems with failure to thrive and multiple internal anomalies can be expected; increased muscle tone, seizures, and uncoordinated swallowing place these patients at high risk for aspiration (swallowing fluid into the lung) which may further increase their risks for breathing problems (apnea). Eye, external ear, inner ear, heart, urinary tract, and brain/spinal cord anomalies are common along with certain tumors (leukemias, neuroblastoma, Wilms). Psychomotor development does occur in patients with trisomy 13/18, with developmental quotients (developmental age divided by chronologic age) averaging 0.18 in trisomy 18 individuals (age 1–232 months) and 0.25 in trisomy 13 individuals (age 1–130 months). Older children responded to words or phrases, communicated with simple words or signs, crawled, used a walker, interacted with others, and achieved some toileting skills.

Preventive medical needs

Crucial perinatal decisions involve the aggressiveness of medical and surgical management. Trisomy 13 and 18 patients are often recognized prenatally, offering the opportunity to counsel the parents concerning delivery and neonatal resuscitation options. Avoidance of Cesarean delivery or extreme resuscitation measures is often appropriate, especially in infants with major organ anomalies who may not survive the infantile period. After birth, evaluation for internal anomalies and agreement on interventional versus palliative care options should be reached with the parents. A reasonable strategy is to recommend simple surgeries and supportive strategies that alleviate suffering or ease management; more elaborate surgery or prolonged intensive care is usually not recommended. Appropriate fluid and nutritional support are always indicated. As with any medical crisis, social and pastoral services should be included as part of the medical counseling. The ~10% of patients surviving infancy will need preventive care including careful monitoring of growth, feeding, and nutrition. Feeding and gastrointestinal specialists may be required to achieve adequate caloric intake in these hypertonic, irritable, and neurologically immature patients. Malformations of the eye, external ear, and inner ear are frequent, emphasizing the need for frequent hearing and vision assessment to ensure maximal function. Urinary tract anomalies are frequent in both trisomies, and liver cancer or Wilms tumor has been encountered in longer survivors with trisomy 18. These risks should be monitored by performing periodic urinalyses and abdominal palpation. The debilitated state of many patients requires vigilance for respiratory infections or osteoporosis, and attention to social or local services such as social work, clergy, occupational or physical therapy, respite, and hospice care. The medical interventions listed on the trisomy 13/18 checklist should obviously be tailored to prognosis, since palliative care is appropriate for patients with severe anomalies.

Family counseling

Parents of children with trisomy have recurrence risks of about 1%, increasing in the usual way with maternal age (2–3% total risk by maternal age 40 years). Parental chromosome studies are required if the infant has translocation 13 or 18, with risks in the 5–10% range if one parent is a balanced translocation carrier. If genetic counseling is not available during the neonatal period, then referral to a genetics clinic is essential. Prenatal diagnosis via chorionic villus sampling or amniocentesis is an option for subsequent pregnancies.

Preventive management of Down syndrome

Description: Clinical pattern caused by extra chromosome 21 material with an incidence of 1 in 800–1000 births.

Clinical: Variable findings include characteristic facial appearance due to flat occiput, up-slanting eyes, epicanthal folds, and shallow nasal bridge; small ears, extra neck folds, single palmar creases, curved fifth fingers, large space/deep crease between first and second toes; hypotonia with head lag and frog-leg posture; hearing/vision, heart, GI, thyroid defects.

Laboratory: The blood chromosome study (karyotype) is definitive, showing extra chromosome 21 due to trisomy (96%), translocation (3%), or mosaicism (1%). Rapid results can be obtained by FISH but need confirmation with a full karyotype.

Genetics: Trisomy 21 is sporadic with approximate 1% recurrence risk that increases with maternal age; parents of children with translocations require chromosome studies and have 10–95% recurrence risks if they carry the translocation present.

Key management issues: Positive attitude with people-first language (child with Down syndrome); neonatal evaluation for hearing, heart defects, and GI anomalies; monitoring for feeding, growth, hearing/vision, thyroid, and cervical spine problems; early intervention and developmental/behavioral monitoring; parental support and parent groups.

Specific growth Charts: Available for height, weight, head circumference and developmental progress (Cronk et al., 1988) or go to (www.ds-health.com) for growth charts, health information, and preventive care guidelines.

Parent information: National Down Syndrome Congress (www.ndsccenter.org), National Down Syndrome Society (www.ndss.org), Down's Syndrome Association (downs-syndrome.org.uk); go to www.downsed.org for information about educating children with Down syndrome or to www.woodbinehouse.com for a good series of books for parents.

Basis for management recommendations: Consensus guidelines from Cooley & Graham (1991), Carey (1992), and Committee on Genetics (2001).

Summary of clinical concerns

General	Learning	Cognitive and learning **differences**, expressive language disorder
	Behavior	Behavior problems (10%) – hyperactivity, oppositional, adjustment, adolescent mental health problems (depression, anxiety)
	Growth	**Feeding problems, short stature, obesity**
Facial	Eyes	**Hyperopia, astigmatism** (70%), **strabismus** (20–40%), **blepharitis** (30–46%)
	Ears	**Small ear canals** (53%), **chronic otitis** (40–60%), cholesteatoma
	Nose	**Shallow nasal bridge** (61%), **sinusitis, chronic nasal discharge**
	Mouth	**Tooth anomalies** (23–47%), **periodontal disease** (90%), **sleep apnea** (31%), protruding tongue
Surface	Neck/trunk	**Lax connective tissue**, inguinal hernias
	Epidermal	**Dry skin**, alopecia, skin rashes
Skeletal	Cranial	Microcephaly, brachycephaly
	Axial	Atlantoaxial or occipitoatlantal instability (2–5%)
	Limbs	Slipped femoral epiphysis, arthritis, joint dislocations
Internal	Digestive	**Neonatal jaundice** (60%), anal stenosis, **constipation** (30%), gastrointestinal anomalies (10–18%), Hirshsprung disease, gastroesophageal reflux, celiac disease
	Pulmonary	Increased severity and frequency of **respiratory infections**
	Circulatory	**Cardiac anomalies** (40–50%), cardiac failure, pulmonary hypertension
	Endocrine	**Hypothyroidism** (22–40%), type I diabetes
	RES	**Frequent infections** (increased 12-fold), neonatal transient myeloproliferative disorder, leukemias (increased 10–20-fold)
	Excretory	Cystitis, renal anomalies
	Genital	**Cryptorchidism** (14–27%), micropenis, infertility
Neural	Central	Early senescence, dementia, **Alzheimer disease**
	Motor	**Hypotonia**, oromotor dysfunction, motor delays
	Sensory	**Vision and hearing deficits** (50–70%)

RES, reticuloendothelial system; **concerns** of frequency >20% are **highlighted**

Key references

Carey, J.C. (1992). Health supervision and anticipatory guidance for children with genetic disorders (including specific recommendations for trisomy 21, trisomy 18, and neurofibromatosis). *Pediatric Clinics of North America* 39:25–53.

Clark, D. & Wilson, G.N. (2003). Behavioral assessment of children with Down syndrome using the Reiss psychopathology scale. *American Journal of Medical Genetics* 118A:210–16.

Committee on Genetics (2001). Health supervision for children with Down syndrome. *Pediatrics* 107:442–9.

Cooley, W.C., Graham, J.M., Jr. (1991). Down syndrome – an update and review for the primary pediatrician. *Clinical Pediatrics* 30:233–53.

Down syndrome

Preventive medical checklist (0–3 years)

Name _____ Birth date __ / __ / __ Number _____

Age	Evaluations: key concerns	Management considerations	Notes
New born ↓ **1 month**	Dysmorphology examination: anomalies ☐ Hearing, vision:[5] deafness, cataracts Color: jaundice, cyanosis Feeding: reflux, poor intake Stooling: anal stenosis, megacolon Heart: murmur, tachycardia Parental adjustment	Karyotype, genetic counseling[1] ☐ ABR ☐ CBC, differential ☐ Feeding specialist; video swallow[3] ☐ Rectal examination ☐ Echocardiogram; cardiology ☐ Family support[4] ☐	Transient myeloproliferative disorder significantly increases risk of later leukemia
2 months ↓ **4 months**	Growth and development[5] Nutrition: feeding, poor intake Stooling: constipation[3] Hearing and vision[2] Eyes, eyelids: blepharitis Neck flexibility[2] Parental adjustment Other:	ECI;[6] Down syndrome charts ☐ Extra feeding;[3] feeding specialist[3] ☐ Rectal examination ☐ ABR[3] ☐ Saline washes;[3] ophthalmology[3] ☐ Anesthesia precautions ☐ Family support[4] ☐ ☐	
6 months ↓ **9 months**	Growth and development[5] Nutrition: feeding, constipation Hearing and vision[2] Eyes, eyelids: blepharitis, strabismus Ears, nose, sinuses: congestion Other:	ECI[6] ☐ Supplements;[3] laxatives;[3] oromotor therapy[3] ☐ ABR[3] ☐ Saline washes;[3] ophthalmology ☐ Nasal saline;[3] ENT, audiology ☐ ☐	
1 year	Growth and development[5] Feeding, stooling: reflux, constipation Thyroid: hypothyroidism Eyes, eyelids: blepharitis, strabismus Ears, nose, sinuses: congestion Neck flexibility Other:	ECI[6] ☐ Supplements;[3] laxatives[3] ☐ T[4], TSH; endocrinology[3] ☐ Saline washes[3] ☐ Nasal saline[3] ☐ Anesthesia precautions ☐ ☐	
15 months ↓ **18 months**	Growth and development[5] Eyes, eyelids: blepharitis, strabismus Feeding, stooling: reflux, constipation Neck flexibility	ECI[6] ☐ Saline washes[3] ☐ Supplements;[3] laxatives[3] ☐ Anesthesia precautions ☐	
2 years	Growth and development[5] Thyroid: hypothyroidism Hearing/vision:[2] strabismus, myopia HEENT: blepharitis, otitis, sinusitis Sleep: sleep apnea[7]	ECI[6] ☐ T[4], TSH;[3] endocrinology[3] ☐ ENT; ophthalmology ☐ Nasal saline;[3] saline eye washes;[3] allergist[3] ☐ Sleep study[3] ☐	
3 years	Growth and development[5] Thyroid: hypothyroidism Hearing/vision:[2] strabismus, myopia Neck flexibility: AOI, AAI HEENT: blepharitis, otitis, sinusitis Skin, hair: dry skin, alopecia Other:	Down syndrome charts; ECI;[6] family support[4] ☐ T4, TSH; endocrinology[3] ☐ Audiology; ENT;[3] ophthalmology ☐ Cervical spine flexion/extension radiographs[1] ☐ Nasal saline;[3] saline eye washes;[3] allergist[3] ☐ Dermatology[3] ☐ ☐	

Down syndrome concerns		Other concerns from history	
Poor feeding, weight gain Vision, hearing deficits Eye (cataracts, strabismus) Chronic otitis, sinusitis Hypothyroidism Jaundice, polycythemia Constipation, anal stenosis	GI anomalies, celiac disease Cardiac anomalies Cryptorchidism, micropenis Hypotonia, seizures Obstructive sleep apnea Atlanto-occipital/axial instability Motor and speech delay	**Family history/prenatal** _____ _____ _____ _____ _____	**Social/environmental** _____ _____ _____ _____ _____

Guidelines for the neonatal period should be undertaken *at whatever age* the diagnosis is made; CBC, contralateral breast cancer; GI, gastrointestinal; TSH, thyroid-stimulating hormone; ABR, auditory brainstem evoked response; AOI, atlanto-occipital instability; AAI, atlanto-axial instability; [1]parental chromosomes only if child has translocation; [2]by practitioner; [3]as dictated by clinical findings; [4]parent group, family/sib, financial, and behavioral issues; [5]consider developmental pediatrician/neurologist/behavior therapist/Down syndrome clinic according to symptoms and availability; [6]early childhood intervention including developmental monitoring and motor/speech therapy; [7]snoring, pause in breathing, daytime sleepiness, unusual sleep positioning.

Down syndrome

Preventive medical checklist (4–18 years)

Name _____ Birth date __ / __ / __ Number _____

Age	Evaluations: key concerns	Management considerations	Notes
4 years ↓ **6 years**	Growth:[1] celiac disease Development:[2] preschool transition[5] Hearing, vision:[2] hearing loss, myopia Thyroid: hypothyroidism Sleep: sleep apnea[7] Skin, hair: dry skin, alopecia Other:	❑ Down syndrome charts;[1] celiac panel[3] ❑ ❑ Family support;[4] preschool program[5] ❑ ❑ Audiology;[3] ophthalmology ❑ ❑ T4, TSH; endocrinology[3] ❑ ❑ ENT;[3] sleep study[3] ❑ ❑ Dermatology[3] ❑ ❑ ❑	
7 years ↓ **9 years**	Growth[1] Development:[1] school transition Hearing, vision:[2] hearing loss, myopia Thyroid: hypothyroidism Nutrition: obesity Neck flexibility[2] Other:	❑ Down syndrome charts[1] ❑ ❑ Family support;[4] school progress[6] ❑ ❑ Audiology;[3] ophthalmology ❑ ❑ T4, TSH; endocrinology[3] ❑ ❑ Dietary counsel; activities; exercise ❑ ❑ Anesthesia precautions ❑ ❑ ❑	
10 years ↓ **12 years**	Growth and development[1] Hearing and vision[2] Nutrition: obesity Sleep: sleep apnea[7] Other:	❑ Celiac panel;[3] school progress[6] ❑ ❑ Audiology;[3] ophthalmology ❑ ❑ Dietary counsel; activities; exercise ❑ ❑ ENT;[3] sleep study[3] ❑ ❑ ❑	
13 years ↓ **15 years**	Growth and development[1] Hearing and vision[2] Puberty; thyroid: hyper- and hypothyroid Nutrition: obesity Neck flexibility: AOI, AAI Other:	❑ Down syndrome charts;[1] school progress[6] ❑ ❑ Audiology;[3] ophthalmology ❑ ❑ T4, TSH; endocrinology[3] ❑ ❑ Dietary counsel; activities; exercise ❑ ❑ Cervical spine flexion/extension radiographs ❑ ❑ ❑	
16 years ↓ **18 years**	Growth and development[1] Puberty; thyroid: hyper- and hypothyroid Nutrition: obesity Skin, hair: dry skin, alopecia Other:	❑ Family support;[4] school progress[6] ❑ ❑ T4, TSH; endocrinology[3] ❑ ❑ Dietary counsel; activities; exercise ❑ ❑ Dermatology[3] ❑ ❑ ❑	
19 years ↓ **23 years**	Adult care transition[5] Hearing/vision:[2] myopia, astigmatism Thyroid: hyper- and hypothyroid Nutrition: obesity Sleep: sleep apnea[7]	❑ Family support;[4] school progress[6] ❑ ❑ ENT; ophthalmology ❑ ❑ T4, TSH; endocrinology[3] ❑ ❑ Dietary counsel; activities; exercise ❑ ❑ ENT;[3] sleep study[3] ❑	
Adult	Adult care transition[5] Hearing/vision:[2] myopia, astigmatism Thyroid: hyper- and hypothyroid Heart: mitral valve prolapse Nutrition: obesity Skin, hair: dry skin, alopecia Other:	❑ Family support[4] ❑ ❑ Audiology;[3] ENT; ophthalmology ❑ ❑ T4, TSH; endocrinology[3] ❑ ❑ Cardiology[3] ❑ ❑ Dietary counsel; activities; exercise ❑ ❑ Dermatology[3] ❑ ❑ ❑	

Down syndrome concerns		Other concerns from history	
Hearing, vision Cataracts, myopia Sinusitis Hypothyroidism Mitral valve prolapse	Obesity, exercise Constipation, celiac disease Seizures, sleep apnea Atlanto-occipital/axial instability Speech, learning, behavior Employment, independent living	**Family history/prenatal** _____ _____ _____ _____	**Social/environmental** _____ _____ _____ _____

Guidelines for the neonatal period should be undertaken *at whatever age* the diagnosis is made; TSH, thyroid-stimulating hormone; AOI, atlanto-occipital instability; AAI, atlantoaxial instability; [1]consider developmental pediatrician/neurologist/behavior therapist/Down syndrome clinic according to symptoms and availability; [2]by practitioner; [3]as dictated by clinical findings; [4]parent group, family/sib, financial, and behavioral issues with later focus on independent living and employment; [5]preschool program including developmental monitoring and motor/speech therapy; [6]monitor individual education plan, educational testing, balance of special education and inclusion, academic progress, behavioral differences, later vocational planning; [7]snoring, pause in breathing, daytime sleepiness, unusual sleep positioning.

Parent guide to Down syndrome

Patients with an entire extra copy of chromosome 21 have a pattern of medical and developmental changes called Down syndrome. Modern medical and educational approaches offer excellent quality of life to persons with Down syndrome, enabling an optimistic outlook for families and their health care professionals.

Incidence, causation, and diagnosis

The extra 21 chromosome may arise by abnormal cell division (non-disjunction) to produce a free-standing chromosome (trisomy 21–96% of cases) or by joining of the extra 21 material to another chromosome (translocation: 2–3% of cases). Patients with mixtures of normal and trisomy 21 cells (mosaic: 1% of cases) may have slightly better outcomes. The incidence of Down syndrome is 1 in 650 to 1 in 1000 live births and shows little variation by ethnic group. Increasing maternal age is a significant risk factor, rising from about 1 in 2000 at age 20 years to 1 in 50 at age 40. The newborn with Down syndrome is often recognized because of an unusual facial appearance and low muscle tone. Characteristic minor anomalies that assist in making the diagnosis include: flat occiput (back of the head), up-slanting eyes, folds at the eye corners (epicanthal folds), white spots in the iris (Brushfield spots), extra neck skin, single creases on the palms, curved fifth fingers (clinodactyly), and a broad space/deep crease between the first and second toes.

Natural history and complications

Improvements in the quality of life enjoyed by individuals with Down syndrome are indicated by the 50% mortality by age 5 in 1965 compared with the 80% survival to age 30 or beyond in 1991. Congenital anomalies or underdevelopment can affect any organ system, including particularly the heart, gastrointestinal tract, eyes, ears, teeth, kidney, and skeleton. A harmless, short-lived proliferation of white blood cells may occur in the neonatal period that increases the later risk for leukemia (<1% lifelong). Neonatal jaundice, feeding problems, and narrowing (stenosis) of the anus may cause painful bowel movements and/or constipation. Respiratory infections are more frequent and severe in children with Down syndrome, including chronic otitis, sinusitis, and pneumonia. Tonsillectomy and adenoidectomy are often required, but these procedures may have postoperative complications. Correctable problems such as obstructive sleep apnea, constipation, wandering eyes (strabismus), thyroid hormone abnormalities, dental anomalies, atlantoaxial (neck spine) instability, and cryptorchidism (undescended testicles) are important not to miss. Developmental delays, learning differences, and speech problems are universal, and there is a 10% risk for behavior and psychiatric problems in older individuals with Down syndrome. Despite neuropathologic changes typical of Alzheimer disease in 100% of individuals over age 35 years, symptomatic memory loss and dementia is much less frequent.

Preventive medical needs

Preventive measures include neonatal evaluation of feeding, growth, bowel function, and heart status via echocardiogram annual thyroid testing, early assessment and yearly monitoring of hearing and vision including referral to a pediatric ophthalmologist by age 6–8 months. Annual thyroid tests, X-rays of the cervical spine at age 3 years and subsequent 10-year intervals, and alertness for sleep apnea are important during childhood. Because of their susceptibility to infection, children and adolescents with Down syndrome should receive all immunizations, including pneumococcal, varicella, and influenza vaccines in children with respiratory difficulties. Red or swollen eyelids (blepharitis) can result in unsightly deformities or damage to the eye surface and is easily prevented by washing them with baby shampoo (or saline, if shampoo is irritating) during baths. Nasal saline drops (two in each nostril, morning and night) prevent drying of the mucosa and help prevent colds and sinusitis that are so common in early childhood. Preventive medical checklists for Down syndrome (pp. 2–3) have been used for over two decades and have been endorsed by organizations such as the American Academy of Pediatrics. Parents should be skeptical about unproven therapies including memory-enhancing drugs (e.g., Piracetam), vitamin supplements, biochemical analyses, "cellular" injections, or "patterning" exercise treatments. Improved outcomes from early childhood intervention and later therapies have been demonstrated in controlled trials.

Family counseling

Genetic counseling is needed for parents of children with Down syndrome and for women of "advanced" maternal age (>35). The recurrence risk for parents who have a child with trisomy 21 is 1% if the mother is under age 35, increasing slightly with maternal age to about 2% at age 40–45 years. Parents of children with translocation Down syndrome should have chromosome studies to see if they carry a balanced translocation – parental carriers can have risks between 5% and 100% to have another child with Down syndrome. Pre-implantation or prenatal diagnostic techniques accurately detect Down syndrome by chromosome studies on fetal cells, but maternal serum assays (α-fetoprotein (AFP), triple test, quad screen) are only useful for screening. Counseling should avoid the use of pejorative terms and promote the use of people-first language ("child with Down syndrome" rather than "Down child"). National and local Down syndrome parent groups are tremendously helpful, and most have parent volunteers that will guide and advocate for new families.

8

Sex chromosome aneuploidy and X-linked mental retardation syndromes

Genes on the X chromosome have important roles in cognitive function, as illustrated by the excess of males with severe mental retardation. Remarkable also are the cognitive and behavioral abnormalities in sex chromosome aneuploidies such as the Klinefelter or XYY syndrome. The striking cognitive disability and psychiatric problems that are shared by many sex chromosome aneuploidy and X-linked mental retardation (XLMR) syndromes provide the rationale for their joint treatment in this chapter. The Turner, Klinefelter, and fragile X syndromes will be discussed in detail.

SEX CHROMOSOME ANEUPLOIDY

Sex chromosome imbalance usually has a milder phenotype than autosomal aneuploidy. Tables 8.1 and 8.2 summarize common sex chromosome aneuploidies in females and males. Mild cognitive disabilities, behavioral disorders, and reproductive problems predominate as complications of sex chromosome aneuploidy. Not listed in the tables are rare mosaic or chimeric individuals (e.g., individuals with mixtures of normal and aneuploid cells) that may cause pseudohermaphroditism or ambiguous genitalia. The presence of Y-chromosome-containing cell lines in individuals without testes should trigger surveillance for intra-abdominal germinal tumors; these occur occasionally in X chromosome deletions (Table 8.1). Multidisciplinary management by urology, gynecology, and endocrinology is recommended in such cases.

Turner syndrome

Terminology

Females with short stature, immature sexual development, and webbed neck exhibit features first described by Bonnevie and Ullrich, later popularized by Turner (Frías et al., 2003; Halac & Zimmerman, 2004). Bonnevie–Ullrich and Ullrich–Turner

Table 8.1. Sex chromosome aneuploidy in females

Disorder	Karyotype	Incidence*	Complications
Turner syndrome	45,X; 45,Xr(X)	1 in 5000	Normal mental development
Del(Xp)	Xpter→p22/p21 Xpter→p12/p11 46,Xi(Xq)	10–50	Variable, mild features of Turner syndrome with short stature, menstrual irregularities, ovarian failure
Del(Xq)	Xq11/q12→qter Xq22/q24→qter	10–50	Variable features of Turner syndrome, gonadoblastoma
Trisomy X (triple X)	47,XXX	1 in 2500	DD (25%), variable menstrual irregularity
Tetrasomy X	48,XXXX	>50	DD (IQ 30–80), menstrual irregularity, radioulnar synostosis, genital a., ovarian dysgenesis
Pentasomy X	49,XXXXX	10–50	DD, FTT, cleft, cardiac a., radioulnar synostosis, club feet, renal hypoplasia, genital a., ovarian dysgenesis

Note:

p, short arm; q, long arm; r, ring; i, isochromosome; DD, developmental disability; FTT, failure to thrive; a., anomalies.

*Reported cases or number per live births.

Source: Schinzel (2001) and Gorlin et al. (2001, pp. 57–69).

syndromes may be encountered as synonyms, but Turner syndrome is widely accepted. After the usual 45,X karyotype was defined in 1959, the minimal criterion for Turner syndrome became the deficiency of all or part of one X chromosome (Jones, 1997, pp. 81–7; Gorlin et al., 2001, pp. 57–62). The majority of patients have a 45,X karyotype or mosaicism with 45,X and 46,XX cell lines. Others have mosaicism involving unusual cell lines – isochromosome Xp or Xq, ring X, Xp, or Xq deletion, and even male (46,XY) karyotypes. Rarely, Turner syndrome will involve smaller deletions of the X chromosome (Table 8.1). The term "male Turner syndrome" has been used imprecisely for Noonan syndrome, but the latter condition is now known to result from single-gene mutations rather than chromosomal changes.

Historical diagnosis and management

Henry Turner described the Turner syndrome phenotype in 1938, and its chromosomal basis was recognized 21 years later. Literature predating the use of hormone replacement therapy in Turner syndrome may exaggerate the severity of growth delay and sexual immaturity.

Table 8.2. Sex chromosome aneuploidy in males

Disorder	Karyotype	Incidence*	Complications
Klinefelter syndrome	47,XXY	1 in 1000	Asthenic habitus, behavior differences, connective tissue laxity, gynecomastia, infertility
XX males	46,XX	1 in 50,000	Similar to Klinefelter syndrome with lesser stature
Klinefelter variant	48,XXYY	1 in 50,000	DD, hypogonadism, aggression
Klinefelter variant	48,XXXY	>50	DD (IQ~50), gynecomastia, radioulnar synostosis, kyphosis, hypogonadism
Klinefelter variant	49,XXXXY	>50	DD (IQ 20–60), FTT, cardiac a., radioulnar synostosis, scoliosis, micropenis, cryptorchidism
XYY syndrome	47,XYY	1 in 2000	Rare anomalies – urinary tract a., inguinal hernias, micropenis, hypospadias, cryptorchidism; behavioral a.
XYYY syndrome	48,XYYY	<10	DD, strabismus, pulmonic stenosis, genital a.
XYYYY syndrome	49,XYYYY	<10	DD, trigonocephaly, scoliosis, hydronephrosis
Del(Yq)	Yq11→qter	10–50	None; rare X–Y translocations may have severe DD, microcephaly, cardiac a., genital a. (Lahn et al., 1994)
Ring(Y)	46,Xr(Y)	<10	Short stature, cryptorchidism, hypospadias

Note:
r, ring; DD, developmental disability; FTT, failure to thrive; a., anomalies.
*Reported cases or number per live births.
Source: Schinzel (2001) and Gorlin et al. (2001, pp. 62–7).

Incidence, etiology, and differential diagnosis

Turner syndrome is very common at conception, with an estimated 1–2% of all conceptions being monosomy X. Up to 98–99% of affected pregnancies abort spontaneously, giving a birth incidence of 1 in 2000–5000 births (Frías et al., 2003). Eighty percent of women with monosomy X inherit their single X chromosome from their mother, but paternal versus maternal origin of the monosomy X makes no difference in phenotype. Diagnosis of Turner syndrome is often delayed, since neonatal features may be subtle or unappreciated. A recent Belgian study indicated an average age at diagnosis of 6.6 years, with 22% of girls diagnosed after age 12 (Massa et al., 2005).

Comparison of patients with X chromosome deletions indicates that deletion of the X short arm produces a more severe Turner phenotype than deletion of the X long arm; haplo-insufficiency of genes on the X short arm are thus important for generating the phenotype, even though the mechanisms of pathogenesis are still unknown. The characteristic webbed neck (pterygium colli) is a manifestation of a jugular lymphatic obstruction sequence that occurs in several conditions. Most similar is the Noonan syndrome of short stature, pterygium colli, broad chest, cardiac anomalies (usually of the pulmonary artery rather than aorta), and genital defects. Noonan syndrome is different in that it affects both sexes, has frequent mental disability, and often exhibits autosomal dominant rather than chromosomal inheritance.

Diagnostic evaluation and medical counseling

A karyotype is definitive and requisite for diagnosis; older patients diagnosed by buccal smear (with absent Barr body should have a karyotype to rule out the presence of a Y chromosome.

The ability to perform rapid screening for 45,X/46,XX or 45,X/46,XY mosaicism using fluorescent *in situ* hybridization (FISH) technology offers the opportunity for non-invasive karyotyping of buccal mucosa, urinary sediment, and peripheral blood in Turner females. When more than one tissue is examined, the frequency of mosaicism (usually XX/XO) in Turner syndrome is as high as 80% (Frías et al., 2003). Extensive search for X/XX mosaicism may be most helpful in older patients regarding their fertility, since growth and developmental outcomes in mosaic patients are not consistently better (Sybert & McCauley, 2004). Gonadal dysgenesis causes infertility in only 75% of mosaic 45,X/46,XX females compared to 95% of 45,X females). Search for the presence of Y chromosome material as part of routine peripheral blood karyotyping is definitely justified, since Y-FISH probes are available in most laboratories (Wiktor & Van Dyke, 2004). Significant numbers of XY cells would indicate higher risks (5–10%) for developing gonadoblastoma or dysgerminoma in the abnormal gonads, and prophylactic gonadectomy (Frías et al., 2003).

Family and psychosocial counseling

Initial counseling should emphasize the normal intellectual prognosis and lifespan expected for women with Turner syndrome. Parents who have a child with monosomy X do not have increased risk for subsequent children with chromosomal anomalies. However, fertile women with mosaicism for 45,X or other abnormal cell lines have an increased risk of chromosomal anomalies in their offspring and should be offered prenatal diagnosis. If there is a structural rearrangement of an

X chromosome in the child – that is, ring(X), marker X, isochromosome Xp or Xq, translocations causing partial monosomy X – then these families should be referred for genetic counseling, parental karyotyping, and FISH studies to evaluate the proportions of X and Y material.

When the diagnosis of Turner syndrome is made during infancy or early childhood, families should be informed about the possibility of growth hormone therapy so they can begin considering the large financial demands of this treatment. Because many women will have some potential for fertility, reproductive assessment with pelvic ultrasound together with counseling regarding pregnancy risks and artificial reproductive technology options is reasonable (Mazzanti et al., 1997). Turner syndrome support groups include the Turner Syndrome Society of the US (www.turner-syndrome-us.org/), Turner Syndrome Support Society of the UK (www.turner-syndrome-us.org/), Turner's Syndrome Society, Canada (www.turnersyndrome.ca/), and Turner Center (http:www.aaa.dk/TURNER/ENGELSK/INDEX.HTM); these support groups are useful in giving parents and affected individuals information about medical decisions, as well as the chance to meet adults with the disorder.

Natural history and complications

With modern preventive and surgical therapy, the survival of Turner patients should be normal. They are slightly smaller at birth, with weight of 2500–2900 g and length of 45–47 cm, and about half will exhibit growth delay by age 2 years (Frías et al., 2003). For other children, statural growth continues along the 3rd centile until puberty. Untreated women will fall 3–4 standard deviations below mean stature for age due to growth deceleration and lack or delay of the pubertal growth spurt; growth can continue into the early 20s for such women. Biosynthetic growth hormone coupled with delay of puberty has increased final height by 8–10 cm in some studies, and growth hormone therapy can be instituted early in children showing significant delays by age 2 years (Frías et al., 2003).

Complications of Turner syndrome include eye, ear, cardiovascular, lymphatic, urinary tract, genital, and autoimmune problems (see checklist). Despite normal or above-average intelligence in many, learning differences regarding numerical abilities, spatial visualization, and motor execution have been described (Ross et al., 1998; Bruandet et al., 2004). The potential learning disabilities, together with the risk of early problems with feeding, hearing and vision warrant referral for early intervention services and estrogen therapy. An echocardiogram and abdominal sonogram to visualize cardiac or urinary tract anomalies (see checklist) are warranted as soon as the diagnosis of Turner syndrome is confirmed.

Cardiac anomalies occur in 20–40% of women with Turner syndrome, most commonly bicuspid aortic valve, coarctation of the aorta, mitral valve prolapse, and pulmonary venous anomalies (Ho et al., 2004). Although the valve changes and coarctation may not be clinically significant, these anomalies predispose to aortic aneurysm and atherosclerosis. There is also a high mortality rate from aortic dissection of women with Turner syndrome who achieve pregnancies with ovum donation, and MRI plus echocardiography offers more complete screening. Ostberg et al. (2004) report results of gadolinium-enhanced 3D MR angiography in Turner females, showing elongation of the transverse arch (49%), aortic coarctation (12%), aberrant right subclavian artery (8%), persistent left superior vena cava (13%), and partial anomalous pulmonary venous return (13%). Cardiac MRI studies are also more sensitive in detecting aortic dilation (Chalard et al., 2005), allowing earlier surgery if it is clinically necessary.

Aortic dilation along with lymphatic and small vessel changes in Turner syndrome may be explained by an underlying defect in mesenchyme. Hemangiomas in the gastrointestinal tract may cause bleeding or protein-losing enteropathy, and hypertension occurs in 40% due to changes in vessels or renal function. Progressive sensorineural hearing loss causes problems in some older children and leads to use of hearing aids in 25% of older women (Frías et al., 2003). Autoimmune disorders are more common, including diabetes mellitus, Hashimoto thyroiditis with hypothyroidism, juvenile idiopathic arthritis, celiac disease, and psoriasis. Strabismus and anterior chamber eye anomalies are increased, including glaucoma. Increased risks for skeletal problems (hip dislocation, scoliosis), and arthritis can lead to decreased exercise and obesity in older patients.

In addition to motor delays and subtle learning differences, Cardoso et al. (2004) reported that 52 of 100 women with Turner syndrome met criteria for a current or a past depressive or anxiety disorder, including 18 with criteria for axis I psychiatric disorder (anxiety, major or minor depression, dysthymia). These women had higher rates of lifetime depression compared with rates in the community but were comparable to gynecologic clinic populations experiencing infertility.

An abundance of infrequent complications have been reported in Turner syndrome, including biochemical abnormalities (reduction in cortical bone mineral density and osteoporosis, aberrant lipid profiles), cancers (verrucous carcinoma of the vulva, colon cancer in a 14-year-old female, ovarian mucinous cystadenoma, nephrogenic adenoma of the bladder), cardiovascular problems (pulmonary hypertension secondary to a parachute-like mitral valve, deep venous thrombosis, aortic dissection), endocrinopathies (primary hyperparathyroidism with osteitis fibrosa cystica), primary ovarian failure gastrointestinal problems (acute necrotizing pancreatitis, cholestatic and vascular liver disease), skeletal defects (wrist anomaly similar to that in Leri–Weill dyschondrosteosis, hemihypotrophy), and neurologic problems (hydrocephalus, intracranial hypertension). Regular, thorough history and physical plus alertness for a wide spectrum of problems are essential for preventive management.

The Turner syndrome preventive medical checklist

Consensus recommendations for the health supervision of children with Turner syndrome are available from the American Academy of Pediatrics (aappolicy. aappublications.org/cgi/reprint/pediatrics – Frías et al., 2003), a Consensus Development Conference from pediatric endocrinologists (2004), and recent reviews (Halac & Zimmerman, 2004). Although the diagnosis is often missed in the nursery, unless characteristic pedal edema is present, karyotyping and possibly pelvic sonography (Mazzanti et al., 1997) are crucial for management once the diagnosis is recognized. Bilateral removal of streak gonads during early childhood is indicated in children with mosaicism for Y-chromosome-containing cells. A second peak in the risk of gonadoblastoma occurs at puberty, so review of diagnostic results and consideration of novel tests to detect Y material should be made in adolescent females. Alertness for tumors should be maintained in all women with Turner syndrome, since gonadoblastoma can arise in 45,X patients without detectable Y chromosome material.

Other problems during infancy and early childhood may include cardiac anomalies, strabismus, chronic otitis, and developmental delay. Peripheral pulses and blood pressures should be checked regularly in patients with Turner syndrome. Early intervention is appropriate for some children along with vision, urinalysis, and blood pressure screening for all. Short stature may be associated with low self-esteem and other behavioral problems in Turner syndrome, justifying early referral to endocrinology for the one-half who fall behind by age 2 years (Frías et al., 2003). Some children may also need plastic surgery evaluation if their pterygium colli, nevi, or keloids are disfiguring.

Improved growth velocity has occurred using oxandrolone and/or growth hormone therapy. Early and prolonged treatment with growth hormone together with low-dose estradiol treatment may offer the best outcome (Ross et al., 1998). American and European studies have reported height gains of 4–8 cm in patients receiving growth hormone, estrogen, and oxandrolone therapy that correlate positively with tall parental stature and negatively with spontaneous rather than induced menarche (Ross et al., 1998; Harris et al., 2004; Parvin et al., 2004). Estrogen treatment is useful in promoting normal puberty and avoiding osteoporosis, and suppression of puberty using gonadotropin-releasing hormone analogs has improved height outcomes (Harris et al., 2004).

Growth hormone therapy appears safe and effective. The National Cooperative Growth Study (NCGS) has now followed treatment in over 47,000 patients over 20 years, with slight increases in intracranial hypertension and slipped capital femoral epiphyses in children with renal disease or Turner syndrome (Wyatt, 2004). This study found sub-optimal adherence to guidelines for monitoring children with Turner syndrome, emphasizing the importance of a checklist approach as recently emphasized by Tyler & Edman (2004). Continued surveillance into adult life was recommended, particularly in children receiving supra-physiologic doses of growth hormone or whose underlying condition increases their risk of adverse effects (e.g., those with Turner syndrome – Harris et al., 2004).

Despite growth hormone therapy, some behavior differences remain. Numerous studies report discrepancies between verbal and performance IQ, with lower scores on tests of visual-motor, visual-spatial, and freedom from distractibility. Bruandet et al. (2004) examined understanding of numerosity and quantity in Turner syndrome, observing impairments in cognitive estimation, subitizing, and calculation. While measures of map reading, figure drawing, geometry, or arithmetic may yield lower-than-average scores in Turner syndrome, many adolescents seem to catch up and perform well academically since a majority graduate from college.

The use of hormone therapy and the potential for egg donation provides a more optimistic outlook for sexual and reproductive function in Turner syndrome. Doerr et al. (2005) found that 44% of women with Turner syndrome had a reduced uterine length and incomplete breast development after estrogen therapy, and that women with 45,X/46,XX mosaicism often had normal uterine sizes. Uterine wall thickness can be used as a predictor of fertility in women with mosaicism. Adult women with Turner syndrome express a more negative body image by comparison to controls, but sexually active women report moderate to high levels of satisfaction and improved body image (Sybert & McCauley, 2004). Anticipatory guidance with hormone therapy can thus have tremendous impact on health and gender function in Turner syndrome.

Klinefelter syndrome

Terminology

Klinefelter syndrome describes males of increased stature with gynecomastia, small testes, and a 47,XXY karyotype. Klinefelter syndrome "variants" include disorders with more severe clinical features and additional X or Y chromosomes as the karyotypes 48,XXXY; 48,XXYY; and 49,XXXXY (Jones, 1997, pp. 72–3; Gorlin et al., 2001, pp. 62–6).

Historical diagnosis and management

Klinefelter described the syndrome in 1942, and the 47,XXY karyotype was reported in 1959. Increased frequency of males with 47,XXY and 47,XYY syndromes have been found in mental or penal institutions, but prospective studies to document such associations have been controversial.

Incidence, etiology, and differential diagnosis

The classic Klinefelter phenotype has a prevalence of 1.18 per 1000, with 80% having karyotypes of 47,XXY, 10% being 46,XY/47,XXY mosaics, and the remainder having multiple X or Y chromosomes (Table 8.2). More than 10% of males presenting with sterility and 3% with breast cancer will have Klinefelter syndrome. The additional X interferes with Leydig cell development in the testis, but the pathogenesis is unknown. The immature body habitus, feminine features (like gynecomastia, high voice, or sparse hair), and sterility reflect androgen deficiency. Differential diagnosis includes males with gonadotropin deficiency and other conditions with a lean, eunuchoid habitus such as homocystinuria or Marfan syndrome.

Higher degrees of aneuploidy for the X and Y chromosomes cause a more severe Klinefelter phenotype. The 48,XXYY (1 in 25,000 births) and 48,XXXY (<1 in 100,000 births) syndromes have more severe mental disability and more severe genital hypoplasia. The 48,XXYY condition is associated with more behavioral problems (aggression, conduct disorders) than other Klinefelter variants. Each is more likely to show gynecomastia and skeletal anomalies like radioulnar synostosis. The 49,XXXXY syndrome occurs in 1 in 85,000 births and has more distinctive dysmorphology than other Klinefelter variants. A round face with ear anomalies, eye defects such as strabismus and later myopia, cleft palate, dental anomalies, cardiac defects including patent ductus arteriosus, and a broad range of skeletal anomalies (scoliosis, kyphosis, cervical vertebral anomalies) are present. The developmental disability, eye, heart, and skeletal defects at low risk in 47,XXY Klinefelter syndrome are thus exaggerated in Klinefelter variants, and these will likely come to attention in early childhood.

Diagnostic evaluation and medical counseling

Discrepancies between the frequency of 47,XXY prenatal diagnoses (153 per 100,000 males after maternal age correction) and prevalence among adult men (40 per 100,000) indicate a significant fraction of males with Klinefelter syndrome are unrecognized (Bojesen et al., 2003). Only 18% of individuals with 47,XXY Klinefelter syndrome will have major medical problems, particularly infertility, explaining why fewer than 10% are diagnosed during childhood (Gorlin et al., 2001, pp. 62–6; Bojesen et al., 2003). The karyotype is diagnostic, and serum testosterone levels should be considered in postpubertal patients. For parents of young children, medical counseling should address the probable sterility and the increased risk of school and behavior problems. Adolescents and adults with Klinefelter syndrome should know about the possible benefits of testosterone supplements and cosmetic surgery.

Family and psychosocial counseling

Klinefelter syndrome, like most results of non-disjunction, is associated with advanced maternal age (Bojesen et al., 2004). Genetic referral is needed for affected individuals and their parents. The recurrence risk of parents will be 1% or less, and family studies are needed only if unusual X or Y chromosome rearrangements are found. Occasional non-mosaic 47,XXY patients have been confirmed as fathers by paternity analysis; such couples warrant the option of prenatal diagnosis because of the increased risk of aneuploid offspring. Parent support groups are available (checklist, part 1), including the Klinefelter Support Group (http://klinefeltersyndrome.org/), American Association for Klinefelter Syndrome and Support – Access (http://www.aaksis.org/index.cfm), Klinefelter Syndrome and Associates (KS & A – www.genetic.org/), and Triplo-X Organization (http://www.triplo-x.org/).

Natural history and complications

Men with Klinefelter syndrome may have the female pattern of enhanced longevity or increased morbidity from infectious, neurologic, circulatory, pulmonary, and urinary tract diseases (Bojesen et al., 2004). A 6-fold increased risk of cerebrovascular disease and a 1–2% incidence of neoplasia has been reported, but whether this increase is caused by hypogonadism) or other factors is presently unknown. Bojesen et al. (2003) found that hypercholesterolemia was present in 57% of Klinefelter patients, correlating with age and the magnitude of androgenic deficit. None had diabetes mellitus in their study, but glycemic values above 100 mg% and obesity were present in 16% versus 10% of controls.

Childhood problems include delayed speech (51%), motor delays (27%), and school maladjustment (44% – Gorlin et al., 2001, pp. 62–6; Visootsak et al., 2001; Manning & Hoyme, 2002; Simpson et al., 2003). Antisocial behaviors including theft or arson, alcoholism, and aggressiveness are described in some reports; others describe XXY men as having similar employment and social status to their peers. Psychiatric disorders such as manic–depressive illness, psychosis, schizophrenia, depression, and anorexia nervosa may be increased (Fales et al., 2003).

Relatively uncommon medical complications include facial defects (iris coloboma, strabismus, choroidal atrophy, cleft palate), cardiovascular anomalies (aortic stenosis, mitral valve prolapse, acute pulmonary embolus, varicose veins with leg ulcers), gastrointestinal disorders (e.g., cholelithiasis), genital anomalies (inguinal hernia, cryptorchidism, hypospadias, micropenis), and neurologic problems (distal muscle weakness or myopathy). Autoimmune diseases such as collagen vascular disease, diabetes mellitus, and aplastic anemia occur along with a list of tumors such as acute lymphoblastic leukemia, myelomonocytic, and chronic myelogenous leukemias, non-Hodgkin lymphoma, adenocarcinoma of the prostate, germinoma of the brain, mediastinal immature teratoma. Precocious puberty has been described as a harbinger for tumor, associated with a germ cell tumor. Osteoporosis occurs in older patients, and trials of ibandronate have improved bone mineral density and bone remodeling.

Klinefelter syndrome preventive medical checklist

Patients with Klinefelter syndrome are rarely recognized in the newborn period unless identified through prenatal diagnosis. Several authors (Visootsak et al., 2001; Manning & Hoyme, 2002; Lanfranco et al., 2004) emphasize the advantages of early diagnosis so psychiatric and/or pharmacologic therapy can be considered when school and behavior problems are recognized. Early care consists of screening for hearing or vision problems, plus physical and occupational therapy assessment for motor and speech delays (see checklist). Auditory evoked-response testing should be performed to rule out nerve deafness. If assessment reveals developmental delays, or if an early intervention program is the best way to obtain assessment, then the child should be referred. Eye and genital anomalies are sometimes found, so these regions should be carefully examined.

Many Klinefelter patients present because of behavior problems, abnormal pubertal development, or infertility. Puberty should be monitored carefully, since both delays and precocious puberty have been reported. Gynecomastia, micropenis, or small testes can be a source of ridicule for teenagers and detract from self-image; breast liposuction and orchiectomy followed by testicular implants can improve self-image and behavior. Testosterone therapy is most beneficial if started at age 11–12 years, and has been associated with better mood, less irritability, and more energy, endurance, and concentration. Depot injection or oral testosterone therapy may be tried, but side effects include priapism, salt and water retention, polycythemia, diabetes mellitus, and, in older patients, prostatic hypertrophy with sudden bladder obstruction. Gynecomastia is usually not benefited by androgen therapy. Priming of external genital development using testosterone may be indicated in males with a small phallus. For all of these reasons, endocrinology referral is strongly recommended.

Artificial reproductive technology now provides options for reproduction in Klinefelter syndrome. Denschlag et al. (2004) report 39 successful pregnancies fathered by non-mosaic Klinefelter patients obtained by extracting sperm cells from testicular tissue and used for intracytoplasmic sperm insemination (ICSI). Lanfranco et al. (2004) emphasize that testosterone replacement has no positive effect on infertility, but intracytoplasmic sperm injection offers an opportunity for procreation even when there are no spermatozoa in the ejaculate. The frequency of chromosomal aneuploidies is higher in spermatozoa from patients with Klinefelter syndrome, so prenatal diagnosis should be considered for these pregnancies.

Many studies indicate that men with Klinefelter syndrome have impaired verbal ability and deficits in executive function. For example, one report showed problems with ordering sets of names by personal characteristics or with responding to stimuli encoded by letters, but normal performance in non-verbal reasoning tasks (Fales et al., 2003). Many of the behavioral and expressive language difficulties respond to the combination of androgen therapy and psychologic help, particularly if treatment begins early (Manning & Hoyme, 2002; Simpson et al., 2003). Besides testosterone replacement for correction of the androgen deficiency, school curricula can be tailored to address learning difficulties, and adolescence can be monitored for learning and behavioral problems (Visootsak et al., 2001; Manning & Hoyme, 2002). Several authors emphasize the importance of the primary-care physician in providing anticipatory guidance and serving as a valuable source of support and advocacy for the family of a boy with Klinefelter syndrome (Visootsak et al., 2001; Manning & Hoyme, 2002; Simpson et al., 2003; Tyler & Edman, 2004).

LESS COMMON SEX CHROMOSOME ANEUPLOIDIES

Triple X syndrome and its variants

As with the Klinefelter spectrum, women with extra X chromosomes have risks for mental disability, eye, skeletal, and genital defects that increase as a progression from 47,XXX to 48,XXXX and 49,XXXXX karyotypes. The "triple X" or 47,XXX karyotype is most common at about 1 in 1200 births and, like its brother 47,XXY disorder, shows influence of maternal age with minimal dysmorphic changes. The 48,XXXX and 49,XXXXX conditions are much less common at less than 1 per 100,000 births, and have higher frequencies of the complications listed below (Jones, 1997, pp. 78–9; Gorlin et al., 2001, pp. 67–8).

The phenotypic changes typically have a normal appearance without congenital anomalies, and the main problems in the triple X spectrum are speech and developmental delay. One patient had a dysgerminoma of the ovary. A higher frequency of behavioral problems ranges from immaturity to psychoses, but their frequencies are difficult to estimate because of ascertainment bias. When the diagnosis is made in older females, screening of for behavioral difficulties with provision of counseling resources may be helpful. Some 47,XXX females have had decreased fertility, so reproductive evaluation and counseling is appropriate for adolescents.

Women with higher degrees of sex chromosome aneuploidy have more severe mental disability (average IQ of 55 in 48,XXX and 30–50 in 49,XXXX aneuploidy). Dental, cardiac, renal, and skeletal (club feet, joint laxity, radioulnar synostosis) occur at higher frequencies in these women, meriting attention to these problems during pediatric care (Table 8.1). Short stature and delayed puberty may occur, particularly in 49,XXXXX women, so endocrinology referral and growth hormone treatment might be considered in those with milder disabilities.

Summary of clinical concerns: Triple X syndrome management considerations

Growth and development: Lower birth weights with tall stature in 47,XXX and failure to thrive in 49,XXXXX, microcephaly rare in 47,XXX but frequent in 49,XXXXX, and mild to moderate mental disability, speech delay correlating with chromosome number: Early childhood intervention with speech therapy, and developmental pediatrics, genetics, and/or neurology according to severity of delays and availability.

Cancer: Low incidence of tumors like dysgerminoma of ovary: Routine abdominal examinations.

Craniofacial: Normal in 47,XXX but micrognathia, cleft palate, dental anomalies, hearing loss, and even facial resemblance to Down syndrome in 49,XXXXX: Feeding specialist, nutrition, audiology, otolaryngology, dentistry, cleft palate team.

Eye: Iris coloboma, ptosis, and strabismus: Ophthalmology.

Cardiac: Defects in 40% of 47,XXXXX including patent ductus arteriosus and ventricular septal defects: Cardiology, echocardiogram needed for those with 48 or 49 chromosomes.

Urogenital: Recurrent urinary infections even in 47,XXX, small kidneys, late-onset menarche, early menopause, ovarian dysgenesis: Monitoring of blood pressure, urinalysis, urology, endocrinology evaluations surrounding puberty.

Skeletal: Club feet, joint laxity, radioulnar synostosis, vertebral defects: Orthopedics, cervical spine films and anesthesia precautions if short neck and marked joint laxity/hypotonia.

Neurologic: Significant mental disability in over 25% of patients with 47,XXX, and 80% of those with 49,XXXXX with average IQ of 55 in 48,XXX and 30–50 in 49,XXXX; behavior differences ranging from immaturity, to learning disorders and psychosis: Neurology, psychiatry, school testing and monitoring of progress.

Parental counseling: Low recurrence risks for parents reflective of maternal age (1–2% over age 37 years). Parent support and information is available at Triplo-X Syndrome Organization (www.triplo-x.org/) and the Turner Center (www.aaa.dk/TURNER/ENGELSK/INDEX.HTM).

47,XYY syndrome

This disorder is often recognized incidentally in normal males or as an unexpected finding during evaluation of learning disabilities. The incidence is 1 in 1000 male live births, which is a small fraction of abundant 47,XYY sperm (1%) in the testis of normal males (Gorlin et al., 2001, pp. 66–7). Higher numbers of Y chromosomes (48,XYYY; 49,XYYYY) have been reported but are extremely rare. As with the triple X spectrum, higher numbers of Y chromosomes exaggerate the frequencies of mental disability, behavior differences, skeletal, and urogenital anomalies cited below.

Summary of clinical concerns: 47,XYY management considerations

Growth and development: Accelerated height growth with 38% being above the 90th centile by age 5 years, lower general (79–89) and verbal IQ: Early childhood intervention for children diagnosed prenatally or during infancy.

Craniofacial: Frequent minor anomalies, larger and subtly malformed teeth, rare facial asymmetry with metopic synostosis and micrognathia in 48,XYYY or 49,XYYYY: Routine audiology and dentistry, craniofacial surgery team if severe asymmetry.

Surface: Higher frequency of acne, rare inguinal hernias: Skin hygiene, dermatology, pediatric surgery if needed.

Cardiac: Pulmonic stenosis in 48,XYYY: Routine cardiac examination with obligate cardiology and echocardiogram for those with 48 or 49 chromosomes.

Urogenital: Rare urinary tract anomalies, cryptorchidism, hypospadias, or small testes with mostly normal genital and reproductive function in 47,XYY: Genital examination, monitoring of blood pressure and urinalysis, endocrinology evaluation surrounding puberty, reproductive counseling because of higher risk for miscarriage and chromosome anomalies (including 47,XYY) in pregnancies conceived by XYY males.

Skeletal: Joint laxity, radioulnar synostosis, scapular winging: Routine skeletal examination, orthopedics if needed.

Neurologic: Significant developmental and behavioral differences, including early clumsiness and fine motor problems, muscle weakness and incoordination, borderline mental disability (IQ 70–90) in 38%, impulsive behavior, and temper tantrums: Behavioral evaluation and counseling resources may help families; often parents have gone through considerable frustration that is clarified by the diagnosis.

Parental counseling: Low recurrence risks for parents. Parent information is available at several websites by searching on 47,XYY syndrome, including the contact a family website (www.cafamily.org.uk/Direct/x15.html).

XLMR SYNDROMES

Male genetic deficiency in humans results in numerous X-linked diseases that arise when the single masculine X chromosome allele is abnormal. Over 450 X-linked disorders are known, of which about half alter development and cause mental deficiency and/or malformation syndromes. Many of these syndromes produce obvious (e.g., Aarskog) or subtle (e.g., Coffin–Lowry or FG) manifestations that allow clinical diagnosis. Particularly challenging are the X-linked conditions that cause

Table 8.3. XLMR syndromes

Syndrome	Locus	Complications other than MR
Opitz GBBB	Xp22	Hypertelorism, hypospadias
Coffin–Lowry	Xp22	Coarse facies, broad fingers, joint laxity
Aarskog–Scott	Xp11	Short stature, hypertelorism, shawl scrotum, joint laxity
Norrie	Xp11	Blindness, hearing loss
Allan–Herndon–Dudley	Xp11–Xq21	Hypotonia, joint contractures
Opitz FG	Xp11–Xq22	Macrocephaly, brain a., gastrointestinal a., deafness
Renpenning	Xp21–Xq22	Short stature, microcephaly
α-thalassemia with MR	Xq13	Microcephaly, genital a., skeletal a., α-thalassemia
Simpson–Golabi–Behmel	Xq24–Xq28	Macrosomia, coarse facies, cardiac a., polydactyly, extra nipples
Borjeson–Forssman–Lehman	Xq26–Xq27	Short stature, obesity, microcephaly, hypogonadism
Fragile X	Xq27	Macrocephaly, long face, large ears, macro-orchidism
Otopalatodigital	Xq27–Xq28	Short stature, prominent brow, skeletal a., deafness
MASA, X-linked hydrocephalus	Xq28	Aphasia, shuffling gait, ataxia, spasticity

Note:

MR, mental retardation; a., anomalies.

Source: Ropers & Hamel (2005).

mental deficiency with minimal morphologic alterations, in that gene mapping and characterization with subsequent DNA diagnosis are the only options for specific diagnosis. More than 30 of these "non-specific" XLMR syndromes are known, of which only the fragile X syndrome is amenable to commercial DNA testing. These non-specific XLMR disorders offer a preview of the many X-chromosomal and autosomal causes of mental deficiency and autism that will be identified once DNA testing for multiple gene abnormalities (i.e., a gene screen) becomes as feasible as the present karyotype for chromosome disorders. Since X-linked conditions with pure mental disability will by definition lack birth defects requiring preventive management, some of the more common syndromes with morphologic or behavioral phenotypes are reviewed here, followed by detailed discussion of the fragile X syndrome (Table 8.3).

Aarskog syndrome

This condition was formally described in 1970 by Aarskog, with most cases exhibiting X-linked inheritance and a few with autosomal-dominant or -recessive inheritance (Jones, 1997, pp. 128–9; Gorlin et al., 2001, pp. 366–8). The diagnosis is dependent on the typical facial appearance, genital anomalies (shawl or saddle-bag scrotum), and joint laxity with ability to extend the fingers in a "swan's neck deformity" position. Female carriers often have some phenotypic features, and the causative X-linked gene has been isolated but is not routinely available for carrier screening (Orrico et al., 2004).

Summary of clinical concerns: Aarskog syndrome management considerations

General: Perinatal vascular accidents with resulting hemiplegia have been reported: Careful monitoring of labor in women at risk because of family history.

Growth and development: Mild short stature with occasional growth hormone deficiency; mild mental disability with attention deficit hyperactivity disorder: Growth and developmental monitoring with consideration of endocrinology for marked short stature, early childhood intervention for more severe joint laxity and/or motor delays, developmental pediatrics if learning disability/ attention deficit hyperactivity disorder.

Ophthalmology: Ptosis, strabismus, or tortuous retinal vessels: Neonatal and yearly ophthalmology assessment.

ENT: Dental enamel hypoplasia.

Cardiac: Occasional defects: Cardiac examination with cardiology referral for positive findings.

Urogenital: Cryptorchidism, shawl scrotum, inguinal hernias: Genital examination with surgery referrals as needed.

Skeletal: Cervical vertebral anomalies in 50% (including odontoid hypoplasia with C1/C2 vertebral subluxation), pectus excavatum: Skeletal examination, cervical spine flexion/extension films at age 3 and subsequent decades, orthopedics.

Parental counseling: Usual risks of X-linked-recessive inheritance with 1/4 chance for an affected male and 1/2 chance for a female carrier if mother known to be carrier by family history – reduce these risks by 2/3 if affected male is first case in family. Parent information can be found by searching on Aarskog syndrome, including a US Aarskog Syndrome Parents Support Group listed on the Family Village website (www.familyvillage.wisc.edu/lib_aars.htm).

Coffin–Lowry syndrome

Coffin–Lowry syndrome has a recognizable phenotype that includes a characteristic facies, strikingly soft and flexible hands, and short fingers. The disorder exhibits X-linked-recessive inheritance with some expression in carrier females (Jones, 1997, pp. 274–7; Gorlin et al., 2001, pp. 1029–32). The causative gene is a ribosomal S6 protein kinase (RSK2) located in the Xp22 chromosome region; it is not available for commercial diagnosis (Facher et al., 2004). Once the clinician is familiar with the condition, the facial appearance with down-slanting palpebral fissures and the characteristic handshake allows a rapid diagnosis. Many patients have been evaluated for hypothyroidism or mucopolysaccharidosis because of their clinical findings in infancy.

Summary of clinical concerns: Coffin–Lowry syndrome management considerations

Growth and development: Short stature with moderate mental disability and speech delay, average male IQ 30–50 with females having milder growth and developmental delay: Growth and developmental monitoring with early childhood intervention with developmental pediatric and genetic follow-up in males.

Craniofacial: Small sinuses, delayed closure fontanel: Cranial evaluation together with monitoring of head size.

ENT: Sensorineural hearing loss, dental malocclusion, hypodontia: Neonatal and annual auditory brainstem evoked response (ABR) and audiology, early dental referral.

Cardiac: Mitral insufficiency: Cardiac examinations, cardiology referral if symptoms.

Urogenital: Cryptorchidism, uterine prolapse, inguinal hernias.

Skeletal: Short sternum, pectus excavatum, scoliosis, kyphosis, flat feet: Skeletal examinations and orthopedic referral when necessary.

Neurologic: Seizures (40%), agenesis of the corpus callosum, cataplexy or drop attacks, hydrocephalus: Monitoring of the head circumference, alertness for manifestations of seizures, head MRI if recurrent seizures or rapid head growth.

Parental counseling: Usual risks of X-linked-recessive inheritance with 1/4 chance for an affected male and 1/2 chance for a female carrier if mother known to be carrier by family history – reduce these risks by 2/3 if affected male is first case in family. Parent information can be found by searching on the syndrome name.

FG syndrome

The FG syndrome of mental disability, absent corpus callosum, unusual facies with a frontal hair whorl, and intestinal anomalies was described in 1974 by Opitz and Kaveggia (Jones, 1997, pp. 280–1; Gorlin et al., 2001, pp. 1137–39). The FG syndrome is somewhat intermediate between XLMR disorders with obvious distinguishing features (e.g., Lesch–Nyhan or Coffin–Lowry syndromes) and the non-specific disorders that present only as developmental delay. Anomalies can be subtle in these non-specific disorders, and it is important to remember the possibility of X-linked inheritance when evaluating male children with developmental delay. The term "FG" represents the initials of the first affected individual.

Genetic mapping and gene characterization are increasingly helpful in sorting out different forms of XLMR, and make possible carrier detection and prenatal diagnosis once a genetic locus is defined. This disorder has been mapped to several different loci on the X chromosome. A thorough family history and genetic counseling are needed, since female carriers have no manifestations of the disease and there is not yet DNA testing available.

Summary of clinical concerns: FG syndrome management considerations

General: Some patients may have a severe and lethal course.

Growth and development: Moderate to severe developmental disability, hypotonia causes early feeding problems and susceptibility to pneumonia: Monitoring for dysphagia and constipation with possible gastroenterology referral, early intervention and speech therapy with later evaluations for school placement.

Eye: Ptosis, strabismus: Ophthalmology examination.

ENT: Micrognathia, sensorineural hearing loss, highly arched or cleft palate, drooling, gingival hyperplasia: Neonatal ABR and audiology monitoring, watch for speech apraxia, chronic otitis, cleft palate team, otolaryngology, and dentistry as appropriate.

Surface: Inguinal and umbilical hernias, keloids after scarring: Regular examinations, urology, pediatric surgery, or dermatology as needed.

Cardiac: Mitral insufficiency: Cardiac examinations, particularly in adolescence and adulthood, cardiology referral if symptoms.

Digestive: Pyloric stenosis, imperforate anus, and malrotation: Monitor feeding and stooling, consider milk of magnesia or other laxatives and gastroenterology referral, imaging studies as needed.

Urogenital: Cryptorchidism, hypospadias: Neonatal examination and urology referral as needed.

Skeletal: Joint contractures, flat feet, genu recurvatum, broad thumbs, and broad halluces: Regular skeletal examinations and orthopedic referral when necessary.

Neurologic: Neonatal hypotonia in 90%, partial to complete absence of the corpus callosum, defects of neuronal migration: Initial cranial MRI scan, later monitoring for seizures with neurology and electroencephalographic studies as needed.

Parental counseling: Usual risks of X-linked-recessive inheritance with 1/4 chance for an affected male and 1/2 chance for a female carrier if mother known to be carrier by family history – reduce these risks by 2/3 if affected male is first case in family. A thorough family history and genetic counseling are needed, since female carriers have no manifestations of the disease.

MASA syndrome and X-linked hydrocephalus

MASA is an acronym for mental retardation, aphasia, shuffling gait, and adducted thumbs. Study of over 100 patients has demonstrated that spasticity is an important part of the phenotype, with males having an average IQ of 50–75 (Macias et al., 1992). Several large families allowed genetic linkage of the MASA syndrome to the Xq28 chromosomal region (Macias et al., 1992). Families with X-linked hydrocephalus and clasped thumbs also showed linkage to Xq28, and it was subsequently recognized that both disorders result from mutations in a neural cell adhesion molecule called L1CAM (Vits et al., 1994). DNA and prenatal diagnosis is now available in a few American and European laboratories (see GeneTests at www.geneclinics.org/), and genetic counseling is an essential part of initial management.

Summary of clinical concerns: MASA syndrome management considerations

Growth and development: Short stature with moderate to severe developmental disability in males, occasional mild disability in female carriers: Early intervention with growth/developmental monitoring, occupational and later speech therapy.

Eye: Strabismus: Ophthalmology at 6 months and yearly through age 3 years.

Skeletal: Kyphosis, lordosis, club feet, flat feet, adducted thumbs: Regular skeletal examinations, skeletal X-rays, and orthopedic referral with positive findings.

Neurologic: Lower limb spasticity, rare brain anomalies (agenesis of corpus callosum), seizures; hydrocephalus is unusual except for allelic X-linked hydrocephalus with severe prenatal onset: Consider head MRI scan, neurology referral, developmental pediatric referral for management of spasticity in severely affected individuals, palliative care for patients with severe X-linked hydrocephalus, less severe cases managed as described for those with hydrocephalus in Chapter 4.

Parental counseling: Mothers of isolated male cases have a 2/3 chance to be carriers with a 1/6 chance for affected males and 1/3 chance for female carriers with each pregnancy, increasing, respectively, to 1/4 and 1/2 chance if they are known to be carriers through symptoms or pedigree structure. Parent information can be found by searching on the syndrome name.

Rett syndrome

Rett syndrome is discussed here because it is representative of X-linked conditions with male lethality (or extreme male severity) and because testing for its causative gene, methyl-CpG-binding protein-2 (MECP2), has unified a broad spectrum of patients with autism, seizures, and variable mental degeneration (Zoghbi & Francke, 2001). The Viennese pediatrician Dr. Andreas Rett recognized the disorder based on two girls with typical behaviors sitting in his waiting room, and DNA studies now suggest an incidence of 1 in 10–15,000 births. The classic phenotype in females is a period of normal development lasting 7–18 months, followed by neurodegeneration that makes parents feel that they have "lost their little girl." Over 1–2 years, the girls regress to dementia, autism, characteristic wringing and clasping hand movements, truncal ataxia, and "acquired" microcephaly. Deceleration of growth, unusual patterns of breathing, sleep disturbances, lower limb spasticity, cold hands and feet due to vasomotor instability, and seizures can accompany the deterioration. Although the neurodegeneration appears to stabilize in some patients, others will have severe behavioral problems (e.g., attention deficit disorder, autism), no language development, and jerky movements resembling those in Angelman syndrome.

MECP2 gene testing is available in several commercial laboratories (see www. geneclinics.org/) and has identified a broad spectrum of patients from females with less degeneration and mild mental disability to surviving males with severe encephalopathy. Affected males and severely affected females may show symptoms from birth, having severe spasticity and motor delays, failure to thrive, and sleep disturbances with no seizures. There is also a preserved speech variant in females with the degeneration and stereotypic hand-washing activities, but the patients stabilize and recover some speech and hand use without growth failure or acquired microcephaly (De Bona et al., 2000).

Summary of clinical concerns: Rett syndrome management considerations

Growth and development: Normal early growth with deceleration in stature and head circumference in concert with degeneration, moderate to severe developmental disability with stabilization in some: Early intervention with monitoring of growth and head circumference, developmental monitoring with early intervention, occupational and speech therapy.

Digestive: Constipation, gastroesophageal reflux: Monitor feeding and stooling, consider anti-reflux therapies, dietician and gastroenterology referral for cachexia and other symptoms.

Neurologic: Progressive truncal and gait ataxia with dystonia and spasticity in lower limbs, sometimes with seizures, abnormal EEG; abnormal behaviors include autism, unusual hand movements (clasping, wringing), sleep disturbances with bruxism, irregular breathing and breath-holding: Neurology with anticonvulsant therapy for seizures, chloral hydrate for agitation, dopa derivatives for rigidity, and melatonin for sleep disturbances (Zoghbi & Francke, 2001).

Parental counseling: Most patients will be new mutations with low recurrence risks for their families, but carrier females without symptoms who transmit the mutant gene to 1/2 of their daughters (classic Rett females) and 1/2 their sons (severely affected non-viable males) have been described. DNA testing of mothers of affected children is therefore indicated. Parent information can be found at the International Rett Syndrome Foundation (www.rettsyndrome.org/), Rett Syndrome Research Foundation (www.rsrf.org/), and Rett Syndrome UK (http://www.rettsyndrome.org.uk/) websites.

The fragile X syndrome

Terminology

Fragile X syndrome refers to a combination of mental and physical abnormalities exhibited by males and females with a fragile site at chromosome band Xq27. "Transmitting males" are asymptomatic males who transmit an X chromosome with the fragile site to their daughters. Female carriers have one normal X chromosome and one X chromosome with the Xq27 fragile site. "Triplet or trinucleotide repeats" refer to three-base pair repeating units that occur in DNA at the fragile site. Males or carrier females with large numbers of triplet repeats (i.e., expanded length of the repeat region) exhibit the phenotype of fragile X syndrome.

Historical diagnosis and management

Fragile X syndrome was first described as an XLMR syndrome by Martin and Bell in 1943, who recognized that affected males had a distinctive appearance with behavioral problems (Jones, 1997, pp. 150–3; Gorlin et al., 2001, pp. 71–5). In the 1960s and 1970s, a specific marker or "fragile" X chromosome was visualized in Martin–Bell patients and shown to depend on culture of lymphocytes in tissue culture medium containing low amounts of folic acid. The ability to confirm clinical suspicion with chromosomal or DNA diagnosis has confirmed the fragile X phenotype of elongated body habitus, prominent jaw, large ears, lax connective tissue, and large testes that Martin & Bell first observed in 1943 (Giangreco et al., 1996; Wiesner et al., 2004).

Incidence, etiology, and differential diagnosis

The incidence of fragile X syndrome is about 1 in 1500 males and 1 in 2500 females, accounting for 30–40% of males with XLMR. After the fragile site focused attention on band Xq27 of the X chromosome, several laboratories isolated a gene from that region called "fragile X mental retardation 1" or "FMR-1," this gene was expressed in brain and testes, and provided a good candidate for the cause of fragile X syndrome. Characterization of DNA near the FMR-1 gene demonstrated a cluster of trinucleotide repeating units that varied in normal individuals but were amplified dramatically in individuals with fragile X syndrome. Males or females with more than 200 triplet repeats exhibited symptoms of Martin–Bell syndrome due to inactivation of the FMR-1 gene. A DNA test based on the enumeration of triplet repeats became available and has replaced less accurate chromosomal analysis for the diagnosis of fragile X syndrome.

Differential diagnosis includes other types of XLMR where there is a family history suggestive of X-linked inheritance. Older patients with the Klinefelter or XYY syndromes may prompt fragile X testing, since the males may be tall and have speech or behavior problems. Cerebral gigantism, with its accelerated early growth and hypotonia, may also be confused with fragile X syndrome (Gorlin et al., 2001, pp. 71–5).

Diagnostic evaluation and medical counseling

All males with significant, unexplained developmental delay should have chromosomal studies including fragile X testing. The cytogenetics laboratory must be alerted to test for fragile X syndrome, since the peripheral blood leukocytes must be cultured in low-folate medium. DNA testing for expanded repeats near the FMR-1 gene is more sensitive and precise; however, it will not screen for other chromosomal disorders in a child with developmental delay. Fragile X DNA testing is best used in a child with disability who has already had a normal karyotype, in potential carrier females assessed because of symptoms or family history, and in family studies to assign recurrence risks based on the identification of asymptomatic "transmitting" males or female carriers. Medical counseling is concerned with planning and services for a child with significant developmental disability.

Family and psychosocial counseling

The genetics of fragile X syndrome are quite complex because standard ratios for X-linked transmission must be modified according to gender and the number of amplified triplet repeats. All affected families must be referred for genetic counseling. Normal individuals have 6–52 triplet repeats, individuals with unstable or "premutations" have 60–200, and individuals with Martin–Bell phenotype have 200–2000. Genesis of the premutation is not understood. Once a premutation of 60–200 repeats is present, further amplication occurs only during female meiosis. The risk of females with premutations depends on their number of triplet repeats – those with 60–80 will have lower risks for an affected male (200–2000 repeats) than those with 150–200 repeats. DNA testing is thus necessary for precise genetic counseling, since recurrence risk and phenotype often depend on the average number of triplet repeats. Prenatal diagnosis by chorionic villus biopsy or amniocentesis is now routine, and blastomere analysis before implantation (BABI) is under development at some centers. BABI and related technologies avoid the dilemma of abortion by selecting blastocysts for implantation that are female or lack high numbers of triplet repeats.

As with other conditions that cause severe to moderate developmental disability, initial psychosocial counseling is important for aiding parental adjustment to the child with fragile X syndrome. Complicating adjustment in some families are the subtle or manifest psychiatric problems in female carriers. Females with less than 200 amplified triplet repeats at the fragile X locus ("premutation") exhibit no behavioral differences from control females having children with disabilities. Females with more than 200 amplified repeats ("full mutation") have a greater frequency of avoidance and mood disorders, and the severity of both behavioral and cognitive problems was correlated with the size of DNA amplification. Hagerman (1997) reviews comparisons of females with fragile X full or premutations to their normal sisters that showed significant attentional difficulties in addition to cognitive and behavioral problems. Although these studies offer slightly differing views of the fragile X phenotype in females, it is clear that female carriers require evaluation for school and behavioral difficulties.

For males and females with fragile X syndrome, discussion of early intervention, speech, child behavior, social, and psychology/psychiatry services should be emphasized, and access to these services facilitated as needed. Parent support groups for fragile X syndrome include the Fragile X Research Foundation (www.fraxa.org/), National Fragile X Foundation (www.fragilex.org/), and a Fragile X E-mail Discussion Group for Parents at www.familyvillage.wisc.edu/lib_frgx.htm.

Natural history and complications

Lifespan should be normal in fragile X syndrome, and large numbers of older individuals have been described (Wiesner et al., 2004). The fragile X checklist, part 1 indicates that there are few medical complications, with most problems caused by the mental disability. Gorlin et al. (2001, pp. 71–5) reported an IQ range of 25–69, with 75% having IQs below 39. Many patients are described as "autistic," with 7–15% of males with autism being positive for fragile X testing. Characteristics such as hand flapping, echolalia, aggressiveness, self-mutilation, and emotional instability are described in males and severely affected female carriers with fragile X syndrome. However, controlled studies have disputed the attribution of specific behavioral phenotypes to individuals with fragile X syndrome. Seizures occur in 15% of affected males, and sleep can be a problem as with other disorders with autistic features. Weiskop et al. (2005) discuss behavioral strategies to improve sleep (specific bedtime routines, reinforcement, effective instructions, partner support) and found a decrease in settling problems, night waking, and co-sleeping by parental report.

Recent studies of academic achievement revealed deficits in all academic skill areas for boys with fragile X syndrome (Roberts et al., 2005). Strengths were in general knowledge and integration of information, while weaknesses were observed in prewriting skills and visual-spatial-processing abilities. Several observers have noted a declining rate of academic growth, particularly in core academic skills like reading and mathematics. Roberts et al. (2005) did not find correlation of academic achievement with non-verbal IQ or repeat number, but did see correlation with autistic behavior and maternal education.

Although most children exhibit rapid growth, a few exhibit early failure to thrive. Predisposing factors may include gastroesophageal reflux, tactile defensiveness or food refusal with inadequate intake, and maternal psychiatric disease. Physical abnormalities include large testes, which usually occur after puberty but can occur even in fetuses. Laxity of connective tissue may produce pectus excavatum, inguinal hernias, flat feet, and mitral valve prolapse. The frequency of mitral valve prolapse ranges from 10% in children to 80% in adults. The palate is high, and overbite or crossbite is common. Both males and females are fertile, although few affected males have children.

Preventive medical checklist for fragile X syndrome

Preventive care is directed toward complications of early growth delay, mental disability, joint laxity, and dentistry (see checklist; Wiesner et al., 2004). Growth charts are available (Butler et al., 1992). Early medical concerns include chronic otitis and myopia or strabismus with the need for neurosensory screening. Mitral valve prolapse can be observed during childhood, and orthopedic problems such as flat feet or scoliosis can occur. Large testes may be noted, and the parents should be reassured that they are not signs of early puberty or sexual dysfunction. Supportive services such as early intervention, occupational therapy, physical therapy, behavioral assessment, and financial/school planning are particularly needed by fragile X families. Because of its association with fragile X expression in cultured cells, oral folic acid (10–50 mg/day) has been given to affected males without proven benefit (Hagerman, 1997). More important may be early recognition of seizures, hyperactivity, or psychiatric disorders that may be amenable to pharmacologic therapy. Carbamezapine has been effective for the treatment of epilepsy, and there is evidence that the incidence and treatment of hyperactivity or psychiatric disorders in fragile X syndrome are similar to those of the general population. It is important to recognize female carriers with fragile X syndrome so that they receive adequate early intervention, school options, social services, and genetic counseling as appropriate. Female heterozygotes may have learning disabilities (15%) or frank mental retardation (35%) in addition to their risk of behavioral problems (Gorlin et al., 2001, pp. 71–5). These risks correlate with the number of repeats demonstrated by DNA analysis.

Preventive management of Turner syndrome

Description: Clinical pattern caused by missing X chromosome material in females, 1 in 2500 births with 10-fold higher incidence at conception.

Clinical: Malformation syndrome in females with neonatal pedal edema, webbed neck, heart anomalies, and later short stature with immature sexual development.

Laboratory: 45,X karyotype in the majority with rarer deletions of Xp or Xq; 1/3 of patients are mosaic.

Genetics: Minimal recurrence risk for parents except in rare cases of translocation; mosaic females who are fertile have an increased risk for chromosomal anomalies in their offspring.

Key management issues: Chromosome studies and possible pelvic ultrasound to define mosaicism and tumor risks; monitoring and therapy for growth and pubertal failure with growth hormone and estrogen; monitoring for eye, ear, thyroid, cardiovascular, lymphatic, urinary tract, genital, and autoimmune problems; alertness for gastrointestinal bleeding, protein-losing enteropathy, or gonadoblastoma in the streak gonad.

Specific growth charts: Lyon et al. (1985).

Parent information: Turner Syndrome Society of the US (www.turner-syndrome-us.org/), Turner Syndrome Support Society of the UK (www.turner-syndrome-us.org/), and Turner's Syndrome Society Canada (www.turnersyndrome.ca/).

Basis for management recommendations: Consensus recommendations of the Committee on Genetics and Section on Endocrinology (2003).

Summary of clinical concerns

General	Learning	Subtle differences (decreased fine motor execution, numerical abilities, spatial visualization)
	Behavior	Depression (10%), anorexia nervosa
	Growth	Short stature
	Tumors	Multiple nevi, hemangiomas, **gonadoblastomas** (25% if Y chromosome)
Facial	Eyes	**Eye anomalies**, cataracts, strabismus (22%)
	Ears	**Chronic otitis** (80%)
	Nose	Choanal atresia (1%)
	Mouth	Oromotor dysfunction, high palate (36%), cleft lip/palate (2–3%)
Surface	Neck/trunk	**"Shield" chest** (53%), **pterygium colli** (46%), altered chest contour
	Epidermal	Cutaneous nevi, seborrhea, facial hirsutism, keloid formation
Skeletal	Cranial	Craniosynostosis
	Axial	Scoliosis, hypoplastic arch of atlas
	Limbs	**Cubitus valgus** (54%), **short metacarpals 4/5** (48%), **osteoporosis** (50%), hip dislocation
Internal	Digestive	GI bleeding, GI lymphangiectasia, diarrhea, protein loss, malabsorption, enteropathy
	Circulatory	Cardiac anomalies (16% – coarctation of aorta, bicuspid aortic valve), **lymphedema** (63–80%), **hypertension** (20%), aortic dilation
	Endorine	**Hypothyroidism** (20–30%), **delayed or absent puberty** (75–90%)
	RES	Autoimmune disorders; diabetes mellitus (adult onset, 5%), ulcerative colitis
	Excretory	Renal anomalies (anomalous ureters, horseshoe kidney, renal aplasia/hypoplasia)
	Genital	**Gonadal dysgenesis, infertility** (95%)
Neural	Central	Rare cognitive disability, subtle learning differences
	Motor	**Hearing deficits (15–45%), visual deficits** (22%)
	Sensory	Subtle differences (decreased fine motor execution, numerical abilities, spatial visualization)

RES, reticuloendothelial system; **concerns** of frequency >20% are **highlighted**

Key references

Consensus Development Conference (2004). Management of Turner's syndrome. *Journal of Pediatric Endocrinology and Metabolism* (Suppl. 2):257–61.

Frías, Davenport, & Committee on Genetics and Section on Endocrinology (2003). Health supervision for children with Turner syndrome. *Pediatrics* 111:692–702.

Lyon, et al. (1985). Growth curve for girls with Turner syndrome. *Archives of Disease in Childhood* 60:932–6.

Turner syndrome

Preventive medical checklist (0–3 years)

Name _____ Birth date ___/___/_____ Number_____

Age	Evaluations: key concerns	Management considerations		Notes
New-born ↓ 1 month	Dysmorphology examination: anomalies Hearing, vision:[2] eye examination Feeding: reflux, poor intake Stooling: diarrhea Heart: murmur, peripheral pulses Urinary tract anomalies Parental adjustment	❑ Karyotype, genetic counseling[1] ❑ ABR; ophthalmology[3] ❑ Feeding specialist; video swallow[3] ❑ Imaging studies; GI specialist[3] ❑ Echocardiogram; cardiology ❑ Abdominal sonogram; urology[3] ❑ Family support[4]	❑ ❑ ❑ ❑ ❑ ❑ ❑	
2 months ↓ 4 months	Growth and development[5] Hearing, vision:[2] strabismus, otitis Feeding: reflux, poor intake Stooling: diarrhea Heart: murmur, peripheral pulses Urinary tract: urinalysis, BP Parental adjustment Other:	❑ Turner growth charts, ECI[6] ❑ ABR;[3] ENT;[3] ophthalmology[3] ❑ Feeding specialist; video swallow[3] ❑ Imaging studies, GI specialist[3] ❑ Echolcardiogram;[3] cardiology[3] ❑ Abdominal sonogram; urology[3] ❑ Family support[4] ❑	❑ ❑ ❑ ❑ ❑ ❑ ❑ ❑	
6 months ↓ 9 months	Growth and development[5] Hearing, vision:[2] strabismus Nutrition: feeding, stooling Heart: murmur, peripheral pulses Urinary tract: urinalysis, BP Other:	❑ ECI[6] ❑ ENT;[3] ophthalmology ❑ Dietician;[3] GI specialist[3] ❑ Echocardiogram;[3] cardiology[3] ❑ Urology[3] ❑	❑ ❑ ❑ ❑ ❑ ❑	
1 year	Growth and development[5] Hearing, vision:[2] strabismus, otitis Thyroid: hypothyroidism Nutrition: feeding, stooling Heart: murmur, peripheral pulses Urinary tract: urinalysis, BP Other:	❑ ECI[6] ❑ ENT;[3] ophthalmology ❑ T4, TSH; endocrinology[3] ❑ Dietician;[3] GI specialist[3] ❑ Echocardiogram;[3] cardiology[3] ❑ Urology[3] ❑	❑ ❑ ❑ ❑ ❑ ❑ ❑	
15 months ↓ 18 months	Growth and development[5] Hearing, vision:[2] strabismus, otitis Feeding, stooling: reflux, constipation Urinary tract: urinalysis, BP	❑ ECI[6] ❑ ENT;[3] ophthalmology[3] ❑ Supplements;[3] laxatives[3] ❑ Urology[3]	❑ ❑ ❑ ❑	
2 years	Growth and development[5] Thyroid: hypothyroidism Hearing/vision:[2] strabismus, myopia Heart: murmur, peripheral pulses Urinary tract: urinalysis, BP	❑ ECI[6] ❑ T4, TSH;[3] endocrinology[3] ❑ Audiology; ENT; ophthalmology ❑ Echocardiogram;[3] cardiology[3] ❑ Urology[3]	❑ ❑ ❑ ❑ ❑	
3 years	Growth and development[5] Thyroid: hypothyroidism Hearing/vision:[2] strabismus, otitis Heart: murmur, peripheral pulses Urinary tract: urinalysis, BP Cosmetic issues: web neck Other:	❑ Turner charts; ECI[6]; family support[4] ❑ T4, TSH; endocrinology[3] ❑ Audiology; ENT; ophthalmology ❑ Echocardiogram;[3] cardiology[3] ❑ Urology[3] ❑ Plastic surgery[3] ❑	❑ ❑ ❑ ❑ ❑ ❑ ❑	

Turner syndrome concerns		Other concerns from history	
Vision, hearing deficits Strabismus, chronic otitis Hypothyroidism High palate, dental anomalies Cardiac anomalies (aorta)	Renal anomalies Duplicated ureters Keloids Gonadoblastoma Learning differences	**Family history/prenatal** _____ _____ _____ _____	**Social/environmental** _____ _____ _____ _____

Guidelines for the neonatal period should be undertaken *at whatever age* the diagnosis is made; ABR, auditory brainstem evoked response; BP, blood pressure; GI, gastroenterology; TSH, thyroid-stimulating hormone; [1]parental chromosomes only if child has translocation, consider FISH for Y chromosome studies on blood and urinary sediment/buccal smear; [2]by practitioner; [3]as dictated by clinical findings; [4]parent group, family/sib, financial, and behavioral issues; [5]consider developmental pediatric or genetics clinic according to symptoms and availability; [6]early childhood intervention including developmental monitoring and motor/speech therapy.

Turner syndrome

Preventive medical checklist (4–18 years)

Name _____ Birth date __/__/____ Number_____

Age	Evaluations: key concerns	Management considerations		Notes
4 years ↓ 6 years	Growth:[1] hormone needs hypotonia Development:[2] preschool transition Hearing, vision:[2] hearing loss, myopia Thyroid: hypothyroidism Heart: aortic dilation Urinary tract: urinalysis, BP Other:	❏ Turner syndrome charts;[1] endocrinology ❏ Family support;[4] preschool program[5] ❏ Audiology,[3] ophthalmology ❏ T4, TSH; endocrinology[3] ❏ Echocardiogram;[3] cardiology[3] ❏ Urology[3] ❏	❏ ❏ ❏ ❏ ❏ ❏ ❏	
7 years ↓ 9 years	Growth[1] Development:[1] school transition[5] Hearing, vision:[2] hearing loss, myopia Endocrine: hormone therapy Heart: aortic dilation Urinary tract: urinalysis, BP Other:	❏ Turner syndrome charts[1] ❏ Family support;[4] school progress[6] ❏ Audiology,[3] ophthalmology ❏ T4, TSH; endocrinology ❏ Echocardiogram;[3] cardiology[3] ❏ Urology[3] ❏	❏ ❏ ❏ ❏ ❏ ❏ ❏	
10 years ↓ 12 years	Growth and development[1] Hearing and vision[2] Endocrine: hormone therapy Nutrition: obesity, diabetes Other:	❏ Celiac panel;[3] school progress[6] ❏ Audiology,[3] ophthalmology ❏ T4, TSH; endocrinology ❏ Dietary counsel; activities; exercise ❏	❏ ❏ ❏ ❏ ❏	
13 years ↓ 15 years	Growth and development[1] Hearing and vision[2] Endocrine: hormone therapy, puberty Nutrition: obesity, teeth Heart: aortic dilation	❏ Turner syndrome charts;[1] school progress[6] ❏ Audiology,[3] ophthalmology ❏ T4, TSH; endocrinology ❏ Diet; activities; exercise; lipid profile ❏ Echocardiogram;[3] cardiology[3]	❏ ❏ ❏ ❏ ❏	
16 years ↓ 18 years	Growth and development[1] Endocrine: hormone therapy, puberty Heart: aortic dilation Urinary tract: urinalysis, glycosuria, BP Other:	❏ Family support;[4] school progress;[6] ❏ T4, TSH; endocrinology, gynecology ❏ Echocardiogram;[3] cardiology[3] ❏ Urology;[3] diabetologist ❏	❏ ❏ ❏ ❏ ❏	
19 years ↓ 23 years	Adult transition: body image, stigmata Hearing/vision:[2] myopia Endocrine: reproductive counsel Nutrition: obesity, teeth Heart: aortic dilation	❏ Psychiatry;[3] cosmetic surgery[3] ❏ ENT;[3] ophthalmology[3] ❏ T4, TSH; endocrinology; gynecology ❏ Diet; activities; exercise; lipid profile; dentistry ❏ Echocardiogram;[3] cardiology[3]	❏ ❏ ❏ ❏ ❏	
Adult	Body image, stigmata, keloids, nevi Hearing/vision:[2] myopia, astigmatism Endocrine: reproductive counsel Heart: aortic dilation Nutrition: obesity, teeth Urinary tract: urinalysis, glycosuria, BP Other:	❏ Psychiatry;[3] cosmetic surgery;[3] dermatology[3] ❏ Audiology;[3] ENT; ophthalmology ❏ T4, TSH; endocrinology; gynecology ❏ Echocardiogram;[3] cardiology[3] ❏ Diet; activities; exercise; lipid profile; dentistry ❏ Urology;[3] diabetologist ❏	❏ ❏ ❏ ❏ ❏ ❏ ❏	Fertile women have risks for aortic aneurysm during pregnancy and for chromosome anomalies in offspring.

Turner syndrome concerns		Other concerns from history	
Hearing loss High palate, dental changes Hypothyroidism Mitral valve prolapse Aortic dilation, aneurysm	Delayed puberty, diabetes mellitus Renal anomalies, hypertension Obesity, exercise, lipid changes Scoliosis, osteoporosis Learning disability, depression	**Family history/prenatal** _____ _____ _____ _____	**Social/environmental** _____ _____ _____ _____

Guidelines for the neonatal period should be undertaken *at whatever age* the diagnosis is made; BP, blood pressure; TSH, thyroid-stimulating hormone; [1]consider developmental pediatric or genetics clinic according to symptoms and availability; [2]by practitioner; [3]as dictated by clinical findings; [4]parent group, family/sib, financial, and behavioral issues with later focus on independent living and employment; [5]preschool program including developmental monitoring and motor/speech therapy if needed; [6]monitor individual education plan, educational testing, maturity according to puberty and hormone therapy, academic progress, behavioral differences, later reproductive counseling regarding fertility testing, artificial reproductive technology.

Parent guide to Turner syndrome

Patients lacking material from one X chromosome have a pattern of short stature, immature sexual development, and webbed neck known as Turner syndrome (Bonnevie–Ullrich or Ullrich–Turner syndromes are synonyms). Literature predating the use of hormone replacement therapy in Turner syndrome may exaggerate the severity of growth delay and sexual immaturity.

Incidence, causation, and diagnosis

Turner syndrome is very common at conception, with 98–99% of affected pregnancies aborting spontaneously. The birth incidence is 1 in 2500 female births, with 1/3 having demonstrable mosaicism (mixture of Turner cells and normal cells). The majority of patients have full 45,X or mosaic (45,X/46,XX) karyotypes, but occasional 45,X/46,XY mosaicism mandates fluorescent *in situ* hybridization (FISH) studies to rule out the presence of a Y chromosome with its higher risk for gonadal tumors. The characteristic webbed neck, unusual puffiness of the dorsa of the feet, and certain gastrointestinal anomalies are due to altered lymphatic drainage. Similar conditions include Noonan syndrome (wrongly called male Turner syndrome) with short stature, web neck, broad chest, heart anomalies, and more likely mental deficiency. Chromosome studies are diagnostic, and all patients should have a FISH studies to rule out the presence of a Y chromosome with its higher risk for gonadal tumors.

Natural history and complications

Children with Turner syndrome are slightly smaller at birth, and statural growth continues along the 3rd centile until puberty. Untreated women will rarely reach a height of 5 feet, but growth hormone, androgen, and estrogen therapy can add several inches to adult height and should be considered as early as age 2 years in girls with severe growth delay. Complications of Turner syndrome include eye, ear, cardiovascular, lymphatic, urinary tract, genital, and autoimmune problems. Mosaic patients will generally have a milder course, except that patients with a Y-chromosome-containing cell line face a 25% risk of the development of a gonadoblastoma tumor in their defective ovary. Biochemical abnormalities include increased risk for osteoporosis (softening of the bones), abnormal blood cholesterol, and lipoprotein profiles. Cardiac anomalies such as coarctation of the aorta and bicuspid aortic valve are sufficiently common that an echocardiogram should be considered during infancy. Although the coarctation may not be clinically significant, these anomalies predispose to aortic aneurysm (ballooning of the aorta) and atherosclerosis (hardening of the arteries). The aortic defects may underlie a general predisposition to vascular anomalies and hemangiomas that in the gastrointestinal tract may cause bleeding or protein-losing enteropathy (diarrhea with low blood proteins). There is increased risk of autoimmune disorders, including hypothyroidism and diabetes mellitus. Obesity can also be a problem, necessitating counsel regarding appropriate diet and exercise. Subtle learning differences can occur, with lower school performance and self-esteem in girls with Turner syndrome. Measures of map reading, figure drawing, geometry, or arithmetic may yield lower-than-average scores in Turner syndrome, but many girls catch up and perform well academically; 80% of the adult women in one study had completed 4 years of college.

Preventive medical needs

Although the diagnosis is often missed in the nursery, unless characterisic pedal edema is present, chromosome studies and possible pelvic sonography are crucial for management once the diagnosis is recognized. Removal of the defective ovaries on both sides during early childhood is indicated in children with mosaicism for Y-chromosome-containing cells. A second peak in the risk of gonadoblastoma occurs at puberty, so review of diagnostic results and consideration of novel tests to detect Y chromosome material should be made in adolescent females. Other problems during infancy and early childhood may include cardiac anomalies, chronic otitis, and developmental delay. The potential learning disabilities, together with possible feeding, hearing or vision problems, warrant referral for early intervention services. Echocardiogram and abdominal sonogram to visualize heart or urinary tract anomalies are warranted as soon as the diagnosis of Turner syndrome is confirmed. Periodic blood pressure determination, urinalysis, cardiology follow-up, and appropriate dental prophylaxis should be performed regularly, since hypertension (high blood pressure) occurs independently of aortic or renal disease. Mosaic women who are fertile face risks for aortic aneurysm during pregnancy. Referral to endocrinology should occur as early as age 2 years, with monitoring of thyroid function, growth hormone, and androgen/estrogen therapies. Some children may also need plastic surgery evaluation if their pterygium colli, nevi (birthmarks), or keloids (excessive scar tissue) are disfiguring. There is clearly excellent potential for cognitive and gender function in Turner syndrome, but health care providers should be alert for signs of school or psychosocial problems due to learning disabilities, poor body image, and depression.

Family counseling

Initial counseling should emphasize the normal intellectual prognosis and lifespan expected for women with Turner syndrome. One of the most difficult implications of the diagnosis is infertility, occurring in 95% of 45,X females and 75% of mosaic 45,X/46,XX females. Having one child with a 45,X karyotype does not confer an increased risk to parents for having subsequent children with chromosomal anomalies. However, fertile women with mosaicism for 45,X or other abnormal cell lines have an increased risk of chromosomal anomalies in their offspring and should be offered prenatal diagnosis. Parent support groups for Turner syndrome (see part 1 of this checklist) provide useful information about medical decisions and behavioral challenges, including the opportunity for younger children to see adult women who can be role models.

Preventive management of Klinefelter syndrome

Description: Clinical pattern caused by an extra X chromosome in males with an incidence of 1.18 per 1000 births.

Clinical diagnosis: Findings are subtle, especially before puberty. Early growth is normal with tall stature manifesting after puberty. Eye anomalies (such as coloboma or strabismus), skeletal anomalies (such as pectus, scoliosis, radioulnar synostosis), gastrointestinal anomalies (such as omphalocele), cardiac anomalies (such as aortic stenosis and later mitral valve prolapse), and genital anomalies (such as cryptorchidism or micropenis) can prompt medical attention. After puberty there is characteristic tall stature with asthenic habitus, small testes, gynecomastia, and sexual immaturity. Development and behavior are usually normal early on with possible motor delays and school problems, later showing dull-normal intelligence, antisocial behaviors, depression, and susceptibility to alcoholism.

Laboratory diagnosis: 80% have the definitive karyotype of 47,XXY, 10% are mosaic 46,XY/47,XXY with milder features, and the remainder have multiple X or Y chromosomes (48,XXXY; 48,XXYY; 49,XXXXY) with more severe mental and physical disabilities.

Genetics: A recurrence risk of 1% or less, with family studies needed only for unusual X or Y chromosome rearrangements.

Key management issues: Monitoring for hearing or vision problems; physical and occupational therapy for motor and speech delays; endocrinology evaluation with possible testosterone therapy, monitoring for school and behavioral problems; those with higher degrees of aneuploidy (48,XXXY; 49,XXXXY) will need more aggressive developmental and school monitoring with early intervention and family supports needed for moderate to severe disabilities.

Growth charts: Regular charts can be used for the expected tall stature.

Parent groups: Klinefelter Support Group (klinefeltersyndrome.org/), American Association for Klinefelter Syndrome and Support – Access (www.aaksis.org/index.cfm), Klinefelter Syndrome and Associates (KS & A – www.genetic.org/), and Triplo-X Organization (www.triplo-x.org/).

Basis for management recommendations: Derived from the complications and references below.

Summary of clinical concerns

General	Learning	Cognitive disability (mean IQ of 90 with 30% below 90), **motor delays** (27%)
	Behavior	Behavioral problems, antisocial behavior, depression, neuroses, psychoses, alcoholism
	Growth	Tall stature (2–5 cm taller than normal males), longer limbs
	Cancer	Cerebral germinoma, mediastinal teratoma, myeloproliferative diseases, breast cancer (66-fold higher than normal men)
Facial	Eyes	Coloboma, choroidal atrophy, strabismus, corneal opacity
	Mouth	Oromotor dysfunction, cleft palate, mandibular prognathism, taurodontism
Surface	Neck/trunk	Pectus excavatum, inguinal hernias, **gynecomastia after puberty** (50%)
	Epidermal	Sparse facial hair, varicose veins
Skeletal	Cranial	Mild microcephaly
	Axial	Scoliosis
	Limbs	Radioulnar synostosis; external rotation of legs, genu recurvatum
Internal	Digestive	Omphalocele
	Circulatory	Cardiac anomalies (aortic stenosis, mitral valve prolapse); varicose veins, leg ulceration
	Endocrine	Growth hormone, testosterone deficiency; diabetes mellitus (8%), **hypercholesterolemia** (50%)
	RES	Autoimmune disorders increased, including lupus erythematosis, diabetes mellitus
	Genital	**Small testes after puberty**, infertility, cryptorchidism, micropenis
Neural	Central	**Cognitive deficits** (30% below IQ 90, more severe in 48,XXXY; 49,XXXXY)
	Motor	Neurogenic amyotrophy, decreased muscle mass
	Sensory	Neurosensory deafness

RES, reticuloendothelial system; **concerns** of frequency >20% are **highlighted**

Key references

Bojesen, et al. (2004). Increased mortality in Klinefelter syndrome. *Journal of Pediatric Endocrinology and Metabolism* 89:3830–4.

Lanfranco, et al. (2004). Klinefelter's syndrome. *Lancet* 364:273–83.

Manning, M. A. & Hoyme, H. E. (2002). Diagnosis and management of the adolescent boy with Klinefelter syndrome. *Adolescent Medicine* 13:367–74.

Tyler & Edman (2004). Down syndrome, Turner syndrome, and Klinefelter syndrome: primary care throughout the life span. *Primary Care* 31:627–48.

Visootsak, et al. (2001). Klinefelter syndrome and its variants: an update and review for the primary pediatrician. *Clinical Pediatrics* 40:639–51.

Klinefelter syndrome

Preventive medical checklist (0–3 years)

Name _____ **Birth date** __/__/___ **Number** _____

Age	Evaluations: key concerns	Management considerations		Notes
Newborn ↓ **1 month**	Dysmorphology examination: anomalies Hearing, vision:[2] deafness, coloboma Feeding: cleft palate, dysphagia Heart: murmur, tachycardia Urogenital: cryptochidism, inguinal hernia Parental adjustment	❑ Karyotype; genetic counseling[1] ❑ ABR ❑ Feeding specialist;[3] cleft palate team[3] ❑ Echocardiogram;[3] cardiology[3] ❑ Endocrinology; urology[3] ❑ Family support[4]	❑ ❑ ❑ ❑ ❑ ❑	
2 months ↓ **4 months**	Growth and development[5] Hearing, vision:[2] deafness, coloboma Nutrition: feeding, poor intake Heart: aortic stenosis Urogenital: cryptochidism, inguinal hernia Parental adjustment Other:	❑ ECI[6] ❑ ABR[3] ❑ Feeding specialist[3] ❑ Echocardiogram;[3] cardiology[3] ❑ Endocrinology; urology[3] ❑ Family support[4] ❑	❑ ❑ ❑ ❑ ❑ ❑ ❑	
6 months ↓ **9 months**	Growth and development[5] Hearing, vision:[2] strabismus, deafness Urogenital: cryptochidism, inguinal hernia Nutrition: feeding Other:	❑ ECI[6] ❑ Audiology; ophthalmology ❑ Endocrinology; urology[3] ❑ Oromotor therapy[3] ❑	❑ ❑ ❑ ❑ ❑	
1 year	Growth and development[5] Hearing, vision:[2] strabismus, deafness Nutrition: feeding Urogenital: hernia, micropenis Other:	❑ ECI[6] ❑ Audiology; ophthalmology ❑ Dietician[3] ❑ Endocrinology; urology[3] ❑	❑ ❑ ❑ ❑ ❑	
15 months ↓ **18 months**	Growth and development[5] Hearing, vision:[2] strabismus, deafness Nutrition: feeding Urogenital: hernia, micropenis	❑ ECI[6] ❑ Audiology; ophthalmology ❑ Dietician[3] ❑ Endocrinology; urology[3]	❑ ❑ ❑ ❑	
2 years	Growth and development[5] Hearing, vision:[2] strabismus, deafness Nutrition: feeding Heart: aortic stenosis, mitral prolapse Urogenital: hernia, micropenis	❑ ECI[6] ❑ Audiology; ophthalmology ❑ Dietician[3] ❑ Echocardiogram;[3] cardiology[3] ❑ Endocrinology; urology[3]	❑ ❑ ❑ ❑ ❑	
3 years	Growth and development[5] Hearing, vision:[2] strabismus, deafness Nutrition: feeding Heart: aortic stenosis, mitral prolapse Urogenital: hernia, micropenis Other:	❑ ECI[6]; family support[4] ❑ Audiology; ophthalmology ❑ Dietician[3] ❑ Echocardiogram;[3] cardiology[3] ❑ Endocrinology; urology[3] ❑	❑ ❑ ❑ ❑ ❑ ❑	

Klinefelter syndrome concerns		Other concerns from history	
		Family history/prenatal	**Social/environmental**
Poor feeding, weight gain Vision, hearing deficits Eye (coloboma, strabismus) Aortic stenosis, mitral prolapse Omphalocele	Inguinal hernia Pectus excavatum Radioulnar synostosis Cryptochidism, micropenis Motor delays	_____ _____ _____ _____	_____ _____ _____ _____

Guidelines for the neonatal period should be undertaken *at whatever age* the diagnosis is made; ABR, auditory brainstem evoked response; [1]Most children will not have congenital anomalies; parental chromosomes only if child has rearrangement or translocation; [2]by practitioner; [3]as dictated by clinical findings; [4]parent group, family/sib, financial, and behavioral issues; [5]consider developmental pediatrician/behavior therapist/genetics clinic according to symptoms and availability; [6]early childhood intervention if motor delays – usually required in 48,XXYY or 49,XXXXY – should include developmental monitoring and motor/speech therapy.

Klinefelter syndrome

Preventive medical checklist (4–18 years)

Name _____ Birth date __/__/__ Number _____

Age	Evaluations: key concerns	Management considerations		Notes
4 years ↓ 6 years	Growth:[1] tall stature hypotonia Development:[2] preschool transition Hearing, vision:[2] hearing loss Heart: aortic stenosis, mitral prolapse Skeleton: scoliosis, pectus Urogenital: hernia, micropenis Other:	❑ Regular charts[1] ❑ Family support;[4] preschool program[5] ❑ Audiology,[3] ophthalmology ❑ Echocardiogram;[3] cardiology[3] ❑ Orthopedics[3] ❑ Endocrinology; urology[3] ❑	❑ ❑ ❑ ❑ ❑ ❑ ❑	
7 years ↓ 9 years	Growth[1] Development:[1] school transition[5] Hearing, vision:[2] hearing loss, amblyopia Nutrition: obesity Skeleton: scoliosis, pectus Urogenital: hernia, micropenis Other:	❑ Down syndrome charts[1] ❑ Family support;[4] school progress[6] ❑ Audiology;[3] ophthalmology[3] ❑ Dietary counsel; activities; exercise ❑ Orthopedics[3] ❑ Endocrinology; urology[3] ❑	❑ ❑ ❑ ❑ ❑ ❑ ❑	
10 years ↓ 12 years	Growth and development[1] Hearing, vision:[2] hearing loss, amblyopia Nutrition: obesity Skeleton: scoliosis, pectus Other:	❑ School progress[6] ❑ Audiology;[3] ophthalmology[3] ❑ Endocrinology; dietary counsel; exercise ❑ Orthopedics[3] ❑	❑ ❑ ❑ ❑ ❑	
13 years ↓ 15 years	Growth and development[1] Hearing, vision:[2] hearing loss, amblyopia Puberty; immaturity Nutrition: obesity Urogenital: hernia, micropenis	❑ School progress[6] ❑ Audiology;[3] ophthalmology[3] ❑ Testosterone levels; endocrinology[3] ❑ Dietary counsel; activities; exercise ❑ Urology[3]	❑ ❑ ❑ ❑ ❑	
16 years ↓ 18 years	Growth and development[1] Hearing, vision:[2] hearing loss, amblyopia Puberty; immaturity Nutrition: obesity Other:	❑ Family support;[4] school progress[6] ❑ Audiology;[3] ophthalmology[3] ❑ Testosterone levels; endocrinology[3] ❑ Dietary counsel; activities; exercise ❑	❑ ❑ ❑ ❑ ❑	
19 years ↓ 23 years	Adult-care transition[5] Hearing, vision:[2] hearing loss, amblyopia Nutrition: obesity Heart: aortic stenosis, mitral prolapse	❑ Family support;[4] school progress[6] ❑ Audiology;[3] ophthalmology[3] ❑ Dietary counsel; activities; exercise ❑ Cardiology[3]	❑ ❑ ❑ ❑	
Adult	Adult-care transition[5] Hearing, vision:[2] hearing loss, amblyopia Infertility, diabetes Scoliosis, mitral valve prolapse Nutrition: obesity Behavior: aggression, depression Other:	❑ Breast and genital examinations ❑ Audiology;[3] ophthalmology[3] ❑ Reproductive options; endocrinology[3] ❑ Orthopedics;[3] cardiology[3] ❑ Dietary counsel; activities; exercise ❑ Psychiatry[3] ❑	❑ ❑ ❑ ❑ ❑ ❑ ❑	

Klinefelter syndrome concerns		Other concerns from history	
Tall stature Vision, hearing deficits Strabismus Aortic stenosis, mitral prolapse Infertility Obesity, exercise	Inguinal hernia Pectus excavatum, scoliosis Radioulnar synostosis Micropenis, sexual immaturity Antisocial behavior, depression Breast cancer, rare cancers	**Family history/prenatal** _____ _____ _____ _____	**Social/environmental** _____ _____ _____ _____

Guidelines for the neonatal period should be undertaken *at whatever age* the diagnosis is made; [1]consider developmental pediatrician/behavior therapist/genetics clinic according to symptoms and availability; [2] by practitioner; [3]as dictated by clinical findings; [4]parent group and behavioral issues with later focus on social adjustment and employment; [5]preschool program including developmental and behavioral monitoring; [6]monitor individual education plan, educational testing, academic progress, behavioral differences, later social and vocational adjustment.

Parent guide to Klinefelter syndrome

In 1942, Klinefelter described a syndrome in males with increased stature, enlarged breasts (gynecomastia), small testes, and an extra X chromosome (chromosome constitution of 47,XXY). Klinefelter syndrome "variants" include disorders with more severe clinical features and additional X or Y chromosomes as in the karyotypes 48,XXXY; 48,XXYY; and 49,XXXXY.

Incidence, causation, and diagnosis

The classic Klinefelter phenotype has a prevalence of 1.18 per 1000, with 80% having karyotypes of 47,XXY, 10% being 46,XY/47,XXY mosaics, and the remainder having multiple X or Y chromosomes. More than 10% of males presenting with sterility and 3% of those with breast cancer will have Klinefelter syndrome. The additional X interferes with male hormone (testosterone) secreting cells in the testis, but the exact mechanism is unknown. The immature body habitus, feminine features (like gynecomastia, high voice, or sparse hair), and sterility reflect testosterone deficiency. Differential diagnosis includes males with pituitary gland dysfunction and certain genetic conditions with a lean, immature body habitus such as homocystinuria or Marfan syndrome. Only 18% of individuals with 47,XXY Klinefelter syndrome will have major congenital anomalies, and most are recognized after puberty. The karyotype is diagnostic, and serum testosterone levels should be considered in postpubertal patients.

Natural history and complications

Individuals with Klinefelter syndrome should have normal life expectancy except for a 6-fold increased risk of cerebrovascular disease (strokes) and a 1.6% lifetime incidence of cancer. Delayed speech is found in 51%, motor delays in 27%, and school maladjustment in 44%. Early onset of puberty has been reported in association with a germ cell tumor. Antisocial behaviors including theft or arson, alcoholism, and aggressiveness are described in some reports; others describe XXY men as having similar employment and social status to their peers. Psychiatric disorders such as manic–depressive illness, psychosis, depression, and anorexia nervosa may be increased. Other medical complications include eye anomalies such as coloboma, strabismus or choroidal atrophy, cleft palate, heart defects like aortic stenosis or mitral valve prolapse, inguinal hernia, and genital anomalies such as cryptorchidism (undescended testes) or small penis. Hearing deficits may occur, although most studies do not document higher numbers of respiratory infections during childhood. Increased frequency of autoimmune diseases such as collagen vascular disease or diabetes mellitus has been reported. Unusual complications include distal muscle weakness and severe varicose veins have been reported.

Preventive medical needs

Children with Klinefelter syndrome are rarely recognized in the newborn period unless identified through prenatal diagnosis. An early diagnosis allows psychologic and/or pharmacologic therapy to be considered when school and behavior problems are recognized. Early preventive care should include screening for hearing or vision problems, plus physical and occupational therapy assessment for motor and speech delays. Auditory evoked-response testing should be performed to rule out nerve deafness. If assessment reveals developmental delays, or if an early intervention program is the best way to obtain assessment, then the child should be referred. Eye and genital anomalies are sometimes found, so these regions should be carefully examined. Many Klinefelter patients present because of behavior problems, abnormal pubertal development, or infertility. Puberty should be monitored carefully, since both delays and precocious puberty have been reported. Gynecomastia, small penis, or small testes can be sources of ridicule for teenagers and detract from self-image; breast liposuction and orchiectomy followed by testicular implants improved self-image and behavior in one patient. Testosterone therapy is most beneficial if started at age 11–12 years. In one study, 77% of 30 adult males benefited from testosterone treatment (average 3.6 years) by showing better mood, less irritability, and more energy, endurance, and concentration. Depot injection or oral testosterone therapy may be tried, but side effects include priapism (persistent penile erection), salt and water retention, polycythemia (thickened blood), diabetes mellitus, and, in older patients, prostatic hypertrophy with sudden bladder obstruction. Gynecomastia is not benefited by androgen therapy, although one study obtained benefit from dihydrotestosterone. Priming of external genital development using testosterone may be indicated in males with a small phallus. For all of these reasons, endocrinology referral is strongly recommended when the diagnosis is made.

Family counseling

For parents of young children, medical counseling should address the probable sterility and the increased risk of school and behavior problems. Adolescents and adults with Klinefelter syndrome should know about the possible benefits of testosterone supplements and cosmetic surgery. The abnormal karyotype in Klinefelter syndrome is associated with advanced maternal age. Genetic counseling is useful for affected individuals and their parents. The recurrence risk for parents of a child with Klinefelter syndrome will usually be 1% or less. Family chromosome studies are needed only if unusual X or Y chromosome rearrangements are found. Occasionally, men with Klinefelter syndrome have been confirmed as fathers by paternity analysis. If they are fertile because of mosaicism (mixtures of normal and Klinefelter cells), these men and their spouses warrant the option of prenatal diagnosis because of the increased risk of chromosome abnormalities in their offspring. Parent support groups are useful for discussion of behavioral management and promoting self-image.

Preventive management of fragile X syndrome

Description: A disorder caused by triplet repeat expansion of the fragile X mental retardation gene, causing mild physical changes with mental disability. The incidence is 1 in 4000 males and 1 in 8000 females.

Clinical: Manifestations include elongated body habitus, prominent jaw, large ears, lax connective tissue, large testes, moderate to severe mental disability, and behavioral differences.

Laboratory: DNA testing reveals 50–200 trinucleotide repeats for asymptomatic males or females with "premutations." >200 repeats for males or females with full mutations; 2/3 of females with full mutations have cognitive disability. The unstable trinucleotide repeats are near the fragile X gene at Xq27, where expansion leads to gene inactivation.

Genetics: Complex inheritance since the premutation expands only during female meiosis; individuals with full mutations simulate classical X-linked-recessive inheritance (25% risk for affected or carrier females to have severely affected sons; premutations may be transmitted to asymptomatic children and become symptomatic in grandchildren (anticipation).

Key management issues: Early intervention and speech therapy for mental disability; monitoring for dental and connective tissue problems (pectus excavatum, mitral valve prolapse, inguinal hernias), family support with behavioral assessments and school planning.

Specific growth charts: Available for height, weight, head circumference (Butler et al., 1992).

Parent information: The National Fragile X Foundation (www.fragilex.org) and the Fragile X Research Foundation Inc. (www.fraxa.org) provide resources, conferences, and networking for parents.

Basis for management recommendations: Consensus guidelines from the Committee on Genetics, American Academy of Pediatrics (1996).

Summary of clinical concerns

General	Learning	**Cognitive disability** (100% – IQ range 25–69; 75% with IQ <40), learning differences, speech problems (stuttering, repetitive phrases, dysfluencies, cluttered speech, rhythmic intonation)
	Behavior	**Aggressiveness** (50%); **autistic features** (25% – poor eye contact, hand-flapping, echolalia), hyperactivity, emotional lability
	Growth	Early failure to thrive or overgrowth with obesity; tall, asthenic habitus in older children
Facial	Face	**Long and narrow face** (60%), prominent jaw
	Eyes	Strabismus (10%), **refractive errors** and myopia (25%), nystagmus
	Ears	Large, decreased cartilage; **chronic otitis media** (85%)
	Mouth	High palate, dental malocclusion
Surface	Neck/trunk	Pectus excavatum, inguinal hernia
	Epidermal	Velvety, lax skin with calluses
Skeletal	Cranial	Macrocephaly, prominent occiput
	Axial	Scoliosis
	Limbs	**Flat feet** (40%), increased joint laxity
Internal	Digestive	Early feeding problems
	Circulatory	**Mitral valve prolapse** (80%), aortic dilation (15%)
	Connective	**Lax joints** (70%)
	Genital	**Macro-orchidism** (40–75%); premature ovarian failure in carrier females
Neural	Central	Abnormal EEG (50%), **seizures** (15–20%), irritability
	Motor	Hypotonia, increased deep tendon reflex
	Sensory	Vision and hearing deficits

Concerns of frequency >20% are **highlighted**

Key references

Butler, et al. (1992). Standards for selected anthropometric measurements in males with the fragile X syndrome. *Pediatrics* 89:1059–62.

Chudley & Hagerman (1987). Fragile X syndrome *Journal of Pediatrics* 110:821–31.

Committee on Genetics, American Academy of Pediatrics (1996). Health supervision for children with fragile X syndrome. *Pediatrics* 98:297–300.

Roberts, J. E., et al. (2005). Academic skills of boys with fragile X syndrome: profiles and predictors. *American Journal of Mental Retardation* 110:107–20.

Fragile X syndrome

Preventive medical checklist (0–3 years)

Name _____ Birth date __/__/__ Number _____

Age	Evaluations: key concerns	Management considerations		Notes
New-born ↓ 1 month	Genetic evaluation: family history Hearing, vision:[2] strabismus Feeding: GE reflux, dysphagia Heart: mitral valve, aortic dilation Joints: club feet, hip dislocation Parental adjustment	❑ DNA testing, genetic counseling[1] ❑ ABR; ophthalmology[3] ❑ Feeding specialist; video swallow[3] ❑ Echocardiogram;[3] cardiology[3] ❑ Orthopedics[3] ❑ Family support[4]	❑ ❑ ❑ ❑ ❑ ❑	
2 months ↓ 4 months	Growth and development[5] Hearing, vision:[2] strabismus, otitis Feeding: GE reflux, high palate Heart: mitral valve, aortic dilation Skeletal: pectus, scoliosis Genitalia: inguinal hernia Parental adjustment Other:	❑ ECI[6] ❑ Ophthalmology,[3] ENT[3] ❑ Feeding specialist[3] ❑ Echocardiogram;[3] cardiology[3] ❑ Orthopedics[3] ❑ Pediatric surgery[3] ❑ Family support[4] ❑	❑ ❑ ❑ ❑ ❑ ❑ ❑ ❑	
6 months ↓ 9 months	Growth: macrocephaly[5] Hearing, vision:[2] strabismus, otitis Feeding: GE reflux, dysphagia Heart: mitral valve, aortic dilation Joints: club feet, hip dislocation Other:	❑ ECI[6] ❑ Ophthalmology,[3] ENT[3] ❑ Feeding specialist[3] ❑ Echocardiogram;[3] cardiology[3] ❑ Orthopedics[3] ❑	❑ ❑ ❑ ❑ ❑ ❑	
1 year	Growth and development[5] Hearing, vision:[2] strabismus, otitis Feeding: GE reflux, high palate Heart: mitral valve, aortic dilation Skeletal: pectus, scoliosis Genitalia: inguinal hernia Other:	❑ Fragile X charts;[5] ECI[6] ❑ Ophthalmology,[3] ENT[3] ❑ Feeding specialist[3] ❑ Echocardiogram;[3] cardiology[3] ❑ Orthopedics[3] ❑ Pediatric surgery[3] ❑	❑ ❑ ❑ ❑ ❑ ❑ ❑	
15 months ↓ 18 months	Growth: macrocephaly[5] Hearing, vision:[2] strabismus, otitis Heart: mitral valve, aortic dilation CNS: seizures, behavior	❑ ECI[6] ❑ Ophthalmology,[3] ENT[3] ❑ Echocardiogram;[3] cardiology[3] ❑ Neurology,[3] behavior specialist[3]	❑ ❑ ❑ ❑	
2 years	Growth and development[5] Hearing, vision:[2] strabismus, otitis Heart: mitral valve, aortic dilation Mouth: dental malocclusion CNS: seizures, behavior	❑ Fragile X charts;[5] ECI[6] ❑ Audiology;[3] ophthalmology[3] ❑ Echocardiogram;[3] cardiology[3] ❑ Dentistry[3] ❑ Neurology;[3] behaviorist[3]	❑ ❑ ❑ ❑ ❑	
3 years	Growth: macrocephaly[5] Hearing, vision:[2] strabismus, otitis Heart: mitral valve, aortic dilation Mouth: dental malocclusion Pectus, scoliosis, inguinal hernia CNS: seizures, behavior Other:	❑ Fragile X charts;[5] ECI[6]; family support[4] ❑ Audiology;[3] ophthalmology[3] ❑ Echocardiogram;[3] cardiology[3] ❑ Dentistry[3] ❑ Orthopedics;[3] pediatric surgery[3] ❑ Neurology,[3] behavior specialist[3] ❑	❑ ❑ ❑ ❑ ❑ ❑ ❑	

Fragile X syndrome concerns		Other concerns from history	
Feeding problems High palate GE reflux Strabismus, nystagmus Serous otitis, hearing loss Joint laxity	Mitral valve prolapse Club foot, hip dislocation Inguinal hernia Hypotonia, seizures Developmental disability Aggression, autism	**Family history/prenatal** _____ _____ _____ _____ _____	**Social/environmental** _____ _____ _____ _____ _____

Guidelines for the neonatal period should be undertaken *at whatever age* the diagnosis is made; GE, gastroesophageal; ABR, auditory brainstem evoked response; [1]consider testing carrier status of female relatives; [2]by practitioner; [3]as dictated by clinical findings; [4]parent group, family/sib, financial, and behavioral issues with particular attention to maternal care in view of possible carrier symptoms (psychosis, mental disability); [5]consider developmental pediatrician/neurologist/geneticist/behavior therapist according to symptoms and availability, especially if seizures; [6]early childhood intervention including developmental monitoring and motor/speech therapy.

Fragile X syndrome

Preventive medical checklist (4–18 years)

Name _____ Birth date __/__/___ Number _____

Age	Evaluations: key concerns	Management considerations		Notes
4 years ↓ 6 years	Growth, head size[5] Development:[2] preschool transition Hearing, vision:[2] myopia, hearing loss Heart: mitral valve, aortic dilation Mouth: dental malocclusion CNS: seizures, behavior Other:	❏ Macrocephaly[1] ❏ Family support;[4] preschool program[5] ❏ Audiology,[3] ophthalmology[3] ❏ Cardiology[3] ❏ Dentistry[3] ❏ Neurology,[3] behavior specialist[3] ❏	❏ ❏ ❏ ❏ ❏ ❏ ❏	
7 years ↓ 9 years	Growth[1] Development:[1] school transition[5] Hearing, vision:[2] myopia, hearing loss Heart: mitral valve, aortic dilation Mouth: dental malocclusion Pectus, scoliosis, inguinal hernia Other:	❏ Fragile X charts[1] ❏ Family support;[4] school progress[6] ❏ Audiology;[3] ophthalmology[3] ❏ Cardiology[3] ❏ Dentistry[3] ❏ Orthopedics,[3] pediatric surgery[3] ❏	❏ ❏ ❏ ❏ ❏ ❏ ❏	
10 years ↓ 12 years	Growth and development[1] Hearing, vision:[2] myopia, hearing loss Heart: mitral valve, aortic dilation CNS: seizures, behavior Other:	❏ Fragile X charts;[1] school progress[6] ❏ Audiology,[3] ophthalmology[3] ❏ Echocardiogram,[3] cardiology[3] ❏ Neurology,[3] behavior specialist[3] ❏	❏ ❏ ❏ ❏ ❏	
13 years ↓ 15 years	Growth and development[1] Hearing, vision:[2] myopia, hearing loss Nutrition, obesity, puberty Pectus, scoliosis, flat feet Mouth: dental malocclusion Other:	❏ Fragile X charts;[1] school progress[6] ❏ Audiology,[3] ophthalmology[3] ❏ Cardiology[3] ❏ Orthopedics[3] ❏ Dentistry[3] ❏	❏ ❏ ❏ ❏ ❏ ❏	
16 years ↓ 18 years	Growth and development[1] Hearing, vision:[2] myopia, hearing loss Nutrition, obesity, puberty Heart: mitral valve, aortic dilation Other:	❏ Family support;[4] school progress[6] ❏ Audiology,[3] ophthalmology[3] ❏ Dietary counsel; activities; exercise ❏ Echocardiogram,[3] cardiology[3] ❏	❏ ❏ ❏ ❏ ❏	
19 years ↓ 23 years	Adult-care transition[6] Hearing, vision:[2] myopia, hearing loss Nutrition: obesity Heart: mitral valve, aortic dilation Pectus, scoliosis, flat feet	❏ Family support;[4] school progress[6] ❏ Audiology,[3] ophthalmology[3] ❏ Dietary counsel; activities; exercise ❏ Cardiology[3] ❏ Orthopedics[3]	❏ ❏ ❏ ❏ ❏	
Adult	Adult-care transition[6] Hearing, vision:[2] myopia, hearing loss Nutrition: obesity Heart: mitral valve, aortic dilation Pectus, scoliosis, flat feet, hernias Mouth: dental malocclusion Other:	❏ Family support[4] ❏ Audiology;[3] ENT; ophthalmology ❏ Dietary counsel; activities; exercise ❏ Echocardiogram,[3] cardiology[3] ❏ Orthopedics,[3] surgery[3] ❏ Dentistry[3] ❏	❏ ❏ ❏ ❏ ❏ ❏ ❏	

Fragile X syndrome concerns		Other concerns from history	
Strabismus High palate Dental anomalies Joint laxity Scoliosis, hernias Club feet, flat feet	Mitral valve prolapse Macro-orchidism Seizures Cognitive disability Speech problems Aggression, autism, outbursts	**Family history/prenatal** _____ _____ _____ _____	**Social/environmental** _____ _____ _____ _____

Guidelines for the neonatal period should be undertaken *at whatever age* the diagnosis is made; [1]consider developmental pediatrician/neurologist/genetics clinic/behavior therapist according to symptoms and availability; [2]by practitioner; [3]as dictated by clinical findings; [4]parent group, family/sib, financial, and behavioral issues with later focus on independent living and employment; [5]preschool program including developmental monitoring, motor/speech therapy, later emphasis on behavior issues; [6]monitor individual education plan, educational testing, balance of special education and inclusion, academic progress, behavioral differences (aggression, autism), later vocational planning.

Parent guide to fragile X syndrome

Fragile X syndrome refers to a combination of mental and physical abnormalities exhibited by males and females with a fragile site at chromosome band Xq27. Affected males were first described as a "Martin–Bell syndrome" with subtle facial changes, lax joints, and striking mental and behavior differences. A "fragile site" on the X chromosome was recognized by chromosome analysis of these males, and the fragility was shown to result from amplified "triplet or trinucleotide repeats" within the chromosomal DNA. These amplified repeats inactivate the nearby fragile X mental retardation 1 (FMR-1) gene, causing the features of fragile X syndrome.

Incidence, causation, and diagnosis

The incidence of fragile X syndrome is about 1 in 3000–4000 males and 1 in 8000 females, and it is the most common of more than 20 disorders that exhibit X-linked inheritance of mental disability. A specific DNA test demonstrating increased numbers of triplet repeats provides a definitive diagnose. Diagnosis can be suspected when the Martin–Bell features of developmental delay, behavior differences, prominent jaw and large ears, and joint laxity, and large testes is recognized. Carrier females may be completely normal or have milder delays with behavior changes including psychosis. Fragile X DNA testing is best used in a child with disability who has already had a normal karyotype, in potential carrier females assessed because of symptoms or family history, and in family studies to assign recurrence risks based on the identification of asymptomatic "transmitting" males or female carriers. Medical counseling is concerned with planning services for a child with significant developmental disability.

Natural history and complications

Lifespan should be normal in fragile X syndrome, and large numbers of older individuals have been described. There are few medical complications aside from problems caused by the mental disability and behavior differences. An IQ range of 25–69, with 50–75% having IQs below 39 is commonly cited. Many patients are described as "autistic," with 7–15% of males with autism being positive for fragile X testing. Characteristics such as hand-flapping, echolalia, aggressiveness, self-mutilation, and emotional instability are described in males and severely affected female carriers with fragile X syndrome. However, controlled studies have disputed the attribution of specific behavioral phenotypes to individuals with fragile X syndrome. Seizures occur in 15% of affected males. Although most children exhibit rapid growth, some have early failure to thrive with gastroesophageal reflux, tactile defensiveness with food refusal, or inadequate intake due to maternal disability or psychiatric disease. Physical abnormalities include large testes, which usually occur after puberty but can occur even in fetuses. Laxity of connective tissue may produce concavity of the chest (pectus excavatum, inguinal hernias, flat feet, and mitral valve prolapse (floppy mitral valve). The frequency of mitral valve prolapse ranges from 6% in children to 80% in adults – symptoms of this anomaly can include palpitations, breathlessness, or panic attacks. The palate is high, and overbite or crossbite of the teeth with malocclusion is common. Both males and females are fertile, although few affected males have children.

Preventive medical needs

Preventive care is directed toward complications of mental disability, joint laxity, and dentistry. Early medical concerns include chronic otitis and myopia or strabismus (wandering eye) with the need for hearing/vision screening. Mitral valve prolapse can be observed during childhood, and orthopedic problems such as flat feet or scoliosis (curved spine) can occur. Large testes may be noted, and the parents should be reassured that they are not signs of early puberty or sexual dysfunction. Supportive services such as early intervention, occupational therapy, physical therapy, behavioral assessment, and financial/school planning are particularly useful for families affected by fragile X syndrome. Early recognition of seizures, hyperactivity, or psychiatric disorders that may be amenable to pharmacologic therapy. Carbamezapine has been effective for the treatment of epilepsy, and there is evidence that the incidence and treatment of hyperactivity or psychiatric disorders in fragile X syndrome are similar to those of the general population. It is important to recognize female carriers with fragile X syndrome: they need evaluation for early intervention, school options, and social services. Female carriers may appear normal and have learning disabilities (15%) or frank mental retardation (35%) in addition to their risk of behavioral problems. Severity in males and females correlates with the amount of triplet repeat amplification that is demonstrated by DNA analysis.

Family counseling

The genetics of fragile X syndrome are quite complex because standard ratios for X-linked transmission must be modified according to gender and the number of amplified triplet repeats. All affected families need genetic counseling to correlate the number of repeats demonstrated by DNA testing with clinical symptoms and risks for offspring. Prenatal diagnosis by chorionic villus biopsy or amniocentesis is now routine, and pre-implantation diagnosis is feasible. As with other conditions that cause severe to moderate developmental disability, psychosocial counseling and parent groups are very helpful for parents adjusting to a diagnosis of fragile X syndrome. Such services may be particularly useful in families with subtle or manifest psychiatric problems in female carriers, including avoidance and mood disorders, attention difficulties, and even frank psychosis.

9

Chromosome microdeletion syndromes

Improvements in chromosome banding allowed detection of small deletions and duplications, beginning with missing small bands on chromosome 13 in certain children with retinoblastoma and on chromosome 15 in certain children with Prader–Willi syndrome. These subtle deletions, called microdeletions, were sometimes not reproducible because banding techniques could vary according to the specimen and laboratory conditions. Fluorescent *in situ* hybridization (FISH) and chromosome painting technologies, using fluorescent DNA probes to highlight specific chromosome regions, improved the characterization of microdeletions and complex rearrangements, revealing a new class of submicroscopic deletions that were not visible by the best-banding techniques. If targeted DNA segment is deleted, then the probe will not yield a fluorescent signal on that chromosome. Chromosome microscopic and submicroscopic deletions cause half (haploid) dosage of autosomal genes within the deleted area, or complete deficiency of genes within deleted regions of the X chromosome in males. The phenotypes of submicroscopic deletions are more easily explained by their haploid or missing genes than are aneuploidies of larger chromosome segments described in Chapters 7 and 8.

Schmickel (1986) coined the term "contiguous gene deletion" to denote composite phenotypes that result when neighboring deleted genes are associated with standard Mendelian diseases. Several examples of these aggregate phenotypes are found with small X chromosome deletions like that causing Duchenne muscular dystrophy, glycerol kinase, and adrenal hypoplasia. Each of these disorders had been described as a separate X-linked-recessive disease, so their concurrence in one patient is caused by deletion of the contiguous genes. In other microdeletions exemplified by the Prader–Willi and Angelman syndromes, several mechanisms including genomic imprinting may act with the deficient gene products to produce the phenotype. Some submicroscopic deletions, and particularly larger chromosomal aneuploidies like 5p− (cri-du-chat syndrome), cannot be explained as simple composites of Mendelian disorders because of the many genes and intragenic regions that are deleted or duplicated.

Table 9.1. Chromosome microdeletion syndromes

Deleted region	Disorder	Incidence*	Complications
7q11	Williams syndrome	1 in 20,000–50,000	Short stature, cognitive disability, hypercalcemia, supravalvular aortic stenosis, hypertension
8q24	TRP syndromes I and II	>100 cases	Short stature, microcephaly, sparse hair, bulbous nose, cardiac a., renal a., joint laxity
11p13	WAGR	>50 cases	Wilms tumor–Aniridia–Genital anomalies–Retardation syndrome
13q14	Retinoblastoma, cognitive disability	>50 cases	Retinoblastoma with or without cognitive disability
15q11q13(pat)	Prader–Willi syndrome	1 in 25,000	Short stature, obesity, cognitive disability, hypogonadism, hyperphagia, hypotonia
15q11q13(mat)	Angelman syndrome	>50 cases	Growth failure, cognitive disability, prominent jaw, gelastic seizures, jerky movements
17p11.2	Smith–Magenis syndrome	>50 cases	Growth failure, cognitive disability, self-mutilation, sleep disturbances
17p13.3	Miller–Dieker syndrome	>50 cases	Lissencephaly, growth and developmental delay
20p11.2	Alagille syndrome	1 in 100,000	Unusual facies, cholestasis, vertebral anomalies, peripheral pulmonary stenosis, embryotoxon of eye
22q11	Shprintzen/DiGeorge	>500 cases	Unusual facies, coloboma, conotruncal defects, hypoparathyroidism, immune deficiency
Xp21	DMD, other problems	>10 cases	Combinations of DMD, chronic granulomatous disease, retinitis pigmentosa, glycerol kinase deficiency, adrenal hypoplasia
Xp22	Kallman syndrome, other problems	<10 cases	Kallman syndrome, chondrodysplasia punctata, steroid sulfatase deficiency

Notes:
TRP, Trichorhinophalangeal; DMD, Duchenne muscular dystrophy; a., anomalies.
*Reported cases or number per live births.

Table 9.1 lists several chromosome microdeletion syndromes along with their major complications. The cytogenetics laboratory must be alerted when such disorders are suspected, since the FISH study must be performed with the appropriate DNA probe. In most of these disorders, understanding of the pathogenesis awaits better characterization of the genes and gene products within the deleted region. This chapter will provide brief discussion of the less common microdeletion syndromes, with more detailed review of the Williams, Prader–Willi, and Shprintzen/DiGeorge syndromes.

RARE CONTIGUOUS GENE DELETION SYNDROMES

Alagille syndrome

Five major features characterize Alagille syndrome that was described in 1987 and is also known as arteriohepatic dysplasia (Jones, 1997, pp. 586–7; Gorlin et al., 2001, pp. 1133–5; Kamath et al., 2004). These include a characteristic facial appearance (95%), cholestasis (91%), posterior embryotoxon of the eye (88%), vertebral defects (87%), and peripheral pulmonic stenosis (85%). The incidence is 1 in 70,000–100,000 births. Submicroscopic deletion of band p12 on the short arm of chromosome 20 is seen in 7–10% of cases, and mutations in the JAGGED signal transduction gene can be found in 70%. Some patients with isolated tetralogy of Fallot may have JAGGED gene mutations, and 10–15% of patients with the Alagille spectrum are due to new mutations.

Summary of clinical concerns: Alagille syndrome management considerations

General: The natural history indicates a shortened lifespan because of nutritional, infectious, cardiovascular, and hepatic diseases; over 25% will die by early adulthood.

Growth and development: Growth retardation (30%) including short stature with bony anomalies, mild developmental disability (20%): Early childhood intervention with speech therapy; endocrinology for severe short stature; developmental pediatrics, genetics, and/or neurology according to severity of delays and availability.

Cancer: Thyroid carcinoma, hepatocarcinoma.

Craniofacial: Deep-set eyes, long nose, prominent ears produce a typical appearance that some attribute to cholestasis.

Eye: Iris stromal hypoplasia, posterior embryotoxon (white line over the limbus), fundus hypopigmentation: Ophthalmology at diagnosis and annually thereafter.

Cardiac: Peripheral pulmonic stenosis, tetralogy of Fallot with multiple vascular anomalies including aortic aneurysms, coarctations: Cardiology and echocardiogram at diagnosis, serially thereafter.

Gastrointestinal: Jaundice, pruritis, xanthomas, and hypercholesterolemia due to chronic cholestasis, with eventual cirrhosis in 10–15%. Lipid abnormalities correlate with the severity of jaundice, and children with early-onset liver disease often require transplantation: Liver function studies, blood lipid profile, gastro-enterology at diagnosis, serially thereafter. Attention to nutrition, pruritus, and portal hypertension can improve quality of life and postpone liver transplantation (Cohran & Heubi, 2003).

Urogenital: Renal artery stenosis, renal hypoplasia, medullary cystic disease: Abdominal ultrasound at diagnosis, monitoring of blood pressure and urinalysis, nephrology, and urology follow-up according to symptoms.

Skeletal: Vertebral defects, rib anomalies, osteoporosis, radioulnar synostosis: Skeletal survey at diagnosis, serial X-rays for osteopenia, orthopedics evaluation, and follow-up for scoliosis.

Neurologic: Cerebrovascular changes including strokes, Moya Moya, cranial artery stenoses, mild mental disability in 15%, school problems: Head MRI and neurology evaluation at diagnosis, serial studies according to symptoms, school and behavioral assessments with careful monitoring of school progress.

Parental counseling: Parents and family members should be examined to distinguish variable expression (50% recurrence risk if parent affected) from new mutations (<1% recurrence risk). DNA testing for JAGGED mutations is available at several American and European laboratories (see GeneTest www.genetests.org), including for prenatal diagnosis. Parent support and information is available at the Alagille Syndrome Alliance (www.alagille.org/) and by searching on the syndrome name.

Angelman syndrome

First described by Dr. Harry Angelman in 1965, his name now replaces the pejorative but descriptive term "happy puppet" syndrome (Williams, 2005). The jerky movements, gelastic (laughing) seizures, aphasia, microcephaly, large mouth, prognathism due to jaw movements, and tongue protrusion with drooling allow clinical recognition in some patients. Patients with Angelman and Prader–Willi syndromes share a common chromosomal deletion at bands 15q11q13 but differ in the paternal origin of the deleted chromosome (Gorlin et al., 2001, pp. 758–60). Genes in the deleted region are subject to genomic imprinting, such that those derived from the mother are expressed differently from those derived from the father. As a result, deletion of maternally derived genes gives rise to the Angelman syndrome phenotype. Sixty-five percent of patients will have a chromosome deletion detected by FISH testing, while another 10% can be diagnosed by DNA testing for abnormal methylation due to uniparental disomy or imprinting mutations. At least 20% of patients with Angelman syndrome have gene mutations detected in research laboratories or no known cause (Jones, 1997, pp. 200–1; Gorlin et al., 2001, pp. 758–60).

Summary of clinical concerns: Angelman syndrome management considerations

Growth and development: Severe mental disability with average IQ below 40 and no speech: Early childhood intervention with rehabilitative and psychosocial services, developmental pediatrics, and/or genetics follow-up according to availability.

Craniofacial: Microbrachycephaly, prognathism because of frequent jaw movements, protrusion of the tongue with drooling, dysphagia due to weak suck, rare cleft lip/palate: Feeding specialist, nutrition, audiology, otolaryngology, dentistry, treatment for sialorrhea (drooling – Boyce & Bakheet, 2005).

Eye: Hypopigmentation of iris and choroids, optic atrophy in 30–40%, strabismus in 40%: Ophthalmology evaluation at diagnosis and annually thereafter; visual assessment important to encourage interactions and diminish autistic and self-mutilative tendencies.

Skeletal: Scoliosis and joint contractures in older children: Orthopedics as necessary.

Neurologic: Hypotonia followed by hypertonia in limbs, seizures in 80%, abnormal sleep patterns, self-mutilation, frequent movements, diffuse brain atrophy by EEG: Head MRI, EEG, and neurology assessment at diagnosis and serially according to symptoms; sleep study and possible melatonin therapy for sleep problems, school testing and monitoring of progress.

Parental counseling: Parents of children with deletion or methylation abnormalities have low (<1%) recurrence risks. Occasional gene mutations have been detected in mothers with resulting 50% recurrence risks, a rare but important concern in families with a compelling clinical diagnosis without cytogenetic/molecular confirmation. Parent support and information is available at Facts about Angelman Syndrome (asclepius.com/angel/asfinfo.html), the Angelman Syndrome Foundation (www.angelman.org/angel/), or by searching on the syndrome name.

Miller–Dieker syndrome and lissencephaly sequence

Miller–Dieker syndrome refers to a spectrum of brain, facial, heart, urogenital, and limb anomalies that result from deletion of chromosomal band 17p13.3. The core features are lissencephaly or smooth brain, and its consequent facial and neurologic features that are referred to as lissencephaly sequence (Jones, 1997, pp. 194–5; Gorlin et al., 2001, pp. 728–30). Isolated lissencephaly is associated with microcephaly, bitemporal hollowing, micrognathia, severe hypotonia with deceased fetal movements, and early dysphagia with seizures; it is associated with mutations in the LIS-1 or XLIS genes, allowing molecular diagnosis in 75% of cases. The 17p13 deletion in Miller–Dieker syndrome encompasses 7 genes in addition to the LIS-1 gene, thus combining lissencephaly sequence with more distinctive craniofacial changes and additional anomalies (Cardoso et al., 2003). The lissencephaly spectrum is quite rare, with about 100 reported cases. Preventive management described here can apply to isolated lissencephaly or its associated syndromes by recognizing that Miller–Dieker and other eponymous conditions will share the severe neurologic consequences with various additional complications.

Summary of clinical concerns: Miller–Dieker, lissencephaly management considerations

General: Pregnancy is complicated by decreased fetal movements and polyhydramnios; lifespan is limited in severe patients or those with larger chromosome deletions, with over half of patients dying during infancy: Family support services and counseling.

Growth and development: Development is severely impaired with feeding problems and growth failure: Discussion of palliative care for severely affected patients; early childhood intervention with rehabilitation services and supportive care; developmental pediatrics, genetics, and/or neurology according to availability.

Craniofacial: The lissencephaly and resulting hypotonia contribute to an abnormal face with bitemporal hollowing, high forehead, anteverted nares, and epicanthal folds; occasional cleft palate: Feeding specialist, nutrition, audiology, otolaryngology, dentistry, cleft palate team.

Cardiopulmonary: Heart defects in 65% including patent ductus arteriosus and ventricular septal defects: Cardiology, echocardiogram at diagnosis and serially according to symptoms.

Urogenital: Renal agenesis, hydronephrosis, urinary tract anomalies, sacral dimples, cryptorchidism, small penis: Urogenital examination and abdominal ultrasound in neonatal period with monitoring of blood pressure, urinalysis, urology, endocrinology evaluations surrounding puberty for those with better function.

Skeletal: Clinodactyly, limb contractures, rare polydactyly: Skeletal and range of movement examination at diagnosis, orthopedics, and occupational therapy as necessary.

Neurologic: Severe hypotonia and seizures caused by lissencephaly, associated brain anomalies including hypoplasia of the cerebellum and corpus callosum: Head MRI, EEG, neurology evaluation at diagnosis with neurology follow-up determined by symptoms.

Parental counseling: No specific support group; abundant information is available by searching on Miller–Dieker syndrome or lissencephaly.

Smith–Magenis syndrome

A syndrome of microcephaly, craniofacial changes, digital anomalies, growth failure, and severe mental disability was described in 1982 (Gorlin et al., 2001, pp. 107–8). The patients have midface hypoplasia, severe speech delay, a hoarse, deep voice, and insensitivity to pain with mutilative behavior. Interesting in view of the associated 17p11.2 deletion are decreased deep tendon reflexes and muscle atrophy; a major locus for Charcot–Marie–Tooth disease has been mapped within the Smith–Magenis deletion region. The incidence is estimated at 1 in 25,000 births, but the paucity of reported cases casts doubt on this figure. Under-ascertainment is probable because facial features may not stand out and DNA analysis is required for the recognition of the deletion in many patients.

Summary of clinical concerns: Smith–Magenis management considerations

Growth and development: Growth is delayed, and growth hormone deficiency has been described along with good response to growth hormone (Spadoni et al., 2004). Moderate to severe developmental disability with behavioral problems including aggression, impulsivity, hyperactivity, and odd habits like placing foreign objects in ear/vaginal orifices: Early childhood intervention with emphasis on behavioral assessments and speech therapy; developmental pediatrics, genetics, and/or neurology according to availability.

Craniofacial: Frontal bossing, synophrys, epicanthal folds, and up-slanting palpebral fissures with a full and tented upper lip, cleft lip/palate in 10%: Feeding specialist, nutrition, dentistry, cleft palate team.

Eye: Strabismus, retinal detachment, myopia: Ophthalmology at diagnosis, annually thereafter.

ENT: Recurrent otitis with ear anomalies and conductive hearing loss, sleep problems: Audiology and otolaryngology upon initial diagnosis and annually thereafter.

Cardiac: Cardiac defects (31%) including more subtle changes like total anomalous pulmonary venous return: Cardiology and echocardiogram at diagnosis.

Urogenital: Urinary tract anomalies such as duplicated collection system: Abdominal ultrasound at diagnosis, monitoring of blood pressure and urinalysis in those with anomalies; urology.

Skeletal: Syndactyly toes 3–4, scoliosis (24%), flat feet (61%): Orthopedics.

Neurologic: Conductive (65%) or sensorineural (35%) hearing loss (sleep disturbance is a striking feature of Smith–Magenis syndrome (Smith et al., 1998b)): Neurology, psychiatry, school testing and monitoring of progress.

Parental counseling: Parent-oriented information is available by searching on the syndrome name; a research and information site is available at Baylor College of Medicine in Houston (http://imgen.bcm.tmc.edu/molgen/lupski/sms/Index-SMS.htm).

Trichorhinophalangeal syndromes

Although trichorhinophalangeal (TRP) type I syndrome was originally thought distinct from TRP type II (Langer–Giedion syndrome), microdeletions or submicroscopic deletions in the chromosome 8q23q24 region have been observed in both conditions. TRP syndrome is probably best viewed as a spectrum extending from the sparse hair, bulbous nose, and normal cognitive function of TRP I to the more striking ectodermal/connective tissue changes seen in TRP II. The clinical spectrum is in turn determined by molecular changes extending from single-gene mutations (in a transcription factor) causing TRP I to deletions of several genes (including an exostosis-producing gene) in patients with larger 8q23q24 deletions and severe phenotype (Jones, 1997, pp. 290–3; Gorlin et al., 2001, pp. 1005–10). Discovery of the TRP I gene allowed study of related conditions and identified a third group within the spectrum that has Langer–Giedion severity without exostoses (Sugio–Kajii syndrome or TRP III; Ludecke et al., 2001).

Summary of clinical concerns: Trichorhinophalangeal syndromes management considerations

Growth and development: Stature below the 3rd centile in 40% of TRP I patients, more severe in TRP II with 60% having microcephaly; normal IQ in TRP I with occasional learning disabilities, mild to moderate disability in TRP II (75%): Developmental monitoring, early childhood intervention in children with multiple exostoses and more severe growth delay, speech evaluation for palatal motility if problems.

Craniofacial: Most patients will have the cognate findings of sparse hair and prominent nasal tip; more severe patients have dental anomalies (malocclusion, supernumerary teeth, missing teeth), submucous cleft palate: Monitoring of hearing and vision, regular dental care, alertness for otitis with referral to otolaryngology as needed.

Eye: Strabismus in 40% of TRP II: Regular vision assessment, ophthalmology at diagnosis in severe patients.

Surface: Sparse hair, redundant skin, multiple nevi, and brittle nails with later complete baldness in males and females: Dermatology, plastic surgery for teen/adult cosmetic concerns.

Reticuloendothelial system (RES): Frequent upper respiratory tract infections surveillance for otitis and upper respiratory infections.

Urogenital: Ureteral anomalies, prune belly, persistent cloaca, uterine anomalies: Abdominal ultrasound at diagnosis in more severe patients, monitoring of blood pressure and urinalysis in all; urology, endocrinology evaluations surrounding puberty.

Heart: Mitral valve prolapse in older or more severe patients as in other disorders with lax connective tissue: Regular cardiac examinations especially in teen/adult years, cardiology referral if signs or symptoms.

Skeletal: Short and irregular digits with diagnostic cone-shaped epiphyses on X-ray; scoliosis, flat feet, lax joints, and generalized arthritis; multiple bony exostoses in type II patients arising at age 3–4 years, and increasing in size and number until puberty: Counsel to favor joint-sparing activities and sports, annual examinations of limbs, hips, and spine; orthopedics consultation for symptoms.

Parental counseling: The spectrum of findings represented as TRP I, II, or III exhibit autosomal-dominant inheritance with a 50% recurrence risk for offspring of affected patients. Those with detectable chromosome 8 deletions have the option of prenatal diagnosis, although their severity may preclude family planning. Commercial DNA testing is not yet available for patients with milder TRP I phenotypes who have normal chromosomes and underlying TRP gene mutations. Parent support and information is available at the Langer–Giedion Support Association (lgsa.net/), where families can read (and should perhaps be forewarned) that the more severe phenotypes may not apply to their case.

Williams syndrome

Terminology

Williams and Beuren separately described children with supravalvular aortic stenosis, unusual facies, and other findings. "Williams syndrome" or "Williams–Beuren" syndrome is the preferred terminology, since supravalvular aortic stenosis is not present in all patients. The "idiopathic hypercalcemia–supravalvular aortic stenosis syndrome" and "elfin facies syndrome" are equivalent terms (Jones, 1997, pp. 118–21; Gorlin et al., 2001, pp. 1032–8).

Historical diagnosis and management

Numerous children with infantile hypercalcemia were described in Great Britain and Switzerland in the early 1950s. Many had feeding problems, constipation, and growth failure; a few developed azotemia and nephrocalcinosis. Concerns about a "milk-alkali" syndrome with excessive vitamin D intake led to changes in dietary recommendations for infants. Study of infantile hypercalcemia delineated a more severe group with persistent problems that probably corresponded to the Williams syndrome patients described by Williams and Beuren.

Early reports of Williams syndrome focused on neonatal hypercalcemia and cardiac anomalies, and it was some time before the full syndrome of mental disability, unusual appearance, and multiple congenital anomalies would be appreciated. Supravalvular aortic stenosis was defined as a unique, autosomal-dominant disorder before its recognition as part of Williams syndrome. Mapping of supravalvular aortic stenosis to a region of chromosome 7 (band q11) that contained the elastin gene led to the characterization of deletions in Williams syndrome.

Incidence, etiology, and differential diagnosis

The incidence depends on the accuracy of diagnosis, but is between 1 in 10,000 and 20,000 live births. Families containing some individuals with supravalvular stenosis and some with Williams syndrome have been reported, suggesting that milder patients may not be recognized. Deletion of one copy of the elastin gene presumably explains the supravalvular aortic stenosis and connective tissue alterations in Williams syndrome, with additional features caused by the deletion of contiguous genes. The chief differential is between other syndromes with developmental disabilities and vascular problems; rubella embryopathy and Alagille syndrome can have pulmonary artery stenoses. Hypercalcemia occurs in hyperparathyroidism and vitamin D intoxication, but these disorders should be easily distinguished by history or physical examination.

Diagnostic evaluation and medical counseling

Neonatal diagnosis of Williams syndrome is difficult unless hypercalcemia is detected. The characteristic face with stellate iris pattern, strabismus, periorbital fullness, thick lips, and long philtrum may not be obvious until early childhood. Chromosome analysis should be performed using FISH to detect 7q11 deletions that occur in 90–95% of patients. Medical counseling should emphasize the risks of ocular, cardiovascular, and renal anomalies, with mention of learning and behavioral problems (see checklist). The hypercalcemia is still not understood; it seems related to defective calcitonin release and diminished response to a calcium load.

Infancy is often difficult because of colic, feeding problems, cardiovascular complications, and even seizures such as infantile spasms. Parents may need considerable support during this period, but can often look forward to a calmer childhood period when the considerable verbal abilities and happy affect of children are quite rewarding.

Family and psychosocial counseling

Although Williams syndrome has exhibited rare parent–child transmission and concordance in identical twins, the recurrence risks for parents of affected children is <1%. Rare families have demonstrated autosomal-dominant inheritance, and referral for genetic counseling is important. Supportive counseling is required for the early feeding problems with colic, vomiting, or constipation; later difficulties with hyperactivity, distractibility, and learning differences may require psychosocial counseling and support. An article written by parents of a child with Williams syndrome provides useful insight for health professionals (Anonymous, 1985). Parent support groups include the Williams Syndrome Association (www.williams-syndrome.org), a Williams Syndrome Comprehensive Website (www.wsf.org/), and the Williams Syndrome Foundation (www.wsf.org/).

Natural history and complications

There are distinct stages in the natural history of Williams syndrome; facial characteristics and medical challenges change considerably with age. Intrauterine growth retardation is common, and the neonatal period may be turbulent with feeding difficulties and hypercalcemia. In one study, a 13.0 mg/dl intravenous pamidronate in a single dose of 1 mg/kg was effective in lowering serum calcium within 48 h, and it remained normal during infancy (Oliveri et al., 2004). The abnormal calcitonin release and high serum calcium may be related to acquired arterial problems such as coarctation of the aorta or later cerebral artery stenoses, but there is not yet evidence that mandates therapy. Infants often have mild flexion contractures and skeletal X-rays may show sclerotic lesions from the hypercalcemia (Gorlin et al., 2001, pp. 1032–8).

Childhood is usually dominated more by behavioral than medical concerns. The loquacious, "cocktail-party" manner and happy affect are attractive, but the accompanying hyperactivity, emotional lability, and excessive anxiety may be taxing (Udwin et al., 1998). Hyperacusis is common, and extreme responses to doorbells or lawnmowers may complicate behavioral management. Microcephaly and developmental delay are usual, with 59% of children having a global IQ under 70. Many children perform at age-appropriate levels in the areas of visual recognition, expressive language, and verbal recall (Udwin et al., 1998). Strengths are in music and language, but tangential reasoning, resistance to change, and autistic tendencies do occur (Gorlin et al., 2001, pp. 1032–8).

Supravalvular aortic or pulmonary stenosis, renal artery stenosis, and hypertension may cause problems in childhood, and sudden death because of coronary artery changes has complicated anesthesia (Medley et al., 2005). Coronary artery stenoses or aneurysms may occur independently of aortic anomalies, and in one patient presented as dysphagia (Mignosa et al., 2004). Wessel et al. (2004) examine the issue of sudden death in Williams syndrome, reviewing data on 293 patients. They recorded 10 total and 5 sudden deaths with an incidence of 1 death per 1000 patient years – a risk comparable to that following surgery for congenital heart disease and at least 25-fold higher than in a normal population. Renal anomalies (nephrocalcinosis, cystic dysplasia, renal failure, small kidney, unilateral renal agenesis) occur in 10–20% and should be monitored from infancy. Hypothyroidism, sometimes compensated with high thyroid-stimulating hormone (TSH) values, occurs in 25% (Gorlin et al., 2001, pp. 1032–8).

Complications in adolescents and adults include obesity (with abnormal glucose tolerance or type II diabetes), gastrointestinal problems (peptic ulcer, cholelithiasis, diverticular disease), cardiovascular disease (mitral valve prolapse, hypertension), decreased bone density, urinary problems (infections, bladder diverticula), sensorineural hearing loss, and frequent psychiatric symptoms (anxiety, impulsivity) requiring multimodal therapy (Cherniske et al., 2004). Hypercalciuria persists in many adult patients, sometimes causing paradoxical release of parathormone. The nephrocalcinosis plus renal artery narrowing in 40% cause hypertension to be a frequent complication, often with onset in the second or third decade (Cherniske et al., 2004). A few patients have had cerebral arterial stenosis with strokes at a young age, but the majority had normal MRI scans. Early graying of the hair, together with occasional Alzheimer-like brain changes in one patient, suggests that aging may be accelerated.

Williams syndrome preventive medical checklist

The Committee on Genetics of the American Academy of Pediatrics (2001a) has published guidelines for preventive management. Renal and cardiac sonography should be performed at the time of diagnosis, and frequent monitoring of arterial status and blood pressure is necessary. Where possible, four-extremity blood pressures should be obtained so peripheral vascular stenoses can be recognized. Although feeding problems, colic, and constipation often complicate early growth, conservative management is indicated since gastrointestinal anomalies are rare. Chronic otitis is a frequent problem, necessitating frequent audiologic assessments and possible referral to otolaryngology. Dental anomalies are frequent, and dentistry with appropriate endocarditis prophylaxis should be an integral part of preventive care. Risks for renal dysfunction and urinary tract infections justify frequent renal function tests, and follow-up renal sonograms should be performed in adolescence or adulthood.

As with other disorders involving neurologic dysfunction, early feeding difficulties are often followed by later inactivity, constipation, and risks for obesity. Early intervention therapies for joint contractures should be followed by alertness for scoliosis and hernias. Performance and behavior in school should be followed, with referral to behavioral specialists as needed. Anxiety may cause peptic ulcer disease, and cholelithiasis should be born in mind as a possibility in patients with abdominal pain. Community care networks are helpful if they can be established for adults with Williams syndrome (Udwin et al., 1998).

Prader–Willi syndrome

Terminology

The first report of Prader–Willi syndrome was by Prader in 1956, but several years elapsed before larger reviews established the full phenotype. Occasionally the syndrome is referred to as Prader–Labhart–Willi syndrome to include the three original authors or as the hypotonia–hypomentia–hypogenitalism–obesity (HHHO) syndrome (Jones, 1997, pp. 202–5; Gorlin et al., 2001, pp. 419–24).

Historical diagnosis and management

The obese, sleepy boy immortalized in the *Pickwick Papers* may have been the first reported case of Prader–Willi syndrome. The condition remains "underdiagnosed and undertreated" (Cassidy, 1987), but consensus diagnostic criteria (Holm et al., 1993) and findings most likely to yield a positive laboratory diagnosis (Whittington et al., 2002) have been defined. The disorder was one of the first examples of a contiguous gene deletion syndrome and, together with Angelman syndrome, is the prototypic clinical example of genomic imprinting in humans (Hall, 1990). Current interest includes the distinctive phases of natural history (see below), the unusual behaviors, and the disordered hypothalamic function exemplified by changes in appetite, temperature regulation, and sleep (Vogels et al., 2004).

Incidence, etiology, and differential diagnosis

The incidence of Prader–Willi syndrome is 1 in 16,000–25,000 births. Occasional familial cases led to suspicion of a genetic etiology, and this was proven when approximately 70% of patients with a classical phenotype were shown to have a deletion on the paternally derived chromosome 15 between bands q13 and q15 (Holm et al., 1993). Many of the remaining 30% will have uniparental disomy for the maternally derived chromosome 15, thus being deficient in paternally derived genes from the 15q13q15 region. Rare patients have normal chromosome 15 structure and origin, but lack mechanisms for DNA methylation that are necessary for establishing the genomic imprint. Cytogenetic FISH testing for 15q11 deletions can be done first, followed by DNA testing for abnormal 15q11 methylation patterns in highly suspect, deletion-negative patients. Prader–Willi syndrome is caused by altered expression of genes within the 15q13q15 region, although the precise genes and mechanisms of dysmorphogenesis have not been defined.

The diagnosis is aided by facial changes including almond-shaped eyes, down-turned corners of the mouth, and bitemporal hollowing. Karyotypic confirmation is especially needed in the infantile period before the development of hyperphagia. Differential diagnosis includes other disorders with neurologic dysfunction, severe hypotonia, and obesity. In the neonatal hypotonic phase, patients with the Prader–Willi syndrome may be confused with those of Down syndrome, Zellweger syndrome, or congenital neuropathies and myopathies. In the childhood obesity phase, disorders such as Cohen syndrome or Bardet–Biedl syndrome might be considered. Rare patients with the fragile X syndrome may exhibit the obesity, hypogonadism, and growth failure of Prader–Willi syndrome (Schrander-Stumpel et al., 1994).

Diagnostic evaluation and medical counseling

Consensus diagnostic criteria have been formulated for Prader–Willi syndrome and include neonatal/infantile hypotonia with its associated facial features, consequent infantile feeding problems, excessive weight gain between ages 1 and 6 years, hypogonadism, global developmental delay/mental disability, and hyperphagia/food obsession (Holm et al., 1993). Minor criteria include decreased fetal movement; unstable, stubborn or oppositional behavior; sleep apnea; short stature; hypopigmentation; small hands and feet; strabismus; thick saliva; problems with speech articulation; and skin picking. Whittington et al. (2002) reviewed infantile cases in the United Kingdom and showed that five clinical features – floppy at birth, weak cry/inactivity, poor suck, feeding difficulties with decreased vomiting, and hypogonadism – were present in 100% of confirmed diagnoses; these features plus thick saliva in the absence of hypogonadism that is hard to appreciate in females were predictive in 92%. Demonstration of deletion or altered imprinting/DNA methylation of chromosome region 15q11 is the keystone of diagnosis, but absence of any one feature mentioned by Whittington et al. (2002) greatly increases the likelihood of a negative laboratory result.

Although early diagnosis of Prader–Willi syndrome confers the anticipation of improved muscle strength and function, the parents face considerable challenges in caring for a child with nutritional, motor, cognitive, and behavioral problems. The greatest emphasis of medical counseling will be weight management, since obesity is a large contributor to morbidity and early mortality. Later issues will include school arrangements, behavior management, and provision for adolescents and adults living in a controlled environment.

Family and psychosocial counseling

From data on more than 1500 families, Cassidy (1987) derived a parental recurrence risk of less than 1 in 1000. Extremely rare cases can have small deletions in the Prader–Willi region that can be transmitted from parent to child, sometimes requiring transmission from females so as to lack the paternal imprint. The vast majority of parents can be reassured about future reproduction without the need for prenatal diagnosis; however, fetal screening is possible for reassurance when deletion or methylation defects are demonstrated. As for other disorders that inflict mental disability, supportive services such as psychology, social work, and grief counseling may be appropriate for some parents. Parent support groups include the Prader–Willi Syndrome Association (www.pwsausa.org/) and the Prader–Willi Syndrome Association UK (http://www.pwsa-uk.demon.co.uk/).

Natural history and complications

Few disorders exhibit the striking phenotypic changes observed in Prader–Willi syndrome. Prenatal hypotonia, decreased movement, and a propensity for breech positioning are followed by neonatal hypotonia that may be severe enough to mimic a congenital myopathy. Infantile hypotonia is associated with a weak suck and poor feeding that produces a "failure to thrive" picture until the change to hyperphagia occurs. Between ages 1 and 4 years, there is a transformation from growth failure to obesity caused by a voracious appetite. Abnormal eating behaviors include stealing food, nocturnal foraging for food, eating inappropriate foods, and binge eating. Morbid obesity may ensue that causes a shortened lifespan in Prader–Willi syndrome because of cardiopulmonary disease (Cassidy, 1987; Jones, 1997, pp. 202–5; Gorlin et al., 2001, pp. 419–24). Patients as old as 71 years have been reported; it is interesting that all older reported patients have been females.

The most taxing complications of Prader–Willi syndrome are developmental and behavioral, but ocular, dental, cutaneous, and genital anomalies occur. Because oculocutaneous albinism occurs in 50% of patients with Prader–Willi syndrome, the misrouting of retinogeniculate-cortical projections as occurs in albinism has been invoked as a cause for strabismus (40–95%). Dental problems include increased caries and enamel hypoplasia, perhaps reflecting the high-carbohydrate diet and decreased, thick saliva in Prader–Willi syndrome (Cassidy, 1987). Rumination occurs in 10–17% of patients, and aspiration pneumonitis must be added to the cor pulmonale, temperature instability, and cardiac arrhythmias that complicate anesthesia in patients with Prader–Willi syndrome. Wilms tumor and myeloid leukemias have been described with a 1.6-fold higher cancer risk in one study (Davies et al., 2003).

Hypogonadotrophic hypogonadism, irregular menses, and infertility are common, joining with hyperphagia, disruption of the sleep cycle, and temperature instability as evidence of hypothalamic dysfunction. Hoybye et al. (2002) documented a mean body mass index (BMI) of $35.6 \, kg/m^2$, increased total body fat, growth hormone deficiency (50%), osteoporosis or osteopenia (75%) in their study of older patients. They concluded that many risk factors for cardiovascular disease were secondary to growth hormone deficiency and emphasized the importance of growth hormone therapy in children and adults with Prader–Willi syndrome. Diabetes mellitus (5–15%) accompanies cardiopulmonary and sleep disturbances secondary to obesity.

Behavior problems dominate the management of Prader–Willi syndrome. Sleep disorders are common, with 50–90% of patients having daytime hypersomnolence. Although frequent snoring and a narrow upper airway occur in these patients, a central nervous system derangement of sleep is as common as obstructive sleep apnea. Sleep problems have been reported in some patients on growth hormone, and sleep studies are recommended before starting therapy. Violent outbursts, temper tantrums, obsessive–compulsive behavior, rigidity, manipulation, and stubbornness are common (Holm et al., 1993); older children and adults exhibit depression, and a "refusal–lethargy syndrome" of hyperkinesis, refusal of food and drink, and soiling. Skin picking with cellulitis and scarring and recurrent nasal bleeding may reflect the obsessive–compulsive and oppositional aspects of the syndrome. Spontaneous psychoses unrelated to other physical or behavioral problems have been reported in Prader–Willi syndrome, but their prevalence is not known.

Developmental delay is most obvious in motor milestones, with sitting at an average age of 12–13 months, walking at 24–30 months, and riding a tricycle at 4.2 years (Cassidy, 1987). Cognitive functions that are independent of hypotonia are less severely delayed, with single words appearing at 21–23 months and sentences at a mean of 3.6 years. Articulation defects are common and the speech often has a nasal quality. Reading is a relative strength, with mathematics and social interactions being weaknesses. Performance in solving mazes or codes was substantially above verbal performance that required auditory processing; this profile may explain the clinical impression that many Prader–Willi patients enjoy puzzles. As noted on the checklist, 40% of patients have a global IQ that is above 70 and in the borderline or normal range. Poor performance in school often reflects specific learning disabilities, distractibility, or behavioral problems.

Preventive medical checklist for Prader–Willi syndrome

When the diagnosis is suspected based on infantile hypotonia, karyotyping and DNA analysis to establish chromosome 15 deletion or uniparental disomy are critical. Early diagnosis is useful, since the inculcation of needed dietary controls is more easily accomplished before the oppositional, stubborn, and obsessive behaviors of later childhood and adolescence are encountered. Close monitoring of feeding is necessary during infancy, since some children require enhanced-calorie formula or gavage feeding. Strabismus, sleep problems, dental anomalies, and early intervention for developmental problems are important aspects of management in early childhood. A sleep study should be considered in all children with Prader–Willi syndrome once the diagnosis is made, and is mandated in those with symptoms of respiratory distress or sleep apnea, before anesthesia, before starting growth hormone therapy, and in older patients with severe obesity. Patients with severe growth delays may benefit by growth hormone therapy as early as 2 years of age, so early referral to endocrinology is useful.

Hyperphagia and morbid obesity are the major issues for later childhood and adolescence, but a wide variety of behavior problems require monitoring. Rumination can lead to gastric contents in the posterior pharynx during anesthesia, and preoperative preparations using anti-reflux medicines, decompression of the gastric contents, and body positioning are recommended for anesthesia. Pharmacologic treatment has been of benefit in skin picking, using drugs such as fluoxetine (Prozac). Serotonergic drugs have also shown promise in controlling appetite, and have had beneficial results in ameliorating hyperphagia, obsessive–compulsive behavior, and self-mutilation in Prader–Willi syndrome. Haloperidol and thioridazine have also had anecdotal success for behavioral control, depression, and anxiety in Prader–Willi syndrome. Periodic evaluation of behavior is an important and involvement of school psychologists and/or behavioral therapists will often be required.

The most successful strategies for weight management involved close supervision to regulate intake and the encouragement of regular exercise (Cassidy, 1987). Patients with Prader–Willi syndrome do not experience satiety and have remarkable resistance to vomiting; unregulated caloric intake can approach 6000 kcal/day (Cassidy, 1987). Restriction of calories to 800–1100 per day in adolescents is usually necessary to achieve weight control. Education of parents and children is vital, and behavioral modification using rewards, restricted access to all food sources, and the promotion of exercise is necessary. Many adolescents and adults do best living in group homes restricted to Prader–Willi syndrome, so a uniform lifestyle can be designed. Despite these efforts, most patients become obese and require monitoring of cardiopulmonary status and blood pressure.

Shprintzen/DiGeorge syndrome and the del(22q) spectrum

Terminology

Shprintzen and colleagues in 1978 described a syndrome with unusual facies, velopalatine insufficiency, and conotruncal anomalies, drawing together observations dating back to 1955 (Jones, 1997, pp. 266–7; Shprintzen, 2000; Gorlin et al., 2001, pp. 907–11). The condition is also known as velocardiofacial syndrome. Some patients with Shprintzen syndrome have the absent thymus and parathyroid glands reported by DiGeorge in 1968. Because a single error in branchial arch development is thought to be involved, the combination of thymic, parathyroid, and conotruncal cardiac anomalies is called DiGeorge sequence or DiGeorge anomaly. Partial monosomy 22 and then subtle deletions in chromosome band 22q11 were demonstrated in DiGeorge sequence. Soon it was demonstrated that some patients with isolated conotruncal cardiac anomalies had a 22q11 microdeletion, and the spectrum of Shprintzen syndrome, DiGeorge, and conotruncal anomaly was denoted as "CATCH 22" – an acronym for *c*ardiac defects, *a*bnormal facies, *t*hymic hypoplasia, *c*left palate, and *h*ypocalcemia that may result from chromosome 22 deletion, but its connotation of "can't win" is not flattering to patients and is replaced here by the Shprintzen/deletion 22 spectrum.

Historical diagnosis and management

Because of subtle manifestations in some patients, Shprintzen syndrome is undoubtedly underdiagnosed. McDonald-McGinn et al. (2001) supported this fact by studying 30 patients identified after diagnosis in a relative: only 6 of 19 adults (32%) and 6 of 11 children (55%) had findings demanding medical attention. These milder patients offer encouragement to the families with newly diagnosed children. The spectrum of problems united by the finding of chromosome 22 deletion, ranging from orofacial and cardiac anomalies to those of brain and behavior, emphasize the breadth of management needed by these patients.

Incidence, etiology, and differential diagnosis

The incidence of deletion 22q11 is estimated at 1 in 5000 live births, and an estimated 50% of these patients will have significant manifestations of the Shprintzen/deletion 22 spectrum. Shprintzen syndrome is in turn estimated to comprise about 8% of patients with syndromic cleft palate. The frequency of chromosome 22 deletion is about 63% in patients with Shprintzen syndrome, 83% in patients with DiGeorge anomaly, and 29% of patients with non-syndromic conotruncal anomalies (Jones, 1997, pp. 266–7; Shprintzen, 2000; Gorlin et al., 2001, pp. 907–11). Differential diagnosis includes other conditions with orofacial and cardiac problems, including the orofacial digital syndromes. The DiGeorge sequence also occurs in *C*oloboma, *H*eart disease, *A*tresia choanae, *R*etarded growth and development, *G*enital anomalies, and *E*ar anomalies (CHARGE) association (see Chapter 5), but the facial characteristics are different from those of Shprintzen syndrome.

Family and psychosocial counseling

Before the discovery of the chromosome 22 deletion, Shprintzen syndrome was considered autosomal-dominant and DiGeorge anomaly sporadic. Isolated conotruncal heart defects were usually multifactorial with a 2–3% recurrence risk, although occasional families would exhibit vertical transmission. Parents of affected children should have FISH analysis for deletion 22q11 because many will not have suggestive physical or psychiatric features (McDonald-McGinn et al., 2001). All families should be referred for genetic counseling. Ryan et al. (1997) reported that 204 of 285 patients (75%) had *de novo* deletions, and that 61 (75%) of the 79 parents with deletions were female.

Individuals with the deletion or a presumptive clinical diagnosis of Shprintzen/deletion 22 spectrum should be given a 50% recurrence risk, with the understanding that affected children will vary in their number and severity of features. Psychosocial counseling may be quite important, since many affected children and occasional parents will have behavior problems ranging from poor social interaction to frank psychosis or phobic responses. Parent information and support can be found at the Velocardiofacial Syndrome Educational Foundation, Inc. (www. vcfsef.org/) and by searching on the various syndrome names.

Natural history and complications

Neonatal complications are particularly important to consider in Shprintzen/deletion 22 syndrome, since their detection and management will have considerable influence on natural history. Cardiac anomalies and dysphagia may be severe and life threatening, and failure to investigate the cardiovascular and gastrointestinal systems can lead to debilitating bronchiectasis or cardiopulmonary failure. The European Collaborative Study (Ryan et al., 1997) found that 8% of 554 patients had died and, of 29 patients whose age of death was known, 25 died within 6 months from congenital heart disease, and 1 from severe immune deficiency. The possibility of DiGeorge sequence must be considered from the perspective of early treatment and modification of the immunization schedule to omit live vaccines.

The natural history of Shprintzen/deletion 22 syndrome has three phases; a turbulent infantile course, with possible cardiac disease, severe dysphagia and reflux, obstructive sleep apnea, and upper respiratory infections; a childhood compromised by hearing, speech, learning, and growth problems: and an adolescence/adulthood challenged by personality, school, and behavioral problems. Growth below the 3rd centile was present in about 1/3 of the European patients (Ryan et al., 1997) and in 10% reported by McDonald-McGinn et al. (2001), but many will catch up in later childhood. Partly responsible are cardiac defects present in about 80% of patients, mostly conotruncal defects including tetralogy of Fallot, ventricular septal defect, interrupted aortic arch, pulmonary atresia/ventricular septal defect, and truncus arteriosus.

Ocular anomalies occur in 70%, including small optic disks and cataracts. Ear, nose, and throat anomalies (in 50%) include cleft palate, submucous cleft, velopharyngeal insufficiency without clefting, and conductive hearing loss. Obstructive sleep apnea is frequent during infancy because the pharynx is hypotonic, and tonsillectomy/adenoidectomy must be approached with caution. Aberrant arterial anatomy may also pose risks for otolaryngologic procedures.

Renal abnormalities occur in 15–35% and include absent, dysplastic, or multicystic kidneys, urinary tract anomalies, and vesicoureteric reflux in 6. Some 203 of 340 had hypocalcemia in the European study, mostly in the neonatal period and often accompanied by seizures (Ryan et al., 1997). Connective tissue problems such as hernias, scoliosis, club feet, increased joint laxity, and costovertebral anomalies occur in 35%. Up to 1/3 of patients may have normal mental development with speech concerns, but patients with mental disability may have brain anomalies such as cerebellar hypoplasia and Chiari malformation. Performance IQ is lower than verbal IQ in patients with Shprintzen syndrome, and hypernasal speech with articulation problems and language delay is common. A characteristic personality has been described with a bland affect, poor social interaction, and impulsive behavior (Gorlin et al., 2001, pp. 907–11). Psychosis and phobic reactions have been seen in some adults.

Preventive medical checklist for Shprintzen/deletion 22 spectrum

The presence of DiGeorge anomaly is essential to suspect and recognize so appropriate surveillance for infections and modification of the immunization schedule can be provided. Risks for upper respiratory infections are increased in most patients, necessitating aggressive treatment of chronic otitis and screening for hearing loss. In patients without overt cleft palate, submucous clefts may occur, with significant risks for otitis and speech problems. Many patients have feeding problems and failure to thrive, so feeding specialists may be needed to accomplish reasonable growth.

Echocardiography, audiography, consideration of obstructive sleep apnea, and close monitoring of feeding and palatal function are important in patients with suspected Shprintzen/deletion 22 spectrum. In the presence of tetany or recurrent infections, chest X-rays, peripheral leukocyte counts, and serum calcium/phosphorus measurements should be obtained to evaluate the presence of DiGeorge sequence. Medical counseling should be optimistic because of the many patients with normal cognitive function or mild disability (McDonald-McGinn et al., 2001).

The care of older children and adolescents should focus on learning disabilities and potential school problems that may be augmented by behavior differences. Attention to speech, language, and hearing should continue, and awareness of the increased joint laxity may influence the recommendations for physical activity.

Preventive management of Williams syndrome

Description: Clinical pattern caused by deletion or mutation of genes within chromosome band 7q11 with an incidence of 1 in 10,000 births.

Clinical diagnosis: Characteristic pattern including neonatal hypercalcemia, characteristic facial appearance, periorbital fullness, prominent lips, stellate irides, early feeding problems and failure to thrive, happy personality in older children, hyperacusis, excellent musical and verbal skills (Udwin & Rule, 1991).

Laboratory diagnosis: Special chromosome Fluorescent *in situ* hybridization (FISH) study demonstrating deletion on chromosome 7q including the elastin gene.

Genetics: Rarely inherited, recurrence risk <1%.

Key management issues: Positive attitude, early intervention, feeding, vision, hearing, heart, renal, and behavioral problems.

Growth charts: Morris et al. (1988).

Parent groups: Parent support groups include the Williams Syndrome Association (www.williams-syndrome.org), a Williams Syndrome Comprehensive Website (www.wsf.org/), and the Williams Syndrome Foundation (www.wsf.org/).

Basis for management recommendations: Committee on Genetics, American Academy of Pediatrics (2001) consensus recommendations (aappolicy.aappublications.org/cgi/content/full/pediatrics;107/5/1192).

Summary of clinical concerns

General	Learning	**Cognitive and learning differences** (97%)
	Behavior	Friendly, loquacious personality; hyperactivity, sensory integration issues
	Growth	**Feeding problems** (71%), **failure to thrive** (81%), **obesity** (21%)
Facial	Eyes	**Oculomotor problems, esotropia** (50%), **hyperopia** (24%)
	Ears	Hyperacusis (95%), **chronic otitis** (43%)
	Nose	Shallow nasal bridge
	Mouth	**Dental malocclusion** (85%), **enamel hypoplasia** (48%), microdontia (55%)
Surface	Neck/trunk	**Pectus excavatum** (40%), **inguinal hernias** (38%), umbilical hernia
	Epidermal	Prematurely gray hair
Skeletal	Cranial	**Microcephaly**, brachycephaly
	Axial	**Kyphosis** (21%), scoliosis
	Limbs	**Contractures or mild joint limitations** (50%); hypoplastic nails
Internal	Digestive	**Early colic and vomiting** (40–67%), **constipation** (43%), peptic ulcer (18%), cholelithiasis (12%), rectal prolapse (12%), diverticulosis
	Pulmonary	Vocal cord paralysis, rare sudden death with anesthesia
	Circulatory	**Cardiac anomalies** (79%), **hypertension** (47–60%), arterial stenoses (18%) including renal artery stenosis
	Endocrine	**Early hypercalcemia** (67%), diabetes mellitus (12%)
	RES	Early susceptibility to respiratory infections, chronic otitis
	Excretory	**Enuresis** (52%), **urinary tract infections** (29%), renal anomalies (18%), nephrocalcinosis, small or asymmetric kidneys
	Genital	Micropenis
Neural	Central	**Hypotonia, motor delays**, cerebral artery stenosis, strokes
	Motor	**Oculomotor problems, esotropia** (50%), **hyperopia** (24%)
	Sensory	**Hyperacusis** (95%), hearing loss, vision loss

RES, reticuloendothelial system; **concerns** of frequency >20% are **highlighted**

Key references

Anonymous (1985). Case history of a child with Williams syndrome. *Pediatrics* 75:962–8.

Committee on Genetics American Academy of Pediatrics (2001). Health care supervision for children with Williams syndrome. *Pediatrics* 107:1192–204.

Morris, et al. (1988). Growth data for Williams syndrome patients, collected with the assistance of the Williams Syndrome National Association. In: *Growth References Third Trimester to Adulthood*, eds R. A. Saul, et al., pp. 128–32. Greenville, SC: Keys Printing.

Udwin, et al. (1998). Community care for adults with Williams syndrome: How families cope and the availability of support networks. *Journal of Intellectual Disability Research* 42:238–45.

Williams syndrome

Preventive medical checklist (0–3 years)

Name _____ Birth date __/__/____ Number_____

Age	Evaluations: key concerns	Management considerations		Notes
New-born ↓ 1 month	Dysmorphology examination: hernias Hearing, vision:[2] esotropia Feeding: reflux, poor intake Heart: aortic, pulmonary stenosis Urinary function: renal anomalies Metabolic: hypercalcemia, renal function Parental adjustment	❑ FISH karyotype; genetic counseling[1] ❑ ABR ❑ Feeding specialist; video swallow[3] ❑ Echocardiogram; cardiology ❑ Renal sonogram; urinary tract studies ❑ Blood calcium; electrolytes; renal functions ❑ Family support[4]	❑ ❑ ❑ ❑ ❑ ❑ ❑	
2 months ↓ 4 months	Growth and development: head size[5] Nutrition: feeding, colic, GE reflux Hearing and vision:[2] esotropia, otitis Urinary function: infection Connective tissue: hernias, contractures Vocal cord paralysis[2] Parental adjustment Other:	❑ ECI[6] ❑ Feeding specialist; GI referral[3] ❑ Ophthalmology; ENT[3] ❑ Urinalysis; BP ❑ Orthopedics[3] ❑ Anesthesia precautions ❑ Family support[4] ❑	❑ ❑ ❑ ❑ ❑ ❑ ❑ ❑	
6 months ↓ 9 months	Growth and development: head size[5] Nutrition: feeding, GE reflux, constipation Hearing and vision:[2] esotropia, otitis Cardiovascular, urinary tract anomalies Vocal cord paralysis[2] Other:	❑ ECI[6] ❑ Feeding specialist; GI referral[3] ❑ Ophthalmology; ENT[3] ❑ Urinalysis; BP; cardiology ❑ Anesthesia precautions ❑	❑ ❑ ❑ ❑ ❑ ❑	
1 year	Growth and development: head size[5] Nutrition: GE reflux, constipation Hearing and vision:[2] esotropia, otitis Cardiovascular, urinary tract anomalies Metabolic: hypercalcemia, renal function Connective tissue: hernias, contractures Other:	❑ ECI;[3,6] family support[3,4] ❑ Dietician;[3] GI referral[3] ❑ Ophthalmology; ENT[3] ❑ Urinalysis; BP; IVP,[3] cardiology ❑ Blood calcium; BUN; creatinine, T4, TSH ❑ Anesthesia precautions ❑	❑ ❑ ❑ ❑ ❑ ❑ ❑	
15 months ↓ 18 months	Growth and development: head size[5] Nutrition: GE reflux, constipation Hearing and vision:[2] esotropia, otitis Urinary function: infection	❑ ECI[6] ❑ Feeding specialist; GI referral[3] ❑ Ophthalmology; ENT[3] ❑ Urinalysis, BP	❑ ❑ ❑ ❑	
2 years	Growth and development: head size[5] Nutrition: GE reflux, constipation Hearing and vision:[2] esotropia, otitis Cardiovascular, urinary tract anomalies Metabolic: hypercalcemia, renal function	❑ ECI;[3,6] family support[3,4] ❑ Dietician;[3] GI referral[3] ❑ Ophthalmology; ENT[3] ❑ Urinalysis; BP; cardiology[3] ❑ Blood calcium; BUN; creatinine, T4, TSH	❑ ❑ ❑ ❑ ❑	
3 years	Growth and development: head size[5] Nutrition: GE reflux, constipation Hearing and vision:[2] esotropia, otitis Cardiovascular, urinary tract anomalies Metabolic: hypercalcemia, renal function Connective tissue: hernias, contractures Other:	❑ ECI;[3,6] family support[3,4] ❑ Dietician;[3] GI referral[3] ❑ Ophthalmology; ENT[3] ❑ Urinalysis; BP; IVP;[3] cardiology ❑ Blood calcium; BUN; creatinine; T4, TSH ❑ Orthopedics;[3] anesthesia precautions ❑	❑ ❑ ❑ ❑ ❑ ❑ ❑	

Williams syndrome concerns		Other concerns from history	
Feeding problems, colic Strabismus, esotropia Chronic otitis, hearing loss Constipation Aortic, pulmonary stenosis	Renal anomalies Inguinal hernias Vascular stenoses Developmental disability Hypotonia Motor and speech delay	**Family history/prenatal** _____ _____ _____ _____ _____	**Social/environmental** _____ _____ _____ _____ _____

Guidelines for the neonatal period should be undertaken *at whatever age* the diagnosis is made; ABR, auditory brainstem evoked response; GE, gastroesophageal; GI, gastrointestinal; IVP, intravenous push; TSH, thyroid-stimulating hormone; BP, blood pressure; BUN, blood–urea–nitrogen; [1]parental chromosomes not necessary; [2]by practitioner; [3]as dictated by clinical findings; [4]parent group, family/sib, financial, and behavioral issues; [5]consider low-calcium diet, developmental pediatrician/neurologist/behavior therapist according to symptoms and availability; [6]early childhood intervention including developmental monitoring and motor/speech therapy.

Williams syndrome

Preventive medical checklist (4–18 years)

Name _____ Birth date __/__/____ Number _____

Age	Evaluations: key concerns	Management considerations		Notes
4 years ↓ **6 years**	Growth, preschool transition[1,5] Nutrition: hypercalcemia, constipation Hearing and vision:[2] hyperacusis, otitis Cardiovascular, urinary tract anomalies Metabolic; hypercalcemia, renal function Connective tissue: hernias, contractures Other:	❑ Family support;[4] preschool program[5] ❑ Dietician;[3] GI referral[3] ❑ Ophthalmology, ENT[3] ❑ Urinalysis; BP; IVP;[3] cardiology ❑ Blood calcium; BUN; creatinine; T4, TSH ❑ Orthopedics;[3] anesthesia precautions ❑	❑ ❑ ❑ ❑ ❑ ❑ ❑	
7 years ↓ **9 years**	Growth, school transition[1,5] Nutrition: hypercalcemia, constipation Hearing, vision:[2] hyperacusis, hyperopia Cardiovascular, urinary tract anomalies Metabolic; hypercalcemia, renal function Skeletal: scoliosis, joint limitation Other:	❑ Family support;[4] school progress[6] ❑ Dietician;[3] GI referral[3] ❑ Audiology; ophthalmology;[3] ENT[3] ❑ Urinalysis; BP; IVP;[3] cardiology ❑ Blood calcium; BUN; creatinine; T4, TSH ❑ Orthopedics;[3] anesthesia precautions ❑	❑ ❑ ❑ ❑ ❑ ❑ ❑	
10 years ↓ **12 years**	Growth and development[1,5] Hearing, vision:[2] hyperacusis, hyperopia Cardiovascular, urinary tract anomalies Metabolic; hypercalcemia, renal function Other:	❑ Family support;[4] school progress[6] ❑ Audiology; ophthalmology;[3] ENT[3] ❑ Urinalysis; BP; IVP;[3] cardiology ❑ Blood calcium; BUN; creatinine; T4, TSH ❑	❑ ❑ ❑ ❑ ❑	
13 years ↓ **15 years**	Growth and development[1,5] Obesity, constipation, puberty Hearing, vision:[2] hyperacusis, hyperopia Urinary function: infection Metabolic; hypercalcemia, renal function Other:	❑ Family support;[4] school progress[6] ❑ Dietician;[3] GI referral;[3] endocrinology[3] ❑ Audiology; ophthalmology;[3] ENT[3] ❑ Urinalysis; BP ❑ Blood calcium; BUN; creatinine; T4, TSH ❑ Endocrinology[3]	❑ ❑ ❑ ❑ ❑ ❑	
16 years ↓ **18 years**	Growth and development[1,5] Obesity, constipation, puberty Hearing, vision:[2] hyperacusis, hyperopia Cardiovascular, urinary tract anomalies Other:	❑ Family support;[4] school progress[6] ❑ Dietician;[3] GI referral;[3] endocrinology[3] ❑ Audiology; ophthalmology;[3] ENT[3] ❑ Urinalysis; BP; IVP;[3] cardiology ❑	❑ ❑ ❑ ❑ ❑	
19 years ↓ **23 years**	Adult-care transition[1,6] Hypercalcemia, obesity, constipation Hearing, vision:[2] hyperacusis, hyperopia Cardiovascular, urinary tract anomalies Metabolic; thyroid, renal function	❑ Family support;[4] school progress[6] ❑ Dietary counsel; activities; exercise ❑ Audiology; ophthalmology;[3] ENT[3] ❑ Urinalysis, BP, IVP;[3] cardiology ❑ BUN; creatinine; T4, TSH	❑ ❑ ❑ ❑ ❑	
Adult	Adult-care transition[6] Neurosensory:[2] hearing, vision, strokes Metabolic, obesity, constipation Cardiovascular, urinary tract anomalies Skeletal: scoliosis, joint limitation GI: cholelithiasis, peptic ulcer Other:	❑ Family support[4] ❑ Audiology; ophthalmology;[3] ENT;[3] neurology[3] ❑ Nutrition; exercise; BUN; creatinine; T4, TSH ❑ Urinalysis; BP; IVP;[3] cardiology ❑ Orthopedics[3] ❑ GI referral[3] ❑	❑ ❑ ❑ ❑ ❑ ❑ ❑	

Williams syndrome concerns		Other concerns from history	
Vision: hyperopia Hearing: hyperacusis Peptic ulcer, cholelithiasis Hypertension, renal failure Urinary tract infections Micropenis	Cardiac defects Hypercalcemia, diabetes mellitus Scoliosis, joint contractures Short stature, obesity Cognitive disability, strokes later Behavior problems	**Family history/prenatal** _____ _____ _____ _____	**Social/environmental** _____ _____ _____ _____

Guidelines for the neonatal period should be undertaken *at whatever age* the diagnosis is made; IVP, intravenous push; BP, blood pressure; TSH, thyroid-stimulating hormone; BUN, blood–urea–nitrogen; GI, gastrointestinal; [1]consider low-calcium diet, developmental pediatrician/pediatric genetics clinic/behavior therapist according to symptoms and availability, and neurologist if symptoms of stroke or cerebral artery stenosis; [2]by practitioner; [3]as dictated by clinical findings; [4]parent group, family/sib, financial, and behavioral issues with later focus on independent living and employment; [5]preschool program including developmental monitoring and motor/speech therapy; [6]monitor individual education plan, educational testing, balance of special education and inclusion, academic progress, behavioral differences, later vocational planning.

Parent guide to Williams syndrome

Williams and colleagues in 1961 described children with supravalvular aortic stenosis (narrowing of the aorta above its valve), unusual facies, high blood calcium during infancy, and developmental disabilities. A region of chromosome 7 containing the elastin gene is deleted in over 90% of children with Williams syndrome. "Williams syndrome" or "Williams–Beuren" syndrome is the preferred terminology, although "idiopathic hypercalcemia–supravalvular aortic stenosis syndrome" and "elfin facies syndrome" are older and equivalent terms.

Incidence, causation, and diagnosis

The incidence depends on the accuracy of diagnosis, but is between 1 in 20,000 and 1 in 50,000 live births. Families containing some individuals with supravalvular stenosis and some with Williams syndrome have been reported, suggesting that milder patients are difficult to recognize. Once the diagnosis is suspected, chromosomal analysis can be performed using fluorescent *in situ* hybridization (FISH) to look for subtle deletions in the 7q11 chromosome region. The chromosome laboratory must be alerted to perform this specific FISH analysis. Over 90% of children with classical Williams syndrome have a detectable 7q deletion; the diagnosis must be clinical in the remaining 10%. Deletion of one copy of the elastin gene presumably explains the supravalvular aortic stenosis and connective tissue alterations in Williams syndrome, with additional features caused by the deletion of nearby genes. Neonatal diagnosis of Williams syndrome is difficult unless hypercalcemia is detected. The characteristic face with unusual (star-like) patterns in the iris, strabismus (wandering eye), fullness of tissues around the eye, thickened lips, and long philtrum (crease from the nose to upper lip) may not be obvious until early childhood.

Natural history and complications

Infancy is often difficult because of colic and feeding problems; parents may need considerable support during this period. Kidney anomalies and infantile spasms can occur. During later childhood, subtle visual abnormalities and learning differences are more problematic. The considerable verbal abilities and happy affect of children with Williams syndrome warrant optimism for the long-term outlook. The facial appearance of individuals with Williams syndrome changes considerably with age. Lifespan may be somewhat decreased because of cardiovascular or renal anomalies, but several studies described adults with excellent quality of life. Behavioral concerns are frequent, including hyperactivity, emotional lability, and excessive anxiety. Hyperacusis (hypersensitive hearing) is common, including extreme responses to sounds like those of doorbells or lawn-mowers. Small head size with developmental delay and decreased IQ is common, but many children perform at appropriate age levels in the areas of visual recognition, expressive language, and verbal recall. Hypercalcemia seems to be an altered response to normal dietary calcium, and low-calcium diets can be considered. Later complications include mitral valve prolapse, peptic ulcer, gall stones, obesity, urinary tract infections with bladder diverticula (outpouchings), and diabetes mellitus. Calcification of the kidney and narrowing of the arteries to the kidney and other organs cause high blood pressure to be a frequent complication, often with onset in the second or third decade. A few patients have had cerebral arterial stenosis with strokes at a young age.

Preventive medical needs

Preventive management should begin at the time of diagnosis, with ultrasound study of the heart and kidneys to document anomalies. Hypertension may be associated with cardiovascular or renal disease, so frequent monitoring of blood pressure is important. Where possible, four-extremity blood pressures should be obtained so peripheral narrowing of the arteries can be recognized. Although feeding problems, colic, and constipation often complicate early growth, conservative management is indicated since gastrointestinal anomalies are rare. Chronic otitis is a frequent problem, necessitating frequent audiologic assessments and possible referral to otolaryngology. Dental anomalies are frequent, and dentistry with appropriate antibiotic prophylaxis to prevent heart infections should be an integral part of preventive care. Renal anomalies and urinary tract infections are sufficiently common to recommend periodic screening of kidney function with blood–urea–nitrogen (BUN) and blood creatinine testing. Teens and adults should be monitored for scoliosis (curved spine) and joint contractures. Obesity is a later problem, as is diabetes mellitus, warranting dietary counsel. Performance and behavior in school should be followed, with referral to behavioral specialists as needed. Anxiety may cause peptic ulcer disease and gall bladder disease should be borne in mind as a possible diagnosis in patients with abdominal pain.

Family counseling

Although Williams syndrome has exhibited rare parent–child transmission and concordance in identical twins, the recurrence risks for parents of affected children is <1%. Affected patients are fertile and may transmit the disorder. It is important to realize that early feeding problems with colic, vomiting, or constipation will improve later. Behavior differences like hyperactivity, distractibility, and learning differences require team management by parents, health care, and school professionals, and parent groups (see part 1 of this checklist) can be extremely useful.

Preventive management of Prader–Willi syndrome

Description: Clinical pattern caused by deletion or altered imprinting of chromosome region 15q11 with incidence of 1 in 10,000–15,000 live births.

Clinical diagnosis: Pattern of manifestations including neonatal hypotonia and hypogonadism with later hyperphagia, obesity, and mental disability. A characteristic appearance may develop with almond-shaped palpebral fissures, down-turned corners of the mouth, small hands, and feet.

Laboratory diagnosis: Chromosome and DNA diagnosis demonstrating microdeletion of band 15q13q15 (~60% of patients), maternal origin of both chromosomes 15 (uniparental disomy, ~25%; or defective DNA methylation, ~5%). The latter test is positive for all three categories.

Genetics: Deletion, uniparental disomy, or defective DNA methylation are sporadic events with a low recurrence risk for parents of affected children.

Key management issues: Monitoring for eye, nutritional, motor, sleep apnea, cognitive, and behavioral problems. Emphasis on weight management is most important in order to avoid morbidity and early mortality from obesity.

Growth charts: Butler & Meaney (1991).

Parent groups: Prader–Willi Syndrome Association (www.pwsausa.org/) and the Prader–Willi Syndrome Association UK (http://www.pwsa-uk.demon.co.uk/).

Basis for management recommendations: Complications below as drawn from Cassidy (1987) and Holm et al. (1993).

Summary of clinical concerns

General	Learning	**Cognitive disability** – normal/borderline (40%), mild (41%), moderate (12%); **learning and speech problems** (100%)
	Behavior	**Eating disorder** (hyperphagia, voracious appetite, binge eating, food foraging), difficult behaviors (stubbornness, tantrums, outbursts), poor self-image, psychoses
	Growth	Early failure to thrive, **short stature**, morbid obesity, inactivity, decreased exercise
	Cancer	Wilms tumor, myeloid leukemia
Facial	Eyes	**Myopia** (25%), **strabismus** (40–95%)
	Nose	Nasal picking with nose bleeds
	Mouth	**Thick and scanty saliva**, **dental malocclusion** (40%), increased caries (44%), enamel hypoplasia
Surface	Epidermal	Deceased pain sensitivity, **hypopigmentation** (50%), skin picking, cellulitis, scarring
Skeletal	Cranial	Microcephaly
	Limbs	Clubfoot (6%), hip dislocation (9%), later scoliosis, and osteoporosis
Internal	Digestive	Thick, decreased saliva; gastroesophageal reflux, aspiration, and gastric distension (especially with anesthesia)
	Pulmonary	Respiratory problems, sleep apnea, anesthesia problems due to obesity or reflux
	Circulatory	Congestive heart failure due to morbid obesity
	Endocrine	Hypothalamic dysfunction, diabetes mellitus (5–15%), **insulin requirement** (66%)
	Genital	Hypogonadism, **cryptorchidism** (80%), micropenis, labial hypoplasia, dysmenorrhea, male and female infertility with gonadotrophin deficiency, oligospermia
Neural	Central	**Sleep disorders** – 50%, including daytime somnulence (50%), snoring (45%), restless sleep (40%), cataplexy (15%), sleep apnea; seizures (16–20%)
	Motor	Hypotonia, decreased muscle mass, weakness, inactivity
	Sensory	Misrouting of retinal–ganglion fibers, visual deficits

Concerns of frequency >20% are **highlighted**

Key references

Butler & Meaney (1991). Standards for selected anthropometric measurements in Prader–Willi syndrome. *Pediatrics* 88:853–60.

Cassidy (1987). Prader–Willi syndrome. Characteristics, management, and etiology. *Alabama Journal of Medical Sciences* 24:169–75.

Holm, et al. (1993). Prader–Willi syndrome: consensus diagnostic criteria. *Pediatrics* 91:398–402.

Hoybye, et al. (2002). Metabolic profile and body composition in adults with Prader–Willi syndrome and severe obesity. *Journal of Clinical Endocrinology and Metabolism* 87:3590–7.

Prader–Willi syndrome

Preventive medical checklist (0–3 years)

Name _____ Birth date __/__/____ Number _____

Age	Evaluations: key concerns	Management considerations		Notes
New-born ↓ 1 month	Newborn examination: anomalies, hypotonia Hearing, vision[2] Feeding: dysphagia, reflux, poor intake Pulmonary: airway, aspiration Genitalia: cryptorchidism Parental adjustment	❏ FISH karyotype; DNA; genetic counseling[1] ❏ ABR ❏ Feeding specialist; video swallow[3] ❏ Chest X-ray; blood gases,[3] apnea monitor[3] ❏ Urology[3] ❏ Family support[4]	❏ ❏ ❏ ❏ ❏ ❏	
2 months ↓ 4 months	Growth and development[5] Hearing and vision:[2] otitis, strabismus Nutrition: feeding, GE reflux Pulmonary: airway, aspiration Skeletal: club feet, hip dislocation Parental adjustment Other:	❏ ECI[6] ❏ Repeat ABR;[3] ophthalmology[3] ❏ Extra feeding;[3] feeding specialist[3] ❏ Apnea monitor; anesthesia precautions ❏ Skeletal X-rays;[3] orthopedics[3] ❏ Family support[4] ❏	❏ ❏ ❏ ❏ ❏ ❏ ❏	
6 months ↓ 9 months	Growth and development[5] Hearing and vision:[2] otitis, strabismus Nutrition: feeding, GE reflux Pulmonary: airway, aspiration Skeletal: club feet, hip dislocation Other:	❏ ECI[6] ❏ Ophthalmology ❏ Extra feeding;[3] feeding specialist[3] ❏ ENT;[3] anesthesia precautions ❏ Skeletal X-rays;[3] orthopedics[3] ❏	❏ ❏ ❏ ❏ ❏ ❏	
1 year	Growth and development[5] Hearing and vision:[2] otitis, strabismus Nutrition: feeding, GE reflux Pulmonary: airway, aspiration Skeletal: club feet, hip dislocation Sleep: sleep apnea[7] Other:	❏ ECI[6] ❏ Ophthalmology ❏ Extra feeding;[3] feeding specialist[3] ❏ ENT;[3] anesthesia precautions ❏ Skeletal X-rays;[3] orthopedics[3] ❏ Sleep study[3] ❏	❏ ❏ ❏ ❏ ❏ ❏ ❏	
15 months ↓ 18 months	Growth and development[5] Nutrition: feeding, GE reflux Growth hormone deficiency Skeletal: club feet, hip dislocation	❏ ECI[6] ❏ Dietician[3] ❏ Endocrinology ❏ Skeletal X-rays;[3] orthopedics[3]	❏ ❏ ❏ ❏	
2 years	Growth and development[5] Hearing and vision:[2] otitis, strabismus Nutrition: feeding, GE reflux Pulmonary: airway, aspiration Sleep: sleep apnea[7]	❏ ECI[6] ❏ Audiology, ophthalmology ❏ Dietician[3] ❏ ENT;[3] anesthesia precautions ❏ Sleep study[3]	❏ ❏ ❏ ❏ ❏	
3 years	Growth and development[5] Hearing and vision:[2] otitis, strabismus Nutrition: hyperphagia, obesity Pulmonary: airway, aspiration Skeletal: club feet, hip dislocation Sleep: sleep apnea[7] Other:	❏ ECI[6]; family support[4] ❏ Ophthalmology ❏ Dietician;[3] endocrinology ❏ ENT;[3] anesthesia precautions ❏ Skeletal X-rays;[3] orthopedics[3] ❏ Sleep study[3] ❏	❏ ❏ ❏ ❏ ❏ ❏ ❏	

Prader–Willi syndrome concerns		Other concerns from history	
Poor feeding (infancy) Hyperphagia (>2 years) Strabismus Decreased salivation Dental anomalies GE reflux, aspiration	Cryptorchidism, micropenis Club feet, hip dislocation Hypotonia Central, obstructive sleep apnea Motor and speech delay Behavioral differences	**Family history/prenatal** _____ _____ _____ _____	**Social/environmental** _____ _____ _____ _____

Guidelines for the neonatal period should be undertaken *at whatever age* the diagnosis is made; ABR, auditory brainstem evoked response; FISH, fluorescent *in situ* hybridization GE, gastroesophageal; [1]DNA methylation study may be needed if FISH (deletion) negative; parental chromosomes not necessary; [2]by practitioner; [3]as dictated by clinical findings; [4]parent group, family/sib, financial, and behavioral issues; [5]consider developmental pediatrician/neurologist/behavior therapist/genetic clinic according to symptoms and availability; [6]early childhood intervention including developmental monitoring and motor/speech therapy; [7]snoring, pause in breathing, daytime sleepiness, unusual sleep positioning (of concern with growth hormone therapy).

Prader–Willi syndrome

Preventive medical checklist (4–18 years)

Name _____ Birth date __/__/___ Number _____

Age	Evaluations: key concerns	Management considerations		Notes
4 years ↓ 6 years	Growth:[1] short stature, obesity Development:[2] preschool transition Hearing, vision:[2] vision loss Nutrition: hyperphagia, obesity Pulmonary: aspiration, sleep apnea Skeletal: scoliosis Other:	❑ Endocrinology ❑ Family support;[4] preschool program[5] ❑ Audiology;[3] ophthalmology ❑ Dietician ❑ ENT;[3] sleep study;[3] anesthesia precautions ❑ Skeletal X-rays;[3] orthopedics[3] ❑	❑ ❑ ❑ ❑ ❑ ❑ ❑	
7 years ↓ 9 years	Growth:[1] short stature, obesity Development:[1] school transition[5] Hearing, vision:[2] vision loss Nutrition: hyperphagia, obesity Pulmonary: aspiration, sleep apnea Skeletal: scoliosis Other:	❑ Endocrinology ❑ Family support;[4] school progress[6] ❑ Audiology;[3] ophthalmology[3] ❑ Dietician ❑ ENT;[3] sleep study;[3] anesthesia precautions ❑ Skeletal X-rays;[3] orthopedics[3] ❑	❑ ❑ ❑ ❑ ❑ ❑ ❑	
10 years ↓ 12 years	Growth and development[1] Hearing and vision[2] Nutrition: hyperphagia, obesity Pulmonary: aspiration, sleep apnea Other:	❑ School progress;[6] endocrinology ❑ Audiology;[3] ophthalmology[3] ❑ Dietician ❑ ENT;[3] sleep study;[3] anesthesia precautions ❑	❑ ❑ ❑ ❑ ❑	
13 years ↓ 15 years	Growth, development;[1] obesity, behavior Hearing and vision[2] Puberty; micropenis, menstruation Pulmonary: aspiration, sleep apnea Skeletal: scoliosis Other:	❑ School progress;[6] dietician ❑ Audiology;[3] ophthalmology[3] ❑ Endocrinology[3] ❑ ENT;[3] sleep study;[3] anesthesia precautions ❑ Skeletal X-rays;[3] orthopedics[3] ❑	❑ ❑ ❑ ❑ ❑ ❑	
16 years ↓ 18 years	Growth, development;[1] obesity, behavior Puberty; micropenis, menstruation Nutrition: obesity Skin: skin picking, scarring Other:	❑ Family support;[4] school progress[6] ❑ Endocrinology[3] ❑ Dietary counsel; activities; exercise ❑ Dermatology[3] ❑	❑ ❑ ❑ ❑ ❑	
19 years ↓ 23 years	Adult-care transition:[6] behavior Hearing/vision[2] Nutrition: obesity Pulmonary: aspiration, sleep apnea Skeletal: scoliosis	❑ Family support;[4] psychiatry[3] ❑ Audiology;[3] ophthalmology[3] ❑ Dietician, activities; endocrinology ❑ ENT;[3] sleep study;[3] anesthesia precautions ❑ Skeletal X-rays;[3] orthopedics[3]	❑ ❑ ❑ ❑ ❑	
Adult	Adult-care transition[6] Hearing/vision[2] Nutrition: obesity Pulmonary: aspiration, sleep apnea[7] Skeletal: scoliosis Skin: skin picking, scarring Other:	❑ Family support;[4] psychiatry[3] ❑ Audiology;[3] ophthalmology[3] ❑ Dietician; activities; endocrinology ❑ ENT,[3] sleep study;[3] anesthesia precautions ❑ Skeletal X-rays;[3] orthopedics[3] ❑ Dermatology[3] ❑	❑ ❑ ❑ ❑ ❑ ❑ ❑	

Prader–Willi syndrome concerns		Other concerns from history	
Hyperphagia, obesity Strabismus Decreased salivation Dental anomalies GE reflux, aspiration Scoliosis	Cryptorchidism, micropenis Menstrual irregularity Central, obstructive sleep apnea Speech, learning, behavior Obesity, exercise Employment, independent living	**Family history/prenatal** _____ _____ _____ _____ _____	**Social/environmental** _____ _____ _____ _____ _____

Guidelines for the neonatal period should be undertaken *at whatever age* the diagnosis is made; GE, gastroesophageal; [1]consider developmental pediatrician/neurologist/behavior therapist/genetic clinic according to symptoms and availability; [2]by practitioner; [3]as dictated by clinical findings; [4]parent group, family/sib, financial, and behavioral issues with later focus on independent living and employment; [5]preschool program including developmental monitoring and motor/speech therapy; [6]monitor individual education plan, educational testing, balance of special education and inclusion, academic progress, behavioral differences, later vocational planning; [7]snoring, pause in breathing, daytime sleepiness, unusual sleep positioning (of concern with growth hormone therapy).

Parent guide to Prader–Willi syndrome

Prader–Willi syndrome was described in 1956 and later discovered to result from missing or altered chromosome material within a region on chromosome 15. Patients have early hypotonia (low muscle tone) that causes facial features such as down-turned corners of the mouth, poor feeding, and failure to thrive. During early childhood, a remarkable change to voracious eating and obesity occurs together with mental disability and behavior differences.

Incidence, causation, and diagnosis

The incidence of Prader–Willi syndrome is 1 in 10,000–15,000 live births. The cause in 70% of patients is a small deletion on the copy of chromosome 15 inherited from the father that is detected by fluorescent *in situ* hybridization, (FISH) study. The remaining 30% of children with Prader–Willi syndrome will have inherited two copies of their mother's chromosome 15 (uniparental disomy) or a chromosome 15 from their father that is dysfunctional in the 15q13q15 region (imprinting mutation). These children must have DNA methylation studies to document abnormal imprinting. The clinical diagnosis is aided by facial changes including almond-shaped eyes, down-turned corners of the mouth, and hollowing at the temples due to hypotonia (low muscle tone). Consensus diagnostic criteria have been formulated for Prader–Willi syndrome and include early hypotonia with feeding problems, excessive weight gain between ages 1 and 6 years with voracious appetite, compatible facial features, underdeveloped genitalia, and global developmental delay/mental disability with behavior differences. Minor criteria include decreased fetal movement; unstable, stubborn or oppositional behavior; sleep apnea (poor sleep due to breathing difficulties); short stature; decreased eye and skin hypopigmentation; small hands and feet; strabismus (wandering eye); thick saliva; problems with speech articulation; and picking at the skin or orifices to produce bleeding and scarring. Deletion or altered imprinting of chromosome 15 is the keystone of diagnosis, provided the clinical features are compatible.

Natural history and complications

Decreased fetal movement, lower birth weights, and breech positioning are common in pregnancy. Low muscle tone after delivery produces a weak suck and poor feeding with a "failure to thrive" picture until overeating begins between ages 1 and 4 years. Abnormal eating behaviors include stealing food, nocturnal foraging for food, eating inappropriate foods, and binge eating. Morbid obesity may ensue that causes a shortened lifespan in Prader–Willi syndrome because of cardiopulmonary disease. The most taxing complications of Prader–Willi syndrome are developmental and behavioral, but eye, dental, skin, and genital problems occur. Dental problems include increased caries and enamel hypoplasia, perhaps reflecting the high-carbohydrate diet and decreased salivation in Prader–Willi syndrome. Regurgitation of food occurs in 10–17% of children, and pneumonias due to aspiration (swallowing of food into the lungs) must be added to the heart failure, temperature instability, and heart irregularities that complicate anesthesia in children with Prader–Willi syndrome. Sleep problems include daytime sleepiness, snoring, narrow upper airway, and abnormal brain regulation of sleep. Violent outbursts, temper tantrums, obsessive–compulsive behavior, rigidity, manipulation, and stubbornness are common. Skin picking with skin infections or scarring and recurrent nasal bleeding may reflect the obsessive–compulsive and oppositional aspects of the syndrome. Speech articulation defects are common, but reading is a relative strength with mathematics and social interactions being weaknesses. Performance in solving mazes or codes was substantially above verbal performance that required auditory processing; this profile may explain the clinical impression that many Prader–Willi patients enjoy puzzles. Over 40% of patients have a global IQ that is above 70 and in the borderline or normal range.

Preventive medical needs

When the diagnosis is suspected based on low muscle tone in infancy, karyotyping and DNA analysis to establish chromosome 15 deletion or uniparental disomy are critical. Early diagnosis is useful for instituting dietary controls and exploring growth hormone therapy that may be used as early as age 2 years. Close monitoring of feeding is necessary during infancy, since some children require enhanced-calorie formula or gavage feeding. Surveillance for strabismus (wandering eye), sleep problems, dental anomalies, or developmental problems are important aspects of management in early childhood, and all children should be referred for early intervention. Regurgitation can bring gastric contents into the throat during anesthesia, even after a 10-h fast; reduction of acid secretion, decompression of the gastric contents, and body positioning to minimize reflux/aspiration are recommended for anesthesia. Prozac or serotonergic drugs may benefit skin picking and obsessive–compulsive behavior, and haloperidol and thioridazine have been used for depression, and anxiety. Since patients do not experience fullness and have remarkable resistance to vomiting; unregulated caloric intake can approach 6000 kcal/day. Calorie restriction to 800–1100 per day in adolescents, behavioral modification using rewards, restricted access to all food sources, promotion of exercise, and family education is vital for weight control. Many adolescents and adults do best living in group homes restricted to Prader–Willi syndrome, so a uniform lifestyle can be designed. Obese patients require monitoring of cardiopulmonary status and blood pressure.

Family counseling

Familial cases are extremely rare, and there is an extremely low recurrence risk for future children. Affected individuals will often be infertile, and there is little experience with their reproduction. As for other disorders that inflict mental disability, supportive services such as psychology, social work, and grief counseling may be appropriate for some parents.

Preventive management of Shprintzen/DiGeorge spectrum

Description: Clinical pattern caused by submicroscopic deletion of chromosome 22 with incidence of 1 in 10,000 births.

Clinical diagnosis: A broad spectrum of manifestations range from isolated conotruncal heart defects to syndrome patterns recognized by DiGeorge and Shprintzen. The former includes absent thymus and hypoparathyroidism with small jaw, the latter long face, narrow palpebral fissures, ear anomalies, and velopalatine incompetence. Some patients have few major anomalies besides their heart defect, and parents discovered through diagnosis in offspring may have no significant abnormalities or mild mental disability/mental illness.

Laboratory diagnosis: Submicroscopic deletion of band 22q11 demonstrated by fluorescent *in situ* hybridization (FISH) technology.

Genetics: Sporadic inheritance with about 10% of cases resulting from parent–child transmission.

Key management issues: Neonatal feeding problems and cardiac anomalies, growth delay with dysphagia and failure to thrive, developmental disability with palatal dysfunction and speech problems, hearing and vision deficits with ear and eye anomalies, immune deficiency with predisposition to infections, internal anomalies of the thyroid, larynx, and kidneys.

Growth charts: None available.

Parent groups: Parent information and support can be found at the Velocardiofacial Syndrome Educational Foundation, Inc. (www.vcfsef.org/) and by searching on the various syndrome names.

Basis for management recommendations: Derived from the complications and references listed below.

Summary of clinical concerns

General	Learning	**Cognitive disability** (40% – verbal IQ 69–87, performance IQ 55–78), **learning differences** (99%), hypernasal speech with hoarse voice, **speech problems** (nasality, articulation)
	Behavior	Behavior problems (bland affect, impulsive behavior, phobias, psychoses)
	Growth	Dysphagia, **failure to thrive** (25%), **short stature** (35%)
Facial	Eyes	**Narrow palpebral fissures with suborbital swelling /"allergic shiners"** (35%), **small optic disks, cataracts** (60%), colobomata (3%), blue sclerae, tortuous retinal vessels
	Ears	**Small auricles** (60%), **chronic otitis** (75%)
	Nose	**Narrow choanae** (75%)
	Mouth	**Cleft palate** (35%), **submucous cleft palate**, **velar paresis** (33%), **hypotonic pharynx** (90%), micrognathia and Robin sequence (17%), dental malocclusion
Surface	Neck/trunk	**Umbilical hernia** (23%), **inguinal hernia** (30%)
Skeletal	Cranial	**Microcephaly** (40%)
	Axial	Scoliosis (15%), **rib and vertebral defects** (35%)
	Limbs	**Slender digits** (60%), increased joint laxity, club feet (10%), rheumatoid arthritis
Internal	Digestive	**Gastroesophageal reflux**, aspiration (90%), dysphagia
	Pulmonary	Stridor (vascular rings, laryngeal webs, laryngeal clefts)
	Circulatory	**Cardiac anomalies** (82% – ventricular septal defects, right-sided aortic arch, tetralogy of Fallot), Raynaud's phenomenon
	Endocrine	Hypocalcemia (10%),* hypothyroidism, Hashimoto thyroiditis
	RES	Thymic aplasia (10%),* immune deficiency (10%),* autoimmune diseases
	Excretory	Ureteral reflux (10%), **renal anomalies** (35%)
	Genital	Hypospadias (10%), cryptorchidism
Neural	Central	Seizures, cognitive disability, **obstructive sleep apnea** (50% of neonates)
	Sensory	Chronic otitis, **conductive hearing loss** (75%), visual deficits

*particularly if DiGeorge anomaly is present; **RES**, reticuloendothelial system; **concerns** of frequency >20% are **highlighted**

Key references

McDonald-McGinn, et al. (2001). Phenotype of the 22q11.2 deletion in individuals identified through an affected relative: cast a wide FISHing net! *Genetics in Medicine* 3:23–9.

Shprintzen (2000). Velo-cardio-facial syndrome: a distinctive behavioral phenotype. *Mental Retardation and Developmental Disabilities Research Reviews* 6:142–7.

Shprintzen/DiGeorge spectrum

Preventive medical checklist (0–3 years)

Name _____ **Birth date** __/__/__ **Number** _____

Age	Evaluations: key concerns	Management considerations	Notes
New-born ↓ 1 month	Dysmorphology examination: anomalies Hearing, vision:[2] deafness, cataracts Feeding: cleft palate, dysphagia Chest: heart defects, absent thymus Urogenital: renal defects; cryptorchidism Skeletal: hernias, spine, club feet Airway: laryngeal defects, sleep apnea	☐ Karyotype, genetic counsel;[1] family support[4] ☐ ☐ ABR; ENT;[3] ophthalmology[3] ☐ ☐ Cleft palate team;[3] video swallow;[3] GI[3] ☐ ☐ Chest X-ray; echocardiogram; cardiology ☐ ☐ Renal sono; urinary tract studies; urology[3] ☐ ☐ Skeletal survey;[3] orthopedics[3] ☐ ☐ Pulmonology;[3] sleep study[3] ☐	Infantile airway problems common with Robin anomaly, sleep apnea, palatal dysfunction, aspiration.
2 months ↓ 4 months	Growth, development:[5] failure to thrive Hearing, vision:[2] deafness, otitis Nutrition: dysphagia, poor intake Heart: ASD, VSD, aortic arch defects Urogenital: renal defects; cryptorchidism Airway: laryngeal defects, sleep apnea[7] Skeletal: vertebral defects, club feet Other:	☐ ECI;[6] family support[4] ☐ ☐ Repeat ABR[3] ☐ ☐ Cleft palate team;[3] video swallow;[3] GI[3] ☐ ☐ Echocardiogram; cardiology ☐ ☐ Renal sono;[3] urinary tract studies;[3] urology[3] ☐ ☐ Pulmonology;[3] sleep study[3] ☐ ☐ Skeletal survey;[3] orthopedics[3] ☐ ☐ ☐	Avoid live vaccines if DiGeorge suspected.
6 months ↓ 9 months	Growth, development:[5] failure to thrive Hearing, vision:[2] deafness, otitis Nutrition: dysphagia, poor intake Cardiovascular, urinary tract anomalies Airway: laryngeal defects, sleep apnea[7] Other:	☐ ECI;[6] family support[4] ☐ ☐ ENT;[3] ophthalmology[3] ☐ ☐ Extra feeding;[3] feeding specialist;[3] GI[3] ☐ ☐ Urinalysis; BP; cardiology;[3] urology[3] ☐ ☐ Pulmonology;[3] sleep study[3] ☐ ☐ ☐	
1 year	Growth, development:[5] failure to thrive Hearing, vision:[2] deafness, otitis Heart, oral, GI, urinary tract defects Thyroid, immune defects Airway: aspiration, sleep apnea[7] Spine, limbs, hernias, neck flexibility Other:	☐ ECI[6] ☐ ☐ ENT; ophthalmology ☐ ☐ Dietician;[3] GI;[3] urinalysis; BP; cardiology[3] ☐ ☐ T4, TSH; endocrinology;[3] immunology[3] ☐ ☐ Pulmonology;[3] sleep study[3] ☐ ☐ Anesthesia precautions; orthopedics[3] ☐ ☐ ☐	
15 months ↓ 18 months	Growth, development:[5] failure to thrive Hearing, vision:[2] deafness, otitis Heart, oral, GI, urinary tract defects Airway: aspiration, sleep apnea[7]	☐ ECI[6] ☐ ☐ ENT; ophthalmology ☐ ☐ Dietician;[3] GI;[3] urinalysis; BP; cardiology[3] ☐ ☐ Pulmonology;[3] sleep study[3] ☐	
2 years	Growth, development:[5] failure to thrive Hearing, vision:[2] deafness, otitis Heart, oral, GI, urinary tract defects Thyroid, immune defects Airway: aspiration, sleep apnea[7]	☐ ECI[6] ☐ ☐ Audiology; ENT; ophthalmology ☐ ☐ Dietician;[3] GI;[3] urinalysis; BP; cardiology[3] ☐ ☐ T4, TSH; endocrinology;[3] immunology[3] ☐ ☐ Pulmonology;[3] sleep study[3] ☐	
3 years	Growth, development:[5] short stature Hearing, vision:[2] deafness, otitis Heart, oral, GI, urinary tract defects Thyroid, immune defects Airway: aspiration, sleep apnea[7] Spine, limbs, hernias, neck flexibility Other:	☐ ECI;[6] family support[4] ☐ ☐ Audiology; ENT; ophthalmology ☐ ☐ Dietician;[3] GI;[3] urinalysis; BP; cardiology[3] ☐ ☐ T4, TSH; endocrinology;[3] immunology[3] ☐ ☐ Pulmonology;[3] sleep study[3] ☐ ☐ Anesthesia precautions; orthopedics[3] ☐ ☐ ☐	

Deletion 22 syndrome concerns		Other concerns from history	
Poor feeding, dysphagia Failure to thrive Palatal clefts, dysfunction Vision, hearing deficits Hypothyroidism Cardiac anomalies Immune deficiencies	Vertebral, rib defects Club feet, scoliosis Renal anomalies, reflux Cryptorchidism, micropenis Hypotonia, seizures, deafness Obstructive sleep apnea Learning disabilities	**Family history/prenatal** _____ _____ _____ _____	**Social/environmental** _____ _____ _____ _____

Guidelines for the neonatal period should be undertaken *at whatever age* the diagnosis is made; ASD, atrial septal defect; VSD, ventricular septal defect; GI, gastrointestinal; BP, blood pressure; T4, thyroid hormone; TSH, thyroid-stimulating hormone; ABR, auditory brainstem evoked response; [1]parental chromosomes if the 22q11 deletion is found; [2]by practitioner; [3]as dictated by clinical findings; [4]parent group, family/sib, financial, and behavioral issues; [5]consider developmental pediatrician/neurologist/behavior therapist/genetic clinic according to symptoms and availability; [6]early childhood intervention including developmental monitoring motor/speech therapy with emphasis on palatal function; [7]snoring, pause in breathing, daytime sleepiness, unusual sleep positioning.

Shprintzen/DiGeorge spectrum

Preventive medical checklist (4–18 years)

Name _____ Birth date __/__/____ Number_____

Age	Evaluations: key concerns	Management considerations		Notes
4 years ↓ 6 years	Growth:[1] short stature Development:[2] preschool transition Sensory, sleep:[2] deafness sleep apnea[7] Heart, oral, GI, urinary tract defects Thyroid, immune, genital defects Spine, limbs, hernias, neck flexibility Other:	❑ Family support[4] ❑ Preschool program[5] ❑ Audiology; ENT; ophthalmology; sleep study[3] ❑ Dietician;[3] GI;[3] urinalysis, BP; cardiology[3] ❑ T4, TSH; endocrinology;[3] immunology[3] ❑ Anesthesia precautions; orthopedics[3] ❑	❑ ❑ ❑ ❑ ❑ ❑ ❑	
7 years ↓ 9 years	Growth[1] Development:[1] school transition Sensory, sleep:[2] deafness sleep Heart, urinary tract defects, obesity Thyroid, immune, genital defects Skeletal: hernias, scoliosis Other:	❑ Family support[4] ❑ School progress[6] ❑ Audiology; ENT; ophthalmology; sleep study[3] ❑ Dietician;[3] urinalysis, BP; cardiology[3] ❑ T4, TSH; endocrinology;[3] immunology[3] ❑ Anesthesia precautions; orthopedics[3] ❑	❑ ❑ ❑ ❑ ❑ ❑ ❑	
10 years ↓ 12 years	Growth and development[1] Sensory, sleep:[2] deafness sleep Heart, urinary tract defects, obesity Thyroid, immune, genital defects Other:	❑ Family support;[4] school progress[6] ❑ Audiology; ENT; ophthalmology; sleep study[3] ❑ Dietician;[3] urinalysis, BP; cardiology[3] ❑ T4, TSH; endocrinology;[3] immunology[3] ❑	❑ ❑ ❑ ❑ ❑	
13 years ↓ 15 years	Growth and development[1] Sensory, sleep:[2] deafness sleep Heart, obesity, precocious puberty Thyroid, immune, genital defects Skeletal: hernias, scoliosis Other:	❑ School progress[6] ❑ Audiology; ENT; ophthalmology; sleep study[3] ❑ Dietician;[3] endocrinology;[3] cardiology[3] ❑ T4, TSH; endocrinology;[3] immunology[3] ❑ Anesthesia precautions; orthopedics[3] ❑	❑ ❑ ❑ ❑ ❑ ❑	
16 years ↓ 18 years	Growth and development[1] Sensory, sleep:[2] deafness sleep Heart, obesity, precocious puberty Thyroid, immune, genital defects Other:	❑ Family support;[4] school progress[6] ❑ Audiology; ENT; ophthalmology; sleep study[3] ❑ Dietician;[3] endocrinology;[3] cardiology[3] ❑ T4, TSH; endocrinology;[3] immunology[3] ❑	❑ ❑ ❑ ❑ ❑	
19 years ↓ 23 years	Adult-care transition[6] Sensory, sleep:[2] deafness sleep Heart, obesity, precocious puberty Thyroid, immune, genital defects Skeletal: hernias, scoliosis	❑ Family support;[4] school progress[6] ❑ Audiology; ENT;[3] ophthalmology; sleep study[3] ❑ Dietician,[3] endocrinology,[3] cardiology[3] ❑ T4, TSH, endocrinology,[3] immunology[3] ❑ Anesthesia precautions, orthopedics[3]	❑ ❑ ❑ ❑ ❑	
Adult	Adult-care transition[6] Sensory, sleep:[2] deafness sleep Heart, obesity, precocious puberty Thyroid, immune, genital defects Skeletal: hernias, scoliosis Behavior: impulsivity, psychoses Other:	❑ Family support[4] ❑ Audiology; ENT;[3] ophthalmology; sleep study[3] ❑ Dietician;[3] endocrinology;[3] cardiology[3] ❑ T4, TSH; endocrinology;[3] immunology[3] ❑ Anesthesia precautions; orthopedics[3] ❑ Behavior therapy; psychiatry[3] ❑	❑ ❑ ❑ ❑ ❑ ❑ ❑	

Deletion 22 syndrome concerns		Other concerns from history	
Short stature Palatal clefts, dysfunction Vision, hearing deficits Hypothyroidism Cardiac anomalies Immune deficiencies Vertebral, rib defects	Scoliosis Renal anomalies, reflux Cryptorchidism, micropenis Seizures, deafness Obstructive sleep apnea Behavior problems, psychosis Cognitive disabilities Employment, independent living	**Family history/prenatal** _____ _____ _____ _____	**Social/environmental** _____ _____ _____ _____

Guidelines for the neonatal period should be undertaken at whatever age the diagnosis is made; GI, gastrointestinal; BP, blood pressure; T4, thyroid hormone; TSH, thyroid-stimulating hormone; [1]consider developmental pediatrician/neurologist/behavior therapist/genetics clinic according to symptoms and availability; [2]by practitioner; [3]as dictated by clinical findings; [4]parent group, family/sib, financial, and behavioral issues with later focus on independent living and employment; [5]preschool program including developmental monitoring and motor/speech therapy; [6]monitor individual education plan, educational testing, balance of special education and inclusion, academic progress, behavioral differences, later vocational planning; [7]snoring, pause in breathing, day time sleepiness, unusual sleep positioning.

Parent guide to Shprintzen/DiGeorge spectrum

Patients reported by DiGeorge (1968) with heart defects, absent thymus, and hypocalcemia and those described by Shprintzen (1978) with unusual facies, velopalatine insufficiency, and conotruncal anomalies were recognized as part of a spectrum when submicroscopic deletions of chromosome 22 were found in both patient groups. The term Shprintzen/DiGeorge spectrum is preferred to the acronym CATCH 22 because of its negative connotation.

Incidence, causation, and diagnosis

Incidence of the Shprintzen/DiGeorge spectrum is 1 in 10,000 births, rising to 1 in 5000 if patients with isolated heart defects with deletion 22 are included. The spectrum comprises about 8% of patients with cleft palate and other anomalies. Adding to this prevalence figure are asymptomatic relatives whose deletion is identified only because they have an affected child. Half-dosage of key genes on chromosome 22 within the deletion are the cause, and current research is examining their mechanisms and variability (most patients have similar extents of deletion). Differential diagnosis includes other conditions with orofacial and cardiac problems, including the genetic conditions called orofacialdigital syndrome. The DiGeorge sequence also occurs in CHARGE association, but the facial appearance is different from that of Shprintzen syndrome.

Natural history and complications

Neonatal complications are particularly important to consider in Shprintzen/DiGeorge/chromosome 22 deletion spectrum, since their detection and management will have considerable influence on prognosis. Cardiac anomalies, palatal dysfunction, dysphagia with aspiration, and obstructive sleep apnea are common in affected neonates, potentially causing debilitating lung disease or heart failure. The natural history of Shprintzen syndrome has three phases; a turbulent infantile course, with possible heart disease, severe dysphagia and reflux, obstructive sleep apnea, and upper respiratory infections; a childhood compromised by hearing, speech, learning, and growth problems; and an adolescence/adulthood challenged by personality, school, and behavioral problems. The mental disability can relate to neuroanatomic changes such as undergrowth of the cerebellum. Patients also have an increased risk of ocular, urinary tract, and genital anomalies, and increased connective tissue laxity confers risks of inguinal hernia in 30% of patients and scoliosis (spinal curvature) in 13–15%. Aberrant anatomy of the arteries of the head and neck has been described, posing risks for surgical procedures of the ear, nose, and throat. Growth is slow early in 35% of children and in two of five adults identified in one study. Learning disabilities are almost universal in Shprintzen syndrome, and significant mental disability occurs in some. Performance IQ is lower than verbal IQ, and hypernasal speech with articulation problems and language delay is common. A characteristic personality has been described, consisting of a bland affect, poor social interaction, and impulsive behavior. Psychosis and phobic reactions occur.

Preventive medical needs

Live vaccines should not be given if DiGeorge anomaly is suspected. Heart ultrasound (echocardiography), assessment of hearing, consideration of obstructive sleep apnea and close monitoring of feeding and palatal function are important during infancy. In the presence of low blood calcium or recurrent infections, chest X-rays, peripheral white blood cell counts, and blood calcium/phosphorus measurements should be obtained to evaluate the presence of DiGeorge anomaly. Medical counseling should be optimistic for most children with Shprintzen/DiGeorge/chromosome 22 deletion spectrum, since ultimate cognitive function ranges from normal to mild/moderate mental disability. Risks for upper respiratory infections are increased in most patients, necessitating aggressive treatment of chronic otitis and screening for hearing loss. Submucous clefts or velopalatine dysfunction may confer significant risks for otitis and speech problems. Many patients have feeding problems and failure to thrive, so feeding specialists may be needed to accomplish reasonable growth. The care of older children and adolescents should focus on learning disabilities and potential school problems, which may be augmented by abnormal behaviors. Attention to speech, language, and hearing should continue, and awareness of the increased joint laxity may influence the recommendations for physical activity. Scoliosis (curved spine) and inguinal hernias occur at increased frequency, and the occurrence of genital anomalies in boys makes it important to monitor puberty.

Family counseling

Before the discovery of the chromosome 22 deletion, Shprintzen syndrome was considered to exhibit autosomal-dominant inheritance and the DiGeorge anomaly to be sporadic (not inherited). Isolated heart defects such as interrupted aortic arch, ventricular septal defects, or tetralogy of Fallot are usually multifactorial with a 2–3% recurrence risk, although occasional families would exhibit vertical transmission. Parents of affected children should have FISH analysis for the chromosome 22 deletion. Parents without clinically suggestive physical or psychiatric features should have FISH analysis since the deletion has been found in apparently normal individuals. All families should be referred for genetic counseling. Individuals with the deletion or a presumptive clinical diagnosis of Shprintzen syndrome should be given a 50% recurrence risk, with the understanding that their affected children will likely vary in the distribution and severity of manifestations. Parents of children with the Shprintzen/DiGeorge spectrum will have recurrence risks <1% providing they do not have the chromosome 22 deletion. Psychosocial counseling may be quite important, since many affected children and occasional parents will have behavior problems ranging from poor social interaction to frank psychosis or phobic responses.

Part IV

Syndromes remarkable for altered growth

Monitoring of growth is a major component of anticipatory guidance in pediatrics, and its abnormalities guide the physician to various categories of disease. It is important to monitor head circumference in addition to height and weight, even beyond the 36 months included on standard charts, because disproportion among height, weight, and head circumference is pivotal in separating nutritional problems from congenital disorders.

For infants and young children with growth delay (failure to thrive), a disproportionately small head circumference can indicate abnormal brain development as seen in fetal alcohol or many genetic syndromes. A head circumference that is closer to the normal range than the length and weight may indicate "head-sparing;" such measures often indicate psychosocial or nutritional deprivation with preferential routing of calories to cerebral development. A normally expanding, proportionately larger head circumference often occurs in children with developmental disabilities like fragile X syndrome, cerebral gigantism, or certain autism spectrum disorders – these disorders may alter the programmed death or "pruning" of brain cells that is so critical for normal development.

The chapters in this section focus on children with constitutional causes of growth deficiency, and it is critical to distinguish those that are proportionately small (see Chapter 10) from those with disproportionate short stature (skeletal dysplasia or dwarfism – see Chapter 11). Single gene causes predominate in both categories, with the congenitally small having syndromes analogous to the chromosome disorders discussed in Chapter 7 and the skeletal dysplasias manifesting very different signs that include large heads with frontal bossing, short limbs, and small or deformed chests and spines. Skeletal dysplasias particularly emphasize the value of preventive management, for anticipation of their sleep, immune, and orthopedic problems can greatly minimize physical disability and preserve their potential for normal intelligence.

10

Syndromes with proportionate growth failure as a primary manifestation

Stature or length, limb segments, and head circumference are proportionate in symmetrical or harmonic growth failure, and disproportionate in asymmetrical or dysharmonic dwarfism. Disproportion of the head, thorax, or limbs often suggests a skeletal dysplasia as will be discussed in Chapter 11. Proportionate growth failure of stature and limbs may be accompanied by a slightly larger head circumference in nutritional deficiencies ("head-sparing") or by a slightly smaller head circumference in some congenital syndromes. Table 10.1 summarizes various syndromes with proportionate growth failure, classifying them by time of onset (prenatal and/or postnatal) and by accompanying changes in head circumference (with or without microcephaly).

Syndromes with symmetrical intrauterine growth retardation include many chromosomal and teratogenic syndromes discussed in Chapters 5–7. Intrauterine growth retardation is a harbinger for congenital disease, and a thorough investigation of maternal health, gestational history, and the fetal karyotype is often indicated. Once disorders such as fetal alcohol syndrome, Cri-du-Chat syndrome, and trisomy 13/18 are excluded by physical and laboratory findings, the clinician should begin considering syndromes with primary growth failure. Since isolated fetal disease (e.g., cardiac anomaly, renal anomaly) rarely produces intrauterine growth failure, a more global process must be suspected. Table 10.1 lists the more common syndromes with growth failure that do not involve obvious karyotypic changes. These disorders will exhibit proportionately small birth measurements and/or symmetrical failure to thrive. Any clinician concerned about shortened limbs, small thorax, frontal bossing with a shallow nasal bridge, or certain skeletal anomalies should obtain a skeletal radiographic survey to evaluate the possibility of a skeletal dysplasia (dwarfism – see Chapter 11).

Follow-up may be necessary to recognize many of the primordial growth failure syndromes listed in Table 10.1. Children with the Russell–Silver, Donahue, Dubowitz, Niikawa, Seckel, or Williams syndrome may not exhibit obvious dysmorphology in the neonatal nursery. Many of the conditions have early feeding problems that may

Table 10.1. Syndromes with growth failure

Syndrome	Incidence*	Frequent abnormalities
Syndromes with prenatal growth retardation, normocephaly		
Russell–Silver	~150 cases	Facial, skeletal, renal, genital
Donohue (leprechaunism)	~30 cases	Facial, epidermal, endocrine, genital
Syndromes with prenatal growth retardation, microcephaly		
Bloom	~130 cases	Facial, vascular, epidermal, skeletal, immune
Dubowitz	~30 cases	Facial, ocular, dental, skeletal, epidermal
Seckel	~30 cases	Ocular, dental, skeletal, genital
Smith–Lemli–Opitz	~50 cases	Facial, ocular, cardiac, GI, skeletal, genital
Syndromes with postnatal growth retardation, normocephaly		
Aarskog	~100 cases	Facial, skeletal, genital
Costello	~50 cases	Facial, cardiac, dental, epidermal
Noonan	1 in 2500	Facial, ocular, dental, cardiac, skeletal, genital
Robinow	~50 cases	Facial, skeletal, genital
Syndromes with postnatal growth retardation, microcephaly		
Brachmann–de Lange	1 in 10,000	Facial, ocular, cardiac, skeletal, GI, immune
Hallermann–Streiff	~150 cases	Facial, ocular, dental, skeletal, genital, epidermal
Niikawa–Kuroki	~150 cases	Facial, cardiac, skeletal, genitourinary
Rubinstein–Taybi	~600 cases	Facial, ocular, cardiac, skeletal, genital
Williams	1 in 25,000	Facial, ocular, dental, cardiac, renal, genital

Notes:

GI, gastrointestinal.

*Cases or per number of live births.

mask the underlying syndrome while gastrointestinal (GI) disorders are evaluated. Some premature infants may be confused with small-for-gestational-age babies until catch-up growth is documented. Hand radiographs to evaluate the bone age may be helpful in evaluating older infants and toddlers with growth failure, since the bone age may be extremely delayed in endocrine problems such as hypothyroidism or growth hormone (GH) deficiency. By age 2–3 years, the evolution of dysmorphology, the presence of developmental delay, the accentuation of microcephaly, or the lack of catch-up growth should identify the child with a primary growth failure syndrome.

Of the disorders with growth failure listed in Table 10.1, most, like the Rubinstein–Taybi syndrome, are rare and will be discussed briefly. Brachmann–de Lange and Noonan syndromes are sufficiently common to warrant detailed preventive management (discussed later in this chapter). The Williams syndrome has been associated with a chromosome microdeletion was discussed in Chapter 9; Smith–Lemli–Opitz syndrome will be discussed in Chapter 19.

Bloom syndrome

Bloom syndrome was first described in 1954 as "congenital telangiectatic erythema resembling lupus erythematosus in dwarfs." This autosomal-recessive syndrome involves pre- and postnatal growth retardation, mild microcephaly, immune deficiency, male hypogonadism, and sensitivity to sunlight producing erythematous malar and upper limb telangiectasia (Jones, 1997, pp. 104–5; Gorlin et al., 2001, pp. 368–72). Chromosomal studies show a high rate of exchange between sister chromatids and breakage leading to unusual rearranged chromosomes. The chromosomal changes are diagnostic, and probably explain the predilection for neoplasia in patients with Bloom syndrome.

Summary of clinical concerns: Bloom syndrome management considerations

Growth and development: Pre- and postnatal growth retardation, mild microcephaly, mild mental disability with behavioral problems secondary to short stature and facial lesions; GH deficiency with response to GH therapy: Monitoring of growth, development, school progress, and social adjustment with referral to early intervention, developmental pediatrics, endocrinology, and behavioral therapy/psychiatry as needed.

Cancer: Neoplasms occur in 30–40%, often in childhood, and include squamous and basal cell carcinomas, leukemias, lymphomas, adenocarcinomas of the gut or breast, and Wilms tumor, often with onset in childhood: Prompt investigation of masses, ulcerated or pigmented skin lesions, anemias, bone or joint pain, asymmetric growth, or unusual GI symptoms.

Craniofacial: Light sensitivity with development of telangiectasia, erythema, and pigmented lesions; vesicles can appear after sunlight exposure: Stringent sun protection.

Cardiac: Occasional cardiac anomalies: Cardiology and echocardiogram if symptoms.

Endocrine: Diabetes mellitus has occurred in about 10% of adolescents and adults: Annual urinalysis, alert for acanthosis nigricans, referral to endocrinology as needed.

Reticuloendothelial system (RES): Patients with frequent infections may have deficient immunoglobulins (IgA, IgG, or IgM) and may be candidates for gamma-globulin injections. Chronic upper respiratory infections often require otolaryngology involvement.

Urogenital: Hypogonadism including small or undescended testes in males and menstrual irregularities in females: Monitor genital development, urology, or endocrinology referral.

Skeletal: Unequal leg lengths, congenital hip dislocation, or club feet: Orthopedics evaluation as needed.

Neurologic: Mild mental disability in 15%, school and self-image problems: School and behavioral assessments with careful monitoring of school progress.

Parental counseling: The syndrome exhibits autosomal-recessive inheritance, with a 25% recurrence risk to parents of affected children. The causative BKM gene has been isolated and DNA diagnosis for some types of Bloom syndrome is available (see GeneTest, www.genetests.org). A negative test result does not eliminate the diagnosis. The American College of Obstetrics and Gynecology (2004) notes availability of carrier testing for Bloom syndrome in Ashkenazi Jews of Eastern European origin, but does not recommend it as it does for Tay–Sachs, Canavan, and cystic fibrosis. Parent support and information is available at several academic sites by searching on the syndrome name, including a registry of mutations (bioinf.uta.fi/BLMbase/index2.html).

Costello syndrome

Initially described in 1977 by Costello, the pattern of manifestations includes normal birth weight with subsequent short stature, normal or large head circumference, skin findings such as papillomas and acanthosis nigricans, curly hair, and joint laxity (Jones, 1997, pp. 124–5). The syndrome will usually present as possible Noonan syndrome because of its similar facial appearance, short stature, and pulmonic stenosis with increased frequency of cardiomyopathy; appearance or recognition of the papillomas around the lips and mouth will lead to the correct diagnosis.

Summary of clinical concerns: Costello syndrome management considerations

Growth and development: Short stature is the norm with occasional GH deficiency; verbal, receptive vocabulary, and adaptive behavior skills are below average but highly variable (Axelrad et al., 2004): In receptive language, level of adaptive behavior functioning, and emotional/behavioral aspects; IQ range from 50 to near normal: Endocrine referral for severe growth delays, early childhood intervention with speech therapy; developmental pediatrics, genetics, and/or neurology according to symptoms and availability.

Cancer: Increased risk for solid tumors: Annual physical examinations.

Craniofacial: Coarsening of facial features with papillomas around lips and mouth: Cosmetic surgery if disfiguring.

Cardiac: Pulmonic stenosis, ventricular septal defects, arrhythmias, cardiomyopathy: Cardiology and echocardiogram at diagnosis followed by annual reassessment.

Skeletal: Connective tissue laxity with risks for hip dislocations, hernias, flat feet, scoliosis, and joint dislocations: Regular skeletal examinations, counsel to avoid high intensity or collision sports, orthopedics referral as needed.

Parental counseling: Inheritance is autosomal dominant with most cases being sporadic (i.e., new mutations). Most parents will have less than a 1% recurrence risk while affected patients may have as high as a 50% recurrence risk. The diagnosis is clinical, and no DNA testing is available. Parent support and information is available at the International Costello Syndrome Support Group (www.costellokids.co.uk/) and by searching on the syndrome name.

Donohue syndrome (leprechaunism)

Initially described in 1948, Donahue syndrome or leprechaunism includes delayed pre- and postnatal growth, decreased subcutaneous tissue, hirsutism, nail hypoplasia, and genital hypertrophy (Jones, 1997, p. 599; Gorlin et al., 2001, pp. 1022–3; Kosztolanyi, 1997). It is caused by homozygous deletion of the insulin receptor gene, and certain symptoms resemble that of severe diabetes mellitus.

Summary of clinical concerns: Donahue syndrome management considerations

General: Premature gestation with death by age 2 years in 60%; administration of insulin-like growth factor and other therapies have not been useful.

Growth and development: Severe growth retardation with progressive marasmus and retarded bone age; motor delays due to muscle wasting: Early childhood intervention with early evaluation and follow-up by endocrinology.

Tumors: Pituitary and pancreatic hyperplasia with nesidioblastosis; ovarian granulose cell tumor in one patient.

Craniofacial: Subcutaneous atrophy of the skin plus hyperinsulinism produces a hirsute and coarse facial appearance.

Surface-skin: Generalized hirsutism with acanthosis nigricans, dysplastic nails.

Endocrine: Hypoglycemia, elevated insulin levels: Monitoring of levels by endocrinology.

Gastrointestinal: Hepatic cholestasis or fibrosis with iron storage, dilated intestines: Monitor liver functions with GI referral for symptom relief.

Urogenital: Glomerular changes in kidney similar to that of diabetes mellitus: Monitor of blood pressure and urinalysis, nephrology, and urology referral for symptoms.

Skeletal: Occipital bony defects, scoliosis, valgus deformities of the lower limbs: Skeletal examinations with X-rays and orthopedics evaluation as needed.

Neurologic: Severe muscle hypoplasia with motor delays.

Parental counseling: Autosomal-recessive inheritance with 25% recurrence risk for parents of affected children. Although mutations in the insulin receptor are well characterized, commercial DNA testing is not yet available to allow prenatal diagnosis. Parent support and information is best obtained searching on "leprechaunism."

Dubowitz syndrome

Dubowitz syndrome was initially confused with Bloom syndrome until it was recognized as a separate entity in 1971 (Jones, 1997, pp. 102–3; Gorlin et al., 2001, pp. 377–99). Manifestations of pre- and postnatal growth failure, microcephaly, high-pitched voice, skin changes (eczematous), cancer predilection, and immune deficiency are shared with Bloom syndrome.

Summary of clinical concerns: Dubowitz syndrome management considerations

Growth and development: Low birth weight with postnatal growth failure and delayed bone age; infantile feeding problems in 75% with vomiting and gastroesophageal reflux; most patients having dull normal intelligence but 10–15% have severe mental disability; delayed speech (60%) and hyperactivity (40%) are common: Neonatal feeding evaluation and feeding specialist/dietician, particularly if cleft palate; early childhood intervention with speech therapy; later assessment for hyperactivity; developmental pediatrics, genetics, and/or neurology follow-up according to availability.

Cancer: Neoplasms have included leukemia, lymphoma, and neuroblastoma: Peripheral blood cell counts should be obtained in children with infectious illnesses or fatigue, since aplastic anemias have also been described.

Craniofacial: Microcephaly and a distinctive facial appearance with ptosis, blepharophimosis, telecanthus, and a high-pitched voice.

ENT: Overt or submucous cleft palate in 35%, external ear malformations with otitis: Audiology and frequent middle ear evaluations; cleft palate team and otolaryngology as needed.

Eye: Strabismus, microphthalmia, tortuous retinal vessels/retinal pigmentation, colobomata; ophthalmology at age 6 months, then annually.

Surface-skin: Eczema: Monitor skin with monteleukast therapy rather than steroid creams that can affect growth.

Cardiac: Rare cardiac defects: Cardiology and echocardiogram if symptoms.

Gastrointestinal: Achalasia, vomiting, GI reflux: Monitor symptoms with gastroenterology referral as necessary.

Urogenital: Hypospadias or cryptorchidism in 70% of males: Newborn and follow-up genital examinations, urology as needed.

RES: Immune deficiency with occasional hypogammaglobulinemia or IgA deficieny: Serum immunoglobulins if frequent infections, immunology referral for abnormalities.

Skeletal: Progressive scoliosis and cervical vertebral anomalies (Swartz et al., 2003): Annual skeletal examinations, anesthesia precautions, consider cervical flexion–extension films to examine neck and occiput at age 2–3 years; neurosurgery and orthopedics evaluation for abnormalities as appropriate.

Neurology: Some patients have had brain anomalies including absent corpus callosum and small anterior pituitary gland: consider head MRI scan and neurology referral in children with severe delays.

Parental counseling: Dubowitz syndrome exhibits autosomal-recessive inheritance, conferring a 25% recurrence risk for parent of affected children. The causative gene is not yet defined, so prenatal diagnosis is not available. Parent information is available at several medical sites accessed by searching on the syndrome name.

Hallermann–Streiff syndrome

Although Hallermann in 1948 and Streiff in 1950 defined the syndrome as a separate entity, François established the diagnostic criteria of microcephaly, cataracts, microphthalmia, sparse hair, skin atrophy, and proportionate growth failure (Jones, 1997, pp. 110–11; Gorlin et al., 2001, pp. 379–82).

Summary of clinical concerns: Hallermann–Streiff syndrome management considerations

Growth and development: Low birth weight (35%) and proportionate short stature (50%), mental disability in 15–30%, hyperactivity in some: Early childhood intervention with speech therapy; evaluation and follow-up by developmental pediatrics, genetics, and/or neurology according to severity of delays and availability.

Craniofacial: Characteristic appearance with sparse hair, small eyes, beaked nose, and small jaw; malformed teeth: Dental evaluation and follow-up together with otolaryngology.

Eye: Ocular anomalies including cataracts and strabismus: Ophthalmology evaluation at 6–8 months with annual follow-up.

ENT: Narrow upper airway with respiratory embarrassment or obstructive sleep apnea: Neonatal otolaryngology referral for inspection of nasopharyngeal anatomy and possible tracheostomy; anesthesia precautions for airway anomalies – rapid induction is not recommended unless the larynx is first visualized, otolaryngologists should be available for emergency tracheostomy is required during surgery, and patients should not be extubated until they are fully awake and functional; audiology and monitoring for otitis.

Pulmonary: Severe pulmonary infections require early and aggressive treatment of respiratory infections.

Cardiac: Septal defects and tetralogy of Fallot in 5%: Cardiology and echocardiogram if symptoms.

RES: Immune deficiencies: Monitoring of immunoglobulin levels, immunization against respiratory illnesses, immunology referral if symptoms.

Urogenital: Cryptorchidism, hypospadias, clitoral enlargement, breast asymmetry: Neonatal examinations and monitoring of puberty, urology, and endocrinology as needed.

Skeletal: Pectus, scoliosis: Regular skeletal examinations, orthopedics evaluation and follow-up for scoliosis.

Neurologic: Obstructive sleep apnea, seizures: Cohen has urged that any child with snoring and daytime somnolence have appropriate sleep studies.

Parental counseling: Sporadic disorder with minimal risk for future pregnancies to parents of affected children. An autosomal-recessive progeria (Hallerman–Streiff syndrome) is similar, but the presence of spastic paraplegia allows differentiation (Gorlin et al., 2001, pp. 379–82). Parent support and information is available at medical sites by searching on the syndrome name.

Niikawa–Kuroki (Kabuki) syndrome

The Niikawa–Kuroki syndrome was first described in Japan, with characteristics likened to a Kabuki theater mask because of the wide palpebral fissures, eversion of the lower eyelids, prominent ears, and down-turned corners of the mouth (Jones, 1997, pp. 116–17; Gorlin et al., 2001, pp. 938–40). The malformation pattern in non-Asian patients is somewhat different, and clinical experience suggests this condition is more common than is suggested by the ~150 cases published to date (Wilson, 1998; Armstrong et al., 2005). There are intriguing associations with X chromosome anomalies and a few patients have had a microduplication of chromosome 8. Armstrong et al. (2005) suggest an abnormality in the interferon pathways may be responsible.

Summary of clinical concerns: Niikawa–Kuroki (Kabuki) syndrome
management considerations

Growth and development: Short stature in 80% with turbulent early course and failure to thrive in many; mild to moderate mental disability in 85%: Feeding specialist and dietician, gastroenterology if gastroesophageal reflux: Early childhood intervention with speech therapy; developmental pediatrics, genetics, and/or neurology according to severity of delays and availability.

Cancer: Neuroblastoma has been described.

Craniofacial: Distinctive facial appearance with wide eyes, down-turned corners of the mouth, prominent external ears; cleft or submucous cleft palate in 30–40%: Cleft palate team, feeding specialists.

ENT: Chronic otitis in 50%, conductive and sensorineural hearing loss with malformations of ear ossicles: Neonatal ABR, regular middle ear examinations,
annual hearing evaluations.

Eye: Strabismus: Ophthalmology at age 6 months and annually thereafter.

Cardiac: P cardiovascular anomaly (26–50%), eripheral coarctations: Cardiology
and echocardiogram at diagnosis, serially thereafter.

Gastrointestinal: Imperforate anus, biliary atresia, diaphragmatic defects less common: Neonatal examination and gastroenterology referral as needed.

RES: Immune deficiency with frequent infections.

Urogenital: Urinary tract anomalies (30%), premature thelarche, ovarian dysfunction:
Abdominal ultrasound at diagnosis, monitoring of blood pressure and urinalysis,
monitor puberty, urology and endocrine follow-up according to symptoms.

Skeletal: Congenital hip dislocation (21%), scoliosis (35%): Skeletal examinations
with orthopedic referral as needed.

Neurologic: Neonatal hypotonia (33%), seizures (29%), microcephaly (36%), hearing loss (26–50%): Neonatal examination with neurology referral as needed.

Parental counseling: Most authors favor autosomal-dominant inheritance with
nearly all patients being new mutations. Parents without clinical signs or symptoms will have a negligible recurrence risk. Parent support and information is
available at the Kabuki Syndrome Network in Canada (www.kabukisyndrome.
com/) with branches underway in several countries.

Robinow syndrome

Children with Robinow syndrome have short stature with an unusual "fetal" face,
mesomelic shortening of the limbs, and genital anomalies (Jones, 1997, pp. 130–1;
Gorlin et al., 2001, pp. 991–95). The face is characterized by a prominent forehead,
wide palpebral fissures, hypertelorism, and micrognathia, giving rise to the term
"fetal face syndrome." Most patients are new mutations reflecting autosomal-
dominant inheritance, but a recessive form has been confirmed by demonstrating
mutations in a signal transduction gene called ROR2 (Jones, 1997, pp. 130–1;
Gorlin et al., 2001, pp. 991–5).

Summary of clinical concerns: Robinow syndrome management considerations

General: Patients with the autosomal-recessive form have risk for sudden death
under age 3 years from cardiopulmonary causes.

Growth and development: Most children have a normal birth weight with mild
delay in postnatal growth and adult short stature, but GH deficiency has been
described; normal intellect in 80%: Early childhood intervention for those with

significant delays, monitoring of growth with endocrinology referral if severely delayed.

Cancer: Thyroid carcinoma, hepatocarcinoma.

Craniofacial: Distinctive facial appearance with midface hypoplasia and small jaw that can lead to anesthesia problems (Sleesman & Tobias, 2003); cleft lip or palate in 10%, dental anomalies in 96%: Anesthesia precautions with emphasis on potential airway problems; cleft palate team if warranted, early and regular dental evaluations.

Cardiac: Cardiac anomalies in 15%: Cardiology and echocardiogram if symptomatic.

Urogenital: Genital anomalies in males (micropenis, 94%; cryptorchidism, 65%) may be severe enough to present as ambiguous genitalia; urinary tract anomalies (29%) such as ureteral duplication, hydronephrosis: Newborn examination with abdominal ultrasound to evaluate urinary tract anomalies; regular genital examinations, blood pressures and urinalyses through puberty and adolescence with referrals to urology and endocrinology as needed.

Skeletal: Characteristic forearm shortening (mesomelia) with short fingers; vertebral and rib anomalies (66%), scoliosis (50%): Skeletal survey at diagnosis, orthopedics evaluation and follow-up for scoliosis.

Parental counseling: Low recurrence risk in most cases, but a 25% recurrence risk should be mentioned because of the recessive form. Parent support and information is available at the Robinow Syndrome Foundation (www.robinow.org/).

Rubinstein–Taybi syndrome

Rubinstein–Taybi syndrome is a sporadic disorder with an incidence of about 1 in 125,000 live births (Jones, 1997, pp. 96–7; Gorlin et al., 2001, pp. 382–7). The syndrome is characterized by mental disability, unusual facies with a prominent nose, and broad thumbs and great toes. Hennekam et al. (1993) described a submicroscopic deletion at chromosome band 16p13.3 that includes a gene encoding a transcriptional regulatory protein. Mutations in the regulatory gene account for 90% of patients, so deletion testing is not very sensitive as a diagnostic test.

Summary of clinical concerns: Rubinstein–Taybi syndrome management considerations

Growth and development: Turbulent infantile course with feeding problems, constipation, and poor weight gain (70–80%); moderate to severe mental disability with average IQ of 51 and severe speech delays; affectionate personality with behavior differences in some: Early intervention with speech therapy, neonatal assessment of feeding with follow-up studies, careful monitoring of school progress with behavioral evaluations as indicated, developmental pediatrics, genetics, and/or neurology according to availability.

Cancer: Predisposition to tumors of the central nervous system including meningioma, leukemia, pheochromocytoma.

Craniofacial: Distinctive facial appearance with prominent nose, down-slanting palpebral fissures, coarsened appearance during infancy: Obstructive sleep apnea due to adenoidal enlargement: Monitor for disordered, restless sleep with unusual positioning, otolaryngology and sleep studies if symptomatic.

Eye: Strabismus, cataracts, colobomata, refractive errors, glaucoma: Ophthalmology at age 6 months with annual follow-up.

Surface: Keloid formation, pigmentary changes.

Cardiopulmonary: Upper respiratory infections with chronic otitis, cardiac defects in 35% (septal defects, coarctation, and pulmonic stenosis), delayed recovery from anesthesia or difficult intubation from pliable trachea: Cardiology and echocardiogram at diagnosis with annual follow-up, aggressive evaluation of respiratory infections, precautions pre- and post-anesthesia.

RES: Immune deficiencies with frequent respiratory infections, particularly otitis and sinusitis.

Urogenital: Adults may have urinary tract infections Renal artery se: Abdominal ultrasound at diagnosis, monitoring of blood pressure and urinalysis, nephrology and urology follow-up according to symptoms.

Skeletal: Broad thumbs and toes are characteristic, but may not be evident until middle childhood; joint laxity, scoliosis, instability of the patellofemoral joints, aseptic necrosis of the hip in adolescence: Hand films when diagnosis is suspected, orthopedics evaluation and follow-up for scoliosis, joint injuries.

Neurologic: Abnormalities on electroencephalogram (EEG), seizures, brain anomalies such as agenesis of corpus callosum, Dandy–Walker malformation: Head MRI and neurology evaluation for children with severe disabilities or seizures.

Parental counseling: Most parents will have low recurrence risks, but occasional dominant transmission has been reported. Fluorescent *in situ* hybridization (FISH) studies are available in several laboratories, but are positive in only 10–15% of valid cases. Parent support and information is available at the Rubinstein–Taybi syndrome (RTS) site (www.rubinstein-taybi.org/) with links to sister organizations in many countries.

Russell–Silver syndrome

Russell–Silver syndrome was described initially by Silver in 1953 and Russell in 1954. Diagnosis is based on the characteristic early growth delay with head-sparing (pseudohydrocephaly), triangular facies, and body asymmetries (Jones, 1997, pp. 96–9; Gorlin et al., 2001, pp. 391–4). The dysmorphologic findings of prominent forehead, triangular face, fifth finger clinodactyly, and café-au-lait spots are non-specific and perhaps best described as a Russell–Silver phenotype rather than a particular syndrome. Reflecting this heterogeneity is the 7–15% of patients that have imprinting changes in genes like growth factor receptor-bound protein 10 on the long arm of chromosome 7 or somatomammotropin hormone 1 on the long arm of chromosome 17.

Summary of clinical concerns: Russell–Silver syndrome management considerations

General: Low birth weight with small placenta; the natural history is very optimistic in most patients, with catch-up growth and normal lifespan.

Growth and development: Early motor delays due to muscle hypoplasia in 35% with most having normal intellect: Early childhood intervention for motor delays is beneficial even though the majority have normal cognitive function.

Cancer: Testicular tumors, craniopharyngioma, and Wilms tumor have been described: Those with hemihypertrophy should have abdominal ultrasound studies performed every 6–12 months.

Craniofacial: Frontal bossing with the appearance of a large head (pseudohydrocephaly) and bluish sclerae; tooth crowding: Early dental assessments and regular care.

Endocrine: Neonatal hypoglycemia may occur from being small-for-gestational age or pituitary anomalies including later GH deficiencies; precocious puberty or premature estrogenization of the vaginal mucosa have been reported: Subcutaneous administration of GH has produced increased height and muscle mass, so endocrinology referral should be initiated by age 2 years for monitoring of growth and puberty.

Urogenital: Cryptorchidism and hypospadias (35%), hydronephrosis, horseshoe kidney, renal tubular acidosis: Serial genital examinations, abdominal ultrasound at diagnosis, monitoring of blood pressure and urinalysis, nephrology and urology follow-up according to symptoms. Close monitoring of puberty and genital development is needed in adolescence.

Skeletal: Congenital asymmetry with limb-length discrepancy (60%), metacarpal bone and phalangeal abnormalities (30%), scoliosis (15%), developmental dysplasia of the hips (5%), and a higher risk of slipped capital femoral epiphysis has been noted (Abraham et al., 2004): Neonatal skeletal examination with monitoring for asymmetry and hip dysplasia, orthopedic referrals for symptoms.

Parental counseling: Parents will have a low recurrence risk, although they should be inspected and questioned about a history of low birth weight, early growth delay since dominant forms have been described. Parent support and information can be found at the Magic Foundation that deals with growth disorders (www.magicfoundation.org) and by searching on the syndrome name.

Seckel syndrome

The report of Seckel syndrome in 1960 emphasized the prominent nose and mid-face that were produced by striking growth retardation and microcephaly (Jones, 1997, pp. 108–9; Gorlin et al., 2001, pp. 387–91; Faivre et al., 2002). Seckel syndrome is now known to be a heterogenous group of conditions categorized as osteodysplastic primordial dwarfisms. The primary cause is under-development of the brain, with secondary microcephaly, mental deficiency, facial changes, and growth deficiencies that reflect the severity of brain maldevelopment. Associated manifestations of the eyes, bone marrow, skeleton, and urogenital system probably are components of specific disorders that fall within the Seckel grouping. These associated manifestations provide a guide to management of the Seckel group provided there is ongoing consideration of related diagnoses (e.g., Dubowitz, Bloom, Cockayne, other syndromes involving altered DNA repair). It is likely that severe congenital brain anomalies that produce microcephaly and its consequent facial/growth changes are grouped under the label of Seckel phenotype.

Summary of clinical concerns: Seckel syndrome management considerations

Growth and development: Low birth weight with average of 1500 g, extreme postnatal growth delay and microcephaly that is proportionate to height in half and even smaller in the other half; moderate to severe mental disability in almost all children defined as Seckel syndrome: Early childhood intervention with monitoring of head circumference for signs of craniosynostosis; developmental pediatrics, genetics, and/or neurology according to severity of delays and availability.

Craniofacial: About 50% will develop craniosynostosis; secondary to microcephaly; dental enamel hypoplasia or malocclusion: Craniofacial clinic referral and operative correction of synostosis should be considered in high-functioning children; early and regular dental evaluations.

Eye: Optic atrophy and retinal degenerations have been described: Regular vision assessments, ophthalmology referral for deficits.

Urogenital: Cryptorchidism, hypospadias, clitoromegaly have been reported: Regular genital examinations, urology referral as needed.

Skeletal: Congenital hip dislocation, changes in limbs and clavicles, other changes in skeletal dysplasias that present with the Seckel phenotype: Neonatal skeletal examination, skeletal survey if altered proportions or suggestions of skeletal dysplasia with the microcephaly; orthopedics referral as necessary.

Neurologic: Brain anomalies are often described and may be the primary cause (pachygyria, heterotopias, agenesis corpus callosum, cerebellar hypoplasia, intracranial aneurysms): Head MRI at the time of diagnosis, neurology evaluation and follow-up.

Parental counseling: Like the Bloom and Dubowitz syndromes, the Seckel group usually exhibits autosomal-recessive inheritance. Parents will have a 25% recurrence risk. All patients should have chromosome studies because of the syndrome variability. Parent-oriented information is available at several medical sites by searching on the syndrome name.

Noonan syndrome

Terminology

Noonan syndrome, first described by the cardiologist Jacqueline Noonan, is a recognizable pattern of short stature, ptosis, hypertelorism, webbed neck, pectus, and hypogonadism (Jones, 1997, pp. 122–3; Gorlin et al., 2001, pp. 1000–5; Jongmans et al., 2005). Resemblance to the phenotype of Turner syndrome and equal affliction of males and females prompted use of the term "male Turner syndrome. The karyotype is normal in Noonan syndrome, and about half the cases are associated with mutations in a protein-tyrosine phosphatase 11 (PTPN11) signal transduction gene (Jongmans et al., 2005). However, the head and neck changes in Noonan syndrome are not specific, deriving from altered lymphatic drainage and cystic hygroma *in utero*. These manifestations may occur together with neurofibromatosis in Watson syndrome, with myopathy and malignant hyperthermia in King syndrome, and together with ichthyosis in cardiofaciocutaneous syndrome (Gorlin et al., 2001, pp. 1000–5). The implied genetic heterogeneity may be emphasized by using the term "Noonan phenotype."

Historical diagnosis and management

The disorder has been recognized since 1883, and more than 300 cases have been reported. The facial appearance of Noonan syndrome changes significantly over time, providing a challenge for early diagnosis.

Incidence, etiology, and differential diagnosis

Noonan syndrome is quite common, having an incidence of 1 in 1000–2500 (Jones,1997; pp. 122–3; Gorlin et al., 2001, pp. 1000–5). The etiology is unknown, although pathogenesis includes an abnormality of fetal lymphatic circulation that produces a cystic hygroma reminiscent of Turner syndrome. The fetal hygroma may cause the postnatal webbed neck, anteverted ear lobes, and chest deformities. Direct transmission from parent to child has been observed in 30% of cases and is consistent with autosomal-dominant inheritance. Genetic linkage studies have been successful in some families and have highlighted one locus on the long arm of chromosome 12.

Differential diagnosis includes the syndromes mentioned above which have Noonan syndrome features plus other findings like café-au-lait spots, myopathy, or ichthyosis. Some cases of Watson syndrome (Noonan-neurofibromatosis features) have alterations of the neurofibromatosis type 1 gene on chromosome 17. The Aarskog syndrome (with short stature and hypertelorism), Costello syndrome with mucosal papillomas (see above), the Williams syndrome (with short stature and coarse facies), and the LEOPARD syndrome with (*L*entigines, *E*lectrocardiographic conduction abnormalities, *O*cular hypertelorism, *P*ulmonary stenosis, *A*bnormalies of the Genitalia, *R*etardation growth, and *D*eafness) may cause confusion. Females with Noonan syndrome may be misdiagnosed as having Turner syndrome until the different heart lesion and the karyotype are appreciated.

Diagnostic evaluation and medical counseling

Although it is expected to be normal, a karyotype should be performed in all but the most typical cases of Noonan syndrome. The heterogeneous Noonan phenotype can be mimicked by several chromosomal disorders including Turner syndrome. A normal lifespan with frequently normal intelligence warrants optimistic medical counseling for the parents of a child with Noonan syndrome. An echocardiogram is needed in early infancy to evaluate the degree of pulmonary valve dysplasia and cardiomyopathy in the 65–85% of patients with congenital heart anomalies. The degree of pulmonary valve dysplasia has significant impact on prognosis, since dilation of severely dysplastic valves is difficult. Although the cardiomyopathy of Noonan syndrome is not associated with sudden death, it can be chronic and lethal.

Family and psychosocial counseling

A thorough history and partial physical examination should be conducted on parents of children with Noonan syndrome to rule out the possibility of parental transmission; parental baby/childhood photographs may be very helpful in this determination. A parent with typical manifestations of Noonan syndrome may exhibit autosomal-dominant transmission with a 50% risk for their child to receive the predisposing gene with each pregnancy. However, only 15–30% of children receiving the gene will exhibit the full phenotype including the mild mental disability. Mothers are three times more likely to transmit the gene, perhaps because many affected fathers have genital anomalies. Recurrence risks to have a child with the full Noonan phenotype can thus be estimated at 1–2% for normal parents with one affected child, 15% when a mother has substantial manifestations (moving towards 25% if she already has an affected child), 15% when a father has substantial manifestations but with decreased chance of conception, and about 5% when a parent has subtle manifestations like shorter stature than family background. Accurate diagnosis to eliminate other disorders like Watson syndrome is crucial for accurate genetic counseling, and evaluation by an experienced clinical geneticist is crucial. Commercial DNA testing is not yet available for pre- or postnatal diagnosis.

Parent representatives are useful in supporting families, both in affirming the significant potential of children with Noonan syndrome and in helping with advocacy for early intervention and school placement. Parent support and information can be found at the Noonan Syndrome Support Group (www.noonansyndrome.org/) and the disorder is included on many medical websites.

Natural history and complications

The major complications of Noonan syndrome involve the heart, eyes, ears, teeth, trunk, coagulation system, and musculoskeletal system, as listed on Part 1 of the checklist. Problems with feeding can be severe, with 24% of patients requiring tube feedings. Although some patients experience motor and speech delays, the outlook for overall intelligence and learning is excellent, with 80–90% having normal intelligence and only 11% requiring special education. Ocular problems such as ptosis, strabismus, and amblyopia, together with chronic otitis media or anomalies of the ear ossicles, may produce vision and hearing impairment. Dental malocclusion is common and cherubism (cystic enlargement of the jaws) is occasionally seen in Noonan syndrome (Gorlin et al., 2001, pp. 1000–5). Affected males may have delayed puberty, delay of sexual function, and usually are fertile unless they have uncorrected cryptorchidism with resulting azoospermia.

The cardiac anomalies in Noonan syndrome often involve the pulmonary valve, as opposed to aortic defects in the Turner or Williams syndromes. Pulmonary hypertension can occur, emphasizing the importance of early cardiac assessment. A bleeding diathesis is present in as many as 56% of patients, and this has been attributed to partial factor XI deficiency. Lymphedema may occur, and spontaneous chylothorax has been treated with prednisone. Autoimmune thyroiditis is common, and there is early hepatosplenomegaly of unknown cause. If these abnormalities reflect a generalized immune dysfunction, then neoplastic defenses seem normal except for rare patients with acute lymphoblastic leukemia or neurogenic tumors. Renal and urinary tract anomalies (10%) can include hydronephrosis, ureteral stenoses, and small/dysplastic kidneys.

Neurologic complications have been reported in single patients with Noonan syndrome, including moya moya disease, cerebral infarction, and progressive hydrocephalus. These may be related to the bleeding diathesis, and complications have been reported after surgeries.

Noonan syndrome preventive medical checklist

Preventive care for patients with Noonan syndrome should begin with an echocardiogram to define the cardiac anatomy, and evaluation of feeding to promote growth during infancy. Chronic otitis, hearing, and visual problems are frequent, so referrals to audiology, ophthalmology, and possibly otolaryngology are recommended. Growth charts are available (Witt et al., 1986) and GH therapy has been effective. Despite the normal intellectual outlook for many children, early intervention with occupational, physical, and speech therapy is recommended because of frequent motor and language delays. Monitoring of thyroid function is recommended because of autoimmune thyroiditis, and occasional children require cervical spine films if they have unusually short or immobile necks. A creatine phosphokinase (CPK) level as a screen for the possibility of malignant hyperthermia, and a bleeding time are recommended before surgery.

Later childhood and adolescent care should be concerned with optimizing school placement and performance; screening for thyroid, vision, or hearing problems; and close monitoring of nutrition and dentistry. Males need evaluations for cryptorchidism, micropenis, and pubertal development to optimize the chances for later fertility. For this reason, and to monitor growth with possible GH therapy, referral to endocrinology should be considered at age 4–6 years.

Brachmann–de Lange syndrome

Terminology

Brachmann–de Lange syndrome combines the name of Cornelia de Lange, an academic pediatrician who described the syndrome in 1933, and W. Brachmann, a young physician-in-training who had reported a case in 1916 (Jones, 1997, 88–91; Gorlin et al., 2001, 372–7). Although Cornelia de Lange named the condition "Typus degenerativus Amstelodamensis," the term "Cornelia de Lange syndrome" or "Brachmann–de Lange syndrome" is now preferred.

Historical diagnosis and management

Awareness of Brachmann–de Lange syndrome was renewed by reports in the 1960s. Severe feeding problems and a propensity for infection undoubtedly led to significant mortality in earlier times.

Incidence, etiology, and differential diagnosis

Although most authors feel that the incidence of Brachmann–de Lange syndrome is underestimated because of early mortality and occasional mildly affected individuals, a birth prevalence of at least 1 in 10,000 is accepted. The majority of cases are sporadic, but four cases of monozygotic twins and several families with vertical transmission favor autosomal-dominant inheritance with a high frequency of new mutations. Although duplication or rearrangement of the distal long arm of chromosome 3 produced a phenotype similar to that of Brachmann–de Lange syndrome, mutations in the nipped-B gene on the chromosome 5 short arm (a gene influencing chromatin condensation) have been detected in several patients (Tonkin et al., 2004). A milder, vertically transmitted form of Brachmann–de Lange syndrome has been linked to the long arm of chromosome 3.

The differential diagnosis of Brachmann–de Lange syndrome includes the fetal alcohol, duplication 3q, and ring 9 syndromes. Growth retardation, problems with feeding, and facial characteristics such as synophrys (fusion of the eyebrows), eye anomalies, thin upper lip, and a long philtrum are seen in the fetal alcohol, dup(3q), and Brachmann–de Lange syndromes. Until commercial DNA testing is available for probable subtypes, the diagnosis of Brachmann–de Lange syndrome is clinical, based on the distinctive facial appearance and pattern of anomalies.

Diagnostic evaluation and medical counseling

The facial appearance is usually sufficient for a diagnosis of Brachmann–de Lange syndrome. Tracheomegaly visualized by radiography may be a diagnostic sign. Chromosomal disorders should be excluded in typical cases, and a thorough gestational history to exclude alcohol exposure is important. Evaluation of feeding and GI function should be performed in early infancy, since 77% of children have problems. In the presence of significant gastroesophageal reflux or vomiting, particularly when accompanied by respiratory distress, chest X-ray and imaging of the GI tract should be performed to rule out pyloric stenosis, intestinal malrotation, or diaphragmatic hernia. Congenital heart disease should also be considered, since it occurs in 13–29% of patients. Cleft lip and palate may also complicate early management. Medical counseling should be concerned with growth, feeding, cardiac, and GI problems, with planning for medical and financial services appropriate for children with significant developmental disability.

Family and psychosocial counseling

Because the disorder is heterogenous, a recurrence risk of 2–5% can be cited (Gorlin et al., 2001, 372–7). There seems to be a mild form that is autosomal dominant with a 50% recurrence risk. Parents will need supportive counseling regarding the risks of mental disability and growth failure, although recent developmental assessment is more positive than that reported previously (Kline et al., 1993b). Parent support groups include the CdlS USA Foundation (www.cdlsusa.org/) and the disorder is listed in many medical website accessed by searching on the syndrome name.

Natural history and complications

Problems with feeding, growth, speech, and mental development dominate the natural history of patients with Brachmann–de Lange syndrome. About 4.5% of children have early deaths due to apnea, aspiration, cardiac anomalies, intracranial bleeding with a risk for brain anomalies, and postoperative events. The intracranial bleeding occurred in a child with thrombocytopenia, a rare complication of Brachmann–de Lange syndrome. There is little information on adolescents or adults, but reports document a milder form of Brachmann–de Lange syndrome with reasonable self-help and communication skills. Eight individuals have been reported with normal intelligence (IQ >70). Nevertheless, most individuals with the syndrome require supervisory care throughout life.

An under-appreciated complication of Brachmann–de Lange syndrome is poor feeding during infancy, often because of gastroesophageal reflux. Cleft or high-arched palate and narrow external auditory canals place children with Brachmann–de Lange syndrome at greater risk of chronic otitis; conductive and/or sensorineural hearing loss is common. Ophthalmologic problems include high myopia, nystagmus, and ptosis that may cause chin lifting to achieve vision. Communication may be impaired by visual or hearing problems, and only 4% of children had low-normal to normal speech by age 4 years. Limb anomalies include small hands and feet, proximally placed thumbs, fifth finger clinodactyly, syndactyly of toes 2/3, and, in about 20%, oligodactyly or phocomelia. Flexion contractures of the elbow are common and the acetabular angle is low with coxa valga. Internal anomalies of the heart, urinary tract and GI tract are common, and genital anomalies include hypospadias, cryptorchidism, bicornuate uterus, and narrow ovaries. A higher risk for malignancies may be present, including adenocarcinoma of the esophagus.

Brachmann–de Lange syndrome preventive medical checklist

Attention to feeding and screening for cardiac and urinary tract anomalies are important for infants with Brachmann–de Lange syndrome. The high frequency of gastroesophageal reflux, and the known deaths from apnea or aspiration mandate observation and counseling regarding early feeding so appropriate medical or surgical treatment is provided. High risks of chronic otitis and hearing loss require careful monitoring of hearing, so patients develop sufficient communication skills to enable placement of the child in a group home rather than a custodial care facility. Other preventive measures in early childhood include urinalysis to rule out urinary tract infection, dental care for the detection and correction of tooth anomalies, and physical/occupational therapy to minimize the effects of contractures and hip malpositioning. In the older child, school performance requires evaluation because of the risks of behavioral (57%) or cognitive (75–100%) dysfunction. Monitoring of puberty is particularly important in males, in whom hypogonadism may cause ostracism, and depilatory treatments may be useful for hypertrichosis. GH deficiency has been reported, and very short individuals should have endocrine evaluation with consideration of GH therapy. Acute monocytic leukemia and Wilms tumor have been reported in single patients, but it is not clear whether these malignancies were coincidental or part of the syndrome. The older individual with Brachmann–de Lange syndrome should certainly have regular hearing and vision assessments, since myopia and hearing loss are common.

Preventive management of Noonan syndrome

Description: Clinical pattern caused by mutations in a PTPN11 signal transduction gene in 50% of cases; incidence is 1 in 1000–2500 affecting both males and females.

Clinical diagnosis: Pattern of manifestations including short stature, ptosis, anteverted ear lobes, connective tissue changes (pectus, hernias, joint laxity), cardiac anomalies (pulmonic stenosis, septal defects), hypogonadism, and learning differences. A similar clinical pattern occurs in conditions such as Watson, LEOPARD, Costello, and Turner syndromes, but chromosome studies are normal.

Laboratory diagnosis: DNA testing is not yet commercially available.

Genetics: Autosomal dominant inheritance with many spontaneous mutations. Parents with the full syndrome have a 15% recurrence risk with each pregnancy to transmit the gene and have it fully expressed, but transmission is less common from affected males. Parents with a few or minor manifestations of the syndrome have a 5% recurrence risk for a fully affected child.

Key management issues: Monitoring for early feeding, growth, vision, hearing, dental cardiac, coagulation, and orthopedic problems. Cognitive disability is usually mild but requires early intervention and school planning.

Growth Charts: Witt et al. (1986).

Parent groups: Noonan Syndrome Support Group (www.noonansyndrome.org).

Basis for management recommendations: Derived from the complications below as documented by Jongmans et al. (2005), Witt et al. (1986).

Summary of clinical concerns

General	Learning	**Cognitive disability** (11–20%) **median IQ 102** (range 64–127), **speech problems** (20%), **verbal/IQ discrepancy** (15%), **learning differences**
	Behavior	Stubborn behavior, increased risk for mood disorders, rare autistic manifestations
	Growth	**Failure to thrive** in early childhood (50%), **short stature** (50%)
	Tumors	Pheochromocytoma, ganglioneuroma, rare acute or chronic leukemias
Facial	Eyes	**Ptosis** (42%), **strabismus** (50%), **refractive errors** (60%) **amblyopia** (31%)
	Ears	Posteriorly rotated ears, anteverted lobules, otitis media with conductive hearing loss
	Mouth	**Feeding problems** (76%), **dental anomalies** (35%)
Surface	Neck/trunk	**Webbing of neck** (23–90%), **pectus** carinatum superiorly, pectus excavatum inferiorly (70%)
	Epidermal	Pigmented nevi, café-au-lait spots (25%), decreased hair growth, curly or sparse hair
Skeletal	Axial	Cervical spine fusion (2%), **vertebral anomalies** (25%), scoliosis (13%)
	Limbs	**Cubitus valgus** (50%), **increased joint laxity** (30%), vertebral and sternal anomalies, club feet (12%), joint contractures
Internal	Digestive	**Dysphagia** (24%), **hepatosplenomegaly** (26%)
	Circulatory	**Cardiac anomalies** (60–70% – pulmonary valve stenosis, atrial septal defect, ventricular septal defects, hypertrophic cardiomyopathy), lymphatic abnormalities (generalized lymphedema, chylothorax, cystic hygroma)
	Pulmonary	Pulmonary lymphangiectasia
	Endocrine	**Antithyroid antibodies** (30%), **hypo- or hyperthyroidism**
	RES	**Abnormal bleeding** (20–56%), severe hemorrhage (3%), metrorrhagia
	Excretory	Renal and urinary tract anomalies (10–20%) including ureteral stenosis, obstructive uropathies, small/dysplastic kidneys
	Genital	**Cryptorchidism** (60–77%), delayed sexual development in males with later azoospermia
Neural	Central	Cerebrovascular anomalies, hydrocephalus, seizures (9%)
	Motor	**Delayed motor skills** (26%)
	Sensory	**Abnormal vision** (55%), mild hearing loss (12–40%), usually conductive

RES, reticuloendothelial system; **concerns** of frequency >20% are **highlighted**

Key references

Jongmans, et al. (2005). Genotypic and phenotypic characterization of Noonan syndrome: New data and review of the literature. *American Journal of Medical Genetics* 134A:165–70.

Witt, et al. (1986). Growth curves for height in Noonan syndrome. *Clinical Genetics* 30:150–3.

Noonan syndrome

Preventive medical checklist (0–3 years)

Name _____ Birth date __/__/____ Number _____

Age	Evaluations: key concerns	Management considerations		Notes
New-born ↓ 1 month	Dysmorphology examination: anomalies Hearing, vision:[2] eye examination Feeding: reflux, poor intake Heart: murmur, cardiomyopathy Urogenital: renal, genital defects Bleeding tendency, lymphatic changes Parental adjustment	❑ Genetic evaluation[1] ❑ ABR, ophthalmology[3] ❑ Feeding specialist; video swallow[3] ❑ Echocardiogram, cardiology ❑ Abdominal sonogram, urology[3] ❑ Surgical precautions, surface examination ❑ Family support[4]	❑ ❑ ❑ ❑ ❑ ❑ ❑	
2 months ↓ 4 months	Growth and development[5] Hearing, vision:[2] strabismus, otitis Feeding: reflux, poor intake Heart: murmur, cardiomyopathy Urogenital: renal, genital defects Bleeding, lymph, muscle changes Parental adjustment Other:	❑ Noonan growth charts, ECI[6] ❑ ABR;[3] ENT;[3] ophthalmology[3] ❑ Feeding specialist; video swallow[3] ❑ Echocardiogram;[3] cardiology[3] ❑ Abdominal sonogram; urology[3] ❑ Clotting factors; CPK before surgery ❑ Family support[4] ❑	❑ ❑ ❑ ❑ ❑ ❑ ❑ ❑	
6 months ↓ 9 months	Growth and development[5] Hearing vision:[2] strabismus Nutrition: feeding; dysphagia Skeletal: neck mobility, pectus, joint laxity Urogenital: renal, genital defects Other:	❑ ECI[6] ❑ ENT;[3] ophthalmology[3] ❑ Dietician;[3] GI specialist[3] ❑ Cervical spine X-rays;[3] orthopedics[3] ❑ Urinalysis, BP; urology[3] ❑	❑ ❑ ❑ ❑ ❑ ❑	
1 year	Growth and development[5] Hearing, vision:[2] strabismus, otitis Nutrition: feeding; dysphagia Thyroid: hyper- or hypothyroidism Heart: murmur, cardiomyopathy Urogenital: renal, genital defects Other:	❑ ECI[6] ❑ ENT;[3] ophthalmology ❑ Dietician;[3] GI specialist[3] ❑ T4, TSH; endocrinology[3] ❑ Cardiology;[3] ❑ Urinalysis, BP; urology[3] ❑	❑ ❑ ❑ ❑ ❑ ❑ ❑	
15 months ↓ 18 months	Growth and development[5] Hearing, vision:[2] strabismus, otitis Nutrition: feeding, dysphagia Urogenital: renal, genital defects	❑ ECI[6] ❑ ENT;[3] ophthalmology[3] ❑ Dietician;[3] GI specialist[3] ❑ Urinalysis, BP; urology[3]	❑ ❑ ❑ ❑	
2 years	Growth and development[5] Hearing, vision, teeth:[2] strabismus, otitis Thyroid: hypothyroidism Bleeding, lymph, muscle changes Skeletal: neck mobility, pectus, joint laxity	❑ ECI[6] ❑ Audiology; ENT,[3] ophthalmology, dentistry ❑ T4, TSH;[3] endocrinology[3] ❑ Clotting factors; CPK before surgery ❑ Cervical spine X-rays;[3] orthopedics[3]	❑ ❑ ❑ ❑ ❑	
3 years	Growth and development[5] Hearing, vision, teeth:[2] strabismus, otitis Thyroid: hyper- or hypothyroidism Heart: murmur, cardiomyopathy Urogenital: renal, genital defects Cosmetic issues: web neck, pectus Other:	❑ Noonan growth charts; ECI[6]; family support[4] ❑ Audiology; ENT; ophthalmology, dentistry ❑ T4, TSH; endocrinology[3] ❑ Cardiology[3] ❑ Urinalysis, BP; urology[3] ❑ Plastic surgery[3]	❑ ❑ ❑ ❑ ❑ ❑	

Noonan syndrome concerns		Other concerns from history	
Failure to thrive, short stature Vision, hearing deficits Strabismus, chronic otitis Hypo- or hyperthyroidism High palate, dental anomalies Bleeding tendency	Cardiac anomalies (pulmonic) Renal, urinary tract anomalies Cryptorchidism Hydrocephalus, seizures Speech problems, hearing loss Mild mental disability	**Family history/prenatal** _____ _____ _____ _____ _____	**Social/environmental** _____ _____ _____ _____ _____

Guidelines for the neonatal period should be undertaken *at whatever age* the diagnosis is made; ABR, auditory brainstem evoked response; BP, blood pressure; GI, gastrointestinal; TSH, thyroid stimulating hormone; CPK, creatine phosphokinase level for possible malignant hyperthermia; [1]clinical genetic evaluation is crucial for correct diagnosis and counseling; [2]by practitioner; [3]as dictated by clinical findings; [4]parent group, family/sib, financial, and behavioral issues; [5]consider developmental pediatric or genetics clinic according to symptoms and availability; [6]early childhood intervention if motor or speech delays with particular alertness for articulation problems.

Noonan syndrome

Preventive medical checklist (4–18 years)

Name _____ Birth date __/__/___ Number _____

Age	Evaluations: key concerns	Management considerations		Notes
4 years ↓ **6 years**	Growth:[1] hormone needs[1] Development:[2] preschool transition Hearing, vision, teeth:[2] dental anomalies Heart: murmur, cardiomyopathy Thyroid, urogenital defects Skeletal: neck mobility, pectus, joint laxity Other:	❑ Noonan syndrome charts;[5] endocrinology[3] ❑ Family support;[4] preschool program[5] ❑ Audiology; ENT;[3] ophthalmology; dentistry ❑ Cardiology[3] ❑ T4, TSH; urinalysis, BP; urology[3] ❑ Cervical spine X-rays;[3] orthopedics[3] ❑	❑ ❑ ❑ ❑ ❑ ❑ ❑	
7 years ↓ **9 years**	Growth:[1] hormone needs Development:[1] school transition[5] Hearing, vision, teeth:[2] myopia Endocrine: hormone therapy Bleeding, lymph, muscle changes Cosmetic issues: web neck, pectus Other:	❑ Noonan syndrome charts;[1] endocrinology[3] ❑ Family support;[4] school progress[6] ❑ Audiology;[3] ophthalmology;[3] dentistry ❑ T4, TSH; endocrinology ❑ Clotting factors; CPK before surgery ❑ Plastic surgery[3] ❑	❑ ❑ ❑ ❑ ❑ ❑ ❑	
10 years ↓ **12 years**	Growth and development[5] Hearing, vision, teeth:[2] myopia Endocrine: hormone therapy, puberty Urogenital: renal, genital defects Other:	❑ School progress[6] ❑ Audiology;[3] ophthalmology;[3] dentistry ❑ T4, TSH; endocrinology ❑ Urinalysis, BP; urology[3] ❑	❑ ❑ ❑ ❑ ❑	
13 years ↓ **15 years**	Growth and development[1] Hearing and vision[2] Endocrine: hormone therapy, puberty Skeletal: neck mobility, pectus, joint laxity Urogenital: renal, genital defects Other:	❑ Noonan syndrome charts;[1] school progress[6] ❑ Audiology;[3] ophthalmology ❑ T4, TSH; endocrinology ❑ Cervical spine X-rays;[3] orthopedics[3] ❑ Urinalysis, BP; urology[3] ❑	❑ ❑ ❑ ❑ ❑ ❑	
16 years ↓ **18 years**	Growth and development[1] Endocrine: hormone therapy, puberty Heart: murmurs, cardiomyopathy Urogenital: renal, genital defects Other:	❑ Family support;[4] school progress;[6] ❑ T4, TSH; endocrinology; gynecology ❑ Echocardiogram,[3] cardiology[3] ❑ Urinalysis, BP; urology[3] ❑	❑ ❑ ❑ ❑ ❑	
19 years ↓ **23 years**	Adult transition: body image, stigmata Hearing and vision[2] Endocrine: reproductive counsel Skeletal: joint laxity, contractures Urogenital: renal defects, fertility	❑ Cosmetic surgery,[3] dermatology[3] ❑ Audiology;[3] ophthalmology ❑ T4, TSH; endocrinology; gynecology ❑ Exercise; activity; physical therapy ❑ Urinalysis, BP; urology[3]	❑ ❑ ❑ ❑ ❑	
Adult	Body image, stigmata, keloids, nevi Hearing/vision:[2] myopia, hearing loss Endocrine: reproductive counsel Heart: murmurs, cardiomyopathy Bleeding, lymph, muscle changes Urogenital: renal defects, fertility Other:	❑ Dentistry; cosmetic surgery;[3] dermatology[3] ❑ Audiology;[3] ENT;[3] ophthalmology[3] ❑ T4, TSH; endocrinology; gynecology ❑ Echocardiogram;[3] cardiology[3] ❑ Clotting factors; CPK before surgery ❑ Urinalysis, BP, urology[3] ❑	❑ ❑ ❑ ❑ ❑ ❑ ❑	

Noonan syndrome concerns		Other concerns from history	
Short stature Refraction errors Chronic otitis, hearing loss Hypo- or hyperthyroidism High palate, dental anomalies Bleeding tendency	Cardiac anomalies (pulmonic) Cardiomyopathy Renal, urinary tract anomalies Cryptorchidism Seizures, stubborn behaviors Learning deficits	**Family history/prenatal** _____ _____ _____ _____ _____	**Social/environmental** _____ _____ _____ _____ _____

Guidelines for the neonatal period should be undertaken *at whatever age* the diagnosis is made; BP, blood pressure; GI, gastrointestinal; TSH, thyroid stimulating hormone; CPK, creatine phosphokinase level for possible malignant hyperthermia; [1]consider developmental pediatric or genetics clinic according to symptoms and availability; [2]by practitioner; [3]as dictated by clinical findings; [4]parent group, family/sib, financial, and behavioral issues with later focus on independent living and employment; [5]preschool program including developmental monitoring and motor/speech therapy if needed; [6]monitor individual education plan, educational testing, maturity according to puberty and hormone therapy, academic progress, behavioral differences, later reproductive counseling regarding fertility testing, artificial reproductive technology.

Parent guide to Noonan syndrome

Noonan syndrome was described in 1963 by Jacqueline Noonan, a pediatric cardiologist. The short stature, widely spaced eyes, forwardly placed ear lobes, webbed neck, chest concavity, and genital underdevelopment prompted use of the term "male Turner syndrome" because of resemblance to women with Turner syndrome. However, both sexes are affected in Noonan syndrome and the karyotype is normal. The "Noonan phenotype" of facial and surface manifestations occurs in several disorders (Watson, King, cardiofaciocutaneous syndromes).

Incidence, causation, and diagnosis

Noonan syndrome is quite common with an incidence of 1 in 1000–2500 live births. The cause in 50% of patients is a mutation in the gene for protein-tyrosine phosphatase 11 (PTPN11). Abnormal lymphatic circulation with a cystic hygroma (swollen neck) causes certain facial features and the web neck. Since there is no laboratory test for Noonan syndrome, the diagnosis is made by recognizing the typical pattern of clinical features. Because so many conditions can resemble Noonan syndrome, clinical genetic evaluation is needed before accepting the diagnosis. Chromosome studies will usually be indicated to rule out other conditions, particularly Turner syndrome with its different heart lesion (coarctation of the aorta rather than pulmonic stenosis) and abnormal karyotype (45,X).

Natural history and complications

Major complications of Noonan syndrome involve the heart, eyes, ears, teeth, trunk, coagulation system, and musculoskeletal system. Feeding problems can be severe, followed by speech articulation difficulties. The outlook for overall intelligence and learning is excellent, with 80–90% having normal intelligence and only 11% requiring special education. Ocular problems such as strabismus, chronic otitis media with hearing loss, and dental anomalies are common. Males may have delayed puberty and sexual function, but usually have normal fertility if their cryptorchidism (undescended testes) is corrected. The cardiac anomalies in Noonan syndrome often involve the pulmonary valve as opposed to aortic defects in the Turner or Williams syndromes. Pulmonary hypertension (high blood pressure) can occur, emphasizing the importance of early cardiac assessment. A bleeding diathesis is present in as many as 56% of patients, and evaluations of clotting factors before surgery is recommended. Swelling of the lower limbs with lymph may occur, and one case of spontaneous leakage of lymph into the chest was treated with prednisone. Autoimmune inflammation of the thryoid gland is common, and there is early enlargement of the liver and spleen without known cause. Rare children have had leukemias or tumors of the nervous system. In a series of 44 patients having abdominal ultrasounds, 11% had kidney anomalies, 53% had enlargement of the spleen, and none had tumors. Neurologic complications have been reported in single patients with Noonan syndrome, including moya moya disease (narrowing of a brain artery), cerebral infarction (death of brain substance due to arterial blockage), and progressive hydrocephalus (accumulation of fluid in a brain cavity).

Preventive medical needs

A normal life span with frequently normal intelligence warrants optimistic medical counseling for the parents of a child with Noonan syndrome. An echocardiogram is needed in early infancy to evaluate the degree of pulmonary valve abnormality and cardiomyopathy (heart muscle weakness) in the 70–90% of patients with congenital heart anomalies. The degree of pulmonary valve abnormality has significant impact on prognosis, since the surgical correction of severely abnormal valves is difficult. The cardiomyopathy of Noonan syndrome is not associated with sudden death but can be lethal. Preventive care for patients with Noonan syndrome should begin with an echocardiogram to define the cardiac anatomy, and evaluation of feeding to promote growth during infancy. Chronic otitis, hearing, and visual problems are frequent, so referrals to audiology, ophthalmology, and possibly otolaryngology are recommended. Despite the normal intellectual outlook for many children, early intervention with occupational, physical, and speech therapy is helpful because of frequent motor and language delays. Monitoring of thyroid function should be performed because of autoimmune thyroiditis, and occasional children require cervical (neck) spine films if they have unusually short or immobile necks. A creatine phosphokinase (CPK) level as a screen for the possibility of muscle abnormality with the potential for severe temperature elevation is recommended before surgery. A bleeding time should also be documented prior to surgery, and appropriate blood replacements made available. Later childhood and adolescent care should be concerned with optimizing school placement and performance. Screening for thyroid, vision, or hearing problems with close monitoring of nutrition and dentistry is also useful. Males need evaluations for cryptorchidism (undescended testicles), for small penis, and for abnormalities in sexual development to optimize the chances for later fertility. For this reason and for concerns about stature or growth hormone therapy, referral to endocrinology should be considered at age 4–6 years.

Family counseling

A thorough history and partial physical examination should be conducted on parents of children with Noonan syndrome to rule out the possibility of parental transmission. Obviously affected parents have a 15% risk with each pregnancy for their child to have full Noonan syndrome; parents with mild features have a 5% risk. Family studies have demonstrated that maternal transmission is 2–3-fold more common than paternal transmission, probably reflecting the hypogonadism and decreased fertility of males with Noonan syndrome.

Preventive management of Brachmann–de Lange syndrome

Description: Clinical pattern caused by mutation of genes including a nipped-B gene on the chromosome 5 with an incidence of 1 in 10,000 births.

Clinical diagnosis: Pattern of manifestations including a characteristic facial appearance with joined eyebrows (synophrys), down-turned corners of the mouth; small hands and feet with potentially missing digits; internal anomalies of the heart, gastrointestinal and urinary systems, growth failure and moderate/severe developmental disability.

Laboratory diagnosis: None; commercial DNA testing for nipped-B mutations not yet available.

Genetics: Sporadic disorder with minimal recurrence risk for most parents; rare milder cases may exhibit autosomal dominant inheritance with a 50% recurrence risk for affected parents.

Key management issue: Monitoring for early feeding problems and gastroesophageal reflux, screening for cardiac and urinary tract anomalies, monitoring of hearing and vision, dental care, physical/occupational therapy to minimize the effects of contractures and hip malpositioning, depilatory treatments for hypertrichosis, early intervention and speech therapy.

Growth Charts: Kline et al. (1993a).

Parent groups: CdlS USA Foundation (www.cdlsusa.org/).

Basis for management recommendations: Derived from the complications below as documented by Kline et al. (1995a, b).

Summary of clinical concerns

General	Learning	**Cognitive disability** (87% with IQ <60), **learning differences** (100%), **speech delay** (75–100%)
	Behavior	Behavior problems (excessive screaming, stereotypic movements, tantrums, biting) dietary behavior problems,
	Growth	**Low birth weight** (72%), **failure to thrive, short stature** (86–96%), **poor feeding** (lack of interest in food, regurgitation, projectile vomiting)
	Tumors	Acute monocytic leukemia Wilms tumor
Facial	Eyes	**Eye anomalies** – 57% (myopia, 60%, ptosis, 45%, nystagmus, 37%)
	Ears	**Narrow ear canals** (30%), **chronic otitis** (60%)
	Nose	Choanal atresia
	Mouth	**Cleft lip/palate** (13–21%), **high palate** (59–86%), **anomalous teeth** (86%)
Surface	Neck/trunk	Nuchal webbing (11–33%), **low hairline** (92%)
	Epidermal	**Hypertrichosis** (78–97%)
Skeletal	Cranial	**Microbrachycephaly** (50–98%)
	Axial	**Limb anomalies** (56–99% – proximal thumbs 80%, reduction defects 20–27%, syndactyly of toes 2–3 86%), contractures (32–84%)
Internal	Digestive	**Gastroesophageal reflux** (27%), **gastrointestinal anomalies** (49–71% – pyloric stenosis, malrotation, diaphragmatic hernia)
	Pulmonary	**Respiratory infections** (25%)
	Circulatory	Cardiac anomalies (13–29% – ventricular septal defect, atrial septal defect, pulmonic stenosis)
	Endocrine	Growth hormone deficiency
	RES	Thrombocytopenia
	Excretory	Ureteral reflux (12%), urinary tract infections
	Genital	Hypospadias (11–33%), **cryptorchidism** (73%)
Neural	Central	Seizures (14–20%)
	Sensory	**Chronic otitis, hearing loss** (20–27%), vision deficits

RES, reticuloendothelial system; **concerns** of frequency >20% are **highlighted**

Key references

Kline, et al. (1993a). Growth manifestations in the Brachmann-de Lange syndrome. *American Journal of Medical Genetics* 47:1042–9.

Kline, et al. (1993b). Developmental data on individuals with the Brachmann-de Lange syndrome. *American Journal of Medical Genetics* 48:1053–8.

Brachmann–de Lange syndrome

Preventive medical checklist (0–3 years)

Name _____ Birth date __/__/____ Number _____

Age	Evaluations: key concerns	Management considerations	Notes
New-born ↓ 1 month	Dysmorphology examination: limb defects Hearing, vision:[2] nystagmus Feeding: reflux, poor intake Airway: choanal atresia, clefts Heart: murmur, cyanosis Urogenital: renal, genital defects Parental adjustment Other:	❑ Genetic evaluation, counseling[1] ❑ ❑ ABR; ophthalmology[3] ❑ ❑ Feeding specialist; video swallow[3] ❑ ❑ Airway patency; ENT[3] ❑ ❑ Echocardiogram; cardiology ❑ ❑ Renal sonogram; genital examination; urology[3] ❑ ❑ Family support[4] ❑ ❑ ❑	
2 months ↓ 4 months	Growth and development: head size[5] Hearing, vision:[2] nystagmus Nutrition: feeding, colic, GE reflux Brain anomalies: hypertonia, seizures Urogenital: renal, genital defects Heart: murmur, cyanosis Parental adjustment Other:	❑ ECI[6] ❑ ❑ Ophthalmology; ENT[3] ❑ ❑ Feeding specialist; GI referral[3] ❑ ❑ Head MRI scan;[3] neurology[3] ❑ ❑ Renal sonogram; genital examination; urology[3] ❑ ❑ Echocardiogram; cardiology ❑ ❑ Family support[4] ❑ ❑ ❑	
6 months ↓ 9 months	Growth and development: head size[5] Hearing, vision:[3] nystagmus Nutrition: feeding, colic, GE reflux Urogenital: renal, genital defects GI system: pyloric stenosis, malrotation Other:	❑ ECI[6] ❑ ❑ Ophthalmology; ENT[3] ❑ ❑ Feeding specialist; GI referral[3] ❑ ❑ Urinalysis, BP; urology[3] ❑ ❑ GI referral[3] ❑ ❑ ❑	
1 year	Growth and development: head size[5] Hearing and vision:[2] nystagmus, otitis Nutrition: feeding, colic, GE reflux Heart: murmur, cyanosis Urogenital: renal, genital defects GI system: pyloric stenosis, malrotation Other:	❑ ECI;[3,6] family support[3,4] ❑ ❑ Ophthalmology; ENT[3] ❑ ❑ Dietician;[3] GI referral[3] ❑ ❑ Cardiology[3] ❑ ❑ Urinalysis, BP; urology[3] ❑ ❑ GI referral[3] ❑ ❑ ❑	
15 months ↓ 18 months	Growth and development: head size[5] Hearing and vision:[2] nystagmus, otitis Nutrition: feeding, GE reflux Urogenital: renal, genital defects	❑ ECI[6] ❑ ❑ Ophthalmology;[3] ENT[3] ❑ ❑ Dietician;[3] GI referral[3] ❑ ❑ Urinalysis, BP; urology[3] ❑	
2 years	Growth and development: head size[5] Hearing and vision:[2] nystagmus, otitis Nutrition: feeding, GE reflux Brain anomalies: hypertonia, seizures GI system: pyloric stenosis, malrotation	❑ ECI;[3,6] family support[3,4] ❑ ❑ Audiology; ophthalmology,[3] ENT[3] ❑ ❑ Dietician;[3] GI referral[3] ❑ ❑ Head MRI scan;[3] neurology[3] ❑ ❑ GI referral[3] ❑	
3 years	Growth and development: head size[5] Hearing and vision:[3] nystagmus, otitis Nutrition: feeding, GE reflux Urogenital: renal, genital defects GI system: pyloric stenosis, malrotation Limb defects, contractures Other:	❑ ECI,[3,6] family support[3,4] ❑ ❑ Audiology; ophthalmology,[3] ENT[3] ❑ ❑ Dietician;[3] GI referral[3] ❑ ❑ Urinalysis, BP; urology[3] ❑ ❑ GI referral[3] ❑ ❑ Orthopedics[3] ❑ ❑ ❑	

de Lange syndrome concerns		Other concerns from history	
Feeding problems, GE reflux Eye anomalies;-nystagmus Otitis media, hearing loss Late tooth eruption Cardiac septal defects Malrotation, pyloric stenosis	Limb deficiencies Ureteral reflux, cryptorchidism Developmental disability Speech delay Self-mutilation, aggression Irritability, seizures	**Family history/prenatal** _____ _____ _____ _____	**Social/environmental** _____ _____ _____ _____

Guidelines for the neonatal period should be undertaken at whatever age the diagnosis is made; ABR, auditory brainstem evoked response; GE, gastrointestinal; GE, gastroenterology; [1]routine chromosome analysis to exclude other syndromes if diagnosis uncertain; [2]by practitioner; [3]as dictated by clinical findings; [4]parent group, family/sib, financial, and behavioral issues; [5]consider developmental pediatrician/neurologist/behavior therapist according to symptoms and availability; [6]early childhood intervention including developmental monitoring and motor/speech therapy.

Brachmann–de Lange syndrome

Preventive medical checklist (4–18 years)

Name _____ Birth date __/__/____ Number _____

Age	Evaluations: key concerns	Management considerations		Notes
4 years ↓ **6 years**	Growth, preschool transition[1,5] Hearing and vision:[2] myopia, glaucoma Nutrition: dysphagia, no food interest Urogenital: renal, genital defects GI system: pyloric stenosis, malrotation Heart: murmur, cyanosis Other:	❑ Family support;[4] preschool program[5] ❑ Ophthalmology; ENT[3] ❑ Dietician;[3] GI referral;[3] dentistry ❑ Urinalysis, BP; urology[3] ❑ GI referral[3] ❑ Cardiology[3] ❑	❑ ❑ ❑ ❑ ❑ ❑ ❑	
7 years ↓ **9 years**	Growth, school transition[1,5] Hearing, vision:[2] myopia, hearing loss Nutrition: dysphagia, no food interest Urogenital: renal, genital defects GI system: pyloric stenosis, malrotation Heart: murmur, cyanosis Other:	❑ Family support;[4] school progress[6] ❑ Audiology; ophthalmology;[3] ENT[3] ❑ Dietician;[3] GI referral;[3] dentistry ❑ Urinalysis, BP; urology[3] ❑ GI referral[3] ❑ Cardiology[3] ❑	❑ ❑ ❑ ❑ ❑ ❑ ❑	
10 years ↓ **12 years**	Growth and development[1,5] Hearing and vision:[2] myopia, glaucoma Nutrition: dysphagia, no food interest Heart: murmur, cyanosis Other:	❑ Family support;[4] school progress[6] ❑ Audiology; ophthalmology;[3] ENT[3] ❑ Dietician;[3] GI referral;[3] dentistry ❑ Cardiology[3] ❑	❑ ❑ ❑ ❑ ❑	
13 years ↓ **15 years**	Growth and development[1,5] Hearing, vision:[2] myopia, hearing loss Nutrition: dysphagia, no food interest Heart: murmur, cyanosi Puberty: genital anomalies Other:	❑ Family support;[4] school progress[6] ❑ Audiology; ophthalmology;[3] ENT[3] ❑ Dietician;[3] GI referral;[3] dentistry ❑ Cardiology[3] ❑ Genital examinations; urology;[3] gynecology[3] ❑	❑ ❑ ❑ ❑ ❑ ❑	
16 years ↓ **18 years**	Growth and development[1,5] Hearing and vision:[2] myopia, glaucoma Nutrition: dysphagia, no food interest Puberty: genital anomalies Other:	❑ Family support;[4] school progress[6] ❑ Audiology; ophthalmology;[3] ENT[3] ❑ Dietician;[3] GI referral;[3] dentistry ❑ Genital examinations; urology,[3] gynecology[3] ❑	❑ ❑ ❑ ❑ ❑	
19 years ↓ **23 years**	Adult care transition[1,6] Hearing, vision:[2] myopia, hearing loss Nutrition: dysphagia, no food interest Heart: murmur, cyanosis Behavior: aggression	❑ Family support[4] ❑ Audiology; ophthalmology;[3] ENT[3] ❑ Dietician;[3] GI referral;[3] dentistry ❑ Cardiology[3] ❑ Behavior therapist[3]	❑ ❑ ❑ ❑ ❑	
Adult	Adult care transition[6] Hearing and vision:[2] myopia, glaucoma Nutrition: dysphagia, no food interest Heart: murmur, cyanosis Behavior: aggression Brain anomalies: hypertonia, seizures Other:	❑ Family support[4] ❑ Audiology; ophthalmology;[3] ENT[3] ❑ Dietician;[3] GI referral;[3] dentistry ❑ Cardiology;[3] ❑ Behavior therapist[3] ❑ Head MRI scan;[3] neurology[3] ❑	❑ ❑ ❑ ❑ ❑ ❑ ❑	

de Lange syndrome concerns		Other concerns from history	
Short stature Myopia, glaucoma Otitis media, hearing loss Late tooth eruption Cardiac septal defects Malrotation, pyloric stenosis	Limb deficiencies Ureteral reflux, cryptorchidism Developmental disability Self-mutilation, aggression Irritability, seizures	**Family history/prenatal** _____ _____ _____ _____	**Social/environmental** _____ _____ _____ _____

Guidelines for the neonatal period should be undertaken at whatever age the diagnosis is made; BP, blood pressure; TSH, thyroid stimulating hormone; GI, gastrointestinal; [1]consider low calcium diet, developmental pediatrician/pediatric genetics/behavior therapist according to symptoms and availability; [2]by practitioner; [3]as dictated by clinical findings; [4]parent group, family/sib, financial, and behavioral issues with later focus on independent living and employment; [5]preschool program including developmental monitoring and motor/speech therapy; [6]monitor individual education plan, educational testing, balance of special education and inclusion, academic progress, behavioral differences, later vocational planning.

Parent guide to Brachmann–de Lange syndrome

Brachmann–de Lange syndrome combines the name of Cornelia de Lange, an academic pediatrician who described the syndrome in 1933, and W. Brachmann, a young physician-in-training who had reported a case in 1916. Awareness of Brachmann–de Lange syndrome was renewed by reports in the 1960s. Severe feeding problems and a propensity for infection undoubtedly led to significant mortality in earlier times.

Incidence, causation, and diagnosis

The incidence is 1 in 10,000. The majority of cases are sporadic, but there is a milder autosomal dominant form. Mutations in the nipped-B gene on the chromosome 5 account for many cases. Growth retardation, problems with feeding, and facial characteristics such as synophrys (fusion of the eyebrows), eye anomalies, thin upper lip, and a long philtrum (crease between the nose and upper lip) are seen in the fetal alcohol, dup(3q), and Brachmann–de Lange syndromes. The diagnosis of Brachmann–de Lange syndrome is clinical, based on the distinctive facial appearance and pattern of anomalies. Chromosomal disorders should be excluded if the diagnosis is not secure.

Natural history and complications

Problems with feeding, growth, speech, and mental development dominate the natural history of patients with Brachmann–de Lange syndrome. Early death occurs in 4.5% due to apnea (cessation of breathing), aspiration (swallowing food into the lungs), heart anomalies, intracranial bleeding, and postoperative events. There is little information on adolescents or adults, but reports document a milder form of Brachmann–de Lange syndrome with reasonable self-help and communication skills. Eight individuals have been reported with relatively normal intelligence (IQ >70). Nevertheless, most individuals with the syndrome require supervisory care throughout life. An under-appreciated complication of Brachmann–de Lange syndrome is poor feeding during infancy, often because of gastroesophageal reflux. Cleft or high-arched palate and narrow external auditory canals place children with Brachmann–de Lange syndrome at greater risk of chronic otitis; conductive and/or sensorineural hearing loss is common. Eye problems include high myopia, nystagmus (stuttering gaze), and ptosis (hooded brows) that may cause chin lifting to achieve vision. Communication may be impaired by visual or hearing problems, and only 4% of children had low-normal to normal speech by age 4 years. Limb anomalies include small hands and feet, proximally placed thumbs, fifth finger curvature, fusing together of toes 2/3, and, in about 20%, absent fingers or hands. Mild flexion contractures of the elbow are common and the hips may be extended in a frog-leg position. Internal anomalies of the heart, urinary tract and gastrointestinal tract are frequent, and genital anomalies include hypospadias, cryptorchidism (undescended testes), and uterine anomalies. A higher risk for malignancies may be present.

Preventive medical needs

Attention to feeding and screening for cardiac and urinary tract anomalies are important for infants with Brachmann–de Lange syndrome. The high frequency of feeding problems and gastroesophageal reflux (77%), and the known deaths from apnea (cessation of breathing) or aspiration (swallowing of food into the lungs), mandate observation and counseling regarding early feeding so appropriate medical or surgical treatment is provided. In the presence of significant gastroesophageal reflux or vomiting, particularly when accompanied by respiratory distress, chest X-ray and imaging of the gastrointestinal tract should be performed to rule out congenital anomalies like pyloric stenosis or intestinal malrotation. Congenital heart disease should also be considered, since it occurs in 13–29% of patients. Cleft lip and palate may also complicate early management. Medical counseling should be concerned with growth, feeding, cardiac, and gastrointestinal problems, with planning for medical and financial services appropriate for children with significant developmental disability. High risks of chronic otitis and hearing loss require careful monitoring of hearing, so children develop sufficient communication skills to facilitate school and home functions. Other preventive measures in early childhood include urinalysis to rule out urinary tract infection, dental care for the detection and correction of tooth anomalies, and physical/occupational therapy to minimize the effects of contractures and hip dislocation. In the older child, school performance requires evaluation because of the risks of behavioral (57%) or cognitive (75–100%) dysfunction. Monitoring of puberty is particularly important in males, in whom hypogonadism may cause ostracism, and depilatory treatments may be useful for increased body hair. Growth hormone deficiency has been reported, and very short individuals should have endocrine evaluation with consideration of growth hormone therapy. Some have recommended against growth hormone therapy unless there is significant hypoglycemia. Acute monocytic leukemia and Wilms tumor have been reported. The older individual with Brachmann–de Lange syndrome should certainly have regular hearing and vision assessments, since myopia and hearing loss are common.

Family counseling

Parents of a child with Brachmann–de Lange syndrome have an empiric recurrence risk of 2–5%. A mild form may be autosomal dominant with a 50% recurrence risk for affected individuals. Parents will need supportive counseling regarding the risks of mental disability and growth failure, although recent developmental assessment is more positive than that reported previously.

11

Syndromes with disproportionate growth failure (dwarfism)

Skeletal dysplasias are distinguished by disproportionate short stature and bony anomalies with more than 100 disorders now recognized. (Jones, 1997, pp. 326–98; Gorlin et al., 2001, pp. 178–280). Several of the more common or prototypic skeletal dysplasias are listed in Table 11.1. Pediatricians become involved with skeletal dysplasia in three ways: With perinatal management of dwarfism recognized by prenatal ultrasound studies, with management of neonatal lethal dysplasias where a diagnosis is essential before death occurs, or with long-term preventive management of children and adults with dwarfism. The importance of diagnostic skeletal radiographs for stillborn or neonatal lethal bone dysplasias cannot be overemphasized.

The early diagnosis and preventive management of skeletal dysplasias can vastly improve the length and quality of life for affected children. General preventive management for skeletal dysplasias is first discussed, including a general checklist that can be used for these disorders. Many of the management considerations on the general skeletal dysplasia checklist are similar to those for achondroplasia, but the broader possibilities for complications mandate that physicians add specific concerns to the general checklist. Brief discussion on the more common skeletal dysplasias follows to facilitate addition of their complications to the general checklist. Achondroplasia and osteogenesis imperfecta are then reviewed in detail.

Skeletal dysplasias – general manifestations and preventive management

Terminology

The terms "dysplasia" indicates abnormal growth and indicates that many defects in the skeletal dysplasias are tissue defects rather than true malformations. The defective cartilage tissue or its subsequent mineralization causes shortening and deformation of the bones with resulting short stature and disproportion. Almost all are due to single gene changes and exhibit Mendelian inheritance, making the Online Mendelian Inheritance in Man (OMIM – http://www.ncbi.nlm.nih.gov/entrez/) and Genetests (www.genetests.org) databases very useful for obtaining

Table 11.1. Skeletal dysplasias and dystrophies

Syndrome	Incidence*	Frequent abnormalities (in addition to dwarfism)
Lethal dwarfisms		
Thanatophoric dwarfism	1 in 25,000	Short limbs, small thorax, craniosynostosis, cleft palate
Short-rib polydactyly syndromes	~50 cases	Short limbs, small thorax, polydactyly, genital a.
Chondrodysplasias		
Achondroplasia	1 in 25,000	Short limbs, frontal bossing, spinal compression, hypotonia
Cleidocranial dysplasia	~700 cases	Macrocephaly, large fontanel, absent clavicles, dental a.
Diastrophic dysplasia	~130 cases	Short limbs, heart a., progressive scoliosis, dislocated hip, cervical spinal cord compression, heart a., speech problems
SED	1 in 100,000	Myopia, vitreoretinal degeneration, scoliosis, odontoid hypoplasia
Chondrodysplasias with unusual features		
Cartilage-hair hypoplasia	~100 cases	Short limbs, immune deficiency, Hodgkin's disease, lymphomas
Ellis–van Crevald syndrome	~250 cases	Short limbs, cardiac a., small nails, genitourinary a.
Chondrodysplasia punctata	~200 cases	Short limbs, cataracts, ichthyosis, ocular a., cardiac a.
Recognized metabolic alterations		
Osteogenesis imperfectas	1 in 20,000	Multiple fractures, blue sclerae, hearing loss, bowed limbs
Pseudohypoparathyroidism	~200 cases	Short digits, hypocalcemia, bowed limbs, hypothyroidism
Hypophosphatasia	1 in 100,000	Craniosynostosis, seizures, eye a., dental a., orthopedic a.
Other skeletal disorders		
Osteopetrosis	~600 cases	Pancytopenia, blindness, deafness, fractures, renal disease (rare)
FOP	~550 cases	Exogenous bone deposition, hearing loss, respiratory failure

Notes:

FOP, Fibrodysplasia ossificans progressiva; SED, Spondyloepiphyseal dysplasia; a., anomalies.

*Cases or per number of live births.

updated clinical and diagnostic information. Because these striking phenotypes were recognized before their molecular bases were known, they were often named by the skeletal parts that were altered. Short limbs are thus described by the segment (rhizo- for root or proximal, meso- for middle, acro- for terminal) or region (diaphysis, metaphysic, epiphyses) that is affected. Affected parts like the skull (cranio-), spine (spondylo-), ribs (costo-), hips (coxo-) or clavicle (cleido-) are then added to produce descriptive names like spondylometaphyseal or costovertebral dysplasia. As with other genetic conditions, diseases named by the regions affected are often heterogenous as indicated by several types of spondylometaphyseal dyplasias (McKusick, Strudwick, etc.).

Incidence, etiology, and differential diagnosis

Skeletal dysplasias have a combined prevalence of 2–4 per 10,000 births (Jones, 1997, pp. 326–98; Gorlin et al., 2001, pp. 178–280). One of the most common is the achondroplasia–hypochondroplasia family with an incidence of 1 in 10,000–15,000. Genetic and phenotypic heterogeneity in many of the skeletal dysplasias are indicated by the fact that achondroplasia, homozygous lethal achondroplasia, milder hypochondroplasia, and severe thanatophoric dwarfism all result from mutations in the fibroblast growth factor-3 receptor gene. Diagnosis of a skeletal dysplasia becomes more secure as one progresses from the clinical description to radiologic evaluation to DNA diagnosis.

Diagnostic evaluation and medical counseling

Skeletal radiography is the cardinal diagnostic study, allowing the recognition of skeletal dysplasia and classification according to affected skeletal regions and accessory anomalies. Although a growing number of skeletal diseases have characterized gene mutations, commercial DNA diagnosis is still scarce. The neonatal lethal dwarfisms are particularly important to recognize, since the clinician will not have the luxury of follow-up X-rays or tissue studies to make a diagnosis. Thanatophoric (death-bringing) dwarfism is the most common example, with an incidence of about 1 in 25,000. These infants have the appearance of severely affected achondroplasts, with frontal bossing, shallow nasal bridge, and short extremities. This disorder exhibits autosomal-dominant inheritance with most cases being new mutations, so parents will have a low recurrence risk for future pregnancies.

Other examples of neonatal-lethal skeletal dysplasias are the short-rib polydactyly syndromes of Saldino–Noonan, Naumoff, and Majewski (Jones, 1997, pp. 326–43; Gorlin et al., 2001, pp. 249–59). These again must be diagnosed through ultrasound and radiographic findings, and all three syndromes exhibit autosomal-recessive inheritance with thoracic dysplasia and neonatal death. Lethal dwarfisms can often be distinguished by their accompanying anomalies, illustrated by cleft lip/palate, cardiac anomalies, pre- or postaxial polydactyly, gastrointestinal anomalies, renal anomalies, and ambiguous or hypoplastic genitalia in the Saldino–Noonan, Naumoff, and Majewski group. Prompting prenatal ultrasound studies may be polyhydramnios or fetal hydrops that occur in several lethal dwarfisms, and serial level II ultrasound studies are imperative once fetal dwarfism is suspected (e.g., Varkey & Jones, 2004). In these and other complex skeletal disorders, the role of primary care is to link prenatal with neonatal studies, coordinate imaging studies and subspecialty consultations to delineate anomaly patterns, and accomplish fetal/neonatal necropsy studies for stillbirths or neonatal deaths. These data will be crucial for determining anticipatory versus palliative management and for assigning diagnosis and recurrence risks for the purposes of genetic counseling. An example is a dwarfism with a snail-like pelvis or Schneckenbecken dysplasia that is clinically similar to thanatophoric dwarfism (Varkey & Jones, 2004); prenatal recognition of dwarfism can prepare the perinatal team to obtain appropriate X-rays and tissue/DNA analysis to distinguish this autosomal-recessive disorder and its 25% recurrence risk.

Family and psychosocial counseling

Diagnosis of lethal dwarfisms is obviously important for medical counseling, allowing planning of palliative care options. Recent publicity regarding a child with thanatophoric dysplasia that was kept alive for many months at parental insistence illustrates this medical dilemma. Non-lethal dwarfisms also require accurate diagnosis and counseling, since the specter of severe short stature has similar impact to the diagnosis of mental disability (see discussion for achondroplasia). Patients with skeletal dysplasias often have risks to transmit their disorder, sometimes in a more severe form as illustrated by homozygous achondroplasia. Correct diagnosis and genetic counseling is thus important for parents and affected individuals. Parent-oriented literature and parent support for diverse skeletal dysplasias is available by searching on the syndrome name or generally through the Little People of America organization (www.lpaonline.org/).

Natural history and complications

Many skeletal dysplasias are compatible with a normal lifespan, but have complications affecting the membranous and cartilaginous bony skeletons, brain, spinal cord, eyes, teeth, heart, and bone marrow (Apajasalo et al., 1998). As a rule, affected children have a head that is large in proportion to the body with platybasia or other cranial deformities; these impose risks for hydrocephalus, foramen magnum/atlanto-axial abnormalities, and spinal cord injury. Bony foramina or inner ear ossicles may be affected, producing hearing and vision problems. Frequent fractures and/or limb deformities often require orthopedic monitoring, and many skeletal disorders are generalized connective tissue diseases with lax joints, easy bruising, bluish sclerae, or mitral valve prolapse. Some skeletal disorders with exuberant or ectopic bone formation will produce bone marrow failure with bleeding or infection. Those with significant short stature require special appliances to aid ambulation, driving, and daily living.

General skeletal dysplasia preventive medical checklist

Preventive management for the skeletal dysplasias is guided by achondroplasia as an example, since much study and success had derived from management of this more common disorder. Early management will be directed at cranial complications such as hydrocephalus, cervicomedullary spinal compression from platybasia, and assurance of good occupational therapy with measures of head support for the relative macrocephaly. The altered skull base often inhibits ear drainage, causing otitis and hearing loss to be concerns in early childhood. Orthopedic management is of obvious importance as the child begins to walk and accessory anomalies (club feet, hip dislocation) and weaker cartilage (increased neck and joint flexibility, scoliosis, flat feet) cause bony deformities. The tracheal cartilage may be affected, combining with narrow nasal passages to cause airway obstruction and risks for sleep apnea.

Common accessory anomalies are eye problems (retinal detachment, cataracts), cleft palate, small jaw, and cervical spine restriction/maldevelopment, emphasizing the need for hearing/vision screening, airway and anesthesia precautions. Sudden deaths from sleep/airway problems or overwhelming infections (as in McKusick spondylometaphyseal dysplasia with T-cell immune deficiencies) are always of concern in the short-limb dwarfisms, and monitoring is additionally important when a specific diagnosis is delayed. Monitoring for airway or cervicomedullary spinal compression problems can be performed by skull tomograms or CT scans to evaluate foramen magnum diameter, sleep studies, or somatic evoked potentials as discussed for achondroplasia. Suspect patients should be followed with apnea monitors and neurosurgical consultation, and live vaccines such as varicella may be postponed if there is concern about immunity.

Later concerns include arthritis and obesity because of physical immobility, and depression may be an issue in adults with significant short stature and disability. Woman with skeletal dyplasia may face risks during pregnancy because of pelvic disproportion, and it is important to remember that some of the collagens important for bone are found in blood vessels, causing arterial changes that can worsen in pregnancy (see osteogenesis imperfecta, below).

Cartilage-hair hypoplasia

Individuals with cartilage-hair hypoplasia may have a normal facial appearance with sparse hair and short, bowed limbs (Jones, 1997, pp. 384–5; Gorlin et al., 2001, pp. 217–19). The disorder is an example of the T- and B-cell immunologic deficiencies that may be associated with short-limb dwarfism and serves to alert physicians to this possibility in all patients with skeletal dysplasia.

Summary of clinical concerns: Cartilage-hair hypoplasia management considerations

Growth and development: Short stature with disproportionately short and bowed limbs, leading to an average height of about 4 ft in males, early hypotonia with normal intellect: A trial of growth hormone in 4 affected children produced modest increase in stature for 1 year but made no difference on final adult height or immune function (Bocca et al., 2004); early intervention and occupational therapy in children with severe hypotonia.

Cancer: There is an increased risk for cancer, with 6% of patients having Hodgkin disease, lymphoma, or leukemia.

Surface-skin: Sparse hair and eyebrows, baldness.

Reticuloendothelial system (RES): Chronic or cyclic neutropenia with accompanying T-cell dysfunction and normal immunoglobulin levels; failure to mount antibody responses to certain antigens, several deaths from overwhelming varicella infection: Avoid live vaccines like small pox, polio; prophylaxis for bacterial infections; treatment with granulocyte colony-stimulating factor improved neutrophil counts and prevented recurrent bacterial respiratory tract infections in one patient (Ammann et al., 2004), and bone marrow transplant was successful in correcting immune problems in two patients (Gorlin et al., 2001, p. 217).

Digestive: Occasional Hirschsprung disease, more extensive aganglionosis, malabsorption, esophageal atresia: Monitor feeding and stooling, gastroenterology referral as needed.

Skeletal: Disproportionate short stature with short limbs, short digits, broad hands, increased joint laxity, scoliosis, lordosis: Skeletal examinations with annual orthopedic evaluation.

Neurologic: Rare unilateral facial nerve palsy, seizures: Neurology evaluation with signs or symptoms.

Parental counseling: The syndrome exhibits autosomal-recessive inheritance, with a 25% recurrence risk to parents of affected children. DNA diagnosis is not available. Parent support and information is available at a Cartilage-Hair Hypoplasia Information site (members.cox.net/chayim76/chh.htm) and at several medical education sites by searching on the syndrome name.

Chondrodysplasia punctata

Patients with radiographic stippling (chondrodysplasia punctata) were first described by Conradi in 1914 and Hünermann in 1931. Chondrodysplasia punctata describes focal or punctate calcifications of infantile cartilage that occur primarily but not exclusively in the epiphyses. The epiphyses do not exhibit clinical abnormalities but appear stippled on X-ray, as if someone dabbed at them with a white paintbrush. As a clinical sign, chondrodysplasia punctata occurs in many disorders including Zellweger syndrome, Smith–Lemli–Opitz syndrome, trisomy 18, fetal warfarin syndrome, or even hypothyroidism. As a disease entity, chondrodysplasia punctata refers to at least four genetically distinct skeletal dysplasias (Wilson et al., 1988).

Autosomal-recessive chondrodysplasia punctata is the most severe, with short limbs, microcephaly, unusual facies (frontal bossing, shallow nasal bridge), bilateral cataracts (80%), ichthyosis or alopecia (27%), and contractures (48%). This disorder is caused by altered biogenesis of peroxisomes (see Chapter 19). Autosomal-dominant chondrodysplasia punctata is milder, with normal limb lengths, mental development, and survival. X-linked dominant chondrodysplasia punctata exhibits unilateral scoliosis (100%), joint contractures (46%), cataracts (46%), and stippling of epiphyses. Ichthyosis or erythroderma (95%) may occur in patches and whorls as predicted by random inactivation of normal/abnormal X chromosome alleles. X-linked recessive chondrodysplasia punctata denotes a small group of male patients who have visible X chromosome deletions. These males have symmetric short stature with typical facial changes (shallow nasal bridge, short nose) and hypoplastic distal phalanges. The disorder results from the deletion of an arylsulfatase gene, and it has been demonstrated that warfarin is an inhibitor of this gene.

Once non-specific stippling has been excluded, the diagnosis of the autosomal-recessive or X-linked-dominant forms of chondrodysplasia punctata is made by the demonstration of plasmalogen or peroxisomal enzyme deficiency. The X-linked recessive form can be recognized by chromosomal or molecular analysis, but the autosomal-dominant form remains a clinical diagnosis. Preventive management should include ophthalmologic and orthopedic follow-up, with recognition that the autosomal-recessive form often involves chronic pulmonary infections that are lethal in early childhood.

Cleidocranial dysplasia

Cleidocranial dysplasia is an autosomal-dominant disorder with short stature and skeletal and oral anomalies. More than 700 cases have been described, including one by Meckel in 1760 and a potentially affected Neanderthal skeleton (Jones, 1997, pp. 408–9; Gorlin et al., 2001, pp. 306–10). Interestingly, the patients and their parents are often unaware of the absent clavicles, despite anomalies of the sternocleidomastoid, trapezius, and pectoralis major muscles.

Summary of clinical concerns: Cleidocranial dysplasia management considerations

Growth and development: Mild short stature leading to an average height of about 5 ft in males; occasional mild mental disability: Developmental, growth, and school monitoring with early intervention and school assessment for those with delays.

Craniofacial: Broad, flat facies with frontal bossing and hypertelorism

ENT: Conductive hearing loss, high palate, dental anomalies such as supernumerary teeth or lack of tooth eruption (Gorlin et al., 2001, pp. 306–10;

Golan et al., 2004). Care should be taken not to extract baby or supernumerary teeth until permanent teeth can be demonstrated.

Digestive: Occasional tresia: Monitor feeding and stooling, gastroenterology referral as needed.

Skeletal: Patients have a large anterior fontanel and relative macrocephaly in the neonatal period; absent clavicles leading to increased range of motion of shoulders and the appearance of a long neck; normal limb lengths with subtle changes in the vertebrae (hemivertebrae), hips, or pelvis (delayed closure of pubic symphysis); Wormian bones of the skull, decreased ossification of the pubis, spina bifida occulta, and cone-shaped epiphyses of the distal phalanges comprise a distinctive radiographic pattern (Gorlin et al., 2001, pp. 306–10): Regular skeletal examinations and skeletal radiographic survey for diagnosis, annual orthopedic evaluation.

Neurologic: Rare syringomyelia: Neurology/neurosurgery evaluation with signs or symptoms.

Parental counseling: The inheritance is autosomal dominant, and parents should be examined for features to determine if they have a 50% versus virtually zero recurrence risk if their child has a new mutation. One form of this heterogeneous condition is caused by mutations in an osteoblast-specific transcription factor (see OMIM – www.ncbi.nlm.nih.gov/entrez/), but DNA diagnosis is not commercially available. Parent information is available at several medical education sites by searching on the syndrome name, included that of FACES-The National Craniofacial Association (www.faces-cranio.org/Disord/CCD.htm).

Diastrophic dwarfism

Diastrophic dwarfism was described in 1960 and consists of short-limb dwarfism with cleft palate and skeletal deformities (Jones, 1997, pp. 376–7; Gorlin et al., 2001, 229–32). A "hitchhiker thumb" and a cystic malformation of the outer ear, together with progressive scoliosis, club feet, and mesomelic (middle limb segment) dwarfism comprise a diagnostic pattern. Diastrophic dwarfism is representative of a family of disorders, all involving mutations in a sulfate transporter protein that brings sulfate into osteoid cells. The rare, lethal dwarfisms atelosteogenesis type II and achondrogenesis type 1B also involve mutations in the sulfate transporter, which is expressed in many tissues but seems most critical for cartilage development. Diastrophic dyplasia is common in Finland, with an incidence of 1 in 30,000.

Summary of clinical concerns: Diastrophic dwarfism management considerations

General: Twenty-five percent of patients die in infancy from respiratory complications.

Growth and development: Short stature with shortening of the middle segment of limbs (mesomelia), with an average height of just below 4 ft in males, normal intelligence: Monitoring of growth as plotted by Makitie & Kaitila (1997), cleft palate team with speech therapy because of problems with articulation.

Craniofacial: Round facies with striking micrognathia and external ear malformations including cystic swelling in 80% of patients that are present between ages 1–2 weeks and 1 month of life.

ENT: Cleft palate (25%) with small jaw (Robin sequence), narrow auditory canals and platybasia may cause frequent otitis media: Cleft palate team where appropriate, initial otolaryngology consultation with annual audiology screening and follow-up.

Pulmonary: Infantile respiratory distress because of micrognathia and tracheomalacia with aspiration pneumonia. A hoarse cry is predictive of laryngeal hypoplasia and early respiratory problems: Careful assessment of the airway in neonates, with interventions ranging from prone positioning to tracheostomy.

Heart: Congenital heart defects: Echocardiogram and cardiology evaluation during infancy with appropriate follow-up.

Skeletal: Severe kyphoscoliosis may cause cervical spine compression; short limbs with deviated thumbs, club feet, dislocation or subluxation of the hips: Initial skeletal radiographic survey can evaluate both cardiac status and bony deformities, with careful evaluation for congenital dislocation of the hip; neonatal skeletal examination and orthopedic consultation, regular orthopedic visits are needed to monitor and treat kyphoscoliosis and prevent compression of the cervical cord.

Neurologic: Progressive cervical kyphosis with compression of the cervical spinal cord: Neurology/neurosurgery evaluation with signs or symptoms; anesthesia precautions with cervical spine flexion/extension films prior to intubation and monitoring of upper airway/pulmonary function.

Parental counseling: The syndrome exhibits autosomal-recessive inheritance, with a 25% recurrence risk to parents of affected children. DNA diagnosis is not available. Parent support and information is available at a Diastrophic Help website (pixelscapes.com/ddhelp/a) and at several medical education sites by searching on the syndrome name.

Ellis–van Crevald syndrome

The most common form of dwarfism among the Amish, Ellis–van Crevald syndrome is an autosomal-recessive disorder that occurs in other populations as well (Gorlin et al., 2001, pp. 239–42). It is recognized by its unusual pattern of short limbs, polydactyly, club feet, natal teeth, ectodermal dysplasia with hypoplastic nails, congenital heart disease, and genitourinary anomalies.

Summary of clinical concerns: Ellis–van Crevald management considerations

Growth and development: Short stature with disproportionately short and bowed limbs, leading to an average height of about 4 ft in males, early hypotonia with normal intellect: Early intervention and occupational therapy in children with severe hypotonia.

Craniofacial: Cataracts, missing or supernumerary teeth. Ophthalmology and dentistry follow-up.

RES: Chronic or and immune problems in two patients (Gorlin et al., 2001, p. 217).

Heart: Cardiac anomalies (50–60%) including single atrium and endocardial cushion defects, significant incidence of sudden cardiac arrest: Early cardiology evaluation with echo- and electrocardiograms.

Skeletal: Disproportionate short stature with short limbs, short digits, broad hands, increased joint laxity, scoliosis, lordosis: Skeletal examinations with annual orthopedic evaluation.

Urogenital: Cryptorchidism, hypospadias, and hydronephrosis: Periodic urinalyses and evaluation of the genitalia.

Parental counseling: The syndrome exhibits autosomal-recessive inheritance, with a 25% recurrence risk to parents of affected children. DNA diagnosis is not available. Parent support and information is available at one and at several medical education sites by searching on the syndrome name, including a site by the Greenberg Center for Skeletal Dysplasias at Johns Hopkins University (www.hopkinsmedicine.org/greenbergcenter/evc.htm).

Fibrodysplasia ossificans progressiva

Most cases of fibrodysplasia ossificans progressiva (FOP) are sporadic, but a few instances of familial transmission have suggested autosomal-dominant inheritance. Congenital malformations include the absence of digits and thumb anomalies, short femora, and small cervical vertebrae. Most of the complications result from ectopic bone formation, including restriction of limb and pectoral girdle motion, chest wall fixation with respiratory failure, traumatic fractures, spinal deformity, encroachment of marrow to cause aplastic anemia, and conductive or sensorineural hearing loss (Gorlin et al., 2001, pp. 312–15). Mental deficiency occurs but is unusual. Altschuler (2004) points out that FOP patients elaborate excess levels of bone morphogenic protein-4 (BMP-4) from their B lymphocytes, that bone marrow transplant halted progression in two patients, and that Rituximab, a monoclonal antibody against B-cells, might offer less risky therapy. Preventive management should concentrate on monitoring of auditory, skeletal and respiratory function, consideration of therapies against B-cell proliferation, and early intervention and inclusive school programs for those with mental disability.

An International Fibrodysplasia Ossificans Progressiva website (www.ifopa.org/) is available for parent/physician information and support.

Hypophosphatasia

Decreased activity of alkaline phosphatase produces an autosomal-recessive disorder with a phenotype similar to that of vitamin D-deficient rickets. The hypophosphatasia results from mutations in the gene for tissue-nonspecific alkaline phosphatase (Jones, 1997, pp. 392–3; Gorlin et al., 2001, pp. 161–3). The severity is variable, with infantile, childhood, and adulthood forms. Prenatal polyhydramnios and severe skeletal changes (craniotabes, thoracic dysplasia typify the short-lived infantile form, while moderately affected infants can present with failure to thrive and irritability due to hypercalcemia. The radiographic changes of rickets may not be recognized until age 2 or 3 years, although the diagnosis can be made based on a low serum alkaline phosphatase level and increased urinary phosphoethanolamine. The adult form may exhibit only osteomalacia and episodes of bone pain leading to bony deformities (genu valgum, osteoporosis). Bone marrow transplantation showed some improvement of symptoms in a severely affected child, although they remained small (Whyte et al., 2003). In milder cases, remissions may occur in later childhood accompanied by increases in alkaline phosphatase activity.

Summary of clinical concerns: Hypophosphatasia management considerations

General: Prenatal polyhydramnios and premature stillborn deliveries; survival is limited to a few days in severe forms. Unexplained fevers with tender bones.

Growth and development: Failure to thrive with irritability, vomiting, polyuria, and constipation that may reflect hypercalcemia: Monitor feeding and growth; early intervention, occupational, and physical therapy.

Craniofacial: Neonatal craniotabes with large anterior fontanel and wide sutures and later craniosynostosis in more severe patients; exophthalmos due to shallow orbits, keratopathy, conjunctival calcification; dental anomalies (premature tooth loss, periodontal disease): Monitoring of head circumference and referral to craniofacial surgery for altered growth or shape; neonatal ophthalmology and early dental evaluations with annual follow-up.

Renal: Decreased renal function with nephrocalcinosis and renal tubular acidosis: Monitor urinalyses and urinary pH, with neonatal and annual evaluations by nephrology.

Skeletal: Short limbs with bowing and metaphyseal changes, thoracic dysplasia with pulmonary restriction, rachitic rosary, osteomalacia with patches of osteoporosis, bone pain; pseudofracture of the femur with loss of mobility in adults, genu valgum: Neonatal skeletal examination and orthopedic evaluation with annual reassessment.

Neurologic: Seizures, intracranial hypertension: Neurology evaluation for signs or symptoms.

Parental counseling: Most cases exhibit autosomal-recessive inheritance with a 25% recurrence risk to parents of affected children. A mild autosomal-dominant form has been reported, so parents should be assessed for signs and symptoms. Commercial DNA diagnosis is not available. Parent support and information is available at the Canadian Hypophosphatasia Contact (www.homestead.com/ hypophosphatasia/), the National Diabetes Insipidus Foundation (www.ndif. org/ index.html), and various medical information sites.

Osteopetrosis

Osteopetrosis includes mild and severe forms with autosomal-recessive or -dominant inheritance (Jones, 1997, pp. 399–411; Tolar et al., 2004). More than 400 cases of the severe, recessive Albers–Schonberg disease have been reported, many dying in infancy or early childhood. Increased bone deposition encroaches on bone marrow and osteal foramina to produce pancytopenia, hepatosplenomegaly, blindness, deafness, and cranial nerve paralysis. Monitoring of vision, hearing, peripheral blood counts, and dental care is important for preventive management. Bone marrow transplant has been helpful in several patients, but calcium diuresis has not been useful. One form of autosomal-recessive osteopetrosis involves a mutation in the gene for carbonic anhydrase. Affected patients have renal tubular acidosis and dull mentality in addition to features of Albers–Schonberg syndrome.

Autosomal-dominant osteopetrosis is more benign, and does not manifest until early childhood. Complications include fractures after minor trauma, conductive hearing loss, ablation of the sinuses, and frequent osteomyelitis of the mandible (necessitating thorough oral examinations at each pediatric visit together with regular dental care). Elevation of acid phosphatase may be a helpful diagnostic screen, and preventive management should focus on audiology and orthopedic assessment. Parent/physician information is available at the Osteoporosis website (www.osteopetrosis.org/) and several medical education or radiology sites by searching on the term "osteoporosis."

Pseudohypoparathyroidism (Albright hereditary osteodystrophy)

Described by Albright and colleagues in 1942, pseudohypoparathyroidism presents with radiographic, renal, and serum calcium changes suggestive of hypoparathyroidism, but involves normal levels of parathormone (Jones, 1997, pp. 446–7; Gorlin et al., 2001, pp. 139–68). The disorder exhibits marked variability, exemplified by patients with normal calcium levels who were once distinguished by the term "pseudo-pseudo-hypoparathyroidism." The variants are mostly caused by mutations in the alpha subunit of GTP-associated Gs protein. Phenotypic variation according to parental origin of the mutation is implied, and genomic imprinting may contribute to the striking clinical variability of the disorder.

Summary of clinical concerns: Pseudohypoparathyroidism management considerations

General: The diagnosis of pseudohypoparathyroidism is based on compatible clinical manifestations plus the laboratory findings of hypocalcemia, hyperphosphatemia, and increased levels of parathormone.

Growth and development: Short stature (60%), mental disability (70% of hypocalcemic patients, 30% of normocalcemic patients): Patients should also have early intervention and speech/physical therapy/occupational therapy to maximize developmental potential.

Craniofacial: Round face with full cheeks, short neck, cataracts in 10–25%, enamel hypoplasia and delayed eruption of the teeth: Periodic ophthalmologic and audiologic evaluations to rule out cataracts and hearing loss, early dental evaluation.

Endocrine: Hypothyroidism, growth hormone deficiency (Germain-Lee et al., 2003): Neonatal and annual endocrine referral, treatment of hypocalcemia in order to avoid seizures or ectopic calcification, annual thyroid hormone levels, evaluation of growth hormone deficiency in those with short stature and consideration of growth hormone therapy.

Skeletal: Short digits with bowing of the long bones, osteopenia with bone cysts: Neonatal and regular skeletal and orthopedic evaluations to recognize early bowing or limb deformities.

Neurologic: Ectopic calcification in the basal ganglia and choroid plexus, spinal stenosis, anosmia (because Gs proteins are involved in olfactory signal transduction), hearing loss: Audiologic evaluations to rule out hearing loss, monitoring of gait and urinary function to exclude spinal stenosis; spinal MRI and neurology evaluation with signs or symptoms.

Parental counseling: Inheritance is usually autosomal dominant, with predominance of affected females, but autosomal-recessive forms have been described. A small deletion in the chromosome 2q37 region has been found in some patients; others have mutations in the Gs alpha gene but DNA diagnosis is not available. Parent information is available at several medical education sites by searching on the syndrome name.

Spondylo(meta)(epi)physeal dysplasias

Spondyloepiphyseal dysplasia (SED) congenita is one in a group of related disorders with flattened vertebrae (spondylo-), metaphyseal, and/or epiphyseal changes that might better be called SE/M/D (Jones, 1997, pp. 358–9; Gorlin et al., 2001, pp. 263–73). Included in this spectrum are spondyloepimetaphyseal dysplasia, Strudwick spondylometaphyseal dysplasia, and lethal hypochondrogenesis; many are caused by mutations in the type II collagen gene. Skeletal changes of the SE/M/D spectrum may even be seen in congenital hypothyroidism or Down syndrome, and its heterogeneity emphasizes the need for early genetic referral for proper diagnosis and counseling.

Summary of clinical concerns: Spondylo(meta)(epi)physeal management considerations

Growth and development: Short stature is severe in most variants with no established therapy; intelligence is almost always normal unless compromised by cord compression or respiratory problems: Monitoring of growth, providing adaptations for severely dwarfed patients; early intervention/school progress monitoring for those with developmental delays or neurologic sequellae.

Craniofacial: Myopia (50%) and retinal detachment, especially in classic SED; cleft or high palate (30–40%): Cleft palate team, monitoring for feeding problems and hearing loss, neonatal and annual ophthalmology examinations.

Heart: Congenital heart defects such as septal defects can be found in some variants like spondyloepimetaphyseal dysplasia: Echocardiogram and cardiology evaluation for signs and symptoms.

Endocrine: Initial thyroid neonatal screen or infantile thyroid functions should be reviewed to exclude hypothyroidism as the cause of bone dysplasia.

Skeletal: Kyphoscoliosis, hypoplasia of the odontoid bone with potential atlantoaxial instability, progressive scoliosis with some types: Skeletal and orthopedic evaluation at diagnosis and monitoring for cervical spine compression, atlantoaxial instability, and spinal deformities with cord compression or thoracic distortion and respiratory problems; cervical spine flexion/extension radiographs and, in patients with severe scoliosis and thoracic deformation, pulmonary function studies prior to anesthesia or sports participation.

Urogenital: Focal glomerular sclerosis and nephrotic syndrome may occur: Monitoring of urinalysis and blood pressure, referral to nephrology.

Neurologic: Sensorineural hearing loss: Neonatal auditory brainstem evoked response (ABR) with follow-up audiology evaluations.

Parental counseling: The incidence of SED is about 1 in 100,000 births, and the entire spectrum perhaps twice that common. Most forms exhibit autosomal-dominant inheritance with minimal recurrence risks for normal parents of affected children. More severe forms may be autosomal recessive with a 25% recurrence risk, so clinical genetic evaluation is needed for accurate counseling. DNA diagnosis is available for certain types using type II collagen gene testing (see www.genetests.org), but a negative test does not exclude the spectrum.

Parent support and information is available at Little People of America (www.lpaonline.org/) and at numerous medical education sites.

Achondroplasia

Terminology

"Achondroplasia," coined by Parrot in 1878, is a well-established but incorrect term, since cartilage is not completely lacking in the disorder (Jones,1997, 346–51; Gorlin et al., 2001, pp. 197–202). Hypochondroplasia is clinically similar to achondroplasia, with a relatively normal face and milder skeletal changes.

Incidence, etiology, and differential diagnosis

The incidence of achondroplasia is between 1 in 16,000 and 1 in 25,000 births, while that for hypochondroplasia is about 10-fold less. Both disorders result from mutations in different portions of the fibroblast growth factor-3 receptor gene. Thanatophoric dysplasia, a lethal form of dwarfism discussed above, comprises a third member of this allelic group (homozygous achondroplasia is the fourth – see Little People of America – www.lpaonline.org/ – and achondroplasias, UK (www.achondroplasia.co.uk/). Discussion with other average-sized parents can be invaluable in fostering acceptance of the child with dwarfism. Some parents will need time before confronting the reality forced by support groups, but also distinctive). Differential diagnosis involves the separation of achondroplasia from other forms of short-limbed dwarfism. Patients with achondroplasia have rhizomelic (proximal) limb shortening, prominent forehead with shallow nasal bridge, and characteristic splayed or "trident" fingers. Skeletal radiographs will demonstrate characteristic changes in the lumbar vertebrae and pelvis (e.g., unusual iliac wings). Thanatophoric dysplasia can be distinguished at birth by its more severe facial changes, limb shortening, and thoracic narrowing which results in death.

Diagnostic evaluation and medical counseling

The diagnosis of achondroplasia is made by clinical examination and skeletal radiographic survey. DNA analysis could be pursued in uncertain cases, but this is not usually required. Inheritance of achondroplasia, hypochondroplasia, and thanatophoric dysplasia is autosomal dominant, with homozygous achondroplasia representing one of the autosomal-dominant conditions where a double dose of the abnormal allele causes a more severe phenotype. About 75% of achondroplastic patients represent new mutations, explaining why the majority of patients have a normal family history. The chief concerns to be mentioned during medical counseling are the average adult height of 110–145 cm and the risks for early hydrocephalus or spinal cord compression. For achondroplasia and particularly hypochondroplasia, medical counseling can be optimistic in view of the normal intelligence, normal lifespan, and remarkable physical adaptation exhibited by these individuals. Individuals with hypochondroplasia do have a 10% incidence of cognitive disability.

Family and psychosocial counseling

The majority of patients with achondroplasia will be born to normal parents, provoking a crisis similar to that surrounding the birth of a child with Down syndrome. Genetic referral is essential for evaluation and counseling. Timely and unrushed explanation of the diagnostic approach is important, followed by supportive counseling once the diagnosis seems probable. For normal parents, the recurrence risk will be negligible but not zero due to the possibility of germinal mosaicism. Couples with achondroplasia have a 50% risk of having a child with achondroplasia, a 25% risk of having a child with lethal homozygous achondroplasia, and a 25% risk of having a normal or "average-sized" child. The diagnosis of achondroplasia is increasingly made by fetal ultrasound, allowing earlier preparation and counseling of the parents.

Positive literature on achondroplasia and other dwarfing conditions is available from the Little the exposure to medical or psychosocial resources and the positive images promoted for their child warrant continued encouragement to realize the advantages offered by parent groups. Most Western countries will have national and local chapters.

Natural history and complications

Although intellectual potential is normal, complications of the central nervous system are of foremost concern for infants with achondroplasia. The large head, platybasia, and small foramen magnum cause these children to be at risk for compression of the brainstem and upper spinal cord (Pauli et al., 1995). The cervicomedullary compression may present as recurrent apnea, central sleep apnea, unusually severe hypotonia and developmental delay, or sudden death (Pauli et al., 1995). This compression may also be associated with hydrocephalus, causing increased intracranial venous pressure from presumed constriction of jugular venous return.

The lower spinal canal is also narrow, producing cord and nerve root compression from vertebral bone spurs, disk prolapse, or deformed vertebral bodies later in life. The interpedicular distances narrow as one progresses to the lower spine, causing kyphosis (20%) and/or scoliosis (7%). Limbs may become bowed due to ligamentous laxity, resulting in genua vara (15%) or varus foot deformity. Patients over age 18 years have histories of ear infections (75–95%) and many (40–70%) had significant hearing loss. Studies of younger patients showed frequencies of conductive hearing loss as great as 50% with mixed or sensorineural hearing loss being less common.

Other complications of achondroplasia include restrictive lung disease with risks for hypoxia or infection, and mild glucose intolerance. Females have an increased incidence of uterine fibroids with menorrhagia, and their narrow pelvis requires delivery by Cesarean section under general anesthesia (Allanson & Hall, 1986). Little has been written about the psychiatric burdens of dwarfism, but anecdotal evidence of depression in these individuals warrants attention to their affect and mood during medical assessments.

In hypochondroplasia, short stature and macrocephaly are less pronounced than in achondroplasia, and there is developmental disability in 10%. Limb bowing and lumbar lordosis also occur, but rarely require treatment. Chronic otitis or hearing loss has not been documented, but Cesarean section may be required for the delivery of pregnant females. Thus, by virtue of early lethality or benign natural history, few preventive measures can be employed for the other allelic disorders of the fibroblast growth factor-3 receptor.

Achondroplasia preventive medical checklist

Preventive management is critical during infancy to prevent major disability or death, which can result from cervicomedullary spinal compression. Clinicians should follow head circumference and motor development, using charts specific for achondroplasia to account for the macrocephaly and motor delay seen in these children (Horton et al., 1978). Parents should be warned about the possibility of spontaneous or sleep-related apnea, and monitors provided when appropriate. If there is apnea or disproportionate variation in head circumference or growth, then structural and functional evaluations of the foramen magnum region are indicated. Skull tomograms or CT scans to evaluate foramen magnum diameter can be compared with age-specific standards (Committee on Genetics, American Academy of Pediatrics, 1995a; Haga, 2004). Sleep studies to evaluate respiratory abnormalities from medullary compression should be performed. Somatic evoked potentials, which measure the time required for back-and-forth impulse transmission through the foramen magnum, may also be helpful in demonstrating functional spinal cord compression. Those children with demonstrated abnormalities should be followed with an apnea monitor and considered for surgery to enlarge the foramen magnum. There is currently some controversy about the timing and utility of surgical intervention (Pauli et al., 1995). The medical advisory board for Little People of America can be helpful in these decisions, and are available for consultation at national conventions.

Another early concern is to begin preventive management for the skeletal system so that later bony deformities, arthritis, and lower spinal cord compressions can be minimized. Because of their disproportionate macrocephaly and joint laxity, children with achondroplasia need additional support during infancy. The head should be supported during handling and devices that artificially prop the infant or give poor support should be avoided. Such devices include umbrella strollers, baby walkers, and certain types of infant swings. Normal infant activity will not cause damage and should not be restricted. The degree of kyphosis and other joint deformities should be monitored during childhood, and aggressive dietary management should be initiated to avoid obesity that predisposes to nerve root compression and degenerative arthritis. A frequency of ear infections and hearing loss that is comparable to that of Down syndrome suggests the same monitoring of auditory function should apply – yearly audiology until the child is 3–4 years old. Newer therapies for dwarfism include growth hormone supplementation and surgical leg-lengthening procedures. Both are expensive, and the latter includes risks of infection or bony deformity. There is evidence of response to growth hormone supplementation.

Osteogenesis imperfecta

Terminology

Sillence and colleagues in 1979 delineated four major types of osteogenesis imperfecta, and more than a dozen additional syndromes include bone fragility as a component feature (Gorlin et al., 2001, pp. 178–99). Most common is type I osteogenesis imperfecta with short stature, fractures, blue sclerae, and normal lifespan. Perinatal lethal osteogenesis imperfecta is designated as type II, with types III (prominent limb bowing) and IV (normal sclerae) being intermediate in severity.

Incidence, etiology, and differential diagnosis

The estimated prevalence of the major types of osteogenesis imperfecta is about 1 in 20,000 individuals (Gorlin et al., 2001, pp. 178–99). Types I, III and IV were long known to exhibit autosomal-dominant inheritance, while type II was considered autosomal recessive. Now it is realized that all major types of osteogenesis imperfecta involve mutations in the genes for type I collagen, with type II osteogenesis imperfecta caused by new mutations in critical regions of the collagen molecule. Occasional type II families in which normal parents have several affected children are thought to represent germinal mosaicism. Differential diagnosis includes numerous syndromes with osteogenesis imperfecta plus unusual features like craniosynostosis (Cole–Carpenter syndrome), microcephaly (Buyse–Bull syndrome), or Marfanoid habitus (Miegel syndrome). These disorders are discussed by Gorlin et al. (2001, pp. 178–99).

Diagnostic evaluation and medical counseling

The presence of osteopenia, fractures, blue sclerae, and hearing loss is strongly suggestive of osteogenesis imperfecta, particularly when there is a family history.

Skeletal radiographs are often diagnostic, but biochemical and molecular analysis of type I collagen provide the most definitive diagnosis when an abnormality can be detected. Although DNA testing can be performed from blood samples, the variety of mutations in the osteogenesis imperfectas is too great to allow comprehensive screening. A better algorithm for testing is to analyze type I collagen synthesis from cultured fibroblasts in the hope of finding deficient or altered $\alpha 1$ or $\alpha 2$ chains. If an abnormality of type I collagen biosynthesis is detected, then mutational screening of appropriate $\alpha 1$ or $\alpha 2$ procollagen gene regions can proceed based on the clinical and biochemical phenotype.

Since mutations in either procollagen gene have been detected in all four types of osteogenesis imperfecta and in two types of Ehlers–Danlos syndrome, clinical correlation is still required for diagnosis and prognosis. Type II osteogenesis imperfecta often produces thickened limb bones that can be recognized by skeletal radiography; early recognition is important because of very short, deformed limbs, and the limited lifespan and developmental potential. Survival of patients with type II osteogenesis imperfecta is often determined by the severity of rib fractures and deformities as related to respiratory sufficiency. The poor outlook for these children is magnified by the demonstration of impaired nerve cell migration in the brain due to prenatal vascular changes (Verkh et al., 1995). Children with type III osteogenesis imperfecta also exhibit increased mortality. Milder disease in children typical of type I or IV osteogenesis imperfecta warrants optimistic medical counseling, particularly since the frequency of fractures decreases after puberty.

Family and psychosocial counseling

Normal parents of children with type II osteogenesis imperfecta have a surprisingly high recurrence risk of 6% based on the incidence of germinal mosaicism. Parents of children with other types of osteogenesis imperfecta should be evaluated carefully, since affected individuals may not exhibit fractures or blue sclerae. Skeletal radiographs may be warranted to separate affected parents with a 50% recurrence risk from unaffected parents with a negligible recurrence risk. Genetic referral and counseling is essential for these families.

Cole (1993) emphasized the psychosocial effects of osteogenesis imperfecta that result from the stigmatization of individuals as different from their peers. The altered lifestyle enforced by brittle bones will depend on the severity of disease and the number of affected family members, and strategies are available to aid families adjust to their social and work environment (Cole, 1993). Parent support and information can be obtained from the Osteogenesis Imperfecta Foundation (www.oif.org/) or Osteogenesis Imperfecta Foundation Europe (www.oife.org/). These parent group organizations are very helpful in providing information on psychosocial adjustment and diagnostic testing.

Natural history and complications

The complications of osteogenesis imperfecta vary greatly by type. Patients with type II disease are often recognized prenatally, and exhibit extremely short stature with multiple prenatal fractures. Their sclerae will be dark gray or blue, and the skeletal and central nervous system complications listed on the checklist are extremely severe. Patients with other types of osteogenesis imperfecta may be difficult to recognize in the neonatal period. Many present in early childhood for evaluation of short stature or recurrent fractures.

The usual phenotype in osteogenesis imperfecta consists of short stature with relative macrocephaly, small nose and chin with blue sclerae and abnormal teeth, joint laxity with dislocations, limb bowing, or kyphoscoliosis, hearing loss that increases with age, and easy bruisability. Less common complications include basilar impression with brainstem damage (Sawin & Menezes, 1997), communicating hydrocephalus with basilar impression of the skull, seizures, aortic root dilatation or mitral valve prolapse, abdominal pain with constipation from acetabular protrusion, and renal calculi. Rarely, patients may have complications typical of weakened connective tissue such as retinal detachment or aortic or cerebral aneurysm.

Osteogenesis imperfecta preventive medical checklist

Preventive management for the osteogenesis imperfectas will primarily focus on the skeletal, nervous, and vascular systems. A complete skeletal radiologic survey should be performed as soon as the diagnosis is suspected, both for diagnosis and to evaluate bony deformities that may require treatment. Key issues in early management include appropriate developmental support in children with propensity to fractures, avoidance of immunization sites in fracture-prone areas, and close monitoring with dentistry for signs of excessive tooth wear or misalignment because of fragile teeth (dentinogenesis imperfecta).

Binder et al. (1993) described the value of comprehensive rehabilitation of children with osteogenesis imperfecta, emphasizing gain of head and trunk control using physical supports such as internal and external bracing. Even children with severe osteogenesis imperfecta, limited by joint contractures, impaired balance, and low endurance, showed continued improvement after 10 years of physical rehabilitation. Referrals to orthopedic and physical medicine should accompany regular pediatric evaluation of skeletal growth and alignment, and early intervention is important for reasons of physical and occupational therapy.

Neurologic complications include communicating hydrocephalus, basilar skull invagination, skull fracture, spinal cord compression, and seizures (Sawin & Menezes, 1997): neurologic assessment should be part of the regular pediatric examination with periodic neurology referrals for patients with severe disease. Symptoms of basilar invagination included headache (76%), lower cranial nerve dysfunction (68%), hyperreflexia (56%), quadriparesis (48%), ataxia (32%), nystagmus (28%), and scoliosis (20%; Sawin & Menezes, 1997). Basilar invagination was a significant cause of death for patients with more severe forms of osteogenesis imperfecta, along with restrictive lung disease and congestive heart failure secondary to severe kyphoscoliosis.

Short stature is the rule for osteogenesis imperfecta, and increased growth velocity after growth hormone therapy in several studies justifies endocrinology referral for children with severe short stature. Early and regular assessment of hearing and vision is also recommended because of sensorineural hearing loss, retinal detachment, and myopia that is frequent in osteogenesis imperfecta. Although congenital heart disease is not common, later aortic dilatation and mitral valve prolapse warrant careful cardiac examination during pediatric follow-up and formal cardiac assessment in adolescence or early adulthood.

Newer therapies for the severe osteoporosis that accompanies osteogenesis imperfecta include intravenous pamidronate and biphosphonates (Dimeglio et al., 2005); calcium should be monitored since hypercalcemia may occur.

Preventive management for skeletal dysplasias

Description: Skeletal dysplasias refer to abnormal growth (dysplasia) of the skeleton, and comprise more than 100 different disorders. Skeletal dysplasias exhibit disproportionate short stature (dwarfism), with an aggregate incidence of at least 1 in 10,000 births.

Clinical: Typical findings include prenatal onset of short length with proportionately larger head size and subsequent short stature. Typical facial changes are present in some types of skeletal dysplasia, including flattening or asymmetry of the skull, large soft spot (fontanel), prominent forehead, shallow nasal bridge, and small or upturned nose. Skeletal findings depend on the type of dysplasia and can include short neck, short trunk, short proximal segments (rhizomelia), middle segments (mesomelia) or tips (acromelia) of the extremities, small or bell-shaped chest, spinal curvature (scoliosis or gibbus), hip deviation or dislocation, bowing at the knees, and short or deviated digits with occasional polydactyly (extra thumb or finger).

Laboratory: The diagnosis is made by skeletal radiologic survey, a series of X-rays covering the entire body so that changes in skull, neck, spine, hips, and extremities can be documented and compared to standard types. The causative genes are known for most skeletal dysplasias, but there are as yet few blood DNA tests available. Testing is available for achondroplasia and its variants.

Genetics: Skeletal dyplasias are usually caused by single gene mutations and can exhibit autosomal-dominant-recessive, or X-linked inheritance. Many, like achondroplasia, are dominant and represent a new mutation in the child and a low recurrence risk for parents. Recessive or X-linked disorders may have a 25% or 1 in 4 recurrence risk for future pregnancies.

Key management issues: Monitoring of head circumference (to exclude hydrocephalus), hearing (because of frequent otitis and conductive hearing loss), sleep (because of spinal cord compression or hydrocephalus with sleep apnea), development (because lax connective tissue and low muscle tone often causes delays), and skeletal growth (because of frequent limb and spinal deformities). Marked motor delays may represent spinal cord compression with exaggerated low muscle tone, particularly in the lower limbs. Early ophthalmology examination is useful for some forms of skeletal dysplasia.

Specific growth charts: Available for height, weight, head circumference for achondroplasia, not for most others.

Parent information: Little People of America (www.lpaonline.org/) has national and local chapters with parent group meetings and excellent resources.

Basis for management recommendations: The Committee on Genetics, American Academy of Pediatrics (1995) has formulated consensus guidelines for achondroplasia that can be followed for similar forms of dwarfism.

Summary of clinical concerns

General	Behavior	Risk for depression in later childhood
	Growth	Short stature (ranging from the low-normal range to 3½–4 ft).
Facial	Eyes	Retinal detachment, cataracts, strabismus in some types
	Ears	Recurrent otitis media
	Nose	Shallow nasal bridge, narrow nasal passages with chronic congestion
	Mouth	Small jaw with Robin anomaly, cleft palate
Surface	Neck/trunk	Short neck, cervical vertebral fusion, neck injury with anesthesia or collision sports
Skeletal	Cranial	Macrocephaly, platybasia, narrow foramen magnum
	Axial	Spinal stenosis, cervical spine anomalies, kyphosis, scoliosis
	Limbs	Rhizomelic shortening, genu vara, joint laxity, arthritis, joint injuries
Internal	Pulmonary	Restrictive disease due to small chest, apnea and tachypnea, pneumonias, tracheal stenosis
	Circulatory	Heart defects in certain types, including arrhythmias
	Endocrine	Growth hormone therapy may be considered
	RES	Immune deficiency with risks for overwhelming viral sepsis, severe varicella
	Excretory	Renal defects including cystic kidneys, urinary tract obstructions
	Genital	Narrow pelvis, uterine fibroids, metrorrhagia
Neural	Central	Altered CSF circulation, hydrocephalus, cervical cord compression, sleep apnea
	Motor	Hypotonia, oromotor dysfunction, motor delays, increased reflexes with cord compression
	Sensory	Vision and hearing deficits

CSF, cerebrospinal fluid; RES, reticuloendothelial system; **concerns** of frequency >20% are **highlighted**

Key references

Apajasalo, et al. (1998). Health-related quality of life of patients with genetic skeletal dysplasias. *European Journal of Pediatrics* 157:114–21.

Committee on Genetics 1994–5, American Academy of Pediatrics (1995). Health supervision for children with achondroplasia. *Pediatrics* 95:443–51.

Sawin & Menezes (1997). Basilar invagination in osteogenesis imperfecta and related osteochondrodysplasias: medical and surgical management. *Journal of Neurosurgery* 86:950–60.

General skeletal dysplasia

Preventive medical checklist (0–3 years)

Name _____ Birth date __/__/____ Number _____

Age	Evaluations: key concerns	Management considerations	Notes
New-born ↓ 1 month	Skeletal examination: head, jaw, spine, limbs Hearing, vision:[2] cataracts, retinoschisis Feeding: poor intake, hypotonia Respiratory: small chest, restricted lungs Heart: murmur, tachycardia Parental adjustment: palliative care	❑ Skeletal survey;[1] DNA studies ❑ ❑ ABR; ophthalmology[3] ❑ ❑ Feeding specialist, video swallow[3] ❑ ❑ Blood gases, chest X-ray, pulmonology[3] ❑ ❑ Echocardiogram;[3] cardiology[3] ❑ ❑ Family support;[4] genetics ❑	A skeletal read by an experienced pediatric radiologist is the key to diagnosis
2 months ↓ 4 months	Growth and development:[5] head size Hearing and vision:[2] otitis, strabismus Feeding: poor intake, hypotonia Skeletal: jaw, thorax, spine, hips, limbs Neck flexibility:[2] C-spine anomalies Spinal compression: sleep apnea[7] Other:	❑ ECI;[6] family support[4] ❑ ❑ ABR;[3] ophthalmology;[3] ENT[3] ❑ ❑ Feeding specialist; video swallow[3] ❑ ❑ Orthopedics;[3] neurosurgery[3] ❑ ❑ Spinal X-rays; anesthesia precautions ❑ ❑ Head, foramen magnum MRI;[3] sleep study[3] ❑ ❑ ENT[3] ❑	Increased reflexes, small foramen magnum, central apnea on sleep study are the best indicators for basilar skull surgery
6 months ↓ 9 months	Growth and development:[5] head size Hearing and vision:[2] otitis, strabismus Skeletal: jaw, thorax, spine, hips, limbs Neck flexibility:[2] C-spine anomalies Spinal compression: sleep apnea[7] Other:	❑ ECI;[6] family support[4] ❑ ❑ Ophthalmology;[3] ENT[3] ❑ ❑ Orthopedics;[3] neurosurgery[3] ❑ ❑ Spinal X-rays;[3] anesthesia precautions ❑ ❑ Head, foramen magnum MRI;[3] sleep study[3] ❑ ❑ ❑	
1 year	Growth and development:[5] head size Hearing and vision:[2] otitis, strabismus Skeletal: jaw, thorax, spine, hips, limbs Neck flexibility:[2] C-spine anomalies Spinal compression: sleep apnea[7] Immunity: poor T-cell function Other:	❑ ECI;[6] family support[4] ❑ ❑ Ophthalmology;[3] ENT[3] ❑ ❑ Orthopedic team; orthotics;[3] neurosurgery[3] ❑ ❑ Spinal X-rays;[3] anesthesia precautions ❑ ❑ Head, foramen magnum MRI;[3] sleep study[3] ❑ ❑ Postpone live vaccines[3] ❑ ❑ ❑	
15 months ↓ 18 months	Growth and development:[5] head size Hearing and vision:[2] otitis, strabismus Skeletal: jaw, thorax, spine, hips, limbs Spinal compression: sleep apnea[7]	❑ ECI;[6] family support[4] ❑ ❑ Ophthalmology;[3] ENT[3] ❑ ❑ Orthopedic team; orthotics;[3] neurosurgery[3] ❑ ❑ Spinal X-rays;[3] anesthesia precautions ❑	
2 years	Growth and development:[5] head size Hearing and vision:[2] otitis, strabismus Skeletal: jaw, thorax, spine, hips, limbs Spinal compression: sleep apnea[7] Neck flexibility:[2] C-spine anomalies	❑ ECI;[6] family support[4] ❑ ❑ ABR[3] ophthalmology;[3] ENT[3] ❑ ❑ Orthopedic team; orthotics;[3] neurosurgery[3] ❑ ❑ Head, foramen magnum MRI;[3] sleep study[3] ❑ ❑ Spinal X-rays;[3] anesthesia precautions ❑	
3 years	Growth and development[5] Hearing and vision:[2] otitis, strabismus Skeletal: jaw, thorax, spine, hips, limbs Spinal compression: sleep apnea[7] Neck flexibility:[2] C-spine anomalies Respiratory: small chest, restricted lungs Other:	❑ ECI;[6] family support[4] ❑ ❑ Repeat ABR[3] ophthalmology;[3] ENT[3] ❑ ❑ Orthopedic team; orthotics;[3] neurosurgery[3] ❑ ❑ Head, foramen magnum MRI;[3] sleep study[3] ❑ ❑ Spinal X-rays;[3] anesthesia precautions ❑ ❑ Blood gases, chest X-ray, pulmonology[3] ❑ ❑ ❑	

Skeletal dysplasia concerns		Other concerns from history	
Poor feeding from hypotonia Small chest, lung disease Vision, hearing deficits Cataracts, strabismus Chronic otitis, Small jaw Cardiac anomalies	Short neck, spinal fusions Limb shortening, bowling Kyphoscoliosis, gibbus Narrow foramen magnum Sleep apnea, airway obstruction Motor and speech delay	**Family history/prenatal** _____ _____ _____ _____	**Social/environmental** _____ _____ _____ _____

Guidelines for the neonatal period should be undertaken *at whatever age* the diagnosis is made; ABR, auditory brainstem evoked response; C-spine, cervical spine; [1]to determine distribution of bony anomalies and type of skeletal dysplasia – may need to repeat at age 6–12 months for diagnosis; lethal dysplasias imply palliative care; [2]by practitioner; [3]as dictated by clinical findings; [4]Little People of America for education, medical consultation, and family adaptation to short stature and/or physical disabilities; genetic counseling; [5]consider developmental pediatrician/neurologist/genetics clinic according to symptoms and availability; [6]early childhood intervention with occupational therapy for children with significant hypotonia; [7]snoring, pause in breathing, daytime sleepiness, unusual sleep positioning.

Skeletal dysplasia

Preventive medical checklist (4–18 years)

Name _____ Birth date __/__/____ Number _____

Age	Evaluations: key concerns	Management considerations		Notes
4 years ↓ **6 years**	Growth:[1] head size Development:[2] preschool transition Hearing and vision:[2] myopia, retinoschisis Skeletal: jaw, neck, thorax, spine, limbs Neck flexibility:[2] C-spine anomalies Spinal compression: sleep apnea[7] Other:	❏ Endocrinology[1,3] ❏ Family support;[4] preschool program[5] ❏ Audiology;[3] ophthalmology;[3] ENT[3] ❏ Orthopedic team; orthotics;[3] neurosurgery[3] ❏ Spinal X-rays;[3] anesthesia precautions ❏ Head, foramen magnum MRI;[3] sleep study[3] ❏	❏ ❏ ❏ ❏ ❏ ❏ ❏	
7 years ↓ **9 years**	Growth:[1] short stature Development:[1] school transition[5] Hearing and vision:[2] myopia, retinoschisis Skeletal: jaw, neck, thorax, spine, limbs Neck flexibility:[2] C-spine anomalies Spinal compression: sleep apnea[7] Other:	❏ Endocrinology[1,3] ❏ Family support;[4] school progress[6] ❏ Audiology;[3] ophthalmology;[3] ENT[3] ❏ Orthopedic team; orthotics;[3] neurosurgery[3] ❏ Anesthesia precautions ❏ Head, foramen magnum MRI;[3] sleep study[3] ❏	❏ ❏ ❏ ❏ ❏ ❏ ❏	
10 years ↓ **12 years**	Growth and development[1] Hearing and vision:[2] myopia, retinoschisis Skeletal: jaw, neck, thorax, spine, limbs Neck flexibility:[2] C-spine anomalies Other:	❏ School progress;[6] endocrinology[1,3] ❏ Audiology;[3] ophthalmology;[3] ENT[3] ❏ Orthopedic team; orthotics;[3] neurosurgery[3] ❏ Anesthesia precautions ❏	❏ ❏ ❏ ❏ ❏	
13 years ↓ **15 years**	Growth and development[1] Hearing and vision:[2] myopia, retinoschisis Puberty, nutrition: obesity Skeletal: jaw, neck, thorax, spine, limbs Spinal compression: sleep apnea[7] Other:	❏ School progress;[6] endocrinology[1,3] ❏ Audiology,[3] ophthalmology ❏ Dietary counsel; activities; exercise ❏ Orthopedic team; orthotics;[3] neurosurgery[3] ❏ Head, foramen magnum MRI;[3] sleep study[3] ❏	❏ ❏ ❏ ❏ ❏ ❏	
16 years ↓ **18 years**	Growth and development[1] Hearing and vision:[2] myopia, retinoschisis Puberty, nutrition: obesity Skeletal: jaw, neck, thorax, spine, limbs Other:	❏ Family support;[4] school progress[6] ❏ Audiology,[3] ophthalmology ❏ Dietary counsel; activities; exercise ❏ Orthopedic team; orthotics;[3] neurosurgery[3] ❏	❏ ❏ ❏ ❏ ❏	
19 years ↓ **23 years**	Adult care transition:[6] body image Hearing and vision:[2] myopia, retinoschisis Activity: obesity, arthritis Skeletal: jaw, neck, thorax, spine, limbs Spinal compression: sleep apnea[7]	❏ Family support;[4] school progress[6] ❏ Audiology,[3] ophthalmology ❏ Dietary counsel; exercise; rheumatology ❏ Orthopedic team; orthotics;[3] neurosurgery[3] ❏ Head, foramen magnum MRI;[3] sleep study[3]	❏ ❏ ❏ ❏ ❏	
Adult	Adult care transition[6] Hearing and vision:[2] myopia, retinoschisis Activity: obesity, arthritis Skeletal: jaw, neck, thorax, spine, limbs Spinal compression: sleep apnea[7] Depression, reproductive concerns Other:	❏ Family support[4] ❏ Audiology,[3] ophthalmology ❏ Dietary counsel; exercise; rheumatology ❏ Orthopedic team; orthotics;[3] neurosurgery[3] ❏ Head MRI;[3] neurosurgery;[3] sleep study[3] ❏ Psychiatry;[3] maternal–fetal medicine[3] ❏	❏ ❏ ❏ ❏ ❏ ❏ ❏	

Skeletal dysplasia concerns		Other concerns from history	
Obesity, activity Vision, hearing deficits Cataracts, strabismus Small chest, lung disease Cardiac anomalies Immune deficiencies	Short neck, spinal fusions Limb shortening, bowing Scoliosis, kyphosis, gibbus Narrow foramen magnum Sleep apnea Arthritis	**Family history/prenatal** _____ _____ _____ _____	**Social/environmental** _____ _____ _____ _____

Guidelines for the neonatal period should be undertaken *at whatever age* the diagnosis is made; [1]to developmental pediatrics or genetics clinic and orthopedic team according to symptoms and availability; [2]by practitioner; [3]as dictated by clinical findings – endocrinology and growth hormone therapy should be considered; [4]Little People of America for education, medical consultation, and family adaptation to short stature and/or physical disabilities; genetic counseling; [5]preschool program including developmental monitoring and motor/speech therapy for those with cognitive delays; [6]monitor individual education and exercise plans, academic progress, behavioral differences including depression, later vocational planning with appliances and supports; [7]snoring, pause in breathing, daytime sleepiness, unusual sleep positioning.

Parent guide to skeletal dysplasias

The term "skeletal dysplasia" refers to abnormal skeletal growth and is a prime characteristic of more than 100 genetic disorders. Skeletal dysplasia refers to the skeleton as a whole, while individual affected bones may be described as "dysostoses." Most patients will have abnormal proportions of trunk and limbs as distinguished by the term "dwarfism." Names for skeletal dysplasias may reflect the physician who recognized them (e.g., Conradi disease) or the skeletal regions affected: chondro- for cartilage, osteo- for bone, cranio- for skull, spondylo- or vertebro- for spine, cleido- for clavicle, costo- for rib, coxo- for hi; rhizo-, meso-, acro- for respective proximal, middle, or distal limb segments; diaphyseal, metaphyseal, epiphyseal for respective shaft, end, or growth plate of a limb bone. Thus a name like spondyloepiphyseal dysplasia (SED) indicates abnormality of the spine and limb growth plates.

Incidence, causation, and diagnosis

The incidence of skeletal dysplasias as a group is at least 1 in 10,000, with achondroplasia (literally, poor cartilage growth) being the most common at about 1 in 20,000 births. Skeletal dysplasias can exhibit autosomal-dominant (e.g., cleidocranial dysostosis), autosomal-recessive (e.g., Jeune syndrome), X-linked-dominant (e.g., Conradi–Hunerman syndrome), or X-linked-recessive inheritance (e.g., oto–palato–digital syndrome). Many have been traced to specific genes that control skeletal growth or formation, like the fibroblast growth factor-3 receptor gene in achondroplasia or the collagen genes in SED or osteogenesis imperfecta. The key to diagnosis is still a skeletal radiographic survey that looks at skull and all bones of the spine, hips, and limbs. In many cases, the skeletal survey will not be diagnostic at young ages, and serial evaluations may be required. If a specific skeletal dysplasia is suspected based on family history or skeletal survey, then DNA analysis can substantiate the diagnosis for those disorders for which genes are characterized.

Natural history and complications

Most children with skeletal dysplasia will have normal intellectual potential, but many will have low muscle tone (hypotonia) as part of their connective tissue problem. Many of the disorders will be like achondroplasia, having a proportionately larger head with prominent forehead (frontal bossing), shallow nasal bridge, and a flattened skull base (platybasia) with a short neck. These changes mandate alertness for neurologic complications from a small foramen magnum (opening in the bottom of the skull that admits the spinal cord) that causes risks for compression of the brainstem and upper spinal cord. Symptoms of upper spinal compression may include apnea (cessation of breathing), during sleep, low muscle tone and developmental delay, or even sudden death. This compression may also be associated with hydrocephalus (accumulation of fluid in brain cavities), causing increased intracranial venous pressure by interference with venous flow out of the brain. Another common problem is a small chest cage because of altered growth of spine and ribs. These children may have difficulty maintaining normal oxygen levels at night or during intercurrent infections, and may need pulmonary function studies. The most obvious complications will be deformities of the affected bones, including the skull (asymmetry), neck (instability of the cervical vertebrae or poor neck mobility), spine (curving as scoliosis or humping as kyphosis or gibbus), hips (dislocations or deviation of the legs outward with subsequent arthritis), and limbs (curvature or contractures that cause deformities). The short stature accompanying many of the disorders may be lessened by growth hormone therapy, and children with milder dysplasias should be evaluated by endocrinology at ages 3–4 years to consider options. A large variety of other organs can be affected in the skeletal dysplasias, including the eyes (cataracts, changes in the retina), nose (small nasal passages with obstruction), ears (otitis, abnormal ear structures), jaw (small with posterior cleft – Robin sequence – that causes breathing problems when supine), heart (various congenital defects), kidneys (cysts or altered urinary tract with frequent infections), and immune system (low cellular immunity causing severe or lethal infections with chicken pox, live vaccines like chicken pox, etc.).

Preventive medical needs

If a specific diagnosis can be determined, then various medical education websites or the Online Mendelian Inheritance in Man database (www.ncbi.nlm.nih.gov/entrez) an define the likely complications for a particular skeletal dysplasia syndrome. Monitoring of early motor development, feeding, and linear growth are obvious strategies, with alertness for brain and upper spinal cord compression, head circumference, and skeletal deformities being more particular to the skeletal dysplasia category. Physicians should consider whether live vaccines like chicken pox should be given, and ask about symptoms of sleep apnea such as gasping, stridor, daytime somnolence, and abnormal sleep positioning. Children with large heads like those with achondroplasia will need additional head support during handling, avoiding devices that artificially prop the infant or give poor support, for example, umbrella strollers, baby walkers, and certain types of infant swings. Normal infant activity will not cause damage and should not be restricted. Alertness for associated malformations of the eyes, ears, heart, and kidneys should be maintained.

Family counseling

Inheritance risks will depend on the specific diagnosis, with 25% recurrence risk as a worst-case scenario for normal parents of an undiagnosed child. Prenatal diagnosis may be available by ultrasound for severe dysplasias, but usually will require DNA testing to be available in early–mid-pregnancy (see www.genetest.org for available testing). The Little People of America organization (www.lpaonline.org/) can be tremendously helpful for parent support, for improving self-image of affected children, for locating expert consultations, and for matching up families with rare dysplasias.

Preventive management for achondroplasia

Description: Achondroplasia and its milder allelic variant hypochondroplasia are patterns of disproportionate skeletal growth (dwarfism) with an incidence of 1 in 16,000–25,000 live births.

Clinical diagnosis: Pattern of skeletal changes including short stature caused by disproportionately short limbs due to small proximal segments (rhizomelia), large heads with prominent forehead (frontal bossing), shallow nasal bridge, small upper chest, deformities of the limbs (bowing) or spine (scoliosis, kyphosis), broad hands with splayed fingers (trident hands), and distinctive features on skeletal X-rays that include narrow thorax, progressively narrowinging tervertebral spaces from thoracic to lumbar vertebrae, rounded (ping-pong paddle) pelvic wings, sharply angled sacro-sciatic notch, and short limbs.

Laboratory diagnosis: DNA analysis to demonstrate characteristic mutations in the fibroblast growth factor-3 receptor

Genetics: Autosomal-dominant inheritance predicting a 50% recurrence risk for affected individuals; achondroplast couples also have a 25% risk for severely affected homozygotes.

Key management issues: Monitor head circumference, muscle tone, and development to recognize cervicomedullary spinal compression; consider head MRI, radiographs to evaluate hydrocephalus, upper spinal compression by foramen magnum audiology and ENT evaluation for hearing and chronic otitis, orthopedic monitoring for limb bowing and scoliosis, dietary counsel and weight control to minimize later arthritis and lower spinal cord compression.

Growth charts: Horton, et al. (1978); Committee on Genetic (1995).

Parent groups: Little People of America (www.achondroplasia.co.uk/), Achondroplasias United Kingdom (www.achondroplasia.co.uk/).

Basis for management recommendations: Consensus guidelines from the Committee on Genetics (1995) and the complications summarized below.

Summary of clinical concerns

General	Aging	Sudden infant death (5%)
	Behavior	Risk for depression in older individuals
	Growth	Short stature (males average 130 cm, females average 123 cm)
Facial	Face	Frontal bossing
	Eyes	Myopia
	Ears	Otitis media (75–97%)
	Nose	Shallow nasal bridge
Surface	Neck/trunk	Neck injuries, cervical cord compression, spinal fusions
Skeletal	Cranial	Macrocephaly, platybasia, narrow foramen magnum, maxillary hypoplasia
	Axial	Spinal stenosis, kyphosis (20%), scoliosis (7%), anterior wedging of vertebral bodies, occipitalization of the first cervical vertebrae, horizontal acetabular margins, acute angle to sacrosciatic notch
	Limbs	Rhizomelic shortening, genu vara (15%) due to lax knee ligaments, short digits, limited elbow extension, generalized joint laxity, arthritis, joint injuries
Internal	Pulmonary	Restrictive disease (<3%), apnea
	Endocrine	Mild glucose intolerance, obesity, modest response to growth hormone therapy
	Genital	Narrow pelvis, uterine fibroids, metrorrhagia, requirements for cesarean section at delivery, increased prematurity in offspring
Neural	Central	Altered CSF circulation, hydrocephalus, cervical cord compression, sleep apnea
	Motor	Delayed milestones
	Sensory	Conductive and sensorineural hearing loss (70–90%)

CSF, Cerebrospinal fluid, **concerns** of frequency >20% are **highlighted**

Key references

Allanson J.E. & Hall J.G. (1986). Obstetric and gynecologic problems in women with chondrodystrophies. *Obstetrics and Gynecology* 67:74–8.

Committee on Genetics, American Academy of Pediatrics (1995). *Pediatrics* 95:443–51; (www.aap.org/policy/).

Haga, N. (2004). Management of disabilities associated with achondroplasia. *Journal of Orthopaedic Science* 9:103–7.

Horton, et al. (1978). Standard growth curves for achondroplasia. *Journal of Pediatrics* 93:435–8.

Pauli, et al. (1995). Prospective assessment of risks for cervicomedullary-junction compression in infants with achondroplasia. *American Journal of Human Genetics* 56:732–44.

Achondroplasia

Preventive medical checklist (0–3 years)

Name _____ Birth date __/__/___ Number _____

Age	Evaluations: key concerns	Management considerations	Notes
Newborn ↓ 1 month	Skeletal examination: head, neck, spine, limbs Hearing, vision:[2] cataracts Feeding: poor intake, hypotonia Respiratory: small chest, restricted lungs Parental adjustment	❑ Skeletal survey;[1] head sonogram ❑ ❑ ABR; ophthalmology[3] ❑ ❑ Feeding specialist; video swallow[3] ❑ ❑ Blood gases; chest X-ray; pulmonology[3] ❑ ❑ Family support;[4] genetics ❑	
2 months ↓ 4 months	Growth and development:[5] head size Hearing and vision:[2] otitis, strabismus Feeding: poor intake, hypotonia Skeletal: neck, spine, limbs, hips Neck flexibility[2] Spinal compression: sleep apnea[7] Other:	❑ Achondroplasia charts; ECI;[6] family support[6] ❑ ❑ ABR;[3] ophthalmology;[3] ENT[3] ❑ ❑ Feeding specialist; video swallow[3] ❑ ❑ Orthopedic team; orthotics;[3] neurosurgery[3] ❑ ❑ Anesthesia precautions ❑ ❑ Head, foramen magnum MRI;[3] sleep study[3] ❑ ❑ ENT[3] ❑	Increased reflexes, small foramen magnum, central apnea on sleep study are the best indicators for basilar skull surgery
6 months ↓ 9 months	Growth and development[5] Hearing and vision:[2] otitis, strabismus Skeletal: neck, spine, limbs, hips Spinal compression: sleep apnea[7] Neck flexibility Other:	❑ ECI;[6] family support[4] ❑ ❑ ABR;[3] ophthalmology;[3] ENT[3] ❑ ❑ Orthopedic team; orthotics;[3] neurosurgery[3] ❑ ❑ Head, foramen magnum MRI;[3] sleep study[3] ❑ ❑ Anesthesia precautions; support head ❑ ❑ ❑	
1 year	Growth and development[5] Hearing and vision:[2] otitis, strabismus Skeletal: neck, spine, limbs, hips Spinal compression: sleep apnea[7] Sleep: sleep apnea[7] Neck flexibility Other:	❑ Achondroplasia charts; ECI;[6] family support[4] ❑ ❑ ABR;[3] ophthalmology;[3] ENT[3] ❑ ❑ Orthopedic team; orthotics;[3] neurosurgery[3] ❑ ❑ Orthopedic team; orthotics[3] ❑ ❑ Head, foramen magnum MRI;[3] sleep study[3] ❑ ❑ Anesthesia precautions; support head ❑ ❑ ❑	
15 months ↓ 18 months	Growth and development[5] Hearing and vision:[2] otitis, strabismus Skeletal: neck, spine, limbs, hips Spinal compression: sleep apnea[7]	❑ ECI;[6] family support[4] ❑ ❑ ABR;[3] ophthalmology;[3] ENT[3] ❑ ❑ Orthopedic team; orthotics;[3] neurosurgery[3] ❑ ❑ Head, foramen magnum MRI;[3] sleep study[3] ❑	
2 years	Growth and development[5] Hearing and vision:[2] otitis, strabismus Skeletal examination: head size, hips, limbs Spinal compression: sleep apnea[7] Neck flexibility	❑ ECI;[6] family support[4] ❑ ❑ ABR;[3] ophthalmology;[3] ENT[3] ❑ ❑ Orthopedic team; orthotics;[3] neurosurgery[3] ❑ ❑ Head, foramen magnum MRI;[3] sleep study[3] ❑ ❑ Anesthesia precautions; support head ❑	
3 years	Growth and development[5] Hearing and vision:[2] otitis, strabismus Skeletal: neck, spine, limbs, hips Spinal compression: sleep apnea[7] Neck flexibility Other:	❑ Achondroplasia charts; ECI;[6] family support[4] ❑ ❑ Audiology; ophthalmology;[3] ENT[3] ❑ ❑ Orthopedic team; orthotics;[3] neurosurgery[3] ❑ ❑ Head, foramen magnum MRI;[3] sleep study[3] ❑ ❑ Anesthesia precautions; support head ❑ ❑ ❑	

Achondroplasia concerns		Other concerns from history	
Poor feeding from hypotonia Small chest, lung disease Vision, hearing deficits Chronic otitis, dental anomalies Cardiac anomalies Short neck, spinal fusions	Limb shortening, bowing Scoliosis, gibbus Narrow foramen magnum Hydrocephalus, sleep apnea Motor and speech delay	**Family history/prenatal** _____ _____ _____ _____ _____	Social/environmental _____ _____ _____ _____ _____

Guidelines for the neonatal period should be undertaken *at whatever age* the diagnosis is made; ABR, auditory brainstem evoked response; [1] to determine distribution of bony anomalies and type of skeletal dysplasia – may need to repeat at age 6–12 months for diagnosis; [2] by practitioner; [3] as dictated by clinical findings; [4] Little People of America for education, medical consultation, and family adaptation; genetic counseling; [5] consider genetics clinic according to symptoms and availability; [6] early childhood intervention with occupational therapy for children with significant hypotonia; [7] snoring, pause in breathing, daytime sleepiness, unusual sleep positioning.

Achondroplasia

Preventive medical checklist (4–18 years)

Name _____ Birth date __/__/___ Number _____

Age	Evaluations: key concerns	Management considerations	Notes
4 years ↓ **6 years**	Growth:[1] short stature, head size Development:[2] preschool transition[5] Hearing: conductive loss, otitis Skeletal examination: spine, limb deformity Spinal compression: sleep apnea[7] Neck flexibility	❑ Adaptation;[6] endocrinology[3] ❑ ❑ Family support;[4] preschool program[5] ❑ ❑ Audiology; ENT[3] ❑ ❑ Orthopedic team; orthotics;[3] neurosurgery[3] ❑ ❑ Head, foramen magnum MRI;[3] sleep study[3] ❑ ❑ Anesthesia precautions ❑	
7 years ↓ **9 years**	Growth:[1] short stature, obesity School transition Hearing: conductive loss, otitis Skeletal examination: spine, limb deformity Spinal compression: sleep apnea[7] Neck flexibility Other:	❑ Achondroplasia charts; dietician; exercise ❑ ❑ School progress[6] ❑ ❑ Audiology; ENT[3] ❑ ❑ Orthopedic team; orthotics;[3] neurosurgery[3] ❑ ❑ Head, foramen magnum MRI;[3] sleep study[3] ❑ ❑ Anesthesia precautions ❑ ❑ ❑	
10 years ↓ **12 years**	Growth:[1] short stature, obesity Hearing: conductive loss, otitis Skeletal examination: spine, limbs, arthritis Spinal compression: sleep apnea[7] Other:	❑ Dietician; adaptation;[6] endocrinology[3] ❑ ❑ Audiology; ENT[3] ❑ ❑ Orthopedic team; orthotics;[3] rheumatology[3] ❑ ❑ Head, foramen magnum MRI;[3] sleep study[3] ❑ ❑ ❑	
13 years ↓ **15 years**	Growth:[1] short stature, obesity Hearing: conductive loss, otitis Skeletal examination: spine, limbs, arthritis Spinal compression: sleep apnea[7] Other:	❑ Achondroplasia charts; adaptation;[6] exercise ❑ ❑ Audiology; ENT[3] ❑ ❑ Orthopedic team; orthotics;[3] rheumatology[3] ❑ ❑ Head, foramen magnum MRI;[3] sleep study[3] ❑ ❑ ❑	
16 years ↓ **18 years**	Growth:[1] short stature, obesity Hearing: conductive loss, otitis Skeletal examination: spine, limbs, arthritis Spinal compression: sleep apnea[7] Other:	❑ Dietician; adaptation[6] ❑ ❑ Audiology; ENT[3] ❑ ❑ Orthopedic team; orthotics;[3] rheumatology[3] ❑ ❑ Head, foramen magnum MRI;[3] sleep study[3] ❑ ❑ ❑	
19 years ↓ **23 years**	Hearing: conductive loss, otitis Nutrition: obesity Skeletal examination: spine, limb deformity Spinal compression: sleep apnea[7] Females: metrorrhagia, pregnancy	❑ Audiology; ENT[3] ❑ ❑ Dietary counsel; activities; exercise ❑ ❑ Orthopedic team; orthotics[3] ❑ ❑ Head, foramen magnum MRI;[3] sleep study[3] ❑ ❑ Gynecology;[3] maternal–fetal medicine[3] ❑	
Adult	Hearing: conductive loss, otitis Nutrition: obesity Skeletal examination: spine, limbs, arthritis Spinal compression: sleep apnea[7] Females: metrorrhagia, pregnancy Adaptation:[6] depression Other:	❑ Audiology; ENT[3] ❑ ❑ Dietary counsel; activities; exercise ❑ ❑ Orthopedic team; orthotics;[3] rheumatology[3] ❑ ❑ Head, foramen magnum MRI;[3] sleep study[3] ❑ ❑ Gynecology;[3] maternal–fetal medicine[3] ❑ ❑ Psychiatry[3] ❑ ❑ ❑	

Achondroplasia concerns		Other concerns from history	
		Family history/prenatal	**Social/environmental**
Short stature Hearing deficits Chronic otitis, dental anomalies Limb shortening, bowing Scoliosis, gibbus Metrorrhagia	Hydrocephalus Narrow foramen magnum Narrow lower spine Sleep apnea Reproductive risks Depression, socialization	_____ _____ _____ _____	_____ _____ _____ _____

Guidelines for the neonatal period should be undertaken *at whatever age* the diagnosis is made; [1] to developmental pediatrics or genetics clinic and orthopedic team according to symptoms and availability – endocrinology and growth hormone therapy should be considered; [2] by practitioner; [3] as dictated by clinical findings; [4] Little People of America for education, medical consultation, and family adaptation to short stature and/or physical disabilities; genetic counseling; [5] preschool program including developmental monitoring and motor/speech therapy for those with cognitive delays, adaptations for short stature; [6] monitor individual education and exercise plans, academic progress, behavioral differences including depression, later vocational planning with appliances and supports; [7] snoring, pause in breathing, daytime sleepiness, unusual sleep positioning.

Parent guide to achondroplasia

The term "achondroplasia" refers to a condition with short stature, distinctive facial appearance, and short limbs. Hypochondroplasia is a similar disorder with a relatively normal face and milder skeletal changes than patients with achondroplasia.

Incidence, causation, and diagnosis

The incidence of achondroplasia is between 1 in 16,000 and 1 in 25,000 births, while that for hypochondroplasia is about 10-fold less. Both disorders result from mutations in different portions of the fibroblast growth factor-3 receptor gene. Patients with achondroplasia have rhizomelic (proximal) limb shortening, prominent forehead with shallow nasal bridge, and splayed or "trident" fingers. The differential is among other skeletal dyspasias with clinical findings and skeletal findings on X-ray making the diagnosis. DNA analysis can be pursued but is not usually required.

Natural history and complications

Normal intellectual potential mandates alertness for neurologic complications in achondroplasia. The large head, flattened base of the skull (platybasia), and small foramen magnum (opening in the bottom of the skull that admits the spinal cord) cause risks for compression of the brainstem and upper spinal cord. Symptoms may include apnea (cessation of breathing), during sleep, low muscle tone and developmental delay, or even sudden death. This compression may also be associated with hydrocephalus (accumulation of fluid in brain cavities), causing increased intracranial venous pressure by interference with venous flow out of the brain. Although all children with achondroplasia have some degree of low muscle tone and developmental delay, these problems are unusually severe in children with spinal cord compression. Changes in the vertebrae can produce spinal curvatures such as gibbus or kyphosis (forward curve) and scoliosis (sideways curve). Limbs may become bowed due to increased joint laxity and low muscle tone (hypotonia), resulting in bow legs or curved feet. Ear infections and significant hearing loss can occur, and studies of children showed frequencies of conductive hearing loss as great as 50%. Females have an increased incidence of uterine fibroids with heavy menstrual periods, and their narrow pelvis requires that delivery be performed by Cesarean section under general anesthesia. In hypochondroplasia, short stature and macrocephaly are less pronounced than in achondroplasia, and there is developmental disability in 10%. Limb bowing and lumbar lordosis also occur, but rarely require treatment. Chronic otitis or hearing loss has not been documented, but Cesarean section may be required for the delivery of pregnant females.

Preventive medical needs

Alertness for brain and upper spinal cord compression is essential, and the head circumference and motor development should be followed using charts specific for achondroplasia. Parents should be warned about the possibility of spontaneous or sleep-related apnea, and monitors provided when appropriate. Sleep disruptions, apnea, or disproportionate head growth require head MRI and select X-rays to evaluate brain and foramen magnum. Sleep studies and somatic evoked potentials, which measure the time required for back-and-forth impulse transmission through the foramen magnum, may be helpful in demonstrating functional spinal cord compression. Those children with demonstrated abnormalities should be followed with an apnea monitor and considered for surgery to enlarge the foramen magnum. There is currently some controversy about the timing and utility of surgical intervention. The medical advisory board for Little People of America can be helpful in these decisions, and are available for consultation at national conventions. Other concerns include preventive management for the skeletal system so that later bony deformities, arthritis, and lower spinal cord compressions can be minimized. Because of their disproportionately large head circumferences and joint laxity, children with achondroplasia need additional support during infancy. The head should be supported during handling and devices that artificially prop the infant or give poor support should be avoided. Such devices include umbrella strollers, baby walkers, and certain types of infant swings. Normal infant activity will not cause damage and should not be restricted. The degree of spinal curvature and other joint deformities should be monitored during childhood, and aggressive dietary management should be initiated in later childhood to avoid obesity that predisposes to nerve root compression and degenerative arthritis. Frequent ear infections and hearing loss mandate yearly hearing tests until the child is 3–4 years old. Newer therapies for dwarfism include growth hormone supplementation and surgical leg-lengthening procedures. Both are expensive, and the latter includes risks of infection or bony deformity.

Family counseling

Inheritance of achondroplasia and hypochondroplasia is autosomal dominant. For normal parents, the recurrence risk will be negligible but not zero due to the possibility that several eggs or sperm carry the achondroplasia mutation (germline mosaicism). Affected children will have a 50% risk for transmission and, if their spouse has achondroplasia, a 50% risk for a child with achondroplasia, a 25% risk for a child with lethal homozygous achondroplasia, and a 25% risk for a normal or "average-sized" child. The diagnosis of achondroplasia is increasingly made by fetal ultrasound, allowing earlier planning for and acceptance of a child with short stature. Positive literature on achondroplasia and other dwarfing conditions is available from the Little People of America. Discussion with other average-sized parents can be invaluable in fostering acceptance of the child with dwarfism. Though viewing adults with dwarfism may be difficult, the exposure to medical or psychosocial resources and the positive images promoted for their child warrant consideration of parent group contact.

Preventive management for osteogenesis imperfecta

Description: A group of disorders with increased bone fragility with incidence about 1 in 20,000 live births.

Clinical diagnosis: Four major phenotypes including type I osteogenesis imperfecta with short stature, fractures, deafness, and blue sclerae; type II with severe dwarfism, thick bones, deformed craniofacies, small chest and infantile death; type III with prominent limb bowing; and type IV with normal sclerae, fractures, and mild limb bowing.

Laboratory diagnosis: Cell culture demonstrating deficiency of type I collagen synthesis, DNA diagnosis defining characteristic mutations in type I collagen (all four clinical types).

Genetics: Autosomal-dominant inheritance with a 50% risk for transmitting the disease. Significant frequencies of germline mosaicism yield a 5–6% risk recurrence risk for normal parents.

Key management issues: Monitoring of skeletal growth and contour with initial skeletal radiologic survey; hearing assessments; avoidance of immunization sites near fractures; dental evaluations for signs of excessive tooth wear or misalignment; comprehensive rehabilitation with physical supports such as internal and external bracing; early intervention is important for reasons of physical and occupational therapy.

Growth charts: None.

Parent groups: Osteogenesis Imperfecta Foundation, Osteogenesis Imperfecta Foundation (www.oif.org/) or Osteogenesis Imperfecta Foundation Europe (www.oife.org/).

Basis for management recommendations: Derived from the complications listed below as documented by Binder et al. (1993).

Summary of clinical concerns

General	General	**Infant mortality** (90% mortality by age 1 month in type II)
	Growth	Short stature
	Tumors	Osteosarcoma
Facial	Eyes	Blue sclerae, embryotoxon, retinal detachment
	Ears	Conductive hearing loss in second, third decades
	Nose	Shallow nasal bridge, narrow nasal passages with chronic congestion
	Mouth	**Dental anomalies** (tooth discoloration, opalescent teeth (type IV), shortened dental roots, mandibular bone cysts)
Surface	Neck/trunk	**Easy bruisability** (75%), hernias
Skeletal	Cranial	**Macrocephaly**, Wormian bones, **platybasia**
	Axial	**Kyphosis, scoliosis** (20%)
	Limbs	**Multiple fractures**, short limbs (type II), limb bowing (type III), joint laxity, joint dislocations
Internal	Pulmonary	Restricted lung volume from rib fractures (type II)
	Circulatory	Aortic root dilatation (12%), mitral valve prolapse (9%)
	Digestive	Abdominal pain, constipation
	Excretory	Renal calculi
	Genital	Narrow pelvis, uterine fibroids, metrorrhagia
Neural	Central	**Basilar impression** (25%), hydrocephaly, cerebral aneurysm, spinal cord compression, seizures
	Motor	Nerve root compressions
	Sensory	**Sensorineural hearing loss** (50%), trigeminal neuralgia

Concerns of frequency >20% are **highlighted**

Key references

Binder, et al. (1993). Comprehensive rehabilitation of the child with osteogenesis imperfecta. *American Journal of Medical Genetics* 45:265–9.

Cole (1993). Psychosocial aspects of osteogenesis imperfecta: an update. *American Journal of Medical Genetics* 45:207–11.

Sawin & Menezes (1997). Basilar invagination in osteogenesis imperfecta and related osteochondrodysplasias: Medical and surgical management. *Journal of Neurosurgery* 86:950–60.

Osteogenesis imperfecta

Preventive medical checklist (0–3 years)

Name _____ **Birth date** ___/___/___ **Number** _____

Age	Evaluations: key concerns	Management considerations		Notes
New-born ↓ 1 month	Skeletal examination: head, spine, limbs Hearing, vision:[2] deafness, blue sclerae Respiratory: small chest, restricted lungs Heart: murmur, tachycardia Parental adjustment	❑ Skeletal survey;[1] orthopedics ❑ ABR; ophthalmology[3] ❑ Blood gases, chest X-ray; pulmonology[3] ❑ ❑ Echocardiogram;[3] cardiology[3] ❑ Family support;[4] genetics	❑ ❑ ❑ ❑	
2 months ↓ 4 months	Growth and development[5] Hearing, vision:[2] deafness, blue sclerae Respiratory: small chest, restricted lungs Skeletal examination: fractures, hips, limbs Hydrocephalus, basilar impression Other:	❑ ECI;[6] family support[4] ❑ ABR;[3] ophthalmology;[3] ENT[3] ❑ Feeding specialist; video swallow[3] ❑ Orthopedics[3] ❑ Head MRI;[3] neurosurgery[3] ❑	❑ ❑ ❑ ❑ ❑ ❑	
6 months ↓ 9 months	Growth and development:[5] head size Hearing, vision:[2] hearing loss Respiratory: small chest, restricted lungs Skeletal examination: fractures, hips, limbs Hydrocephalus, basilar impression Other:	❑ ECI;[6] family support[4] ❑ Ophthalmology;[3] ENT[3] ❑ Feeding specialist; video swallow[3] ❑ Orthopedics[3] ❑ Head MRI;[3] neurosurgery[3] ❑	❑ ❑ ❑ ❑ ❑ ❑	
1 year	Growth and development:[5] head size Hearing, vision:[2] hearing loss Respiratory: small chest, restricted lungs Skeletal examination: fractures, hips, limbs Hydrocephalus, basilar impression Neck flexibility Other:	❑ ECI;[6] family support[4] ❑ Ophthalmology;[3] ENT[3] ❑ Feeding specialist; video swallow[3] ❑ Orthopedics[3] ❑ Head MRI;[3] neurosurgery[3] ❑ Anesthesia precautions ❑	❑ ❑ ❑ ❑ ❑ ❑ ❑	
15 months ↓ 18 months	Growth and development:[5] head size Hearing, vision, teeth[2] Skeletal examination: head size, hips, limbs Hydrocephalus, basilar impression	❑ ECI;[6] family support[4] ❑ Dentistry; ophthalmology;[3] ENT[3] ❑ Orthopedics[3] ❑ Head MRI;[3] neurosurgery[3]	❑ ❑ ❑ ❑	
2 years	Growth and development:[5] head size Hearing, vision, teeth[2] Skeletal examination: head size, hips, limbs Hydrocephalus, basilar impression Neck flexibility	❑ ECI;[6] family support[4] ❑ Dentistry; ophthalmology;[3] ENT[3] ❑ Orthopedics[3] ❑ Head MRI;[3] neurosurgery[3] ❑ Anesthesia precautions	❑ ❑ ❑ ❑ ❑	
3 years	Growth and development:[5] head size Hearing, vision, teeth[2] Skeletal examination: head size, hips, limbs Hydrocephalus, basilar impression Neck flexibility Other:	❑ ECI;[6] family support[4] ❑ Dentistry; ophthalmology;[3] ENT[3] ❑ Orthopedics[3] ❑ Head MRI;[3] neurosurgery[3] ❑ Anesthesia precautions ❑	❑ ❑ ❑ ❑ ❑ ❑	

Osteogenesis imperfecta concerns		Other concerns from history	
Vision, hearing deficits Small chest, lung disease Dental anomalies Joint laxity, hernias Aortic dilation	Mitral valve prolapse Progressive scoliosis Short neck, spinal fractures Limb bowing Narrow foramen magnum	**Family history/prenatal** _____ _____ _____ _____	**Social/environmental** _____ _____ _____ _____

Guidelines for the neonatal period should be undertaken *at whatever age* the diagnosis is made; ABR, auditory brainstem evoked response; [1]to confirm diagnosis, type, and distribution of fractures; [2]by practitioner; [3]as dictated by clinical findings; [4]Parent group for education, medical consultation, and family adaptation; genetic counseling; [5]consider developmental pediatrician/neurologist/genetics clinic according to symptoms and availability; [6]early childhood intervention with occupational therapy for children with significant bone abnormalities, deafness, bowed limbs with motor delays.

Osteogenesis imperfecta

Preventive medical checklist (4–18 years)

Name _____ Birth date __/__/___ Number_____

Age	Evaluations: key concerns	Management considerations		Notes
4 years ↓ 6 years	Growth:[1] head size Development:[2] preschool transition Hearing, vision, teeth[2] Skeletal examination: scoliosis, hips, limbs Hydrocephalus, basilar impression Aortic dilation, mitral valve prolapse Other:	❏ Family support;[4] preschool program[5] ❏ Dentistry; ophthalmology;[3] ENT[3] ❏ Orthopedics[3] ❏ Head MRI;[3] neurosurgery[3] ❏ Cardiology;[3] echocardiogram[3] ❏ ❏	❏ ❏ ❏ ❏ ❏ ❏ ❏	
7 years ↓ 9 years	Growth and development:[5] head size Hearing, vision, teeth[2] Skeletal examination: scoliosis, hips, limbs Hydrocephalus, basilar impression Aortic dilation, mitral valve prolapse Neck flexibility Other:	❏ Family support;[4] school progress[6] ❏ Dentistry; ophthalmology;[3] ENT[3] ❏ Orthopedics[3] ❏ Head MRI;[3] neurosurgery[3] ❏ Cardiology;[3] echocardiogram[3] ❏ Anesthesia precautions ❏	❏ ❏ ❏ ❏ ❏ ❏ ❏	
10 years ↓ 12 years	Growth and development[1] Hearing, vision, teeth[2] Skeletal examination: scoliosis, hips, limbs Hydrocephalus, basilar impression Other:	❏ Family support;[4] school progress[6] ❏ Dentistry; ophthalmology;[3] ENT[3] ❏ Orthopedics[3] ❏ Head MRI;[3] neurosurgery[3] ❏	❏ ❏ ❏ ❏ ❏	
13 years ↓ 15 years	Growth and development[1] Hearing, vision, teeth[2] Skeletal examination: scoliosis, limbs, hernias Hydrocephalus, basilar impression Aortic dilation, mitral valve prolapse Other:	❏ Family support;[4] school progress[6] ❏ Dentistry; ophthalmology;[3] ENT[3] ❏ Orthopedics[3] ❏ Head MRI;[3] neurosurgery[3] ❏ Cardiology;[3] echocardiogram[3] ❏	❏ ❏ ❏ ❏ ❏ ❏	
16 years ↓ 18 years	Growth and development[1] Hearing, vision, teeth[2] Skeletal examination: scoliosis, limbs, hernias Hydrocephalus, basilar impression Other:	❏ Family support;[4] school progress[6] ❏ Dentistry; ophthalmology;[3] ENT[3] ❏ Orthopedics[3] ❏ Head MRI;[3] neurosurgery[3] ❏	❏ ❏ ❏ ❏ ❏	
19 years ↓ 23 years	Adult care transition[6] Hearing, vision, teeth[2] Skeletal examination: scoliosis, limbs, hernias Hydrocephalus, basilar impression	❏ Family support[4] ❏ Dentistry; ophthalmology;[3] ENT[3] ❏ Orthopedics[3] ❏ Head MRI;[3] neurosurgery[3]	❏ ❏ ❏ ❏	
Adult	Adult care transition[6] Hearing, vision, teeth[2] Skeletal examination: scoliosis, limbs, hernias Hydrocephalus, basilar impression Aortic dilation, mitral valve prolapse Other:	❏ Family support[4] ❏ Dentistry; ophthalmology;[3] ENT[3] ❏ Orthopedics[3] ❏ Head MRI;[3] neurosurgery[3] ❏ Cardiology;[3] echocardiogram[3] ❏	❏ ❏ ❏ ❏ ❏ ❏	

Osteogenesis imperfecta concerns		Other concerns from history	
Vision, hearing deficits Small chest, lung disease Dental anomalies Joint laxity, hernias Aortic dilation	Mitral valve prolapse Progressive scoliosis Short neck, spinal fractures Limb bowing Narrow foramen magnum	**Family history/prenatal** _____ _____ _____ _____	**Social/environmental** _____ _____ _____ _____

Guidelines for the neonatal period should be undertaken *at whatever age* the diagnosis is made; [1] consider neurologist/genetics clinic according to symptoms and availability; [2] by practitioner; [3] as dictated by clinical findings; [4] parent group, family/sib, financial, and behavioral issues with later focus on independent living and employment; [5] preschool program including monitoring for self-image problems and physical disabilities due to fractures; [6] monitor individual education plan, educational testing, academic progress, behavioral differences due to self-image problems, later vocational planning.

Parent guide to osteogenesis imperfecta

There are four major types of osteogenesis imperfecta, and more than a dozen additional syndromes include bone fragility as a component feature. Most common is type I osteogenesis imperfecta with short stature, fractures, blue sclerae, and normal life span. Perinatal lethal osteogenesis imperfecta is designated as type II, with types III (prominent limb bowing) and IV (normal sclerae) being intermediate in severity.

Incidence, causation, and diagnosis

The estimated prevalence of the major types of osteogenesis imperfecta is about 1 in 20,000 individuals. Differential diagnosis includes numerous syndromes with fragile bones and other unusual features. The presence of thin or deformed bones, fractures, blue sclerae (whites of the eyes), and hearing loss is strongly suggestive of osteogenesis imperfecta, particularly when there is a family history. Skeletal X-rays are often diagnostic, but biochemical and DNA testing for collagen abnormalities provide the most definitive diagnosis when they reveal an abnormality. Although DNA testing can be performed from blood samples, the variety of mutations in the osteogenesis imperfectas is too great to allow comprehensive screening. A better method for testing is to analyze collagen synthesis in cultured fibroblasts from skin biopsy. If an abnormality of collagen synthesis is detected in skin fibroblasts, then DNA testing for collagen gene abnormalities can be tried. Since mutations in type I collagen genes have been detected in all four types of osteogenesis imperfecta and in two types of Ehlers–Danlos syndrome, clinical correlation is still required for diagnosis and prognosis. Type II osteogenesis imperfecta is lethal and its thickened limb bones are often recognized by prenatal ultrasound. Children with type III osteogenesis imperfecta also exhibit increased mortality. Milder disease in children typical of types I or IV osteogenesis imperfecta warrants optimistic medical counseling since the frequency of fractures decreases after puberty.

Natural history and complications

The complications of osteogenesis imperfecta vary greatly by type. Patients with type II disease are often recognized prenatally, and exhibit extremely short stature with multiple prenatal fractures. Their sclerae (whites of the eyes) will be dark gray or blue, and the skeletal and central nervous system complications are extremely severe. Patients with other types of osteogenesis imperfecta may be difficult to recognize in the neonatal period. Many present in early childhood for evaluation of short stature or recurrent fractures. The usual phenotype in osteogenesis imperfecta consists of short stature with a relatively large head (macrocephaly), small nose and chin with blue sclerae and abnormal teeth, joint laxity with dislocations, limb bowing, spinal curvature (kyphoscoliosis), hearing loss that increases with age, and easy bruisability. Less common complications include brainstem damage or hydrocephalus (accumulation of fluid in brain cavities) due to skull abnormalities, seizures, dilation of large arteries (aortic aneurysm) or mitral valve prolapse, abdominal pain with constipation from protrusion of the hips into the abdomen, and kidney stones. Rarely, patients may have complications typical of weakened connective tissue such as retinal detachment or dilations of the aorta or cerebral arteries.

Preventive medical needs

Preventive management for the osteogenesis imperfectas will primarily focus on the skeletal, nervous, and vascular systems. A complete skeletal radiologic survey should be performed as soon as the diagnosis is suspected, both for diagnosis and to evaluate bony deformities that may require treatment. Key issues in early management include appropriate developmental support in children with propensity to fractures, avoidance of immunization sites in fracture-prone areas, and close monitoring with dentistry for signs of excessive tooth wear or misalignment because of fragile teeth (dentinogenesis imperfecta). Children with osteogenesis imperfecta should have a comprehensive rehabilitation program, emphasizing gain of head and trunk control using physical supports such as internal and external bracing. Even children with severe osteogenesis imperfecta, limited by joint contractures, impaired balance, and low endurance, show continued improvement after 10 years of physical rehabilitation. Referrals to orthopedic and physical medicine should accompany regular pediatric evaluation of skeletal growth and alignment, and early intervention is important for reasons of physical and occupational therapy. Neurologic assessment should be part of the regular pediatric examination, with periodic neurology referrals for patients with severe disease. Symptoms of skull compression of the brain included headache (76%), facial weaknesses due to cranial nerve dysfunction (68%), increased deep tendon reflexes (56%), weakness in the extremities (48%), unsteady gait and coordination (32%), trembling eye movements (nystagmus – 28%), and spinal curvature (20%) in one study. Short stature is the rule for osteogenesis imperfecta, and growth hormone therapy did increase growth velocity in several children. Early and regular assessment of hearing and vision is also recommended because of sensorineural hearing loss, retinal detachment, and myopia that is frequent in osteogenesis imperfecta. Later heart problems (aortic dilation and mitral valve prolapse) warrant cardiac assessment. Newer therapies for the severe osteoporosis that accompanies osteogenesis imperfecta include intravenous pamidronate and biphosphonates.

Family counseling

Normal parents of children with the severe type II osteogenesis imperfecta have a surprisingly high recurrence risk of 6% due to sperm or eggs that carry the mutation. Parents of children with other types of osteogenesis imperfecta should be evaluated carefully, since affected individuals may not exhibit fractures or blue sclerae. Skeletal radiographs may be warranted to separate affected parents with a 50% recurrence risk from unaffected parents with a negligible recurrence risk.

12

Overgrowth syndromes

Syndromes with increased growth are listed in Table 12.1. Several, including Beckwith–Wiedemann syndrome, exhibit increased fetal growth with a high birth weight. Others, like cerebral gigantism or Sotos syndrome, are more remarkable for accelerated postnatal growth. Often there is neuropathology manifested by macrocephaly, dilated ventricles, structural brain anomalies, or early hypotonia. Predisposition to neoplasia accompanies many overgrowth disorders, exemplified by the occurrence of Wilms tumor in Beckwith–Wiedemann, Sotos, and hemi-hyperplasia syndromes. Accelerated skeletal maturation during childhood is also common, suggesting that growth factors acting early in life provide a common pathogenetic mechanism.

Overgrowth is also found in certain chromosomal disorders (e.g., fragile X syndrome), metabolic disorders (e.g., pseudohypoparathyroidism and the mucopolysaccharidoses), or hamartosis syndromes that also have predisposition to cancer (e.g., neurofibromatosis type 1). These disorders are discussed in other chapters. Obesity may also be considered a form of overgrowth, and increased caloric intake may produce increased statural growth and skeletal maturation during childhood. The growth acceleration induced by hyperphagia is usually transient, however, as exemplified by the short adult stature in Prader–Willi syndrome. Here syndromes with sustained growth acceleration due to unknown etiologies are discussed, including detailed consideration of Beckwith–Wiedemann syndrome.

Börjeson–Forssman–Lehmann syndrome

Börjeson–Forssman–Lehmann syndrome is an X-linked-recessive disorder that involves facial, skeletal, and genital anomalies in addition to mental disability. Overgrowth in this condition consists mainly of obesity, since 80% of patients eventually display short stature (Gorlin et al., 2001, pp. 426–7) Skeletal anomalies include thickened calvaria, narrow spinal canal, epiphyseal dysplasia, and short distal phalanges. Neurologic problems include microcephaly, hypotonia, seizures (50%), and, in the eye, nystagmus and ptosis. Certain of the genital anomalies (small

Table 12.1. Overgrowth syndromes

Syndrome	Inheritance	Incidence[a]	Frequent abnormalities in addition to overgrowth
Hemihyperplasia	S	>200 cases	Asymmetry, neoplasms
Beckwith–Wiedemann	AD[b]	1 in 17,000	Cerebral, facial, cardiac, visceromegaly, GI, skeletal, endocrine, urinary tract, genital
Perlman		~30 cases	Visceromegaly, renal hamartomas, nephroblastomatosis, Wilms tumor
Sotos	S	>200 cases	Macrocephaly, hypotonia, accelerated osseous maturation
Weaver	AD	~20 cases	Macrocephaly, characteristic facies, accelerated osseous maturation developmental disability, joint contractures, hernias
Marshall–Smith	S	~20 cases	Macrocephaly, hypotonia, accelerated osseous maturation, failure to thrive, early death
Simpson–Golabi–Behmel	XLR	~30 cases	Macrocephaly, polydactyly, vertebral anomalies, cardiac conduction defects, genitourinary anomalies, early death
Cohen	AR	~80 cases	Microcephaly, hypotonia, obesity, ocular anomalies, tall stature, genital anomalies, happy affect
Börjeson–Forssman–Lehmann	XLR	~20 cases	Macrocephaly, hypotonia, obesity, hypogonadism

Notes:

S, sporadic; AD, autosomal dominant; AR, autosomal recessive; XLR, X-linked recessive; GI, gastrointestinal.

[a] Cases or per number of live births.

[b] With variable penetrance and genomic imprinting.

penis, atrophic testes) may reflect pituitary dysfunction, with later alterations in puberty (delay, immaturity, gynecomastia). Female heterozygotes may have mild mental disability and ovarian failure. Preventive management should include early intervention, nutritional counseling to minimize obesity, regular ophthalmologic evaluations, and monitoring of puberty with possible referral to endocrinology for hypogonadism. Physician and parent-oriented may be found on the web by searching on the syndrome name.

Cohen syndrome

Cohen syndrome is an autosomal-recessive disorder that includes hypotonia, obesity, facial anomalies, chorioretinal dystrophy, and skeletal anomalies (Jones, 1997, pp. 206–7; Gorlin et al., 2001, pp. 424–6).

Summary of clinical concerns: Cohen syndrome management considerations

Growth and development: Overgrowth (20%) or short stature (68%), propensity for obesity: Early childhood intervention and preschool programs, dietician and nutritional counseling for prevention of obesity; monitoring of growth with consideration of growth hormone therapy or appetite suppressants.

Craniofacial: The facial appearance includes down-slanting palpebral fissures, prominent incisors, open mouth, and a short philtrum. Because patients with hypotonia often keep their mouths open, this non-specific characteristic has undoubtedly led to many reported cases that do not actually have the syndrome.

Eyes: Chorioretinopathy with altered electroretinograms: All patients should have a baseline ophthalmologic evaluation.

ENT: Chronic otitis media: Annual audiology screening with otolaryngology consultation as needed.

Heart: Congenital heart defects (10%): Cardiology evaluation with echocardiography if cardiac symptoms detected.

Coagulation: Schlictemeier et al. (1994) reported a patient with cerebral thrombosis and a coagulation disorder involving protein S and C deficiencies who had several features of Cohen syndrome: Clotting factors may be obtained before surgery.

Skeletal: Hyperextensible joints with narrow hands and fingers (Gorlin et al., 2001, pp. 349–50): Activity should be encouraged because of the propensity to obesity, but high intensity sports should be avoided.

Genital: Delayed puberty (80%) with occasional early puberty in females, cryptorchidism (31%): Urology and endocrinology evaluations with symptoms.

Neurologic: Hypotonia (92%), microcephaly (50–60%) or occasional macrocephaly, mental disability (IQ 30–80), and seizures (6%); several observers have described a happy, pleasant affect, but more careful study has demonstrated significant behavior problems involving anxiety, social interactions, and autistic features (Howlin et al., 2005): Neurology evaluation with signs or symptoms, behavior therapy as needed.

Parental counseling: Parents should be counseled for a 25% recurrence risk when the diagnosis is secure; physician and parent-oriented information is available on the web by searching on the syndrome name, and there is a support group that can be accessed by residents of British Columbia.

Hemihyperplasia (hemihypertrophy)

Gorlin et al. (2001, pp. 405–8) stressed the use of hemihyperplasia rather than hemihypertrophy because the disorder may be limited to a single tissue (i.e., bone) rather than involving overgrowth of multiple tissues. The hallmark of hemihyperplasia is asymmetry of the face or limbs. Most children exhibit asymmetry at birth, but discrepancies in limb lengths may not be noticed until later childhood or during puberty. Recent studies suggest that some forms of hemihyperplasia have changes in DNA methylation that also occur in the Beckwith–Wiedemann syndrome (Martin, R. A., et al., 2005), and there are occasional familial cases.

Many tissues and regions may be abnormal in association with hemihyperplasia, even in children with isolated asymmetry. Abnormalities of the skin (nevi, hemangiomas, ichthyosis), eye (strabismus), mouth (enlarged teeth or tongue), heart (congenital defects), limbs (macrodactyly, polydactyly, clubfoot, hip dysplasia), viscera (hepatic cysts, polycystic kidneys), genitalia (hypospadias, cryptorchidism), and the central nervous system (macrocephaly, mental deficiency, seizures) may be seen (Gorlin et al., 2001, pp. 405–8). Of particular importance are neoplasms such as Wilms tumor, adrenocortical carcinoma, hepatoblastoma, and neuroblastoma, which occur in 3.8% of patients with hemihyperplasia.

Preventive management should include periodic measurement of limb girths and lengths, early intervention, and ophthalmologic referral. The predisposition to tumors warrants surveillance similar to that recommended for Beckwith–Wiedemann syndrome: abdominal ultrasound as soon as the diagnosis is established and followed at 3–6 months intervals until skeletal growth has ceased. Additional preventive measures should include orthopedic monitoring for scoliosis or disturbances in gait, cardiac evaluation with specialty referral if a murmur is detected, and regular dental care.

Marshall–Smith syndrome

This rare syndrome consists of accelerated skeletal maturation with facial and skeletal changes (Jones, 1997, pp. 162–3; Gorlin et al., 2001, pp. 415–7). The clinical course is severe, with hypotonia, failure to thrive, and death before age 3 years in most cases. Facial anomalies include prominent forehead, shallow orbits, large-appearing eyes with blue sclerae and macrocorneae, prominent eyebrows, high-arched palate, unusual ears, and micrognathia. Some patients have a small nose with choanal atresia, and there may be stridor because of a small larynx or laryngomalacia. The extremities and fingers appear long, and patients have unusual posturing with extension of the neck and scoliosis. Several reports of long-term survivors exist and Diab et al. (2003) report osseous fragility in a 7-year-old female with fractures. Occasional anomalies include cardiac defects (patent ductus arteriosus, atrial septal defect), inflammatory rectal polyp and hematochezia, umbilical hernia or omphalocele, and pachygyria of the brain. Preventive management should focus on early intervention for motor and speech delay, hearing and audiology testing, cardiac evaluation with echocardiographic studies if surgery is required, and a baseline head MRI scan to define brain anomalies. Long-term survivors with Marshall–Smith syndrome have been reported.

Perlman syndrome

Perlman syndrome involves a combination of fetal gigantism, renal hamartomas, nephroblastosis, and Wilms tumor. Several authors have emphasized more common urogenital involvement in Perlman than in Beckwith–Wiedemann syndrome, and certain cases exhibit autosomal-recessive inheritance (Gorlin et al., 2001, p. 403). Preventive management should follow the same strategy as outlined in the checklist for Beckwith–Wiedemann syndrome, which does emphasize early abdominal sonograms and monitoring of urinalysis and blood pressure. A 25% recurrence risk should be mentioned to parents whose child is more compatible with autosomal-recessive Perlman syndrome.

Simpson–Golabi–Behmel syndrome

This X-linked recessive overgrowth disorder was first reported by Simpson and colleagues in 1973 and further delineated by Opitz, Golabi, Rosen, and Behmel (Jones, 1997, pp. 168–9; Gorlin et al., 2001, pp. 417–9). After genetic mapping localized the gene for Simpson–Golabi–Behmel syndrome to the Xq26 region, alterations in the glypican-3 gene were characterized (Cohen, 2003). The glypican-3 gene encodes an extracellular proteoglycan that is expressed in embryonic mesoderm. Alterations in glypican 3 may cause accelerated growth because it forms a complex with insulin-like growth factor 2.

Summary of clinical concerns: Simpson–Golabi–Behmel management considerations

General: The neonatal course is turbulent, with an infant mortality rate of 50% due to cardiac defects, cor pulmonale, respiratory infections, or severe hypoglycemia: Neonatal assessment of blood glucose, cardiopulmonary, and urinary tract status. Because of the high rate of infant mortality, baseline electro-, echocardiogram, skeletal radiologic survey, and abdominal ultrasound can be justified.

Growth and development: Affected children have high birth weights with subsequent overgrowth and mild mental deficiency: Early childhood intervention and preschool programs, dietician and nutritional counseling for prevention of obesity; monitoring of growth with consideration of growth hormone therapy or appetite suppressants.

Eyes: Coloboma, strabismus: All patients should have a baseline ophthalmologic evaluation with annual monitoring.

ENT: Cleft palate, macroglossia: Monitoring for feeding problems with management by a cleft palate team, annual audiology screening with otolaryngology consultation as needed.

Surface-trunk: Inguinal or umbilical hernias: Serial examinations with surgical consultation as needed.

Heart: Congenital heart defects (50%): Baseline cardiology evaluation with echocardiography and monitoring as needed.

Skeletal: Short neck, vertebral anomalies with scoliosis, pectus excavatum: Annual skeletal examinations, orthopedic evaluation; patients with a short, broad neck or with torticollis should have cervical spine films during infancy or early childhood. Adolescents should be monitored for scoliosis and other skeletal deformities.

Gastrointestinal: Intestinal malrotation and diaphragmatic hernia have been reported (Gorlin et al., 2001, pp. 417–9).

Urogenital: Cystic kidneys, urinary tract anomalies, and cryptorchidism: Initial renal sonogram, monitoring of blood pressure and urinalysis, nephrology and urology referral for symptoms.

Parental counseling: Parents should be counseled for potential 25% recurrence risks if mother is known to be a carrier through an affected brother or prior affected child. For isolated cases, there is a two-thirds chance that mother is a carrier, reducing the recurrence risk to one-sixth or 16%. Laboratories in St. Louis and the Netherlands offer DNA testing (see www.genetests.org for update), but a mutation may not be found in some patients. Physician and parent-oriented information is available by searching on the syndrome name.

Weaver syndrome

Weaver syndrome is a very rare condition with overgrowth, accelerated skeletal maturation, and distinctive facies (Jones, 1997, pp. 158–61; Gorlin et al., 2001, pp. 413–5). The syndrome has been described in siblings, but most cases have been sporadic. Mutation of the NOD-1 gene has been described in some children with Weaver syndrome, a gene that is frequently mutated in Sotos syndrome (see below). Opitz et al. (1998) review the similarities of Weaver and Sotos syndrome, suggesting that children with Sotos syndrome are more predisposed to cancer with dramatically accelerated dental maturation. Children with Weaver syndrome may have neuroblastoma (one case report), with more frequent contractures. Opitz et al. (1998) were prescient in suggesting the similar features of these disorders could result from allelic heterogeneity.

Typical craniofacial changes of Weaver syndrome include macrocephaly, flattened occiput, hypertelorism, small palpebral fissures, bulbous nasal tip, and abnormal ears. Complications include brain anomalies (cysts of the septum pellucidum, dilated ventricles), delayed motor development, difficulty in swallowing and feeding, skeletal anomalies such as clubfoot or flat feet, and inguinal or umbilical hernia. Preventive management should include early intervention, evaluation of feeding, evaluation for limb deformities (including checking for hemihyperplasia since neuroblastoma has been reported), and monitoring of nutrition since some children exhibit a voracious appetite.

Parents can be advised of a minimal recurrence risk but informed of rare reports of affected siblings. Numerous laboratories will test for NOD-1 gene mutations (see genetests.org), but this testing is directed towards Sotos syndrome without guarantee that the different alleles in Weaver syndrome will be detected.

Beckwith–Wiedemann syndrome

Terminology

Beckwith in 1963 and Wiedemann in 1964 reported several patients with macroglossia, omphalocele, and visceromegaly that comprise Beckwith–Wiedemann syndrome (Jones, 1997, pp. 164–7; Gorlin et al., 2001, pp. 399–408).

Incidence, etiology, and differential diagnosis

The incidence of Beckwith–Wiedemann syndrome is about 1 in 15,000 births (Weng et al., 1995). The disorder is usually sporadic, but occasional familial transmission is now explained by autosomal-dominant inheritance subject to incomplete penetrance and genomic imprinting. Rare cases of Beckwith–Wiedemann syndrome resulted from a duplication of the chromosome 11p15 region, while others involved a deletion of this same region. It was soon demonstrated that the duplications always involved the paternally inherited chromosome 11, while deletions involved the maternally inherited chromosome (Weng et al., 1995). The implied alteration of parental imprinting has been confirmed by showing that the insulin-like growth factor-2 gene within the chromosome 11p15 region is expressed aberrantly in patients with Beckwith–Wiedemann syndrome. The number of genes involved and the pathogenesis by which altered gene expression produces the syndrome remain to be defined.

Differential diagnosis includes other disorders with high birth weight, particularly diabetic embryopathy. The latter condition may also produce neonatal polycythemia, hypoglycemia, and hypocalcemia; it should be excluded by maternal history or evaluation. Children with mucopolysaccharidosis often have visceromegaly, increased early growth, and large tongues, but only the most severe forms would present neonatally. Skeletal survey and urine mucopolysaccharide/oligosaccharide screens should differentiate these disorders from Beckwith–Wiedemann syndrome. Infantile hypothyroidism can present with umbilical hernia and macroglossia. Wilms tumor with renal and genital abnormalities (Drash syndrome) can be discriminated by the presence of mutations in the WT-1 Wilms tumor gene.

Diagnostic evaluation and medical counseling

Monitoring of blood glucose should be performed in the infantile period, and a routine karyotype is worthwhile to detect the minority of Beckwith–Wiedemann children with overt chromosomal anomalies. About 15% of cases will exhibit autosomal-dominant inheritance, another 15–20% paternal uniparental disomy for chromosome 15, and others will have submicroscopic deletions on the paternal copy of that chromosome (Gorlin et al., 2001, pp. 399–408). Fluorescent *in situ* hybridization (FISH) studies for microdeletion and DNA testing for imprinting alterations is available at several academic laboratories (see www.genetests.org). The constellation of macrosomia, glabellar hemangioma, ear pits, and abdominal wall anomaly allows a definitive clinical diagnosis in most cases.

Family and psychosocial counseling

Except for those with unrecognized hypoglycemia or respiratory insufficiency due to macroglossia, the excellent prognosis for infants with Beckwith–Wiedemann syndrome warrants optimistic medical counseling. Because of the complex inheritance, a careful family history complete with parental birth weights and neonatal histories is important. Adults have few manifestations of the syndrome, so childhood histories and photographs are useful to exclude the diagnosis. For sporadic cases with normal parents, a 5% recurrence risk is appropriate, based on the possibility of imprinting/transmission effects. There is little information on reproduction of affected individuals, but the autosomal-dominant form often manifests in offspring of affected or "carrier" females. Increasing use of artificial reproductive technology (approaching 1–2% of pregnancies in industrialized countries) may be associated with an increased risk for imprinting defects such as Beckwith–Weidemann and Angelman syndromes (Maher, 2005).

Parental support is most crucial during the neonatal and infantile periods, when the children may undergo operations or evaluation for respiratory insufficiency (Kamata et al., 2005). Parent information support is available at the Beckwith–Wiedemann Support Network (beckwith-wiedemann.org/) and many websites accessed by searching on the syndrome name.

Natural history and complications

The complications of Beckwith–Wiedemann syndrome derive from anomalies in the orofacial, cardiac, abdominal, gastrointestinal, endocrine, and skeletal regions or systems (Jones, 1997 pp. 164–7; Gorlin et al., 2001, pp. 399–405). Affected pregnancies may be accompanied by proteinuric hypertension, preterm labor, or polyhydramnios, and there have been molar changes in placentas. The birth weight is usually high, followed by increased postnatal growth in 33–88% of patients and hemihyperplasia in 24–33% (see checklist).

The facial appearance is distinctive with a glabellar hemangioma, malar flattening, and a large tongue. Omphalocele and intestinal stenoses or atresias are the most dramatic neonatal anomaly; one infant had meconium ileus scrotal rupture caused by omphalocele and jejunal atresia. Macroglossia is a frequent and severe neonatal problem that may cause respiratory obstruction, hypoxemia, apnea, feeding problems, and speech difficulties. Kamata et al. (2005) report the utility of polysomnograpy assessment and surgical treatment for obstructive apnea, pointing out that it is not only due to macroglossia. Neonatal hypoglycemia relates to pancreatic islet cell hyperplasia, and there is a general visceromegaly, including nephromegaly. Cardiac anomalies have included septal defects, aortic coarctation and pulmonic stenosis, and generalized cardiomegaly. Less frequent complications include seizures, hydrocephalus, umbilical and inguinal hernias, cleft palate, polydactyly, and urinary tract anomalies. A wide variety of tumors can occur, including lymphoma, neuroblastoma, perineurioma, ganglioneuroma, epicardial angiofibroma, and hepatoblastoma. The risk of tumors is less than 10% overall, but 40% of those with tumors have hemihyperplasia as opposed to 13% overall (Gorlin et al., 2001, p. 402). Over 90% of tumors are intra-abdominal, and children with nephromegaly also have higher risks for tumors.

Once neonatal metabolic and morphologic abnormalities have been treated, the outlook for growth and development in the Beckwith–Wiedemann syndrome is excellent. Most patients have normal intelligence, but 12% have mild mental deficiency with or without microcephaly. Rarely, hypothyroidism may occur with low levels of thyroxine-binding globulin.

Beckwith–Wiedemann syndrome preventive medical checklist

In the newborn period, abdominal and renal ultrasounds should be obtained to assess bowel atresias or stenoses, cystic kidneys, and ureteral obstruction that occasionally presents as the "prune belly" anomaly. Weng et al. (1995) recommended a baseline abdominal CT scan followed by abdominal ultrasound studies every 3 months up until ages 5–7 years, then every 6 months until skeletal growth is complete. Serum alpha-fetoprotein (AFP) measurements have been elevated in the presence of tumors or hypothyroidism, and yearly measurements are recommended (Weng et al., 1995). Abdominal palpation is also important, and some advocate training parents to perform this evaluation. Urinalysis may reveal tumor cells, and is indicated for surveillance of nephroblastoma (Wilms tumor) as well as for monitoring of infections in patients with urinary tract anomalies. Early detection of tumors is associated with favorable outcomes, with reports of disease-free survival rates of 100% after 9 years (average age at diagnosis is 3.5 years). This success underlines the recommendations for ultrasound screening of the liver, urinary tract, and adrenal glands every 3–6 months.

Although the macroglossia of Beckwith–Wiedemann syndrome often resolves without visible sequellae in the adult, surgical interventions may be helpful in preventing dental problems or respiratory obstruction (Kamata et al., 2005). Partial glossectomy may lessen the degree of severity of anterior open bite, dental malocclusion, mandibular prognathism, speech articulation problems, and cosmetic concerns. Infantile tracheostomy may be needed for severe macroglossia, but tonsillectomy and adenoidectomy is more often indicated for relief of upper airway obstruction during childhood.

The expected normal intelligence diminishes the need for special school and financial planning by families affected with the Beckwith–Wiedemann syndrome, but early intervention is still useful to monitor growth, development, hearing, and speech problems. Occasional children will have feeding difficulties, developmental delay (especially speech problems), and failure to thrive because of macroglossia, while others will have borderline mental disability. Most children will probably be discharged from early intervention services after demonstrating normal physical and intellectual development.

Sotos syndrome

Terminology

Sotos syndrome, also known as cerebral gigantism, was originally described in five children with overgrowth, macrocephaly acromegaloid features with advanced bone age, hypotonia, and a distinctive facial appearance in early childhood (Jones, 1997, pp. 154–7; Gorlin et al., 2001, pp. 408–10).

Incidence, etiology, and differential diagnosis

The incidence of Sotos syndrome is unknown, but the >200 reported cases suggest a prevalence of at least 1 in 20,000–30,000 individuals. Only about half of the cases reviewed by four clinical geneticists (Cole & Hughes, 1994) proved to have the disorder, so DNA testing for mutations in the NOD-1 gene (positive in 75% of cases) is useful for problem cases (see www.genetests.org). In a study of 59 patients (Cecconi et al., 2005), all patients with NOD-1 gene mutations had the typical facial gestalt of Sotos syndrome but not necessarily macrocephaly or rapid early growth, and those with NOD-1 gene deletions were more likely to have congenital heart defects. Other overgrowth syndromes including Nevo syndrome and familial macrocephaly may be confused with Sotos syndrome (Cole & Hughes, 1994); Weaver syndrome is very similar and can be caused by allelic mutations in the NOD-1 gene. Any condition with early growth acceleration may prompt consideration of the disorder, but the striking neonatal hypotonia and characteristic facial appearance should exclude other possibilities in the differential.

Diagnostic evaluation and medical counseling

The diagnosis of Sotos syndrome is clinical through noting the pattern of neonatal hypotonia; the distinctive facial appearance with dolichocephaly, prominent forehead, oval-shaped face, down-slanting palpebral fissures, and hypertelorism; the large hands and feet; the pre- and postnatal growth acceleration. A karyotype may be considered in patients with cognitive disability as overgrowth can be seen in certain chromosomal disorders; NOD-1 gene testing can also be performed. Hand radiographs to verify an accelerated bone age offers an additional diagnostic criterion. Medical counseling can be optimistic since most children do better than their early hypotonia and motor delay might predict. The cognitive potential may also be underestimated because the over-sized child appears so much older than their actual age.

Family and psychosocial counseling

Most cases are sporadic, and the few literature reports of autosomal-dominant or -recessive inheritance were not thought convincing by Cole & Hughes (1994). The elevated paternal age would be consistent with a new autosomal-dominant mutation, and it will be interesting to monitor offspring of the affected patients that have been registered for study (Cole & Hughes, 1994). The recurrence risk is extremely low for parents whose child has verified Sotos syndrome, and no sibships suggestive of germline mosacism have been documented. Parent support groups include Sotos Syndrome Support Association (www.well.com/user/sssa/), Sotos Syndrome Support Group of Canada (www.sssac.com/), and Height Matters, UK – information about growth disorders and their treatment (www.heightmatters.org.uk/website/).

Natural history and complications

Despite their increased size at birth, the incidence of forceps (7.5%) or Cesarean section (7.5%) deliveries does not seem increased in children with Sotos syndrome despite their large head size. Obstetric complications are therefore unlikely causes of the neonatal hypotonia with subsequent motor, speech, and cognitive delays. Birth length is more increased than weight, and over 50% have a large head circumference at birth. The head circumference quickly joins the height and weight in being over the 97th centile in most children, although adult height is channeled back towards the mean in females because of early puberty.

Medical complications include early feeding problems due to hypotonia with 40% requiring tube feedings (Cole & Hughes, 1994). Problems relating to the early hypotonia may include strabismus, chronic otitis, constipation, clumsiness (with an increased frequency of fractures), and orthopedic problems such as flat feet or scoliosis. Eye anomalies (cataracts, strabismus, nystagmus, myopia); congenital heart defects (patent ductus arteriosus, septal defects); urological anomalies; and malignancies (neuroblastoma, hepatocellular carcinoma, non-Hodgkins lymphoma, leukemia and osteochondroma) also occur at increased frequency (Cole & Hughes, 1994; Gorlin et al., 2001, pp. 408–10). Posterior spinal fusion has been successful in treating scoliosis. Neurologic findings include paradoxically brisk deep tendon reflexes and brain anomalies including dilated cerebral ventricles (without functional hydrocephalus), anomalies of the corpus callosum, and periventricular leukomalacia. The range of developmental quotients in 41 children was 40–129, with a mean of 78 (Cole & Hughes, 1994). No specific language deficits have been defined, but range of behavioral problems have been reported by teachers and parents including tantrums, withdrawal, sleep difficulties, and hyperactivity. Behavioral problems may not exceed those of comparably delayed and over-sized children.

Sotos syndrome preventive medical checklist

Recommendations for preventive management include attention to feeding and stooling problems in the first year; ophthalmologic, urologic, and cardiac assessment during early infancy; early intervention with physical, speech, and occupational therapy; monitoring of growth, hearing, and skeletal development in early childhood through adolescence; and school planning with anticipation of potential behavioral problems (due to inappropriate expectations or actual hyperactivity). The low frequency and different types of tumors do not lend themselves to the regimen of abdominal ultrasounds followed for Beckwith–Wiedemann syndrome, but physicians and parents should be alert for symptoms.

Preventive management of Beckwith–Wiedemann syndrome

Description: An overgrowth syndrome with prominent tongue, ear creases, and omphalocele due to gene mutations, deletions, or altered imprinting of the chromosome 11p15 region, with an incidence of 1 in 12,000 births.

Clinical diagnosis: Pattern of manifestations including large birth weight, facial hemangiomas, ear creases, macroglossia, omphalocele, and visceromegaly; later overgrowth with predisposition to abdominal tumors and hemihypertrophy.

Laboratory diagnosis: Neonatal hypoglycemia is frequent, with some cases due to uniparental inheritance or chromosomal rearrangement in the 11p15 region.

Genetics: Multifactorial disorder with minimal recurrence risk; genetic factors indicated by occasional concordant twins.

Key management issues: Neonatal monitoring of blood glucose, serial abdominal/renal ultrasounds and serum alpha-fetoprotein measurements to screen for urinary tract anomalies and tumors, routine abdominal palpation and urinalysis to screen for tumors and urinary infections, monitoring for respiratory obstruction with aggressive treatment of hypoxemia (partial glossectomy, tonsillectomy, adenoidectomy, tracheotomy), early intervention to monitor growth, development, hearing, and speech problems.

Growth charts: None.

Parent groups: Beckwith–Wiedemann Support Group (Beckwith–Wiedemann.org/).

Basis for management recommendations: Complications documented below as documented by Weng et al. (1995). The timing of abdominal ultrasound examinations is particularly controversial, with recommendations ranging from annually to every 3 months.

Summary of clinical concerns

General	Learning	Cognitive disability (4–12%)
	Growth	**Large birth weight** (39–77%), **macrosomia** (33–88%), **hemihyperplasia** (24–33%)
	Tumors	Abdominal (4–7.5% – Wilms tumor, hepatoblastoma, adrenocortical carcinoma)
Facial	Facies	Maxillary hypoplasia, flat nasal bridge, prognathism
	Ears	**Ear pits, creases** (66–76%), chronic otitis
	Mouth	Oromotor dysfunction, **macroglossia** (82–100%), cleft palate (2.5%), adenoidal hypertrophy
Surface	Neck/trunk	**Diastasis recti** (33%), **umbilical hernia** (24–49%), pectus carinatum, pectus excavatum, prune belly due to renal malformations
	Epidermal	**Nevus flammeus** (63%)
Skeletal	Limbs	Advanced bone age, polydactyly (4%), hemihyperplasia, polydactyly
Internal	Digestive	**Visceromegaly** (57%), **omphalocele** (34–76%), imperforate anus, malrotation (5%)
	Pulmonary	Hypoventilation, hypoxia
	Circulatory	Cardiac defects (6.5–18% – atrial septal defect, ventricular septal defect, patent ductus arteriosus, hypoplastic left heart, tetralogy of Fallot)
	Endocrine	**Hypoglycemia** (30–63%), pancreatic islet hyperplasia, **hypocalcemia** (4.6%)
	Res	Polycythemia (20%)
	Excretory	**Renal anomalies** (59–100%), **nephromegaly** (45%), renal diverticula, hydronephrosis (7%), obstructive uropathy, urinary tract infections
	Genital	Hypospadias, cryptorchidism, bicornuate uterus
Neural	Central	Seizures, hydrocephalus
	Motor	Occasional motor delays
	Sensory	Conductive hearing loss

RES, reticuloendothelial system; **concerns** of frequency >20% are **highlighted**

Key references

Cohen, M. M., Jr. (2003). Mental deficiency, alterations in performance, and CNS abnormalities in overgrowth syndromes. *American Journal of Medical Genetics* 117C:49–56.

Kamata, S. et al. (2005). Assessment of obstructive apnea by using polysomnography and surgical treatment in patients with Beckwith–Wiedemann syndrome. *Journal of Pediatrics Surgery* 40:E17–19.

Weng, E.Y. et al. (1995). Beckwith–Wiedemann syndrome. An update and review for the primary pediatrician. *Clinical Pediatrics* 34:317–32.

Beckwith–Wiedemann syndrome

Preventive medical checklist (0–3 years)

Name _____ Birth date __ / __ / ____ Number _____

Age	Evaluations: key concerns	Management considerations		Notes
New-born ↓ 1 month	Dysmorphology examination: anomalies Hearing, vision:[2] hearing loss Feeding, airway: obstruction, palate Heart: septal defects, tetralogy Urinary function: renal anomalies Metabolic: hypoglycemia, renal function Parental adjustment	❑ FISH or DNA studies; genetic counseling[1] ❑ ABR ❑ Feeding specialist; video swallow;[3] ENT[3] ❑ Echocardiogram; cardiology ❑ Renal sonogram; urinary tract studies ❑ Blood calcium, electrolytes; renal functions ❑ Family support[4]	❑ ❑ ❑ ❑ ❑ ❑ ❑	
2 months ↓ 4 months	Growth and development[2] Hearing, vision:[2] hearing loss Feeding, airway: obstruction, palate Urinary function: infection Metabolic: hypoglycemia, renal function Skeletal: asymmetry, hernias Parental adjustment Other:	❑ ECI[6] ❑ ABR;[3] ENT[3] ❑ Feeding specialist; video swallow;[3] ENT[3] ❑ Urinalysis, BP ❑ Blood glucose; electrolytes; renal functions ❑ Abdominal examination; sonogram; orthopedics[3] ❑ Family support[4] ❑	❑ ❑ ❑ ❑ ❑ ❑ ❑ ❑	Consider abdo-minal sonogram every 3 months, especially in those with hemi-hyperplasia
6 months ↓ 9 months	Growth and development[2] Hearing, vision:[2] hearing loss Feeding, airway: obstruction, palate Cardiovascular, urinary tract anomalies Skeletal: asymmetry, hernias Other:	❑ ECI[6] ❑ ENT[3] ❑ Feeding specialist; video swallow;[3] ENT[3] ❑ Urinalysis, BP; cardiology ❑ Abdominal examination, sonogram; orthopedics[3] ❑	❑ ❑ ❑ ❑ ❑ ❑	
1 year	Growth and development[2] Hearing, vision:[2] hearing loss Feeding, airway: obstruction, palate Cardiovascular, urinary tract anomalies Metabolic: hypercalcemia, renal function Skeletal: asymmetry, pectus Other:	❑ ECI;[3,6] family support[3,4] ❑ ENT[3] ❑ Feeding specialist, video swallow;[3] ENT[3] ❑ Urinalysis, BP, IVP;[3] cardiology ❑ Blood glucose; BUN; creatinine; T4, TSH ❑ Abdominal examination, sonogram; orthopedics[3] ❑	❑ ❑ ❑ ❑ ❑ ❑ ❑	
15 months ↓ 18 months	Growth and development[2] Cardiovascular, urinary tract anomalies Metabolic: hypercalcemia, renal function Skeletal: asymmetry, pectus	❑ ECI[6] ❑ Urinalysis, BP, IVP;[3] cardiology ❑ Blood glucose, BUN, creatinine, T4, TSH ❑ Abdominal examination, sonogram; orthopedics[3]	❑ ❑ ❑ ❑	
2 years	Growth and development[2] Hearing, vision:[2] hearing loss Cardiovascular, urinary tract anomalies Metabolic: hypercalcemia, renal function Skeletal: asymmetry, pectus	❑ ECI,[3,6] family support[3,4] ❑ ENT[3] ❑ Urinalysis; BP; IVP;[3] cardiology ❑ Blood glucose; BUN; creatinine; T4, TSH ❑ Abdominal examination, sonogram; orthopedics[3]	❑ ❑ ❑ ❑ ❑	
3 years	Growth and development[2] Hearing, vision:[2] hearing loss Cardiovascular, urinary tract anomalies Thyroid, renal functions, tumor detection Skeletal: asymmetry, pectus Neuromuscular: seizures Other:	❑ ECI;[3,6] family support[3,4] ❑ ENT[3] ❑ Urinalysis, BP; IVP;[3] cardiology ❑ AFP; BUN; creatinine; T4, TSH ❑ Abdominal examination, sonogram; orthopedics[3] ❑ Neurology[3] ❑	❑ ❑ ❑ ❑ ❑ ❑ ❑	

Beckwith–Wiedemann concerns		Other concerns from history	
Hypoglycemia, hypocalcemia Polycythemia Feeding problems Macroglossia, macrosomia Airway obstruction Omphalocele, umbilical hernia	Cardiac anomalies Urogenital anomalies Hemihyperplasia Abdominal tumors Obstructive apnea Seizures, motor delays	**Family history/prenatal** _____ _____ _____ _____	**Social/environmental** _____ _____ _____ _____

Guidelines for the neonatal period should be undertaken *at whatever age* the diagnosis is made; FISH, fluorescent *in situ* hybridization; ABR, auditory brainstem evoked response; AFP, alpha-fetoprotein level; BP, blood pressure; TSH, thyroid stimulating hormone; BUN, blood urea nitrogen; IVP, intravenous pyelogram or other urinary tract studies; [1]parental chromosomes or DNA studies not necessary; [2]by practitioner; [3]as dictated by clinical findings; [4]parent group, family/sib, financial, and behavioral issues; [5]developmental pediatrician/neurologist/genetics clinic according to symptoms and availability; [6]early childhood intervention including developmental monitoring and motor/speech therapy in the minority with developmental delays.

Beckwith–Wiedemann syndrome

Preventive medical checklist (4–18 years)

Name _____ Birth date __ / __ / __ Number _____

Age	Evaluations: key concerns	Management considerations	Notes
4 years ↓ 6 years	Growth, preschool transition[1,5] Hearing, vision:[2] hearing loss Cardiovascular, urinary tract anomalies Thyroid, renal functions, tumor detection Skeletal: asymmetry, pectus Neuromuscular: seizures Other:	❑ Family support;[4] preschool program[5] ❑ Audiology; ENT[3] ❑ Urinalysis; BP; IVP;[3] cardiology ❑ AFP; BUN; creatinine; T4, TSH ❑ Abdominal examination, sonogram; orthopedics[3] ❑ ❑ Neurology[3] ❑	❑ Consider ❑ abdominal ❑ sonogram ❑ every 3 months, ❑ especially in ❑ those with hemi- hyperplasia
7 years ↓ 9 years	Growth, school transition[1,5] Hearing, vision:[2] hearing loss Cardiovascular, urinary tract anomalies Metabolic, thyroid, renal function Skeletal: asymmetry, pectus Neuromuscular: seizures Other:	❑ Family support;[4] school progress[6] ❑ Audiology; ENT[3] ❑ Urinalysis; BP; IVP;[3] cardiology ❑ AFP; BUN; creatinine; T4, TSH ❑ Abdominal examination, sonogram; orthopedics[3] ❑ ❑ Neurology[3] ❑	❑ ❑ ❑ ❑ ❑ ❑
10 years ↓ 12 years	Growth and development[1,5] Cardiovascular, urinary tract anomalies Thyroid, renal functions, tumor detection Skeletal: asymmetry, pectus Other:	❑ Family support;[4]school progress[6] ❑ Urinalysis; BP; IVP;[3] cardiology ❑ AFP; BUN; creatinine; T4, TSH ❑ Abdominal examination, sonogram; orthopedics[3] ❑ ❑	❑ ❑ ❑
13 years ↓ 15 years	Growth and development[1,5] Cardiovascular, urinary tract anomalies Thyroid, renal functions, tumor detection Skeletal: asymmetry, pectus Puberty: cryptorchidism, uterine anomaly Other:	❑ Family support;[4] school progress[6] ❑ Urinalysis; BP; IVP;[3] cardiology ❑ AFP; BUN; creatinine; T4, TSH ❑ Abdominal examination, sonogram; orthopedics[3] ❑ ❑ Endocrinology;[3] urology ❑	❑ Abdominal ❑ sonograms ❑ can be stopped ❑ after skeletal ❑ development complete
16 years ↓ 18 years	Growth and development[1,5] Hearing, vision:[2] hearing loss Cardiovascular, urinary tract anomalies Skeletal: asymmetry, scoliosis Other:	❑ Family support;[4] school progress[6] ❑ Audiology; ENT[3] ❑ Urinalysis; BP; IVP;[3] cardiology ❑ Orthopedics[3] ❑	❑ ❑ ❑ ❑
19 years ↓ 23 years	Adult care transition[1,6] Cardiovascular, urinary tract anomalies Thyroid, renal functions, tumor detection Skeletal: asymmetry, scoliosis Neuromuscular: seizures	❑ Family support;[4] school progress[6] ❑ Urinalysis; BP; IVP;[3] cardiology ❑ AFP; BUN; creatinine; T4, TSH ❑ Orthopedics[3] ❑ Neurology[3]	❑ ❑ ❑ ❑ ❑
Adult	Adult care transition[6] Hearing, vision:[2] hearing loss Cardiovascular, urinary tract anomalies Thyroid, renal functions, tumor detection Skeletal: asymmetry, scoliosis Neuromuscular: seizures Other:	❑ Family support[4] ❑ Audiology; ENT[3] ❑ Urinalysis; BP; IVP;[3] cardiology ❑ AFP; BUN; creatinine; T4, TSH ❑ Orthopedics[3] ❑ Neurology[3] ❑	❑ ❑ ❑ ❑ ❑ ❑

Beckwith–Wiedemann concerns		Other concerns from history	
Airway obstruction Conductive hearing loss Malocclusion, overbite Macrosomia Cardiac anomalies Urinary tract anomalies	Cryptorchidism Hemihyperplasia, scoliosis Abdominal tumors Obstructive apnea Seizures, motor delays Learning differences	**Family history/prenatal** _____ _____ _____ _____	**Social/environmental** _____ _____ _____ _____

Guidelines for the neonatal period should be undertaken *at whatever age* the diagnosis is made; AFP, alphafetoprotein level; BP, blood pressure; TSH, thyroid stimulating hormone; BUN, blood urea nitrogen; IVP, intravenous pyelogram or other urinary tract studies; GI, gastrointestinal; [1]consider low calcium diet, developmental pediatrician/pediatric genetics/behavior therapist according to symptoms and availability; and neurologist if symptoms of stroke or cerebral artery stenosis; [2]by practitioner; [3]as dictated by clinical findings; [4]parent group, family/sib, financial, and later focus on independent living and employment for the minority with disabilities; [5]preschool program including developmental monitoring and motor/speech therapy for minority with disabilities; [6]monitor individual education plan, educational testing, academic progress, later vocational planning in those with mental disability.

Parent guide to Beckwith–Wiedemann syndrome

Beckwith in 1963 and Wiedemann in 1964 reported several patients with macroglossia (large tongue), omphalocele (outpouching of intestines from the abdomen), and large organs that comprise Beckwith–Wiedemann syndrome.

Incidence, causation, and diagnosis

The incidence of Beckwith–Wiedemann syndrome is about 1 in 12,000 live births. Beckwith–Wiedemann syndrome can result from duplication, deletion, gene mutation, or altered imprinting of the chromosome 11p15 region. The paternal copy of chromosome 11 is usually altered, resulting in increased amounts of an insulin-like growth factor that causes increased growth and enlargement (hyperplasia) of various internal organs or limbs. The diagnosis is usually obvious clinically, but chromosome and DNA testing can be performed for confirmation. Differential diagnosis includes other disorders with increased birth weight, enlarged organs, and skeletal changes. Infants of diabetic mothers may have similar neonatal manifestations with polycythemia (thickened blood), hypoglycemia (low blood sugar), and hypocalcemia (low blood calcium). Other similar conditions can include mucopolysaccharidoses with large organs, increased early growth, and large tongue or infantile hypothyroidism with umbilical hernia (pouch at the belly button similar to omphalocele) and a large tongue. The constellation of large size, birth mark over the nose (glabellar hemangioma), characteristic dimples behind the ear, and a pouch through the abdominal wall allows a definitive clinical diagnosis of Beckwith–Wiedemann syndrome in most cases.

Natural history and complications

The complications of Beckwith–Wiedemann syndrome derive from anomalies in the orofacial, cardiac, abdominal, gastrointestinal, endocrine, and skeletal regions or systems. Affected pregnancies may be accompanied by high blood pressure, premature labor, or excess amniotic fluid, and the placenta may appear abnormal. The birth weight is usually high, followed by increased postnatal growth in 33–88% of patients and enlargement of one side of the body in 24–33%. Macroglossia (large tongue) is a frequent and severe neonatal problem that may cause respiratory obstruction, low oxygenation, cessation of breathing (apnea), feeding problems, and speech difficulties. Low blood sugar (hypoglycemia) during infancy relates to enlargement of the pancreatic islet cells that produce insulin; there is general enlargement of the organs including the kidney. Heart defects have included septal defects, aortic coarctation and pulmonic stenosis, and generalized cardiomegaly (heart enlargement). Less frequent complications include seizures, hydrocephalus (accumulation of fluid in brain cavities), umbilical and inguinal hernias, cleft palate, extra fingers, and urinary tract anomalies. Of most concern for preventive management are the risks of abdominal tumors and of underoxygenation or breathing problems from tongue obstruction. Children with large kidneys may have higher risks for tumors. Once neonatal metabolic and morphologic abnormalities have been treated, the outlook for growth and development in the Beckwith–Wiedemann syndrome is excellent. Most patients have normal intelligence, but 12% have mild mental deficiency.

Preventive medical needs

In the newborn period, ultrasound of the abdomen should be performed to assess bowel anomalies, kidney anomalies, or obstruction of the urine flow that occasionally presents as the "prune belly" anomaly. Most studies recommended a baseline abdominal CT scan followed by abdominal ultrasound studies every 3 months up until ages 5–7 years, then every 6 months until skeletal growth is complete at about age 14–15 years. Serum alpha-fetoprotein (AFP) measurements have been elevated in the presence of tumors or hypothyroidism, and yearly measurements are recommended. Abdominal palpation is also important, and some advocate training parents to perform this evaluation. Urinalysis may reveal tumor cells, and is indicated for surveillance as well as for monitoring of infections in patients with urinary tract anomalies. Treatment of tumors often has an excellent outcome, underlining the recommendations for ultrasound screening of the liver, urinary tract, and adrenal glands every 3–6 months. Partial tongue resection may lessen the degree of dental·and jaw changes. Respiratory obstruction and decreased oxygenation from macroglossia can be significant, so referral to a multidisciplinary craniofacial surgery team should be considered. Infantile tracheostomy, anterior tongue reduction, or tonsillectomy and adenoidectomy may be helpful for upper airway obstruction/apnea, tooth misalignment, speech problems, and cosmetic improvements. The expected normal intelligence diminishes the need for special services in Beckwith–Wiedemann syndrome, but early intervention is still useful to monitor growth and speech. Occasional children will have feeding difficulties, developmental, and growth delay (especially speech problems) because of macroglossia, while others will have borderline mental disability.

Family counseling

Except for those with unrecognized hypoglycemia or respiratory insufficiency due to macroglossia, the excellent prognosis for infants with Beckwith–Wiedemann syndrome warrants optimistic medical counseling. Because of the complex inheritance, a careful family history complete with parental birth weights and neonatal histories is important. Adults have few manifestations of the syndrome, so childhood histories and photographs are useful to exclude the diagnosis. For sporadic cases with normal parents, a 5% recurrence risk is appropriate, based on the possibility of imprinting/transmission effects. There is little information on reproduction of affected individuals, but women with the syndrome have a higher risk for transmission than men. Parental support is most crucial during the neonatal and infantile periods, when the children may undergo operations or evaluation for respiratory insufficiency.

Preventive management of sotos syndrome

Description: A pattern of early rapid growth, large head, oval-shaped face, neonatal hypotonia, and moderate to mild learning disabilities with an a prevalence of 1 in 20,000–30,000.

Clinical diagnosis: Pattern of manifestations including neonatal hypotonia, pre- and postnatal overgrowth, macrocephaly, characteristic facial appearance (frontal bossing, sparse frontal hair, down-slanting palpebral fissures, prominent jaw), accelerated bone age, and cognitive disability.

Laboratory diagnosis: Mutations in the NOD-1 gene can be demonstrated in 75% of individuals.

Genetics: Sporadic occurrence with minimal recurrence risk for parents of affected children; risks for affected individuals to transmit the syndrome are presumed low but not defined.

Key management issues: Monitoring of feeding and stooling during the first year; ophthalmologic, urologic, and cardiac assessment during early infancy; early intervention, monitoring of growth, hearing, and skeletal development; and school planning with anticipation of potential behavioral problems.

Growth charts: Growth profiles are presented by Cole & Hughes (1994).

Parent groups: Sotos Syndrome Support Association (www.well.com/user/sssa/), Sotos Syndrome Support Group of Canada (www.sssac.com/), and Height Matters, United Kingdom / information about growth disorders and their treatment. (www.heightmatters.org.uk/website/).

Basis for management recommendations: Derived from the complications below as documented by Cole & Hughes (1994).

Summary of clinical concerns

General	Learning	**Cognitive disability** (IQ range 40–129, mean 78), learning differences
	Behavior	**Hyperactivity** (38%), **tantrums, withdrawal**
	Growth	Accelerated growth with macrocephaly and macrosomia
	Tumors	Neuroblastoma, hepatocellular carcinoma, lymphomas, acute lymphatic leukemia
Facial	Facies	Frontal bossing, high hairline, oval shape, ocular hypertelorism, down-slanting palpebral fissures, pointed chin
	Eyes	Strabismus, cataracts, nystagmus, glaucoma
	Ears	**Chronic otitis** (72%)
	Mouth	High palate, early tooth eruption, **worn and discolored teeth** (75%), drooling
Surface	Epidermal	Sparse frontal hair (98%), thin or brittle nails (58%)
Skeletal	Cranial	**Macrocephaly** (50% at birth, virtually 100% later), dolichocephaly
	Axial	Kyphoscoliosis (8%)
	Limbs	Joint laxity, **flat feet** (46%), **accelerated bone age** (84%), **large hands and feet** (80%), hip dislocation
Internal	Digestive	**Poor feeding** (40% tube feeding as neonates), constipation, functional megacolon
	Circulatory	Cardiac anomalies (15% – patent ductus arteriosus, atrial septal defect)
	Endocrine	Glucose intolerance (14%)
	Excretory	Ureteral reflux, urinary tract infections
Neural	Central	**Seizures** (50%, often with fevers), brain anomalies (**ventricular dilation**, 63%, anomalies of the corpus callosum, generous extracerebral fluid spaces, periventricular leukomalacia)
	Motor	**Neonatal hypotonia** (88%), muscle weakness, **brisk reflexes** (78%), **poor coordination** (100%)
	Sensory	Hearing and vision deficits

Concerns of frequency >20% are **highlighted**

Key references

Cole & Hughes (1994). Sotos syndrome: a study of the diagnostic criteria and natural history. *Journal of Medical Genetics* 31:20–32.

Finegan et al. (1994). Language and behavior in children with Sotos syndrome. *Journal of American Academy of Child and Adolescent Psychiatry* 33:1307–15.

Sotos syndrome

Preventive medical checklist (0–3 years)

Name _____ **Birth date** __ / __ / __ **Number** _____

Age	Evaluations: key concerns	Management considerations	Notes
New-born ↓ 1 month	Dysmorphology examination: head size, facies ☐ Hearing, vision:[2] cataracts Feeding: hypotonia Heart: septal defects, patent ductus Neuro: brain anomalies, seizures Skeleton: hip dislocation Parental adjustment	DNA studies if needed; genetic counseling[1] ☐ ABR; ophthalmology ☐ Feeding specialist[3] ☐ Echocardiogram;[3] cardiology[3] ☐ Cranial sonogram; neurology[3] ☐ Skeletal examination, X-rays; orthopedics[3] ☐ Family support[4] ☐	
2 months ↓ 4 months	Growth and development:[2] head size Hearing, vision:[2] cataracts Feeding, stooling: hypotonia, constipation Neuro: brain anomalies, seizures Skeleton: hip dislocation Parental adjustment Other:	☐ ECI[6] ☐ ABR;[3] ophthalmology[3] ☐ Feeding specialist;[3] laxatives ☐ Head MRI;[3] neurology[3] ☐ Skeletal examination, X-rays; orthopedics[3] ☐ ☐ Family support[4] ☐	
6 months ↓ 9 months	Growth and development:[2] head size Hearing, vision:[2] strabismus, otitis Feeding, stooling: hypotonia, constipation Tumors: Wilms, neuroblastoma Skeleton: hip dislocation Other:	☐ ECI[6] ☐ ENT;[3] ophthalmology[3] ☐ Feeding specialist;[3] laxatives ☐ Abdominal examination, sonogram[3] ☐ Skeletal examination, X-rays; orthopedics[3] ☐ ☐	
1 year	Growth and development[2] Hearing, vision:[2] strabismus, otitis Feeding, stooling: hypotonia, constipation Neuro: brain anomalies, seizures Tumors: Wilms, neuroblastoma Skeleton: hip dislocation Other:	☐ ECI;[3,6] family support[3,4] ☐ ENT;[3] ophthalmology[3] ☐ Feeding specialist;[3] laxatives ☐ Head MRI;[3] neurology[3] ☐ Abdominal examination, sonogram[3] ☐ Skeletal examination, X-rays; orthopedics[3] ☐ ☐	
15 months ↓ 18 months	Growth and development[2] Hearing, vision:[2] strabismus, otitis Feeding, stooling: hypotonia, constipation Neuro: brain anomalies, seizures	☐ ECI[6] ☐ ENT;[3] ophthalmology[3] ☐ Feeding specialist;[3] laxatives ☐ Head MRI;[3] neurology[3]	
2 years	Growth and development[2] Hearing, vision:[2] strabismus, otitis Feeding, stooling: hypotonia, constipation Neuro: brain anomalies, seizures Skeleton: hip dislocation	☐ ECI[3,6] ☐ ENT;[3] ophthalmology[3] ☐ Feeding specialist;[3] laxatives ☐ Head MRI;[3] neurology[3] ☐ Skeletal examination, X-rays; orthopedics[3] ☐	
3 years	Growth and development[2] Hearing, vision:[2] strabismus, otitis Feeding, stooling: hypotonia, constipation Neuro: seizures, incoordination Tumors: Wilms, neuroblastoma Skeleton: hip dislocation Other:	☐ ECI;[3,6] family support[3,4] ☐ ENT;[3] ophthalmology[3] ☐ Feeding specialist;[3] laxatives ☐ Head MRI;[3] neurology[3] ☐ Abdominal examination, sonogram[3] ☐ Skeletal examination, X-rays; orthopedics[3] ☐ ☐	

Sotos syndrome concerns		Other concerns from history	
Poor feeding in infancy Overgrowth High palate, drooling Eye anomalies (strabismus) Chronic otitis Cardiac anomalies	Hip dislocation Urinary tract anomalies Hypotonia, macrocephaly Tumors: Wilms, neuroblastoma Developmental delays	**Family history/prenatal** _____ _____ _____ _____	**Social/environmental** _____ _____ _____ _____

Guidelines for the neonatal period should be undertaken *at whatever age* the diagnosis is made; ABR, auditory brainstem evoked response; AFP, alpha-fetoprotein level; BP, blood pressure; TSH, thyroid stimulating hormone; BUN, blood urea nitrogen; [1]DNA studies for NOD-1 gene mutations may confirm diagnosis; usually sporadic but parental examinations necessary; [2]by practitioner; [3]as dictated by clinical findings; [4]parent group, family/sib, financial, and behavioral issues; [5]developmental pediatrician/neurologist/genetics clinic according to symptoms and availability; [6]early childhood intervention including developmental monitoring and motor/speech therapy in the minority with developmental delays.

Sotos syndrome

Preventive medical checklist (4–18 years)

Name _____ Birth date __/__/____ Number _____

Age	Evaluations: key concerns	Management considerations		Notes
4 years ↓ **6 years**	Growth, preschool transition[1,5] Hearing, vision:[2] strabismus, glaucoma Constipation, glucose intolerance Neuro: seizures, incoordination Tumors: Wilms, neuroblastoma Skeleton: flat feet, scoliosis Other:	❑ Family support;[4] preschool program[5] ❑ ENT;[3] ophthalmology[3] ❑ Laxatives; urinalysis; GI;[3] endocrinology[3] ❑ Head MRI;[3] neurology[3] ❑ Abdominal examination, sonogram[3] ❑ Skeletal examination, X-rays; orthopedics[3] ❑	❑ ❑ ❑ ❑ ❑ ❑	
7 years ↓ **9 years**	Growth, school transition[1,5] Hearing, vision:[2] strabismus, glaucoma Constipation, glucose intolerance Neuro: seizures, incoordination Tumors: Wilms, neuroblastoma Skeleton: flat feet, scoliosis Other:	❑ Family support;[4] school progress[6] ❑ ENT;[3] ophthalmology[3] ❑ Laxatives; urinalysis; GI;[3] endocrinology[3] ❑ Head MRI;[3] neurology[3] ❑ Abdominal examination, sonogram[3] ❑ Skeletal examination, X-rays; orthopedics[3] ❑	❑ ❑ ❑ ❑ ❑ ❑	
10 years ↓ **12 years**	Growth and development[1,5] Hearing, vision:[2] strabismus, glaucoma Constipation, glucose intolerance Neuro: seizures, incoordination Other:	❑ Family support;[4] school progress[6] ❑ ENT;[3] ophthalmology[3] ❑ Laxatives; urinalysis; GI;[3] endocrinology[3] ❑ Head MRI;[3] neurology[3] ❑	❑ ❑ ❑ ❑	
13 years ↓ **15 years**	Growth and development[1,5] Hearing, vision:[2] strabismus, glaucoma Constipation, glucose intolerance Neuro: seizures, incoordination Tumors: Wilms, neuroblastoma Other:	❑ Family support;[4] school progress[6] ❑ ENT;[3] ophthalmology[3] ❑ Laxatives; urinalysis; GI;[3] endocrinology[3] ❑ Head MRI;[3] neurology[3] ❑ Abdominal examination, sonogram[3] ❑	❑ ❑ ❑ ❑ ❑	
16 years ↓ **18 years**	Growth and development[1,5] Hearing, vision:[2] strabismus, glaucoma Constipation, glucose intolerance Tumors: Wilms, neuroblastoma Other:	❑ Family support;[4] school progress[6] ❑ ENT;[3] ophthalmology[3] ❑ Laxatives; urinalysis; GI;[3] endocrinology[3] ❑ Abdominal examination, sonogram[3] ❑	❑ ❑ ❑ ❑	
19 years ↓ **23 years**	Adult care transition[1,6] Hearing, vision:[2] strabismus, glaucoma Constipation, glucose intolerance Neuro: seizures, incoordination Tumors: Wilms, neuroblastoma	❑ Family support;[4] school progress[6] ❑ ENT;[3] ophthalmology[3] ❑ Laxatives; urinalysis; GI;[3] endocrinology[3] ❑ Head MRI;[3] neurology[3] ❑ Abdominal examination, sonogram[3]	❑ ❑ ❑ ❑ ❑	
Adult	Adult care transition[6] Hearing, vision:[2] strabismus, glaucoma Constipation, glucose intolerance Neuro: seizures, incoordination Tumors: Wilms, neuroblastoma Skeleton: flat feet, scoliosis Other:	❑ Family support[4] ❑ ENT;[3] ophthalmology[3] ❑ Laxatives; urinalysis; GI;[3] endocrinology[3] ❑ Head MRI;[3] neurology[3] ❑ Abdominal examination, sonogram[3] ❑ Skeletal examination, X-rays; orthopedics[3] ❑	❑ ❑ ❑ ❑ ❑ ❑	

Sotos syndrome concerns		Other concerns from history	
High palate, dental problems Eye anomalies (strabismus) Chronic otitis, hearing loss Septal defects, patent ductus Scoliosis, flat feet	Urinary tract anomalies Tumors (Wilms, neuroblastoma) Macrocephaly, overgrowth Developmental delays Hyperactivity	**Family history/prenatal** _____ _____ _____ _____	**Social/environmental** _____ _____ _____ _____

Guidelines for the neonatal period should be undertaken *at whatever age* the diagnosis is made; GI, gastrointestinal; [1]consider developmental pediatrician/pediatric genetics/neurologist/behavior therapist according to symptoms and availability; [2]by practitioner; [3]as dictated by clinical findings; [4]parent group, family/sib, financial, and later focus on independent living and employment for the minority with disabilities; [5]preschool program including developmental monitoring and motor/speech therapy for minority with disabilities; [6]monitor individual education plan, educational testing, academic progress, later vocational planning in those with mental disability.

Parent guide to sotos syndrome

Sotos syndrome, also known as cerebral gigantism, was originally described in five children with overgrowth, large heads, advanced bone age, low muscle tone, and a distinctive facial appearance in early childhood.

Incidence, causation, and diagnosis

The incidence of Sotos syndrome is unknown, but the >200 reported cases suggest a prevalence of at least 1 in 20,000–30,000 individuals. Only about half of the cases reviewed by four clinical geneticists proved to have the disorder, and DNA testing for mutations in the NOD-1 gene (found in 75% of patients) may be helpful in confirming the diagnosis. The advanced paternal age together with sporadic occurrence (no family history) suggests the possibility of a new genetic mutation in most children. Other overgrowth syndromes such as Nevo or Simpson–Golabi–Behmel syndrome may be confused with Sotos syndrome, as may families that have large heads. Some cases of Weaver syndrome also have mutations in the NOD-1 gene and are therefore allelic with Sotos syndrome (different expression of same gene defect). Any condition with early growth acceleration may prompt consideration of the disorder, but the striking low muscle tone in infancy, the characteristic facial appearance, and the accelerated bone development (i.e., early appearance of teeth) usually allow a definitive diagnosis. The diagnosis of Sotos syndrome is clinical through noting the pattern of low muscle tone in infancy; the distinctive facial appearance with elongated head, prominent forehead, oval-shaped face, down-slanting palpebral fissures, and widely spaced eyes; the large hands and feet; the large birth weight and subsequent rapid growth. Chromosome and fragile X DNA studies may be considered in children with mental disability as overgrowth can be seen in certain chromosomal disorders or in fragile X syndrome. Hand X-rays to verify an accelerated bone age offers an additional diagnostic criterion. Medical counseling can be optimistic since most children do better than their early hypotonia and motor delay might predict. The cognitive potential may also be underestimated because the over-sized child appears so much older than their actual age.

Natural history and complications

The incidence of forceps (7.5%) or cesarean section (7.5%) deliveries does not seem increased in children with Sotos syndrome despite their large head size. Obstetric complications are, therefore, unlikely causes of the neonatal hypotonia (low muscle tone) with subsequent motor, speech, and cognitive delays. Birth length is more increased than weight, and over 50% have a large head circumference at birth. The head circumference quickly joins the height and weight in being over the 97th centile in most children, although adult height is channeled back towards the mean in females because of early puberty. Medical complications include early feeding problems due to hypotonia with 40% requiring tube feedings. Problems relating to the early hypotonia may include strabismus, chronic otitis, constipation, clumsiness (with an increased frequency of fractures), and orthopedic problems such as flat feet or scoliosis (spinal curvature). Eye anomalies (cataracts, strabismus, nystagmus, myopia); congenital heart defects (patent ductus arteriosus, septal defects); urological anomalies; and malignancies (neuroblastoma, hepatocellular carcinoma, non-Hodgkins lymphoma, leukemia and osteochondroma) also occur at increased frequency. Posterior spinal fusion was successful in one case of scoliosis (spinal curvature). Neurologic findings include paradoxically brisk deep tendon reflexes and brain anomalies including dilated cerebral ventricles (cavities within the brain), anomalies of the corpus callosum, and decreased brain matter around the ventricles (periventricular leukomalacia). The range of developmental quotients in 41 children was 40–129, with a mean of 78. No specific language deficits have been defined, but range of behavioral problems have been reported by teachers and parents including tantrums, withdrawal, sleep difficulties, and hyperactivity (38%). Behavioral problems may not exceed those of comparably delayed and over-sized children.

Preventive medical needs

Recommendations for preventive management include attention to feeding and stooling problems in the first year; ophthalmologic, urologic, and cardiac assessment during early infancy; early intervention with physical, speech, and occupational therapy; monitoring of growth, hearing, and skeletal development in early childhood through adolescence; and school planning with anticipation of potential behavioral problems (due to inappropriate expectations or actual hyperactivity). The low frequency and different types of tumors do not lend themselves to the regimen of abdominal ultrasounds followed for Beckwith–Wiedemann syndrome, but physicians and parents should be alert for symptoms.

Family counseling

Most cases are sporadic and represent new mutations in the NOD-1 or other genes as supported by the elevated paternal age that is consistent with new autosomal-dominant mutations. Parents should be examined and their childhood photographs reviewed since many affected individuals may have excellent function as adults; those with early large size, large head size, and suggestive facial appearance will have a 50% recurrence risk with each pregnancy, as will affected children when they are adults. The recurrence risk is extremely low for asymptomatic parents whose child has verified Sotos syndrome.

13

Hamartosis syndromes

Hamartomas are overgrowths of normal tissue. They are similar to tumors in their potential for continuous growth and in their lack of normal tissue organization (dysplasia). Hamartomas are different from choristomas, which are composed of tissue that is alien to its body region, and from teratomas, which are true neoplasms arising from embryonic cells. Hamartosis syndromes, epitomized by neurofibromatosis (NF), are characterized by hamartomas, dyshormonic growth, and neoplastic potential (Table 13.1; Jones, 1997, pp. 495–540; Gorlin et al., 2001, pp. 428–93; Roach & Miller, 2004).

In general, hamartosis syndromes affect the central nervous system (seizures, brain tumors, neurosensory abnormalities), oral cavity (tumors, nevi), heart (tumors), skeleton (limb length discrepancies, scoliosis, bony deformities), and epidermis (nevi, café-au-lait spots, surface tumors). Hamartosis syndromes are often associated with high risk of cancer, and produce physical deformities that require supportive counseling and family support. The more common syndromes (Gardner syndrome, NF-1, and tuberous sclerosis) exhibit autosomal-dominant inheritance that is compatible with the causative gene being a tumor suppressor. The cloning and characterization of the responsible gene has provided strong support for this hypothesis in all three syndromes. Since several of the genetic hamartomatous syndromes have high rates of new mutation, it was predicted in the last edition of this book that apparently sporadic disorders such as the Klippel–Trenaunay–Weber or Proteus syndromes (Table 13.1) would prove to be single-gene mutations as well. Mutations in the tumor suppressor phosphatase and tensin homologue (PTEN) gene have been found in patients with a Proteus-like syndrome (Gorlin et al., 2001, p. 481), and mutations in a VG5Q gene encoding an angiogenic factor have been discovered in the Klippel–Trenaunay–Weber syndrome that is sometimes misdiagnosed as Proteus (see Online Mendelian Inheritance in Man (OMIM) www. ncbi.nlm.nih.gov/entrez/). Somatic mosaicism for these dominant mutations undoubtedly contributes to the highly variable phenotypes of these disorders (Hall, 1988) suggested that the latter conditions may represent somatic mutations, accounting for the variable distributions of lesions and the lack of familial transmission.

Table 13.1. Hamartosis syndromes

Syndrome	Incidence*	Inheritance	Complications
Basal cell carcinoma (Gorlin)	~500 cases	AD	Nevoid basal cell carcinomas, eye anomalies, jaw cysts, skeletal changes (scoliosis), other cancers
Bannayan–Riley–Ruvalcaba	~100 cases	AD	Macrocephaly, lipomas, hemangiomas, intestinal polyps, joint laxity, penile spots
Epidermal nevus	~100 cases	AD	Epidermal nevi, hemangiomas, café-au-lait spots, colobomata, nystagmus, hemihyperplasia, limb deformities, cognitive disability, seizures
Gardner (familial polyposis of the colon)	1 in 12,000	AD	Skin cysts, bony osteomas, colonic polyps, colon cancer, retinal changes, adrenal, hepatic and thyroid cancers
Klippel–Trenaunay–Weber (and Sturge–Weber) angiomatosis	~1000 cases	S	Hemangiomas, skeletal asymmetry, eye anomalies, limb anomalies; seizures, cerebrovascular anomalies, and cognitive disability with Sturge–Weber angiomatosis
Mafucci	~150 cases	S	Hemangiomas, enchondromas, skeletal deformities, other cancers
NF-1	1 in 2500	AD	Café-au-lait spots, neurofibromas, skeletal anomalies, seizures, cognitive disability
NF-2	1 in 100,000	AD	Hearing loss due to acoustic neuromas
Peutz–Jeghers	~300 cases	AD	Skin and mouth pigmentation, intestinal polyposis, cancer
Tuberous sclerosis	1 in 10,000	AD	Hypomelanotic nodules, facial angiofibromas, intracranial ependymomas and astrocytomas, cardiac rhabdomyomas, renal angiomyolipomas, seizures, cognitive disability

Notes:
AD, autosomal dominant; S, sporadic.
*Cases or per number of live births.

Bannayan–Riley–Ruvalcaba syndrome

The combination of macrocephaly with hemangiomas, lipomas, and pigmented macules described by authors such as Bannayan, Myhre, Riley, Ruvalcaba, Smith, and Zonana is now recognized as one autosomal condition with striking variability (Jones, 1997, pp. 522–3; Gorlin et al., 2001, pp. 410–12). This variability is further expanded by the finding that some patients with Bannayan–Riley–Ruvalcaba syndrome have mutations in the PTEN tumor suppressor gene mentioned above;

some authors suggest the term PTEN hamartoma-tumor syndrome (PHTS) for this spectrum that may include atypical cases of Proteus syndrome (Waite & Eng, 2002).

Summary of clinical concerns: Bannayan–Riley–Ruvalcaba management considerations

Growth and development: Overgrowth with macrocephaly, hypotonia and mild mental disability: Early childhood intervention and preschool programs, monitoring of head circumference.

Cancer: Intestinal polyps occur in 45% and malignant tumors (thyroid or breast cancers) have also been noted. Although most of the tumors are benign lipomas, hemangiomas, or lymphangiomas, they may grow aggressively and erode normal tissues: Prompt investigation of masses, asymmetric growth, or unusual gastrointestinal symptoms.

Eyes: Ophthalmologic examination may be helpful diagnostically, showing visible corneal nerves and prominent Schwalbe lines.

Skeletal: Connective tissue laxity with scoliosis, flat feet, and joint dislocations: Regular skeletal examinations, orthopedics referral as needed.

Gastrointestinal: Malignant transformation of intestinal polyps has not been reported, but they may be associated with anemia and melena or protein-losing enteropathy: Monitoring of the hematocrit to rule out anemia.

Endocrine: Autoimmune thyroiditis can in some families: Monitoring of thyroid functions.

Genital: Enlarged testes with pigmented macules on the penis may provide subtle aids to diagnosis in affected males.

Neurologic: Hypotonia, mental disability and seizures in 25%. Many patients have had abnormal muscle biopsy with fat accumulation in type I fibers, and report of a long-chain fatty acid oxidation defect in one patient further broadens the Bannayan–Riley–Ruvalcaba spectrum.

Epidermal nevus or Schimmelpenning syndrome

A pattern of sebaceous nevi with anomalies of the central nervous system, eye, and skeletal system were described by Schimmelpenning in 1957, and a confusing nomenclature has attended description of over 100 sporadic cases. Gorlin et al. (2001, pp. 485–8) and Jones (1997, pp. 500–1) suggest the eponym as a unbiased name, particularly because not all linear nevi that characterize the disorder have true sebaceous elements. Jadassohn was an early contributor to this literature, and other names like Fuerstein, Mims, and Solomon are associated. Happle (2004) also favors the Schimmelpenning eponym, and emphasizes that epidermal nevi occur in several disorders like Proteus syndrome, CHILD syndrome (a condition with ichthyosis and limb asymmetry) and in association with lipoepidermoid cysts of the eye or ipsilateral hypoplasia of the breast.

Frequent complications of Schimmelpenning syndrome include cognitive disability, seizures, facial asymmetry, ocular anomalies, oral lesions, and skeletal anomalies (Jones, 1997, pp. 500–1; Gorlin et al., 2001, pp. 485–8). There is a clear correlation between epidermal nevi on the head and complications of the central nervous system. Preventive management should begin with focus on early intervention and supportive counseling appropriate for a disorder with a 50% risk for significant mental disability. Modern surgery offers excellent options and outcomes for treatment of these invasive nevi (Margulis et al., 2003), so early referral to plastic surgery and dermatology is paramount. Periodic vision screening and ophthalmology visits are needed to detect the 33% of patients that have ocular anomalies. Regular monitoring of growth and skeletal development should be conducted, since congenital anomalies of the vertebrae and limbs occur, along with hemihyperplasia and scoliosis secondary to asymmetry. Oral inspection and dental care should include surveillance for clefts or hypoplastic teeth. Neoplasms occur with increased frequency, including Wilms tumor, gastric carcinoma, breast cancer, and astrocytoma.

Gardner syndrome and other hereditary polyposis syndromes

Pediatric health care providers will definitely encounter children with Gardner syndrome, based on its prevalence of 1 in 1400–12,000 individuals (Gorlin et al., 2001, pp. 437–44). Major features of Gardner syndrome include adenomatous polyps of the colon, osteomas of the facial bones, epidermoid cysts and fibrous hyperplasia of the skin, eye changes (congenital hypertrophic retinal pigment epithelium), and multiple changes in the teeth and jaw.

Summary of clinical concerns: Gardner and hereditary polyposis management considerations

General: In the case of Garner syndrome, pediatricians and dentists can make this diagnosis based on dental changes like supernumerary, impacted, or unerupted teeth (Buch et al., 2001). In other polyposis syndromes, pigmentary lesions (Bannayan–Riley–Ruvalcaba, Peutz–Jeghers syndromes), skin papules/fibromas (Cowden, Torre–Muir syndromes), or macrocephaly/alopecia (Cronkhite–Canada syndrome) may prompt recognition during childhood.

Cancer: The most serious complication is the development of cancer within the colon polyps, affecting 50% of patients by age 30 years and virtually 100% by later middle age. Tumors of the central nervous system (glioma, medulloblastoma), viscera (adrenal or hepatocarcinoma), and bones (osteosarcoma, chondrosarcoma) also occur, making Gardner syndrome representative of a group of hamartoneoplastic syndromes that include intestinal polyposis and cancer predisposition (Gorlin et al., 2001, pp. 440–1). All of these polyposis syndromes are likely due to heterozygous mutations, presenting as sporadic cases or with obvious vertical transmission. Malignant lesions of these disorders usually occur in early to late adulthood: Regular physical examinations should be emphasized in the transition to adult care because of the many types and locations of neoplasms that occur in polyposis syndromes.

Gastrointestinal: In Gardner syndrome, only 5% of patients experience malignant degeneration of intestinal polyps before puberty; recognition of accessory features is thus important for pediatric diagnosis: Effective management has been designed for Gardner and other polyposis syndromes once the diagnosis is made. Non-steroidal anti-inflammatory drugs have been shown to shrink the size of polyps and delay malignant transformation; better screening through stool DNA studies and colonoscopy is now available. Some patients still opt for a total colectomy, while others are willing to undergo regular colonoscopy and anti-inflammatory drug therapy with excision of polyps.

Parental counseling: Pediatric recognition is extremely important because early diagnosis can initiate family studies and effective preventive management. DNA diagnosis is available for several of these conditions (see www.genetests.org), illustrated by the familial adenomatous polyposis (FAP) gene where particular alleles correlate with isolated polyposis or the broader anomalies of Gardner syndrome. Early recognition of affected children allows testing of parents and other family members to identify those with 50% risks for genetic transmission plus high cancer risk. Once the primary care physician has raised the concern and referred the family to gastroenterology, surgery, and genetics for counseling and management, the accompanying problems can be addressed – by dentistry, orthopedics, and ophthalmology in the case of Gardner syndrome. Parent information is available at the Network for Peutz–Jeghers and Juvenile Polyposis Syndromes (www.epigenetic.org/~pjs/homepage.html) and an information site for Peutz–Jeghers Syndrome (www.epigenetic.org/~pjs/homepage.html).

Nevoid basal cell carcinoma (Gorlin) syndrome

Over 500 cases of Gorlin syndrome have been described, and it accounts for about 20% of patients who develop basal cell carcinomas of the skin before age 20 years and for 1 in 200 patients who develop them at any age (Jones, 1997, pp. 528–9; Gorlin et al., 2001, pp. 444–53; Gorlin, 2004). The disorder exhibits autosomal-dominant inheritance and is due to mutations in the PTCH gene at chromosome region 9q23–q31; basal cell carcinomas have a double (homozygous) mutation at the PTCH locus, following the classic one-hit for susceptibility, two-hit for cancer model of the

Knudson hypothesis. DNA testing is available to distinguish affected individuals with a 50% risk for transmission from asymptomatic parents with a virtually 0% risk of transmission (see www. genetests.org). The pediatrician and pediatric dentist have important opportunities for early diagnosis through the findings of supernumerary or unerupted teeth and jaw cysts (Buch et al., 2001). Early recognition is important because sun protection and topical treatment with isotretinoin and 5-fluorouracil show promise for long-term suppression of the basal cell carcinomas.

Facial, ocular, oral, and skeletal changes predominate in the nevoid basal cell carcinoma syndrome, but the manifestations are protean and can affect most organ systems. Nevoid basal cell carcinomas are the distinguishing feature of the condition, appearing sometimes at birth but usually between puberty and 35 years of age (Gorlin, 2004). There is a distinctive facies in 70% of patients, caused by prominence of the forehead and supra-orbital ridges with hypertelorism. Eye anomalies include cataracts, glaucoma, and colobomata with occasional retinitis pigmentosa and detachment. Oral changes include cysts in the jaws (keratocysts), which often develop in the first decade of life. Central nervous system changes such as hydrocephalus or agenesis of the corpus callosum are rare, and there is a 3% incidence of mental deficiency (Gorlin, 2004).

Gorlin syndrome has few manifestations in childhood, although central nervous system anomalies causing hydrocephalus have been reported. Nevoid basal cell carcinomas may be present before puberty, but they rarely cause problems. It is after adolescence that regular dermatologic evaluations are needed to identify the surprisingly few tumors that become invasive. Although the nevoid tumors occur in areas unexposed to the sun, full protection from sunlight and from other sources of radiation is an obvious recommendation for affected children. Damage from sunlight may be evident in a study showing earlier onset and greater multiplicity of the tumors for patients in Australia compared to those in England. Other preventive measures include regular ophthalmology and dentistry examinations, evaluation of skeletal growth with referral to orthopedics if scoliosis or bony deformities occur, and referral for early intervention/rehabilitative services for the unusual patient with mental disability. As is common in precancerous syndromes, other neoplasms can occur and include medulloblastomas, ovarian or cardiac fibromas, fibrosarcomas after radiation therapy, and a variety of visceral cancers (Gorlin et al., 2001, pp. 444–53; Gorlin, 2004; Jone, 1997).

Klippel–Trenaunay–Weber (and/or Sturge–Weber, Parkes–Weber) syndromes

Multiple hemangiomas with skeletal asymmetry are characteristic of Klippel–Trenaunay–Weber syndrome (Jones, 1997, pp. 512–3; Cohen, 2000; Gorlin et al.,

2001, pp. 454–5). Over 1000 cases have been described, but an incidence figure has not been determined. Mental development is usually normal unless the craniofacies is involved, when the disorder blends with Sturge–Weber syndrome.

Summary of clinical concerns: Klippel–Trenaunay/Sturge–Weber management considerations

General: The complications of Klippel–Trenaunay–Weber and its related disorders are highly variable and depend on the areas of vascular enlargement.

Growth and development: In those with the typical Sturge–Weber facial hemangioma, 30% have mental disability. Those with seizures have a higher risk of developmental delay (43% versus 0% in those without seizures), special education requirements (71% versus 0%), and emotional or behavioral problems (85% versus 60%). Employability was also decreased in those with seizures (46% versus 78%), but the overall frequency of self-sufficiency (39%) and marriage (55%) provides an optimistic outlook for patients with Sturge–Weber syndrome. Those with somatic rather than facial hemangiomas typical of Klippel–Trenaunay–Weber syndrome usually have normal intelligence: Monitoring of development, with prompt early intervention referral of those with Sturge–Weber facial hemangiomas. The number and severity of neurologic abnormalities will determine the requirements for subsequent medical, rehabilitative, and scholastic evaluations.

Craniofacial: Cranial findings in patients with Klippel–Trenaunay–Weber syndrome are quite similar to those of Sturge–Weber angiomatosis, and there is clear overlap of these two disorders and the Parkes–Weber syndrome. Oral anomalies (gingival angiomas, abnormal tooth eruption, macrodontia) are common: Neurology referral of those with Sturge–Weber hemangiomas as discussed below, serial dental evaluations.

Eye: Anomalies include glaucoma with buphthalmos and choroidal angioma when the Sturge–Weber nevus is present: Early and serial ophthalmology evaluations with pressure measurements.

Skeletal: Parkes–Weber syndrome has similar limb enlargements that are warm to the touch because of arteriovenous fistulae while Sturge–Weber and Klippel–Trenaunay–Weber syndrome have venous malformations and (unique to the latter disorder) lymphatic malformations found in (Cohen, 2000; Gorlin et al., 2001, pp. 454–5). Limb hypertrophy may lead to scoliosis: Annual skeletal examinations and orthopedic referral when skeletal asymmetry is noted. No increased risk of neoplasia has been described, perhaps because limb hypertrophy rather than hemihyperplasia is involved.

Other visceral: Visceral hemangiomatosis can affect the lungs, gastrointestinal tract, and urinary tract, and protein-losing enteropathy due to intestinal lesions has occurred: Imaging studies of internal organs are not indicated unless symptoms are noted.

Vascular: Bleeding can occur in any vascular organ including internal surfaces as illustrated by the occurrence of hemoptysis (Ghosh et al., 2004). Major complications include limb or digital enlargement with edema (84%), varicose veins (36%), and malformations of deep veins such as the popliteal (51%), femoral (16%), iliac (3%), and inferior vena cava (1%). Lymphatic abnormalities with edema and digital anomalies suggestive of embryonic circulatory defects (syndactyly, polydactyly) are also seen. Patients with severe vascular distortions are at risk for bleeding from platelet trapping (Kasabach–Merritt syndrome) or cellulites: Physical examination with imaging studies of affected regions, being alert for internal complications and for problems due to abnormal venous or lymphatic drainage. Cohen (2000) emphasizes the importance of scanning vascular lesions by MRI with gadolinium enhancement to distinguish vascular from lymphatic lesions, and of aggressive cranial and bone imaging to define cerebral and interosseous lesions.

Neurologic: When a nevus flammeus is found over the trigeminal nerve distribution, with or without hemangiomas elsewhere in the body, the Sturge–Weber pattern of angiomatosis should be suspected. Angiomas of the leptomeninges usually occur on the ipsilateral side, and concurrent cerebrovascular anomalies (46%) and/or intracranial calcifications (57%) may be present (Gorlin et al., 2001, pp. 454–64). In patients with radiographic evidence of cortical calcification, about 87% had seizures, 97% a port-wine nevus, and 14% died from their disease over a follow-up period of at least 10 years.

Parental counseling: All three disorders are sporadic with few familial instances, and the finding of an up-regulated VG5Q angiogenic factor in a Klippel–Trenaunay–Weber patient offers a route for better clinical and molecular delineation of these disorders (Tian et al., 2004). Many instances may arise by somatic rather than germ-line mutation, explaining their sporadic occurrence and frequent segmental distribution (Hall, 1988). A virtually zero recurrence risk can be given to parents of affected children. There are several websites listing information for physicians and parents that can be accessed using the syndrome names, and a site designed by the affected professional golfer Casey Martin can provide inspiration for families: (www.linksplayers.com/PLAYER_PROFILES/Casey_Martin/casey_martin.html).

Mafucci syndrome

Mafucci syndrome, like Klippel–Trenaunay–Weber syndrome, involves multiple hemangiomas with risk of skeletal deformities (Gorlin et al., 2001, pp. 460–1). In addition, there are multiple enchondromas of bone and associated other neo-plasms. The enchondromas appear between ages 1 and 5 years, producing greater deformity than is seen in the Klippel–Trenaunay–Weber syndrome, including risk of limb fractures. Beyond surveillance for bleeding or platelet depletion, there is little preventive management for Mafucci syndrome other than surgical referral to manage the cosmetic, vascular, and skeletal complications. Malignant neoplasms have included angiosarcoma, fibrosarcoma, pancreatic and hepatic carcinomas, and brain tumors.

Peutz–Jeghers syndrome

The combination of melanotic nodules on the lips and intestinal polyposis charac-terizes Peutz–Jeghers syndrome. It is an autosomal-dominant disorder with an increased risk of cancer (Jones, 1997, pp. 520–1; Gorlin et al., 2001, pp. 476–80; Schreibman et al., 2005). The oral pigmentation most frequently involves the lips (98%), but also is seen on the buccal mucosa (88%), palate (less common), or tongue (rare). Pigment also appears on the skin, varying from a few macules to large pig-mented areas. The polyps are benign hamartomas that occur in the jejunum (65%), ileum (55%), large intestine (36%), stomach (23%), or duodenum (15%). More than 70% of patients experience some type of symptom (pain, melena) from the polyps, with an age of onset between a few weeks and 82 years (mean age, 29 years). The skin and oral pigmentation is usually present during infancy, but may appear as late as the eighth decade.

Preventive management of Peutz–Jeghers syndrome should include a thorough evaluation of the gastrointestinal tract once the diagnosis is made. The intestinal polyps are hamartomas rather than cancers, but malignant transformation has been clearly documented. While earlier authors recommended removal of polyps only if they were responsible for intussusception, current policy is to surgically excise them when feasible. Endoscopic techniques have greatly lessened the need for repeated abdominal surgery, and most recommend "top and tail" endoscopy to be performed every 2 years, with removal of polyps greater than 0.5 cm in size (Schreibman et al., 2005). Unfortunately, there is also increased risk of neoplasm at other sites, including ovarian, breast, testicular or pancreatic cancers. Since these tumors occur at high frequency (10–14% risk of ovarian tumors in females), abdominal ultrasound screening every 3–6 months should be considered in these patients. Pelvic examination, cervical smear, and breast and testicular examina-tions should also be performed annually after age 30 years.

Peutz–Jeghers syndrome is caused by mutations in the serine–threonine kinase STK11 gene, and DNA testing is available at several laboratories to identify affected individuals with high risks of cancer and a 50% risk of transmission to offspring.

Parent information is available at the Network for Peutz–Jeghers and Juvenile Polyposis Syndromes (www.epigenetic.org/~pjs/homepage.html) and an information site for Peutz–Jeghers Syndrome (www.epigenetic.org/~pjs/homepage.html).

Proteus syndrome

In 1979 Cohen and Hayden first described a syndrome that Wiedemann would name Proteus after the Greek God who could change shape (Gorlin et al., 2001, pp. 480–4). As the name implies, the patients may suffer considerable distortions in appearance due to localized overgrowth and hamartomas. Hemangiomas, lipomas, and lymphangiomas may occur, and fibrous growths on the foot may form the characteristic "moccasin" lesion that is preserved in the skeleton of Joseph Merrick, the "Elephant Man." Other complications include increased growth, strabismus, skeletal abnormalities such as scoliosis, kyphosis, dislocated hips, and striking overgrowth of digits or toes. Mental deficiency (55%) and seizures (13%) also occur (Gorlin et al., 2001, pp. 480–4). Preventive management should consist of early intervention and developmental assessment, ophthalmology referral during the first year, evaluation of skeletal growth for orthopedic problems, and periodic examinations to detect early cancers. Neoplasms of the parotid gland, testis, and breast have been reported, and more evidence of carcinogenesis can be anticipated in this unusual hamartosis syndrome. All cases have been sporadic, with minimal recurrence risks for parents of affected children. A Proteus-like condition has been associated with mutations in the PTEN tumor suppressor gene, but routine DNA testing is not yet available.

Neurofibromatosis-2

As discussed in Gorlin et al. (2001, pp. 469–76), several types of NF can be distinguished according to the type and distribution of hamartomatous lesions. Neurofibromatosis-1 (NF-1) is a common and well-known disorder (see below), while neurofibromatosis-2 (NF-2) is rare (incidence 1 in 40,000–100,000 births) and notable for the presence of vestibular schwannomas along the eighth cranial nerve. The term "acoustic neuroma" has been discarded because the tumors derive from Schwann cells and are distributed along the vestibular branch of the eighth nerve.

Summary of clinical concerns: Neurofibromatosis-2 management considerations

General: The café-au-lait spots and neurofibromata associated with NF-1 can also occur in NF-2, but Lische nodules in the eye and axillary freckling are uncommon. Baser et al. (2002) suggest that NF-2 be considered in any child presenting with the above-mentioned tumors, and point out that the various diagnostic criteria are only 90% sensitive.

Tumors: About 20% of patients with NF-2 present with tumors during childhood, including vestibular schwannoma, meningioma, spinal or cutaneous neurofibroma/schwannoma.

Eyes: Cataracts (50% of patients) may occur at a young age, and these plus the unique ophthalmologic finding of epiretinal membranes provide helpful criteria for diagnosis: Regular ophthalmology examinations on symptomatic children and asymptomatic children with affected parents.

Neurologic: Vestibular schwannomas cause the most severe problems in the disorder. The usual presentation is hearing loss noted in late adolescence or early adulthood. Patients with vestibular schwannomas many also have unilateral hearing loss (93%), tinnitus (60%), poor balance (35%), aural fullness (24%), and headache (5%); – (Jones, 1997, pp. 508–9; Gorlin et al., 2001, pp. 469–76). Variability in the time of presentation mandates early and frequent auditory evoked response and audiology screening once the diagnosis of NF-2 is made, along with annual MRI scan of the brain to measure the tumor size. Children with an affected parent but without hearing deficits can wait until age 10 years for the head MRI so that anesthesia can be avoided. When a vestibular schwannoma is documented, surgery is usually indicated except in debilitated patients. Many patients with vestibular schwannomas will require limited surgery to debulk the lesions, and the preservation of hearing after surgery correlates with tumor size. Referral to neurology, neurosurgery, and otolaryngology is crucial, and better outcomes have been demonstrated at special clinics or centers (Baser et al., 2002). Follow-up is critical, with brain imaging and hearing tests as frequently as every 3 months, depending on the patient's age and the rate of tumor progression.

Parental counseling: A Merlin tumor suppressor gene is mutated in NF-2, and DNA testing is available to help with uncertain diagnoses (see www.genetests.org). Like NF-1, NF-2 is an autosomal-dominant disorder with a 50% recurrence risk for affected individuals, and those who receive a mutant allele have a 95% risk for clinical manifestations (penetrance). Since affected individuals may have few cutaneous lesions, children of a parent with NF-2 (i.e., those at 50% risk) may deserve a baseline head MRI scan and annual hearing assessments until their genetic status is defined by DNA testing. Conversely, parents of affected individuals should also be warned about the symptoms, even though there is a substantial new mutation rate of 50%. Support groups may help patients deal with the prospects and complications (facial nerve palsies, distortions in appearance) of frequent surgery. They may be located through the National Neurofibromatosis Foundation (www.nf.org/), Neurofibromatosis, Inc. (www.nf.org/), Acoustic Neuroma Association (www.anausa.org) and the British Acoustic Neuroma Association (www.ukan.co.uk/bana).

Neurofibromatosis-1

Terminology

Although the disorder was first described in 1849, von Recklinghausen's identification of neural elements in NF-1 gained him credit for recognizing the disease in 1882 (Jones, 1997, pp. 508–9; Gorlin et al., 2001, pp. 469–76). The classical description was of NF-1 with multiple café-au-lait spots and neurofibromas, which accounts for 90% of all cases. NF-2 with schwannomas (acoustic neuromas) discussed above, NF-3 (Riccardi type) with multiple brain tumors of early and lethal onset, NF-3 (intestinal type) with intussception and obstruction, and NF-5 (segmental NF) that likely represents somatic mutations causing NF-1. Isolation of the genes responsible for type 1 (neurofibromin gene on chromosome 17) and type 2 (merlin tumor suppressor on chromosome 22) has established these disorders as separate entities (Ward & Gutmann, 2005). The large size and multiplicity of mutations in the neurofibromin gene limits its diagnostic use and the ability to determine if other NF types are merely variable expressions of NF-1.

Incidence, etiology, and differential diagnosis

The prevalence of NF-1 is between 1 in 2500 and 1 in 3000 births, with about 50% representing new mutations. The disorder exhibits autosomal-dominant inheritance with virtually 100% penetrance if findings such as café-au-lait spots are scored. The responsible gene has been cloned and encodes a protein called neurofibromin; neurofibromin is homologous to components of the G-protein signal transduction pathway and seems to function as a tumor suppressor. Large deletions of the gene are common, as detected by fluorescent *in situ* hybridization (FISH), and these patients often have additional dysmorphology and more café-au-lait spots than others with NF-1 (Ward & Gutmann, 2005). The germ-line mutation of one neurofibromin allele (one-hit) may cause a proliferation of skin (café-au-lait spots) or Schwann cells (neurofibromas), since the second normal neurofibromin allele is retained in neurofibromas. Loss of heterozygosity (second hit) causes certain of the malignant tumors associated with NF-1.

The differential diagnosis is between other hamartoses such as Bannayan–Riley–Ruvalcaba syndrome (macrocephaly, lipomas, pigmented lesions), LEOPARD syndrome (*L*entigines, *E*lectrocardiographic conduction abnormalities, *O*cular hypertelorism, *P*ulmonary stenosis, *A*bnormalities of the Genitalia, *R*etardation of growth, and *D*eafness) with multiple lentigines, or Proteus syndrome with lipomas, epidermal nevi, and asymmetric gigantism of the limbs or face. Cohen (1987) presented compelling evidence that Joseph Merrick, the "Elephant Man," had Proteus syndrome rather than NF-1 (see above). This distinction is reassuring to patients with a common disease (NF-1), although the severe deformities of

Joseph Merrick remain a worrisome symbol for patients with the extremely rare Proteus syndrome. Among the other forms of NF, NF-2 is important to differentiate because of its different preventive management oriented toward vestibular schwannomas (see above). Autosomal-dominant café-au-lait spots without other findings of NF-1 and the clinical pattern of Noonan syndrome with findings of NF-1 (Watson syndrome) can result from mutations within the neurofibromin gene.

Diagnostic evaluation and medical counseling

Crowe and colleagues in 1956 developed a criterion of six café-au-lait spots larger than 1.5 cm when selecting patients for their classic study of NF-1 (Gorlin et al., 2001, pp. 469–76). This criterion is widely accepted for a diagnosis of the disease, although six spots more than 0.5 cm diameter before puberty is accepted. A broader criterion lists the requisite number of café-au-lait spots as one of seven findings, any two of which would confirm the clinical diagnosis of NF-1. The other findings included:

1 two neurofibroma or one plexiform neuroma;
2 axillary or inguinal freckling;
3 optic glioma;
4 two or more Lisch nodules;
5 a distinctive osseous lesion (e.g., pseudoarthrosis);
6 a first-degree relative with NF.

Molecular testing for the more common NF-1 mutations is commercially available at several laboratories (see www.genetests.org), but is not sufficiently sensitive to be useful for diagnosis.

In asymptomatic patients, optimistic medical counseling is warranted based on the 40% of patients with NF-1 who never have complications. However, a milder disease course involving pigmented lesions can quickly change to one with incapacitating neurologic deficits from encroaching tumors. It is thus important to inform patients about the risks of learning disabilities, of neurologic deficits or asymmetries secondary to tumor growth, and of vascular lesions with hypertension. Realistic mention of complications should aid in accomplishing the regular physical examinations that are the crux of preventive management of NF-1.

Family and psychosocial counseling

A common scenario for this autosomal-dominant disease with a 50% new mutation rate is for normal couples to have a child affected with NF-1. If one parent has macrocephaly or other findings suggestive of NF, then examination for café-au-lait spots, head MRI scan, and ophthalmology slit-lamp examination for Lisch spots may detect the diagnosis. Individuals with the disease have a 50% risk to transmit the disorder with each pregnancy, and variable expressivity dictates that mildly affected parents may have severely affected offspring and vice versa. Most states have active NF organizations that can be helpful for family counseling and support, particularly in relieving the specter of deformity that may dominate lay images of the disease. Parent support and information are available at the National Neurofibromatosis foundation (www.nf.org/) and Neurofibromatosis, Inc. (www.nf.org/).

Natural history and complications

As mentioned above, 40% of patients avoid complications beyond café-au-lait spots. The diagnosis may be difficult to recognize in the neonatal period, and most individuals with NF-1 avoid early complications. Macrocephaly is relatively common (30%), and seizures or hydrocephalus may occur. The asymmetry and disfigurement of plexiform neuromas that occur in about 30% of children may cause difficult management problems when the tumors cannot be surgically dissected free of nerve roots. Cutaneous findings are significantly associated with enhanced mortality in NF-1, both in children and adults. Of 703 patients followed for 2.4 years, including 405 (57.6%) children, 40 patients died (mostly due to sarcomas); adults were 3.6 times more likely to have subcutaneous neurofibromas and 5.6 times more likely to be male while childhood mortality was associated with facial plexiform neurofibromas and pruritus (Khosrotehrani et al., 2005).

Optic gliomas are common in NF-1, and are often multifocal. Fortunately, the tumors are less invasive of the optic nerves than optic gliomas in patients without NF-1. Equally troubling are spinal neurofibromas that may recur in patients with NF-1, especially those affecting the cervical spine. NF-1 commonly affects the skeleton, with dislocations, pseudoarthroses, scoliosis, and underdevelopment of the maxilla and mandible being common. The long bones may contain cyst-like lesions that are useful for diagnosis but seem not to cause pain or fractures. Vascular lesions such as renal artery stenosis and congenital cardiac lesions do occur, and hypertension may be a problem during adulthood. Some patients develop arteriovenous fistulae of the spinal column, adding another reason for vigilance concerning neck or back pain and altered gait. Scoliosis may occur from bone lesions or dystrophic vertebrae.

About 40% of NF-1 patients have cognitive disability, with speech delay and selective learning differences. The children may also have neurosensory deficits from optic glioma (4%) or aural neurofibromas. Neurofibromas of the external ear canal and pinna are found in 5% of patients with NF-1, but tumors invading the vestibule and causing hearing loss are rare compared to such events in NF-2. NF-1 patients are at risk for neoplasms in most body regions, with examples of benign (neurofibromas), malignant by position (plexiform neurofibromas), or true malignant tumors (neurofibrosarcomas, Wilms tumor, leukemias, pancreatic or adrenal carcinomas).

Neurofibromatosis-1 preventive medical checklist

Health care recommendations for NF have been endorsed by the Committee on Genetics, American Academy of Pediatrics (1995b). Although some authors have recommended brain imaging studies as soon as the diagnosis of NF-1 is made, the general consensus is to await such symptoms as seizures, increased head circumference, or precocious puberty before obtaining a head MRI scan. Since there is increased risk for optic gliomas and other intracranial tumors, and since benign or malignant tumors can arise in many other body locations, aggressive radiologic evaluations should be pursued when changes are revealed by periodic history review and physical examination. Once tumors such as optic gliomas or acoustic neuromas are discovered, their management will depend on their rate of growth and the disability inflicted on the patient. Since these tumors are usually multifocal, surgical intervention should be saved for symptoms of severe neurosensory dysfunction or of increased intracranial pressure. Debulking operations may have some role in cranial nerve tumors, but conservative approaches aimed at preserving nerve function are particularly important for children.

Regular physical examinations noting the distribution of café-au-lait spots and neurofibromas are useful, including drawings or photographs of lesions. Because neurosensory or skeletal alterations may be harbingers of tumor growth, regular hearing/vision assessment by the physician with annual ophthalmology and audiology screening is recommended through adulthood. Puberty is particularly important to monitor, since precocious puberty and accelerated tumor growth during puberty are established phenomena. Lesions may also grow during pregnancy.

Early intervention, speech evaluation, and preschool evaluation of cognitive performance are important because of the frequent occurrence of learning disabilities in NF-1 (Gorlin et al., 2001, p. 471). About 8% will have an IQ less than 70, and 25% will have some type of learning difference. Skeletal asymmetry and scoliosis may compromise motor function, and job training is important in patients with cognitive disabilities. Hypertension may occur through a narrowing of the renal artery or pheochromocytomas, so annual monitoring of blood pressure is also recommended. A NF clinic in reasonable proximity is an excellent resource for the coordinated subspecialty management that NF-1 patients may require.

Tuberous sclerosis

Terminology

The term "tuberous sclerosis" was coined in 1880 by Bourneville (Jones, 1997, pp. 506–7; Gorlin et al., 2001, pp. 488–93). The fibrotic tumors in brain ("tubers") cause seizures and mental retardation that, together with "adenoma sebaceum," comprise the classic diagnostic recognized by Vogt in 1908. In fact, the term "adenoma sebaceum" is incorrect, because the facial lesions are actually angiofibromas. "Epiloa" is also an outdated term derived from Greek roots meaning epilepsy and mindlessness. Clinical findings in tuberous sclerosis include reddish-yellow plaques on the forehead ("forehead plaque"), leathery plaques in the lumbosacral area ("shagreen patches"), and diffuse regions of skin hyper/hypopigmentation ("confetti skin lesions"). The variability of clinical findings and evidence of genetic heterogeneity in tuberous sclerosis have led to the term "tuberous sclerosis complex" (Gorlin et al., 2001, pp. 488–93; Roach & Sparagana, 2004).

Incidence, etiology, and differential diagnosis

Depending on the rate of clinical detection, the incidence of tuberous sclerosis is 1 per 6000–10,000 births. Tuberous sclerosis is an autosomal-dominant disorder, and genetic linkage studies have identified a TSC1 gene (85% of cases) at chromosome band 9q34 and a TSC2 gene (15% of cases) at 16p13.3. The TSC1 gene is a growth suppressor and the TSC2 gene is a G-protein active in signal transduction – both roles similar to those of neurofibromin. DNA testing is available for both genes (see www.genetests.org), but low sensitivity mandates a clinical diagnosis in most cases. Contiguous gene deletion of TSC2 and the nearby polycystic kidney disease gene has caused early and severe renal cystic disease in some patients with tuberous sclerosis.

The major clinical findings of seizures, facial angiofibromas, ungual fibromas, hypopigmented macules, cardiac or renal tumors, and neural (brain, retina) hamartomas comprise a distinctive clinical picture for tuberous sclerosis. Differential diagnosis would include other disorders with brain and skin lesions, such as Sturge–Weber angiomatosis or NF, congenital infection with toxoplasma or cytomegalovirus, and facial xanthomas or milia.

Diagnostic evaluation and medical counseling

Diagnostic criteria for tuberous sclerosis have been formulated by several consensus conferences summarized by Roach & Sparagana (2004). A major problem with the diagnosis in childhood is that features such as facial angiofibromas, ungual fibromas, renal angiomyolipomas, and even calcified subependymal nodules may not be present during infancy. Periodic diagnostic assessment is thus required for individuals at risk. With this caveat in mind, major diagnostic criteria for tuberous sclerosis are listed in Table 13.2. Some findings require histologic and/or radiographic confirmation before qualifying as criteria, while others (facial angiofibromas, ungual fibromas, retinal astrocytomas, shagreen patches, or hypomelanotic nodules) can be diagnosed only by physical examination. For a definite diagnosis, two major features or one major feature plus two minor features are required (Gorlin et al., 2001, p. 488; Roach & Sparagana, 2004). Patients with fewer features can be considered as probable or suspect for tuberous sclerosis, with the implication

Table 13.2. Diagnostic criteria for tuberous sclerosis

Major features
Facial angiofibromas or forehead plaque
Nontraumatic ungual or periungual fibroma
Hypomelanotic macules
Shagreen patch (connective tissue nevus)
Multiple retinal nodular hamartomas
Cortical tuber
Subependymal nodule or giant cell astrocytoma
Cardiac rhabdomyoma, single or multiple
Lymphangiomyomatosis
Renal angiomyolipoma

Secondary features
Multiple, randomly distributed pits in the dental enamel
Hamartomatous rectal polyps
Bone cysts
Cerebral white matter radial migration lines
Gingival fibromas
Nonrenal hamartoma
Retinal achromatic patch
"Confetti" skin lesions
Multiple renal cysts

Source: Roach & Sparagana (2004).

that younger patients need careful follow-up. Examination with ultraviolet light A (Wood's lamp) is much more sensitive in detecting the white macules in light-skinned people.

Medical counseling must take into account the 60–80% of patients that have mental or learning disabilities, but many affected individuals are asymptomatic. Brain involvement with tumors, heterotopias, seizures, and developmental disability often accompanies the presentation in early childhood, and these patients will require the full spectrum of psychosocial and medical counseling appropriate for children with severe handicaps. Behavioral abnormalities such as childhood autism or later schizophrenia are frequent, and changes in behavior should be mentioned as a mandate for brain imaging.

Family and psychosocial counseling

Affected individuals will have a 50% risk of transmitting tuberous sclerosis with each pregnancy. The difficulty in genetic counseling is to distinguish whether parents of an obviously affected child are themselves affected. Asymptomatic but affected individuals had positive findings by skin examination (96%), cranial CT scan (67%), skull radiographs (46%), hand/foot radiographs (39%), fundoscopic examination (33%), and renal ultrasound study (30%) according to the study of Cassidy et al. (1983). Thorough ascertainment of family members has revised prior estimates of the new mutation rate from 70% to about 50%, and germ-line mosaicism (producing more than one affected child to normal parents is sufficiently common (6%) to warrant mention.

Considerable psychosocial support is needed for families with severely affected infants, since these children will have extensive mental and physical disabilities. Patients with facial lesions (facial angiofibromas, forehead plaques) may require cosmetic surgery, dermatologic treatment, and psychiatric support because of their altered appearance. Parent and physician information can be found at the Tuberous Sclerosis Alliance (www.tsalliance.org/), the Tuberous Sclerosis Association UK (www.tuberous-sclerosis.org/), and Tuberous Sclerosis International (www.stsn. nl/tsi/tsi.htm).

Natural history and complications

Complications of tuberous sclerosis affect the nervous system most severely with seizures in 88–93%, mental deficiency in 60–80%, and intracranial calcifications in 56% (Jones, 1997, pp. 506–7; Gorlin et al., 2001, pp. 488–93; Roach & Sparagana, 2004). Tonic–clonic (41%) and infantile spasms (30%) are the most common types of seizures, but myoclonic, absence, and akinetic seizures also occur. Seizures have an early onset, with 20% starting before age 3 months, 50% starting before age 3–7 months, and only 5% occurring after age 5 years. Cranial calcification of subependymal hamartomas is progressive, with 15% of patients by age 1 year, 35% by age 5 years, and 50–60% by age 14 years exhibiting this finding. Behavioral changes are common, including hyperactivity (28%), impaired social interaction (43%), repetitive behaviors (25%), and aggressive behaviors with attacks on other people (28%) or self-injury (29%).

Other symptomatic findings include intracranial hypertension from cranial giant cell astrocytomas that occur in 6–14% of patients (Roach & Sparagana, 2004). Cardiac rhabdomyomas occur in 30–67% of patients, and symptomatic infants have significant mortality. These cardiac tumors may also resolve over time. Endocrine abnormalities rarely occur, but can include acromegaly or precocious puberty. Cystic disease of the lung (honeycomb lung) occurs predominantly in females, causing symptoms after the third decade with a 5-year mortality rate of 67%.

Lesions of tuberous sclerosis that are generally asymptomatic include the hypomelanotic macules, facial angiofibromas, and ungual fibromas of the skin; renal angiomyolipomas or cysts; and miscellaneous hamartomas in organs such as pancreas, liver, and testes. Retinal hamartomas are of two types, presenting as gray-yellow

semitranslucent lesions (55%) or opaque, nodular lesions (45%). Some patients
have both types, but few have visual problems. The phalanges and, less frequently,
the long bones may exhibit asymptomatic cysts or periosteal new bone formation
on radiographs. Some patients have overgrowth of one digit, and one presented
with an acromegaly.

Tuberous sclerosis preventive medical checklist

Preventive management of tuberous sclerosis will be directed toward early evaluation
of neurologic, ophthalmologic, cardiac, dermatologic, and developmental problems
(Jones, 1997, pp. 506–7; Gorlin et al., 2001, pp. 488–93; Roach & Sparagana, 2004).
If the disease is recognized at birth, head ultrasound or MRI studies can be justified to determine the presence and size of ependymomas or giant cell astrocytomas. Changes in behavior, alterations in head circumference, and symptoms of
intracranial hypertension warrant additional head MRI studies, and contrast may
be helpful in recognizing the more troublesome giant cell astrocytomas. The latter
tumors should be removed when accessible, particularly if they are expanding or
symptomatic (Roach & Sparagana, 2004). Epilepsy begins early and takes many
forms, so pediatric neurology referral is important for diagnosis and treatment.
Anticonvulsant therapy tends to be complex, and surgical treatment has a role in
severe cases. Sleep disturbances are frequent in patients with epilepsy, so sleep studies may be considered. The high risk of mental disability justifies early intervention
with regular speech, occupational, and physical therapy assessments. Financial, psychosocial, and genetic counseling should be facilitated and re-emphasized in subsequent visits; thorough educational evaluations and job training are also essential.

Preventive management for problems outside the nervous system should include
a cardiac evaluation with ultrasound as soon as the diagnosis is made. Renal ultrasound to detect angiomyolipomas or cysts can also be justified at the time of diagnosis, and should be repeated to monitor tumors and cysts or after episodes of
hematuria. Referral to urology is useful for enlarging cysts or other renal symptoms, since decompression of the cysts has been associated with reversal of hypertension and renal failure. Colon carcinoma has occurred, and some patients have
had a high frequency of intestinal polyps. It is, therefore, wise to alert adult patients
to report hematochezia and recognize that oral, gastric, and intestinal hamartomas
occur in these patients. Retinal hamartomas can also progress. Regular evaluation
of the heart, limbs, skin, and oral cavity is indicated, along with periodic referrals
to neurology, ophthalmology, and dentistry. These same management strategies
should extend through adolescence, with vigilance for precocious puberty. The
occurrence of cystic lung disease in adulthood warrants periodic chest radiographs
and auscultation after age 20 years. Anticipation of airway lesions or seizures is
important during anesthesia for patients with tuberous sclerosis.

Preventive management of neurofibromatosis-1

Description: A pattern of neurologic and skin changes ranging from multiple café-au-lait spots to multisystem problems, occurring in 1 in 2500–3000 live births.

Clinical diagnosis: Criterion include six spots café-au-lait more than 0.5 cm diameter before puberty, two neurofibroma or one plexiform neuroma, axillary or inguinal freckling, optic glioma, two or more Lisch nodules, or osseous lesions such as pseudoarthroses.

Laboratory diagnosis: Mutations in the neurofibromin gene can cause neurofibromatosis-1 (NF-1) or multiple café-au-lait spots; DNA testing is not very sensitive (e.g., frequently normal in patients with NF-1), nor is it usually predictive of severity.

Genetics: Autosomal-dominant inheritance with 50% of patients representing new mutations. Normal parents of affected individuals have low (<1%) recurrence risks, those with NF-1 have a 50% risk for transmission with each pregnancy.

Key management issues: Regular physical examinations documenting the location and size of café-au-lait spots and neurofibromas; brain scanning for findings such as seizures, increasing head circumference, or precocious puberty; aggressive radiologic evaluations for skeletal, gait, or movement changes; monitoring of puberty, skeletal growth, and blood pressure; early intervention, speech evaluation, and preschool evaluation of cognitive performance.

Growth charts: None available.

Parent groups: National Neurofibromatosis Foundation – NF (www.nf.org); Neurofibromatosis Inc. (www.nfinc.org/); The Neurofibromatosis Association UK (www.nfauk.org/). Neurofibromatosis information page from National Institutes of Health (www.ninds.nih.gov/disorders/neurofibromatosis/neurofibromatosis.htm).

Basis for management recommendations: Guidelines endorsed by the Committee on Genetics, American Academy of Pediatrics (1995).

Summary of clinical concerns

General	Learning	**Cognitive disability** (40%; 8–9% with IQ < 70), **learning differences** (25%), **speech problems** (30–40%)
	Behavior	Short stature
	Growth	Neurofibromas (15%), skin angiomas (53%), malignancy of various types (6%), neurofibrosarcomas (3–12%)
Facial	Eyes	Eye anomalies (congenital glaucoma, corneal opacity, retinal detachment, optic atrophy, ptosis), **Lisch nodules** (28%), strabismus, proptosis
	Mouth	**Oral changes** (66% – oral neurofibromas, macroglossia, large lingual papillae, malpostioned teeth)
Surface	Epidermal	Café-au-lait spots (99%), axillary freckling (81%), pruritis
Skeletal	Cranial	**Macrocephaly** (30%), craniofacial deformities
	Axial	Scoliosis (5%)
	Limbs	Pseudoarthrosis (3%), hemihyperplasia, dislocations (hip, radius, ulna)
Internal	Digestive	Constipation (10%)
	Circulatory	Pulmonary stenosis, aortic stenosis, renal artery stenosis (2%)
	Endocrine	Precocious puberty
Neural	Central	Hydrocephalus (1%), seizures (5%)
	Motor	**Plexiform neuromas** (30%)
	Sensory	Optic glioma (4%), visual deficits

Concerns of frequency >20% are **highlighted**

Key references

Committee on Genetics, American Academy of Pediatrics (1995). Health supervision for children with neurofibromatosis. *Pediatrics* 96:368–71.

Roach & Miller, eds (2004). Neurocutaneous Disorders. Cambridge UK: Cambridge University Press.

Ward & Gutmann (2005). Neurofibromatosis 1: From lab bench to clinic. *Pediatric Neurology* 32:221–8.

Neurofibromatosis-1

Preventive medical checklist (0–3 years)

Name _____ Birth date __ / __ / ___ Number _____

Age	Evaluations: key concerns	Management considerations	Notes
New-born ↓ 1 month	Dysmorphology: anomalies Examination nerves, bones, skin, eyes Hearing, vision:[2] nerve changes Head: macrocephaly, asymmetry Feeding: reflux, poor swallow Heart: valve stenoses, coarctation Parental adjustment	❑ Related syndromes, genetic counseling[1] ❑ ❑ Neurology;[3] dermatology;[3] orthopedics[3] ❑ ❑ ABR; opthalmology[3] ❑ ❑ Head sonogram, MRI[1] ❑ ❑ Feeding specialist; video swallow[3] ❑ ❑ Echocardiogram;[3] cardiology[3] ❑ ❑ Family support[4] ❑	
2 months ↓ 4 months	Growth and development:[5] head size Hearing, vision:[2] hearing loss, strabismus Head: macrocephaly, asymmetry Feeding: reflux, poor swallow Heart: arteries, skin: new lesions Skeleton: dislocations, hemihypertrophy Parental adjustment Other:	❑ ECI;[6] monitor for seizure symptoms ❑ ❑ ABR;[3] opthalmology[3] ❑ ❑ Head sonogram, MRI[1] ❑ ❑ Feeding specialist; video swallow[3] ❑ ❑ Cardiology;[3] BP; dermatology[3] ❑ ❑ Orthopedics[3] ❑ ❑ Family support[4] ❑ ❑ ❑	
6 months ↓ 9 months	Growth and development:[5] head size Hearing, vision:[2] hearing loss, strabismus Heart: arteries, skin: new lesions Skeleton: dislocations, hemihypertrophy Other:	❑ ECI;[6] monitor for seizure symptoms ❑ ❑ ABR;[3] ophthalmology[3] ❑ ❑ Cardiology;[3] BP; dermatology[3] ❑ ❑ Orthopedics[3] ❑ ❑ ❑	
1 year	Growth and development:[5] head size Hearing, vision:[2] hearing loss, strabismus Skin: pruritis, new lesions Heart: arteries Skeleton: dislocations, hemihypertrophy Head: macrocephaly, asymmetry Other:	❑ ECI;[6] monitor for seizure symptoms ❑ ❑ ABR;[3] ophthalmology[3] ❑ ❑ Dermatology[3] ❑ ❑ Cardiology[3] ❑ ❑ Orthopedics[3] ❑ ❑ Repeat MRI[3] ❑ ❑ ❑	
15 months ↓ 18 months	Growth and development:[5] head size Skin: pruritis, new lesions Heart: arteries Skeleton: dislocations, hemihypertrophy	❑ ECI;[6] monitor for seizure symptoms ❑ ❑ Sunscreen, dermatology[3] ❑ ❑ BP; cardiology[3] ❑ ❑ Orthopedics[3] ❑	
2 years	Growth and development:[5] head size Hearing, vision:[2] hearing loss, strabismus Skin: pruritis, new lesions Heart: hypertension, defects, heart block Skeleton: dislocations, hemihypertrophy	❑ ECI;[6] monitor for seizure symptoms ❑ ❑ Audiology, ophthalmology ❑ ❑ Sunscreen, dermatology[3] ❑ ❑ BP; cardiology[3] ❑ ❑ Orthopedics[3] ❑	
3 years	Growth and development:[5] head size Hearing, vision:[2] hearing loss, proptosis Nutrition: intake, malpositioned teeth Skin: pruritis, new lesions Heart: hypertension, defects, heart block Skeleton: dislocations, hemihypertrophy Other:	❑ ECI;[6] monitor for seizure symptoms ❑ ❑ Audiology; ophthalmology ❑ ❑ Dietician;[3] dentistry ❑ ❑ Sunscreen; dermatology[3] ❑ ❑ BP; cardiology[3] ❑ ❑ Orthopedics[3] ❑ ❑ ❑	

Neurofibromatosis-1 concerns		Other concerns from history	
Poor feeding, poor weight gain Vision, hearing deficits Eye (proptosis, strabismus) Dental anomalies Cardiac anomalies Hypertension	Café-au-lait, axillary freckling Joint dislocations Hemihypertrophy Hydrocephalus, seizures Motor and speech delay Various tumors	**Family history/prenatal** _____ _____ _____ _____ _____	**Social/environmental** _____ _____ _____ _____ _____

Guidelines for the neonatal period should be undertaken *at whatever age* the diagnosis is made; ABR, auditory brainstem evoked response; BP, blood pressure; [1]consider other conditions with café-au-lait spots such as NF–Noonan (Watson) syndrome; head MRI controversial – may be done as baseline or postponed until symptoms; [2]by practitioner; [3]as dictated by clinical findings; [4]parent group, social, and behavioral issues; [5]consider developmental pediatrician/neurologist/neurofibromatosis clinic according to symptoms and availability; [6]early childhood intervention if motor delay, including developmental monitoring and motor/speech therapy.

Neurofibromatosis-1

Preventive medical checklist (4–18 years)

Name _____ Birth date __ / __ / ___ Number _____

Age	Evaluations: key concerns	Management considerations		Notes
4 years ↓ 6 years	Growth and development:[5] head size Development:[2] preschool transition Hearing and vision[2] Face: neuromas, skin: pruritis Heart: hypertension, defects, heart block Skeleton: asymmetries Other:	☐ ECI;[6] monitor for seizure symptoms ☐ Family support;[4] preschool program[5] ☐ Audiology;[3] ophthalmology ☐ Head MRI;[3] sunscreen, dermatology[3] ☐ BP; cardiology[3] ☐ Orthopedics[3] ☐	☐ ☐ ☐ ☐ ☐ ☐ ☐	
7 years ↓ 9 years	Growth and nutrition[1] Development:[1] school transition[5] Hearing and vision[2] Face: neuromas, skin: pruritis Heart: hypertension, defects, heart block Skeleton: asymmetries Other:	☐ Family support;[4] school progress[6] ☐ Audiology;[3] ophthalmology ☐ Head MRI;[3] sunscreen, dermatology[3] ☐ BP; cardiology[3] ☐ Orthopedics[3] ☐ ☐	☐ ☐ ☐ ☐ ☐ ☐ ☐	
10 years ↓ 12 years	Growth and nutrition[1] Face: neuromas, skin: pruritis, fibromas Heart: hypertension, defects, heart block Skeleton: scoliosis, asymmetries Other:	☐ School progress[6] ☐ Head MRI;[3] sunscreen, dermatology[3] ☐ BP; cardiology[3] ☐ Orthopedics[3] ☐	☐ ☐ ☐ ☐ ☐	
13 years ↓ 15 years	Growth and nutrition[1] Hearing and vision[2] Skin: pruritis, neurofibromata Heart: hypertension, defects, heart block Skeleton: scoliosis, asymmetries Other:	☐ School progress[6] ☐ Audiology;[3] ophthalmology ☐ Head MRI;[3] sunscreen, dermatology[3] ☐ BP; cardiology[3] ☐ Orthopedics[3] ☐	☐ ☐ ☐ ☐ ☐ ☐	
16 years ↓ 18 years	Growth and nutrition[1] Face: neuromas, skin: pruritis, fibromas Heart: hypertension, defects, heart block Skeleton: scoliosis, asymmetries Other:	☐ Family support;[4] school progress[6] ☐ Head MRI;[3] sunscreen, dermatology[3] ☐ BP; cardiology[3] ☐ Orthopedics[3] ☐	☐ ☐ ☐ ☐ ☐	
19 years ↓ 23 years	Adult care transition[6] Hearing and vision[2] Face: neuromas, skin: pruritis, fibromas Heart: hypertension, defects, heart block Skeleton: scoliosis, asymmetries	☐ Family support;[4] school progress[6] ☐ Audiology;[3] ophthalmology ☐ Head MRI;[3] sunscreen, dermatology[3] ☐ BP; cardiology[3] ☐ Orthopedics[3]	☐ ☐ ☐ ☐ ☐	
Adult	Adult care transition[6] Hearing and vision[2] Face: neuromas, skin: pruritis, fibromas Heart: hypertension, defects, heart block Skeleton: scoliosis, asymmetries Other:	☐ Family support[4] ☐ Audiology[3], ophthalmology ☐ Head MRI;[3] sunscreen, dermatology[3] ☐ BP; cardiology[3] ☐ Orthopedics[3] ☐	☐ ☐ ☐ ☐ ☐ ☐	

Neurofibromatosis-1 concerns		Other concerns from history	
Facial asymmetry Vision, hearing deficits Dental anomalies Cardiac anomalies (rare) Hypertension Café-au-lait, fibromas	Scoliosis, asymmetries Hemihypertrophy Hydrocephalus, seizures School problems Learning disabilities Various tumors	**Family history/prenatal** _____ _____ _____ _____	**Social/environmental** _____ _____ _____ _____

Guidelines for the neonatal period should be undertaken *at whatever age* the diagnosis is made; BP, blood pressure; [1]consider developmental pediatrician/neurofibromatosis clinic/behavior therapist/genetics clinic according to symptoms and availability; [2]by practitioner; [3]as dictated by clinical findings; [4]parent group, social, and behavioral issues; [5]preschool program including developmental monitoring and motor/speech therapy; [6]monitor individual education plan, educational testing, academic progress, behavioral differences, later vocational planning.

Parent guide to neurofibromatosis-1

Although the disorder was first described in 1849, von Recklinghausen's identification of neural elements in neurofibromatosis gained him credit for recognizing the disease in 1882. The classical description was of type 1 neurofibromatosis with multiple café-au-lait spots (brown, oval spots on the skin) and neurofibromas (wart-like tumors on the skin), which accounts for 90% of all cases. Neurofibromatosis-2 with acoustic neuromas (tumors on the nerve to the ear) is the other more common form of neurofibromatosis.

Incidence, causation, and diagnosis

The prevalence of neurofibromatosis-1 is between 1 in 2500 and 1 in 3000 births, with about 50% representing new mutations. The responsible gene encodes a protein called neurofibromin and is located on chromosome 17. The differential diagnosis is between other benign tumor disorders (hamartoses) such as Bannayan–Riley–Ruvalcaba syndrome (large head, fatty tumors, pigmented spots), Watson syndrome with short stature and pulmonic stenosis, LEOPARD syndrome with multiple freckles, or Proteus syndrome with more severe tumors and distortions (Joseph Merrick, the "Elephant Man," had the latter). One can also have multiple café-au-lait spots without having neurofibromatosis-1 due to changes in a different gene. The criterion of six café-au-lait spots larger than 1.5 cm is widely accepted for a diagnosis of the disease, although six spots more than 0.5 cm diameter before puberty is also accepted. A National Institutes of Health Consensus Development Conference established a broader criterion, wherein the requisite number of café-au-lait spots was one of seven findings, any two of which would confirm the clinical diagnosis of neurofibromatosis-1. The other findings included: (1) two neurofibroma or one plexiform neuroma (a large, spreading neural tumor under the skin), (2) axillary or inguinal freckling, (3) optic glioma (tumor of the nerve leading to the eye), (4) two or more Lisch nodules (brown spots in the iris of the eye, (5) a distinctive bony lesion like fusion of the radius and ulna or a false joint (pseudoarthrosis), and (6) a first-degree relative (parent, child, sibling) with neurofibromatosis. DNA tests to confirm the diagnosis is available but not very sensitive since each family has a different mutation and it is not economical to screen the entire neurofibromin gene.

Natural history and complications

As many as 40–85% of patients avoid complications beyond café-au-lait spots. Most individuals with neurofibromatosis-1 do not have problems in early childhood. Large head circumference is relatively common (30%), and seizures or hydrocephalus (accumulation of fluid in brain cavities) may occur. Plexiform neuromas (thick facial tumors), optic gliomas (tumors of the nerve to the eye) and spinal neurofibromas (within the cord) can occur in neurofibromatosis-1; they are often multifocal (in multiple locations) and difficult to remove. Skeletal problems include dislocations, pseudoarthroses (false joints), scoliosis (spinal curvature), and cyst-like lesions of the long bones. Blood vessel lesions such as narrowing of the artery to the kidney and heart defects do occur, leading to hypertension (high blood pressure). Mild mental disability occurs in 8–9%, with motor/speech delays and learning differences in 25%. The children may also have neurosensory deficits from tumors on the nerves to the eyes or ears. Neurofibromatosis-1 patients have low risks for tumors in most body regions, being malignant by position (not cancer but disruptive) or true malignant tumors (e.g., neurofibrosarcomas, Wilms tumor, leukemias).

Preventive medical needs

Recommendations for preventive care in neurofibromatosis have been proposed by the American Academy of Pediatric. Although some authors have recommended brain imaging studies as soon as the diagnosis of neurofibromatosis-1 is made, the general consensus is to await such symptoms as seizures, increased head circumference, or early puberty before obtaining a head MRI scan. Since there is increased risk for optic nerve and other intracranial tumors, and since benign or malignant tumors can arise in many other body locations, aggressive imaging studies should be pursued when changes are revealed by periodic history review and physical examination. Since these tumors are usually multifocal, surgical intervention should be saved for symptoms of severe neurosensory dysfunction or of increased pressure within the cranium. Conservative surgical approaches aimed at preserving nerve function are particularly important for children. Because changes in vision, hearing, or bones may be harbingers of tumor growth, regular hearing/vision assessment by the physician with annual ophthalmology and audiology screening is recommended through adulthood. Puberty is particularly important to monitor, since early puberty and accelerated growth during puberty are observed. Early intervention, speech evaluation, and preschool evaluation of cognitive performance are indicated in those with delays, and potential hypertension from vascular narrowing or tumor pressure mandates annual monitoring of blood pressure.

Family counseling

In asymptomatic patients, optimistic medical counseling is warranted based on the majority of patients with neurofibromatosis-1 who never have complications. Normal couples who have a child affected with neurofibromatosis-1 will have minimal recurrence risks (<1%), but if one parent has a large head or other findings suggestive of neurofibromatosis, then detailed examination should be made. Affected individuals will have a 50% chance to transmit the gene with each pregnancy, but their affected offspring can be more or less severe.

Preventive management of tuberous sclerosis

Description: A pattern of neurologic and skin changes that includes "ash-leaf" spots, seizures, and mental disability occurring in 1 in 8000–23,000 live births.

Clinical diagnosis: Manifestations include fibrotic tumors in brain ("tubers") that cause seizures and mental disability, adenoma sebaceum on the face, hypopigmented ("ash leaf" spots best seen with a Woods lamp, reddish-yellow plaques on the forehead ("forehead plaque"), leathery plaques in the lumbosacral area ("shagreen patches"), and diffuse regions of skin hyper/hypopigmentation ("confetti skin lesions").

Laboratory diagnosis: Mutations in the tuberin gene can be identified in some patients.

Genetics: Affected individuals will have a 50% risk of transmitting tuberous sclerosis with each pregnancy; parents may require renal and cardiac ultrasound studies to discern if they are subclinically affected.

Key management issues: Monitoring for neurologic, ophthalmologic, cardiac, dermatologic, and developmental problems, head MRI studies for changes in behavior, alterations in head circumference, or symptoms of intracranial hypertension, echocardiographic and renal ultrasound studies to detect angiomyolipomas or cysts, referral to urology for new or persisting renal symptoms, early intervention with school planning.

Growth charts: None.

Parent groups: The Tuberous Sclerosis Alliance (www.tsalliance.org/), The Tuberous Sclerosis Association UK (www.tuberous-sclerosis.org/), and Tuberous Sclerosis International (www.stsn.nl/tsi/tsi.htm).

Basis for management recommendations: Derived from the complications below as documented by Roach & Sparagana (2004).

Summary of clinical concerns

General	Learning Behavior Tumors	**Cognitive disabilit**y (60–80%), learning differences, **speech problems** (69%) **Autism** (25–40%), schizophrenia Multiple hamartomas, astrocytomas (6–14%), colon carcinoma, renal carcinoma, Wilms tumor
Facial	Eyes Mouth	**Retinal hamartomas** (50–87%) **Enamel pits** (70–90%), fibromas of mucosa (11%)
Surface	Epidermal	**White nevi, ash-leaf spots** (82%), **facial angiofibromas** (old term = adenoma sebaceum: 70–85%), poliosis (white hair – 20%), **shagreen patches** (36%)
Skeletal	Cranial Limbs	Thickened calvarium, frontal bone exostoses **Phalangeal cysts** (60%), periosteal new bone formation, digital gigantism, periungual fibromas (15–20%)
Internal	Pulmonary Digestive Circulatory Endocrine Renal	Pulmonary lymphangio-myomatosis (2–3%) Angiomas of liver and spleen, colonic polyps **Cardiac rhabdomyomas** (30–67%); **Wolf–Parkinson–White syndrome** (20%) Precocious puberty, hamartomas of the thyroid, pancreas Renal angiomyolipomas (50–65%), renal carcinoma (2%)
Neural	Central Sensory	**Subependymal and cerebellar nodules (tubers)**, **ventricular dilation** (50%), **brain calcifications** (35%), **seizures** (88–93%), increased intracranial pressure Hearing and vision loss

Concerns of frequency >20% are **highlighted**

Key references

Cassidy et al. (1983): Family studies in tuberous sclerosis. Evaluation of apparently unaffected parents. *Journal of American Medical Association* 249:1302–4.

Roach & Sparagana (2004). Diagnosis of tuberous sclerosis complex. *Journal of Child Neurology* 19:643–9.

Tuberous sclerosis

Preventive medical checklist (0–3 years)

Name _____ Birth date __ / __ / ____ Number _____

Age	Evaluations: key concerns	Management considerations		Notes
New-born ↓ 1 month	Dysmorphology: anomalies Hearing, vision:[2] retinal changes Neuro: seizures, hydrocephalus Heart, kidneys: rhabdomyomas Skeleton: cysts, sclerotic lesions Skin: ash-leaf spots, fibromas Parental adjustment	❑ Genetic counseling[1] ❑ ABR; ophthalmology ❑ Head sonogram, MRI/CT;[1] neurology[3] ❑ Abdominal sonogram; echocardiogram ❑ Skeletal examination, X-rays[3] ❑ Skin examination; dermatology[3] ❑ Family support[4]	❑ ❑ ❑ ❑ ❑ ❑ ❑	
2 months ↓ 4 months	Growth and development:[5] head size Hearing, vision:[2] retinal changes Neuro: seizures, sleep apnea Heart, kidneys: tumors, cysts Skeleton: cysts, sclerotic lesions Skin: ash-leaf spots, fibromas Parental adjustment Other:	❑ ECI;[6] monitor for seizure symptoms ❑ ABR;[3] ophthalmology[3] ❑ Head sonogram,[3] MRI/CT;[1] neurology[3] ❑ Abdominal sonogram;[3] echocardiogram[3] ❑ Skeletal examination, X-rays[3] ❑ Skin examination, dermatology[3] ❑ Family support[4] ❑	❑ ❑ ❑ ❑ ❑ ❑ ❑ ❑	Patients with seizures may have anesthesia risks
6 months ↓ 9 months	Growth and development:[5] head size Hearing, vision:[2] retinal changes Neuro: seizures, sleep apnea Skeleton: cysts, sclerotic lesions Skin: ash-leaf spots, fibromas Other:	❑ ECI;[6] monitor for seizure symptoms ❑ ENT;[3] ophthalmology[3] ❑ EEG;[3] polysomnography;[3] neurology[3] ❑ Skeletal examination, X-rays[3] ❑ Skin/UV examination; dermatology[3] ❑	❑ ❑ ❑ ❑ ❑ ❑	
1 year	Growth and development:[5] head size Hearing, vision:[2] retinal changes Neuro: seizures, sleep apnea Heart, kidneys: tumors, arrhythmias Skeleton: cysts, overgrowths Skin: ash-leaf spots, fibromas Other:	❑ ECI;[6] monitor for seizure symptoms ❑ ENT;[3] ophthalmology[3] ❑ EEG;[3] Head MRI;[3] neurology[3] ❑ EKG, CXR, BP, urinalysis ❑ Skeletal examination, X-rays[3] ❑ Skin examination; dermatology[3] ❑	❑ ❑ ❑ ❑ ❑ ❑ ❑	
15 months ↓ 18 months	Growth and development:[5] head size Hearing, vision:[2] retinal changes Neuro: seizures, sleep apnea Skeleton: cysts, sclerotic lesions	❑ ECI;[6] monitor for seizure symptoms ❑ ENT;[3] ophthalmology[3] ❑ EEG;[3] polysomnography;[3] neurology[3] ❑ Skeletal examination, X-rays[3]	❑ ❑ ❑ ❑	
2 years	Growth and development:[5] head size Hearing, vision:[2] retinal changes Neuro: seizures, sleep apnea Skeleton: cysts, sclerotic lesions Skin: ash-leaf spots, fibromas	❑ ECI;[6] monitor for seizure symptoms ❑ Audiology; ophthalmology[3] ❑ EEG,[3] Head MRI;[3] neurology[3] ❑ Skeletal examination, X-rays[3] ❑ Skin examination; dermatology[3]	❑ ❑ ❑ ❑ ❑	
3 years	Growth and development:[5] head size Hearing, vision:[2] retinal changes Neuro: seizures, sleep apnea Heart, kidneys: tumors, arrhythmias Skeleton: cysts, sclerotic lesions Skin: ash-leaf spots, fibromas Other:	❑ ECI;[6] monitor for seizure symptoms ❑ Audiology; ophthalmology[3] ❑ EEG;[3] polysomnography;[3] neurology[3] ❑ EKG, CXR, BP, urinalysis ❑ Skeletal examination, X-rays[3] ❑ Skin examination; dermatology[3] ❑	❑ ❑ ❑ ❑ ❑ ❑ ❑	

Tuberous sclerosis concerns		Other concerns from history	
Facial angiofibromas Retinal hamartomas Dental enamel pits Cardiac tumors, arrhythmias Renal tumors, rare cancer Renal cysts	Ungual fibromas Limb overgrowth Seizures Intracranial calcifications Developmental disability Learning differences	**Family history/prenatal** _____ _____ _____ _____	**Social/environmental** _____ _____ _____ _____

Guidelines for the neonatal period should be undertaken *at whatever age* the diagnosis is made; ABR, auditory brainstem evoked response; EEG, electroencephalogram; UV, ultraviolet (Wood's) lamp; EKG, electrocardiogram; CXR, chest X-ray; BP, blood pressure; [1]consider parental evaluation by retinal and skin examination, imaging of head, heart, and kidney before genetic counseling; head MRI controversial – may be done as baseline or postponed until symptoms; [2]by practitioner; [3]as dictated by clinical findings; [4]parent group, social, and behavioral issues; [5]consider developmental pediatrician/neurology/genetics clinic according to symptoms and availability; [6]early childhood intervention if motor delay, including developmental monitoring and motor/speech therapy.

Tuberous sclerosis

Preventive medical checklist (4–18 years)

Name _____ **Birth day** __/__/__ **Number** _____

Age	Evaluations: key concerns	Management considerations		Notes
4 years ↓ **6 years**	Growth and development:[5] head size Development:[2] preschool transition Hearing, vision:[2] retinal changes Neuro: seizures, sleep apnea Heart, kidneys: tumors, arrhythmias Skeleton: teeth, cysts, overgrowths Other:	❑ ECI;[6] monitor for seizure symptoms ❑ Family support;[4] preschool program[5] ❑ Audiology; ophthalmology[3] ❑ EEG;[3] head MRI;[3] neurology[3] ❑ EKG; CXR; cardiology;[3] BP, urinalysis ❑ Dentistry, X-rays;[3] orthopedics[3] ❑	❑ ❑ ❑ ❑ ❑ ❑ ❑	Patients with seizures may have anesthesia risks
7 years ↓ **9 years**	Growth and nutrition[1] Development:[1] school transition[5] Hearing, vision:[2] retinal changes Neuro: seizures, sleep apnea Skeleton: teeth, cysts, overgrowths Skin: ash-leaf spots, fibromas Other:	❑ Family support;[4] school progress[6] ❑ Audiology; ophthalmology[3] ❑ EEG;[3] polysomnography;[3] neurology[3] ❑ Dentistry; X-rays;[3] orthopedics[3] ❑ Skin examination; dermatology[3] ❑ ❑	❑ ❑ ❑ ❑ ❑ ❑ ❑	
10 years ↓ **12 years**	Growth and nutrition[1] Hearing, vision:[2] retinal changes Neuro: seizures, sleep apnea Heart, kidneys: tumors, arrhythmias Other:	❑ School progress[6] ❑ Audiology; ophthalmology[3] ❑ EEG;[3] head MRI;[3] neurology[3] ❑ EKG; CXR; cardiology;[3] BP, urinalysis ❑	❑ ❑ ❑ ❑ ❑	
13 years ↓ **15 years**	Growth, nutrition, puberty[1] Hearing, vision:[2] retinal changes Neuro: seizures, sleep apnea Skeleton: teeth, cysts, overgrowths Skin: ash-leaf spots, fibromas Other:	❑ School progress[6] ❑ Audiology; ophthalmology[3] ❑ EEG;[3] polysomnography;[3] neurology[3] ❑ Dentistry; X-rays;[3] orthopedics[3] ❑ Skin examination; dermatology[3] ❑	❑ ❑ ❑ ❑ ❑ ❑	
16 years ↓ **18 years**	Growth, nutrition, puberty[1] Hearing, vision:[2] retinal changes Neuro: seizures, sleep apnea Heart, kidneys: tumors, arrhythmias Other:	❑ Family support;[4] school progress;[6] ❑ Audiology; ophthalmology[3] ❑ EEG;[3] head MRI;[3] neurology[3] ❑ EKG; CXR; cardiology;[3] BP, urinalysis ❑	❑ ❑ ❑ ❑ ❑	
19 years ↓ **23 years**	Adult care transition[6] Hearing, vision:[2] retinal changes Neuro: seizures, sleep apnea Skeleton: teeth, cysts Skin: ash-leaf spots, fibromas	❑ Family support;[4] school progress[6] ❑ Audiology; ophthalmology[3] ❑ EEG;[3] polysomnography;[3] neurology[3] ❑ Dentistry, X-rays;[3] orthopedics[3] ❑ Skin examination; dermatology[3]	❑ ❑ ❑ ❑ ❑	
Adult	Adult care transition[6] Hearing, vision:[2] retinal changes Neuro: seizures, sleep apnea Heart, kidneys, lungs Skeleton, skin: teeth, fibromas, cysts Tumors: colon, renal cancers Other:	❑ Family support[4] ❑ Audiology; ophthalmology[3] ❑ EEG;[3] Head MRI;[3] sleep study;[3] neurology[3] ❑ EKG; CXR;[3] BP, urinalysis; PFTs ❑ Dentistry; dermatology;[3] X-rays;[3] orthopedics[3] ❑ Monitor for hematochezia, hematuria ❑	❑ ❑ ❑ ❑ ❑ ❑ ❑	

Tuberous sclerosis concerns		Other concerns from history	
Facial angiofibromas Retinal hamartomas Dental enamel pits Cardiac tumors, arrhythmias Renal abnormalities Pulmonary cysts	Ungual fibromas Limb overgrowth Seizures Intracranial calcifications Developmental disability Learning differences	**Family history/prenatal** _____ _____ _____ _____	**Social/environmental** _____ _____ _____ _____

Guidelines for the neonatal period should be undertaken *at whatever age* the diagnosis is made; ABR, auditory brainstem evoked response; EEG, electroencephalogram; UV, ultraviolet (Wood's) lamp; BP, blood pressure; EKG, electrocardiogram; CXR, chest X-ray; PFTs, pulmonary function tests; [1]consider developmental pediatrician/neurology/behavior therapist/genetics clinic according to symptoms and availability; [2]by practitioner; [3]as dictated by clinical findings; [4]parent group, social, and behavioral issues; [5]preschool program including developmental monitoring and motor/speech therapy; [6]monitor individual education plan, educational testing, academic progress, behavioral differences, later vocational planning.

Parent guide to tuberous sclerosis

The term "tuberous sclerosis" was coined in 1880 by Bourneville. The fibrotic tumors in brain ("tubers") cause seizures and mental retardation that, together with "adenoma sebaceum," comprise the classic diagnostic recognized by Vogt in 1908. "Epiloa" is also an outdated term derived from Greek roots meaning epilepsy and mindlessness. The variability of clinical findings and evidence of genetic heterogeneity in tuberous sclerosis have led to the term "tuberous sclerosis complex."

Incidence, causation, and diagnosis

The incidence is 1 per 6000–10,000 births. Tuberous sclerosis is an autosomal-dominant disorder that can result from mutations in a TSC1 gene on chromosome 9 (85% of patients) or a TSC2 gene on chromosome 16 (15% of patients). These genes are similar to the neurofibromin gene that is responsible for neurofibromatosis in that they regulate growth and tumor formation. The major clinical findings of seizures, facial angiofibromas (reddish tumors that look like acne), ungual fibromas (tumors under the nail), hypopigmented macules (white spots), heart or kidney tumors, and neural (brain, retina) tumors comprise a distinctive clinical picture for tuberous sclerosis. Differential diagnosis would include other disorders with brain and skin lesions, such as Sturge–Weber angiomatosis or neurofibromatosis, congenital infection with Toxoplasma or cytomegalovirus, and individuals with fatty tumors on their face. A major problem with the diagnosis in childhood is that features such as facial angiofibromas (acne-like tumors that used to be called adenoma sebaceum), nail and kidney tumors, and even brain calcifications may not be present during infancy. Patients with fewer features can be considered as probable or suspect for tuberous sclerosis and followed medically with examinations like the Wood's lamp ultraviolet light for detecting white spots.

Natural history and complications

Complications of tuberous sclerosis affect the nervous system most severely with seizures in 88–93%, mental deficiency in 60–80%, and intracranial calcifications in 56%. Tonic–clonic (41%) and infantile spasms (30%) are the most common types of seizures, but other types occur. Seizures have an early onset, with 20% starting before age 3 months, 46% starting before age 3–7 months, and only 4% occurring after age 5 years in a survey of 300 affected families. Behavioral changes were common in one study, including hyperactivity (28%), impaired social interaction (43%), repetitive behaviors (25%), and aggressive behaviors with attacks on other people (28%) or self-injury (29%). Other symptomatic findings include intracranial hypertension from benign brain tumors that occur in 6–14%. Heart muscle tumors occur in 30–67% of patients, and symptomatic infants can have significant mortality with outflow blockage and arrhythmias. The cardiac tumors may also resolve over time. Cystic disease of the lung (honeycomb lung) occurs predominantly in females, causing symptoms after the third decade with a five-year mortality rate of 67%. Some patients have tumors of the back of the eye (retinal tumors), but few have visual problems. The bones of the digits and, less frequently, the long bones may exhibit asymptomatic cysts or new bone formation on x-rays. Some patients have overgrowth of one digit.

Preventive medical needs

Preventive management of tuberous sclerosis will be directed toward early evaluation of neurologic, ophthalmologic, cardiac, renal, dermatologic, and developmental problems. If the disease is recognized at birth, head ultrasound or MRI studies can be justified to determine the presence and size of tumors. Changes in behavior, alterations in head circumference, and symptoms of intracranial hypertension (e.g., headaches) warrant additional head MRI studies, and contrast may be helpful in recognizing more troublesome tumors. Epilepsy begins early and takes many forms, so pediatric neurology referral is important for diagnosis and treatment. Anticonvulsant therapy tends to be complex, and surgical treatment has a role in severe cases. Sleep disturbances appear frequent in patients with epilepsy, so sleep studies may be considered. The high risk of mental disability justifies early intervention with regular speech, occupational and physical therapy assessments. Financial, psychosocial, and genetic counseling should be facilitated and re-emphasized in subsequent visits; thorough educational evaluations and job training are also essential. Other preventive measures should include monitoring for cardiac symptoms such as outflow tract blockage or arrhythmias, abdominal ultrasound to detect renal tumors with monitoring of blood pressure and urinalysis (for hematuria), alertness for abdominal masses or bloody stools as signs of cancer. The occurrence of cystic lung disease in adulthood warrants periodic chest X-rays and examination after age 20 years. Anticipation of airway problems or seizures is important during anesthesia for patients with tuberous sclerosis.

Family counseling

Brain involvement with tumors, seizures, mental disability (60–80% of patients), and behavior differences such as autism require early intervention, monitoring of school progress, and vocational therapy/assisted living for those with handicaps. Affected individuals will have a 50% risk of transmitting tuberous sclerosis with each pregnancy, and ophthalmology examinations plus brain/heart/kidney imaging may be required to exclude the diagnosis in asymptomatic individuals. Parents who have no signs of tuberous sclerosis after complete evaluation can be assigned a lower recurrence risk of 5–6% that covers the possibilities of incomplete penetrance (gene present but no symptoms) or germline mosaicism (gene present in several eggs or sperm). Families with severely affected infants will benefit from support groups, and adolescents with facial lesions (facial angiofibromas, forehead plaques) may benefit from cosmetic surgery, dermatologic treatment, and psychiatric support because of their altered appearance.

Part V

Management of craniofacial syndromes

14

Craniosynostosis syndromes

Premature fusion of the cranial sutures occurs as a single anomaly or as a primary event in more than 90 craniosynostosis syndromes (Jones, 1997, pp. 412–30; Gorlin et al., 2001, pp. 654–704). Craniosynostosis also occurs as a secondary or occasional event in conditions such as rickets or thalassemia, resulting in an aggregate frequency of 0.4–0.6 per 1000 births. Preventive care is particularly important in the craniosynostosis syndromes, since altered cranial growth can have a severe impact on cognitive, visual, and auditory functions. Patients with fused cranial sutures share many problems with impact on surgical and preventive management regardless of their specific syndrome diagnosis. For this reason, a common craniosynostosis checklist is provided in this chapter that can be used for the Saethre–Chotzen, Apert, Crouzon, Pfeiffer, and Carpenter syndromes. The craniosynostosis checklist can also be used for less common disorders if their unique features are added to the appropriate places on the checklist.

Patients with significant cranial asymmetry (plagiocephaly) and suspected synostosis should be promptly referred to a craniofacial surgery team, since early treatment may avoid the need for surgery or prevent severe complications. Substantial experience with craniofacial surgery has defined team approaches, defined standards (American Cleft Palate-Craniofacial Association, 1993) and resolved complications (Goodrich, 2004); the remarkable ability to normalize facial structure in children with anomalies must rank with the greatest achievements in medicine.

Of recent interest is the influence of local imbalance of skull growth surrounding the fused suture rather than overall constriction of cranial volume (craniostenosis) due to craniosynostosis (Sgouros, 2005). Patients with Apert syndrome actually have increased skull volume, but their regional synostosis (due to genetic tissue alterations) may act with raised intracranial pressure, intracranial venous hypertension, and other brain anomalies (e.g., hindbrain hernia, hydrocephalus) to produce altered skull shape and neural complications. Current surgical techniques aimed at overall expansion of cranial volume offer some prevention, but surgical

Table 14.1. Craniosynostosis syndromes

Syndrome	Incidence*	Inheritance	Accessory findings
Antley–Bixler	10–20 cases	AR	Midface hypoplasia, radiohumeral synostosis, heart a., genital a.
Apert	1 in 100,000	AD	Midface hypoplasia, syndactyly
Baller–Gerold	10–20 cases	AR	Radial ray a., imperforate anus
Carpenter	~50 cases	AR	Preaxial polydactyly, obesity, short stature, mental deficiency
Crouzon	1 in 25,000	AD	Ocular proptosis, shallow orbits
Jackson–Weiss	~100 cases	AD	Short first metatarsal bones
Pfeiffer	~100 cases	AD	Broad thumbs and toes, syndactyly
Saethre–Chotzen	>1 in 25,000	AD	Facial asymmetry, ptosis, brachydactyly, syndactyly

Note:

* Cases or per number of live births.

AD, autosomal dominant; AR, autosomal recessive; a., anomalies.

and tissue therapies focused on the defective sutural region(s) could offer less invasive and more physiologic therapy (Sgouros, 2005).

Cohen (1995) has emphasized the fundamental principle that it is the pattern of accessory malformations, *not* the affected sutures, that allows differentiation among the craniosynostosis syndromes (Table 14.1). For example, patients with the Apert, Pfeiffer, or Crouzon syndrome may have premature synostosis of the coronal sutures, but the digital syndactyly (Apert), broad thumbs (Pfeiffer), or normal hand findings (Crouzon) guide the diagnosis (Table 14.1). Families with craniosynostosis syndromes often exhibit variable expressivity with one or multiple sutures affected. When several sutures are fused, patients present with the severe Kleebattschädel or clover-leaf skull anomaly (Gorlin et al., 2001, pp. 654–704).

Despite their clinical delineation as discrete syndromes, molecular analysis indicates that seemingly different craniosynostosis phenotypes may be caused by mutations in the same gene. Mutations in the fibroblast growth factor receptor 2 (FGFR2) gene have been described in Apert, Crouzon, Jackson–Weiss, and Pfeiffer syndromes (Cohen, 1995; Aleck, 2004). In some instances, identical FGFR2 mutations are found in traditionally discrete syndromes. Variable expressivity or second-site mutations are postulated to explain why the same FGFR2 gene mutation produces limb anomalies in one patient but not in another.

Antley–Bixler syndrome

Antley–Bixler syndrome is a multiple-system disorder involving craniosynostosis, limb anomalies, urogenital anomalies, and congenital cardiac defects (Jones, 1997, pp. 428–9; Gorlin et al., 2001, pp. 671–2). Although mutations in the gene for fibroblast growth factor-2 were reported, a more likely cause is altered steroidogenesis that would explain the male hypogonadism and female virilization seen in some patients. Elevated excretion of pregnenolone, progesterone, and metabolites associated with the classical 17- and 21-hydroxylase deficiencies are caused by mutations in a cytochrome P450 molecule (Fluck et al., 2004). Several instances of consanguinity support autosomal-recessive (AR) inheritance, and this is more consistent with a cytochrome P450 rather than fibroblast growth factor mutation.

The clinical course of Antley–Bixler syndrome can be quite severe because of infantile respiratory obstruction with death in early childhood for 55% of patients. Craniofacial anomalies are often quite severe due to synostosis of the coronal and lambdoidal sutures (Gorlin et al., 2001, pp. 671–2), with a large anterior fontanel, frontal bossing, midface hypoplasia, choanal atresia, and shallow nasal bridge produce a distinctive facies with a high incidence of respiratory obstruction. The skeleton is abnormal, with thin, gracile bones, frequent fractures, bowing of the limbs, deformed chest cage, narrow pelvis, vertebral anomalies, and congenital hip dislocations. Urogenital anomalies may include renal aplasia/duplication, ureteral obstruction, vaginal atresia, and fused labia minor. Other anomalies include radiohumeral synostosis, imperforate anus, cardiac defects, and lumbar meningomyelocele. Some patients have severe renal and anal anomalies.

Preventive management will include multidisciplinary craniofacial assessment with definition of airway function. Otolaryngology, maxillofacial surgery, plastic surgery, and neurosurgery evaluations are important for the treatment of possible craniosynostosis, choanal atresia, and airway compromise. Assessment of thoracic morphology may be useful in aiding respiratory function. Screening for congenital dislocation of the hips, skeletal radiographic survey, and orthopedic evaluation should also be considered during infancy. Additional neonatal evaluations should include echocardiography, renal ultrasound, and examination of the genital and perineal areas for anomalies. Apnea is the usual cause of death, so tracheostomy and apnea monitoring may be needed if home care can be achieved. The long-term prognosis is not established, but the many complications warrant early intervention and nutrition services.

Apert syndrome

Apert syndrome consists of craniosynostosis and syndactyly of the hands and feet (Table 14.1). It is an autosomal-dominant (AD) disorder that occurs in 1.5 per

100,000 newborns and is caused by mutations in the FGFR2 gene (Jones, 1997, pp. 418–19; Gorlin et al., 2001, pp. 654–8).

Summary of clinical concerns: Apert syndrome management considerations

Growth and development: Cohen & Kreiborg (1993) reported a unique growth pattern for patients with Apert syndrome, consisting of increased size of all parameters at birth, deceleration of linear growth during childhood, and deceleration of the head circumference from above the 50th centile at birth to within or at 2 standard deviations in young adulthood. Despite modern surgery, there is a significant incidence of mental disability in Apert syndrome with 50% of children having IQ less than 70 in one study and an average IQ of 74 in another (Gorlin et al., 2001, p. 655). Da Costa et al. (2005) report one patient with global dysfunction and a second with normal IQ but neuropsychologic deficits typical of anterior brain functions. Such region-specific cognitive alterations emphasize potential focal effects of synostosis as hypothesized above by Sgouros (2005): Careful observation of feeding and growth followed by early childhood intervention with later school monitoring for neurosensory and cognitive problems.

Cranial: Premature fusion of the coronal sutures and the absence of true sagittal suture formation cause a deformed cranium with midface hypoplasia. Upward growth of the cranium produces a "tower skull" (acrocephaly), and there is midface hypoplasia due to malformation of the sphenoid bones and the cranial base (see checklist). Infants have a huge fontanel, extending from the lower forehead to the occiput.

Eyes: Optic atrophy, proptosis with keratitis, or strabismus occur: Regular eye examinations with inspection of the corneae and fundi.

Nose: The nasal bridge is depressed and the nasal septum may be deviated. Stenosis or atresia of the posterior choanae may occur and produce respiratory distress or cor pulmonale in the young child.

Mouth: Palatal anomalies (cleft soft palate, highly arched palate) together with maxillary retrusion and prognathism cause dental misalignment. Dental eruption may also be delayed and maxillary hypoplasia can produce crowded teeth: Patients with excessively noisy breathing in association with poor weight gain deserve urgent evaluation. A surgical team as described below is ideal with palatal anomalies, including regular dental care.

ENT: Patients with Apert syndrome are at risk of upper and lower airway obstruction. Upper airway compromise is caused by reduced oro- and nasopharyngeal dimensions, causing symptoms of obstructive sleep apnea and cor pulmonale. Moore (1993) reported that upper airway obstruction is more common in Crouzon and Pfeiffer syndromes than in Apert syndrome. Otitis media and congenital fixation of the stapedial foot plate are common causes of hearing loss: Management is ideally coordinated with a multidisciplinary craniofacial surgery team if it is available; plastic surgery, otolaryngology, maxillofacial surgery, and neurosurgery should evaluate craniofacial morphology and airway function. Regular auditory evoked response and audiology monitoring are required, and surgical treatment including uvulopalatopharyngoplasty, palatal splits, or adenotonsillectomy may be considered for patients with conductive hearing loss and airway obstruction.

Pulmonary: Lower airway obstruction can result from tracheal stenosis and lack of tracheal distensibility, causing difficulty in clearing secretions and possible damage from tracheal suctioning.

Skeletal: Cervical spine fusions occur in 68% of patients with Apert syndrome, involving the lower spine (C5–C6) rather than the upper cervical spine fusions as seen in Crouzon syndrome. There is progressive calcification and fusion of the cervical spine and limb bones in Apert syndrome. Radiography of the cervical spine should be part of the initial diagnostic evaluation. Because cervical vertebral fusions may further compromise the upper airway, cervical spine films are recommended before attempting intubation for general anesthesia. Periodic evaluation for symptoms of cervical spine compression (neck pain, torticollis, altered gait or urination) is also recommended.

Neurologic: Hydrocephalus due to increased intracranial pressure can cause developmental disabilities: Surveillance for hydrocephalus and signs of increased intracranial pressure is important pre- and post-operatively. Impaired absorption of cerebrospinal fluid may explain hydrocephalus in about 25% of patients after operation, and this complication may contribute to the cognitive deficits mentioned above. Management before and after craniofacial surgery should include the coordination of brain imaging and neurosensory studies.

Parental counseling: Genetic counseling should distinguish affected individuals with a 50% recurrence risk from new mutations whose parents will have a 2–3% recurrence risk because of possible germline mosaicism. Parent information can be found at the Children's Craniofacial Association (www.apert.org/apert.htm) and at several educational sites by searching on the syndrome name.

Baller–Gerold syndrome

Baller–Gerold syndrome is an AR condition with variable craniosynostosis, growth deficiency, malformed ears, cleft or highly arched palate, radial ray reduction defects, cardiac anomalies, renal anomalies, and imperforate anus (Jones, 1997, pp. 430–1; Gorlin et al., 2001, pp. 654–8). Craniosynostosis often involves a single suture and is usually milder than encountered in Apert or Crouzon syndrome. Brain anomalies such as microgyria have occurred, and mental deficiency is described in the majority of cases. Appropriate preventive management requires an extensive diagnostic evaluation including radiographic survey of the cranium and appendicular skeleton, echocardiography and renal sonography for the evaluation of internal anomalies, and examination of the limbs and perineal area to rule out radial and anal anomalies. Sudden infant death has been described, so evaluation of the upper airway and respiratory function is important in the neonatal and infantile periods.

Carpenter syndrome

Although first described in 1903 by Carpenter, Temtamy presented a comprehensive review that delineated the Carpenter syndrome in 1966 (Jones, 1997, pp. 425–6; Gorlin et al., 2001, pp. 666–8). The chief findings are craniosynostosis, preaxial polydactyly of the feet, short stature, obesity, and mental deficiency. Optic anomalies (microcornea, corneal opacity, optic atropy) and cardiac anomalies (septal defects, tetralogy of Fallot, transposition of the great arteries) are common. Occasional patients have had urinary tract (hydronephrosis, hydroureter) or genital anomalies (cryptorchidism), and inguinal hernias have occurred. Mental deficiency is common, and cerebellar tonsillar herniation may contribute (Fearon et al., 2001); some patients have normal intelligence with early surgery and some without. External ear anomalies may be associated with conductive hearing loss.

Preventive management of Carpenter syndrome should begin with multidisciplinary evaluation for craniofacial surgery, including imaging studies of the brain, heart, and renal system. Alertness for early respiratory obstruction and serial imaging should be performed in symptomatic or deteriorating patients to identify cerebellar tonsillar herniation that can be ameliorated by surgery (Fearon et al., 2001). Periodic urinalyses and blood pressures should be performed because of the increased risk of urinary tract anomalies. Initial and periodic neurosensory assessments should be conducted, along with early intervention services and psychosocial counseling appropriate for children with disabilities.

Crouzon syndrome

A syndrome of craniosynostosis, maxillary hypoplasia, and shallow orbits with proptosis was described by Crouzon in 1912 (Jones, 1997, pp. 420–1; Gorlin et al., 2001, pp. 658–9). The disorder has an incidence of 1.5 per 100,000 births and exhibits AD inheritance with 50–60% of cases representing new mutations. Mutations have been defined in the FGFR2 gene, but identical mutations may cause a phenotype of Crouzon syndrome in one patient and Pfeiffer syndrome in another despite more usual correlations of syndrome and altered receptor domain.

Coronal, sagittal, and lambdoidal synostoses are most common, occurring in 75% of cases. Many patients will experience airway obstruction during infancy, and may require tracheostomy (Sirotnak et al., 1995). The midface hypoplasia produces shallow orbits with a risk of exposure keratitis to the protruding eyes. Midface hypoplasia contributes to the development of highly arched or cleft palate (3% of patients), and probably explains the frequency of conductive hearing deficit (55%), mouth breathing (32%), and tooth crowding. Deviation of the nasal septum is found in 33% of patients, and there may be jugular foramina synostosis. Cervical vertebral fusions account for 83% of cervical spine anomalies, with fusion of the C2–C3 vertebrae occurring in about 20% of patients. The limbs are usually not affected, but radioulnar synostosis has been described.

Preventive management should follow the craniosynostosis checklist with attention to proptosis and airway obstruction that may result from midface hypoplasia. Early assessment of craniosynostosis, ear, and eye abnormalities should be coordinated through a craniofacial surgical team, and all families should have genetic evaluation and counseling. Surveillance for airway obstruction, sleep apnea, cervical spine anomalies (particularly before anesthesia), exposure keratitis due to proptosis, and neurosensory deficits is particularly important. Although many patients have normal cognitive outcomes, evaluation of developmental progress should be performed during early pediatric visits and appropriate early intervention services provided for those patients with delay.

Jackson–Weiss syndrome

Jackson–Weiss syndrome can be described as the facies of Crouzon syndrome with foot anomalies (Gorlin et al., 2001, pp. 688–9). There is phenotypic overlap with Pfeiffer and Saethre–Chotzen syndromes, and all three AD syndromes have been attributed to mutations in the FGFR2 gene (Aleck, 2004). The foot abnormalities include broad great toes, syndactyly of toes 2 and 3, and fusions of the metatarsal bones. The midface hypoplasia causes proptosis, and there may be hypertelorism.

Preventive management of patients with Jackson–Weiss syndrome will be similar to that of patients with Crouzon syndrome described below, with screening for ophthalmologic or auditory problems and craniofacial evaluation for reconstructive and dental problems. Most reported families exhibit normal intelligence with variable expression of the limb anomalies. Precautions concerning airway management and post-operative hydrocephalus will be similar to those for Apert and Crouzon syndromes, but early intervention services will usually not be needed.

Pfeiffer syndrome

The Pfeiffer syndrome of craniosynostosis with broad thumbs and broad great toes was described in 1964 (Jones, 1997, pp. 416–17; Gorlin et al., 2001, pp. 659–62). It is an AD condition, with major findings including maxillary hypoplasia, mandibular prognathism, ocular proptosis, short fingers and toes, fused cervical and lumbar vertebrae, and occasional mental deficiency. Cervical spine fusion was common and complex in one series of patients with Pfeiffer syndrome, and sacrococcygeal anomalies also occurred. Less common complications include optic nerve hypoplasia or coloboma, hearing deficits, supernumerary teeth, and other skeletal anomalies (club feet, radioulnar or radiohumeral synostosis, short humeri). Bilateral coronal synostosis with tower skull is most common, but unilateral synostosis with cranial asymmetry can occur. Multiple sutural fusion producing the clover-leaf skull anomaly has also been described. Some patients with Pfeiffer syndrome have severe ocular proptosis, and these patients often have an early death.

Preventive management should begin in the neonatal period with thorough craniofacial and skeletal evaluations. Brain MRI scanning and skeletal radiographic survey should be considered based on physical findings. Ophthalmologic referral and auditory evoked response studies will be needed during infancy to rule out optic atrophy, strabismus, and hearing loss. If motor milestones are delayed, referral for early intervention should be considered. As with other craniosynostosis syndromes, regular dental care is needed for the evaluation of tooth crowding and supernumerary teeth. Evaluation of neck mobility and cervical spine fusion should be performed before surgery, and the potential for lumbar vertebral fusion warrants surveillance for back pain or gait disturbances that might indicate cord compression.

Saethre–Chotzen syndrome

Recognized by Saethre in 1931 and Chotzen in 1932, Saethre–Chotzen syndrome has a very broad pattern of malformations including craniosynostosis, facial asymmetry with unilateral ptosis, and partial cutaneous syndactyly (Jones, 1997, pp. 412–15; Gorlin et al., 2001, pp. 664–6). Saethre–Chotzen syndrome has an estimated incidence of 1 in 25,000 births, and exhibits AD inheritance and is caused by a TWIST transcription factor gene on chromosome 7.

The diagnosis of Saethre–Chotzen syndrome is based on clinical examination and radiographic findings. Cranial radiographs and imaging studies will determine the extent and distribution of craniosynostosis, and reveal unusual complications such as hydrocephalus. Examination of the extremities will discover brachydactyly or partial syndactyly that distinguish the disorder from Apert, Crouzon, or Pfeiffer syndrome (Table 14.1).

Summary of clinical concerns: Saethre–Chotzen syndrome management considerations

Growth and development: Short stature with normal development: Monitoring of growth and head circumference.

Craniofacial: Facial asymmetry, low frontal hairline, low set ears, cleft palate; craniosynostosis most frequently in the coronal or metopic suture – often asymmetric and sometimes not present until later life (de Heer et al., 2004): Initial brain imaging and skull radiographs are recommended once craniosynostosis is suspected; multidisciplinary evaluation by a craniofacial surgery team including hearing, vision, feeding, cranial, and cosmetic management. Many children may benefit from helmets to correct cranial asymmetry if management is initiated during infancy.

Eyes: Ptosis or strabismus of the eyes, blepharophimosis: Careful eye assessment at diagnosis, referral to ophthalmology for symptoms; inspection of the eyes for irritation and keratitis due to protrusion and exposure; protective drops and irrigation may be required.

ENT: Cleft palate, dental anomalies including tooth crowding, enamel hypoplasia, or malocclusion: Cleft palate team as part of craniofacial surgery management, attention to early feeding and nutrition, early and regular dentistry.

Heart: Rare congenital heart lesions: Cardiology referral if murmurs or symptoms.

Urogenital: Occasional cryptorchidism, renal defects: Urinalysis, genital examination, urology referral if symptoms.

Skeletal: Syndactyly, brachydactyly, clinodactyly, asymmetry of digits, broad great toes and thumbs, defects of the cervical or lumbar spine: Initial skeletal examination with radiography as appropriate; anesthesia precautions prefaced by cervical spine X-rays; monitoring for scoliosis with appropriate orthopedic referral. If cervical spine anomalies are detected, then lateral radiographs for atlantoaxial instability should be obtained in the 3–5-year-old age range. Many patients have had progressive joint fusions and restrictions, so range-of-motion evaluation should be part of regular examinations.

Neurologic: Occasional mild mental deficiency and epilepsy, but mental development is usually normal. The degree and extent of sutural fusion will determine whether the orbits, optic nerves, conjunctiva, or auditory nerves are compressed, with risk of vision and hearing loss; deterioration or appearance of focal neurologic signs, gait changes may indicate cerebellar tonsillar herniation: Monitoring of hearing and vision, early audiology and ophthalmology assessments; neurology/ neurosurgery evaluation if not part of craniofacial surgery team.

Parental counseling: The low risk for mental deficiency warrants optimistic counseling, and a good cosmetic outcome can be anticipated with modern surgery. Normal parents of children with Saethre–Chotzen syndrome will have a minimal recurrence risk, although germinal mosaicism has been described. Affected patients will have a 50% recurrence risk, and TWIST gene testing or linkage studies are available for prenatal diagnosis (see www.genetests.org). All families should be referred for genetic counseling, which will attend to possible guilt on the part of parents who transmit their disease. Parent support and information is available at the World Craniofacial syndrome (www.worldcf.org/chotzen.cfm) or at numerous sites maintained by craniofacial centers (by searching on the syndrome name).

Preventive management for Craniosynostosis syndromes

Description: Premature fusion of the cranial sutures (craniosynostosis) can present as an isolated anomaly or as part of over 90 syndromes. The combined incidence of craniosynostosis disorders is about 0.4–0.6 per 1000 births, and presence and nature of associated anomalies determines the precise diagnosis rather than the particular suture(s) involved.

Clinical diagnosis: Craniosynostosis with facial changes (Crouzon syndrome), with syndactyly (Apert syndrome), with broad thumbs (Pfeiffer syndrome), with digital anomalies (Saethre–Chotzen syndrome), or with polydactyly (Carpenter syndrome) is characteristic of the more common craniosynostosis syndromes. A fused suture can be palpated as a ridge or deduced by compensatory skull growth upwards (acrocephaly or tower skull with coronal synostosis), backwards (dolichocephaly with sagittal synostosis), sidewards (trigonocephaly from a prow-shaped metopic synostosis or plagiocephaly with unilateral fusion), or as bulging between multiple synostoses (clover-leaf skull with several fusions). Accompanying changes in the sphenoid bone and basilar skull often produce midface hypoplasia, shallow orbits, proptosis, and a prominent nose.

Laboratory diagnosis: Several craniosynostosis syndromes have been associated with mutations in the fibroblast growth factor-2 gene, the TWIST gene, or even to P450 mutations (Antley–Bixler syndrome), and DNA diagnosis is available for the more common syndromes (see www.genetests.org).

Genetics: Apert, Crouzon, Saethre–Chotzen, Pfeiffer syndrome, and many isolated craniosynostoses exhibit autosomal dominant inheritance, requiring parental examination to distinguish those with a 50% recurrence risk from those whose children represent new mutations (2–3% recurrence risk because of possible germline mosaicism). Carpenter syndrome is an autosomal recessive disorder with a 25% recurrence risk.

Key management issues: Multidisciplinary management by a craniofacial surgery team; monitoring for hydrocephalus, airway obstruction, sleep apnea, and growth failure; screening of hearing, vision, and dental status; protection from exposure keratitis in protruding eyes; screening for cervical spine fusion/instability; range-of-motion evaluations for joint fusions and restrictions; orthopedic, cardiac, and urogenital assessment in some patients, early intervention for potential neurosensory and cognitive problems.

Growth charts: Mostly not available, but Cohen and Kreiborg have reported growth patterns for Apert syndrome.

Parent information: World Craniofacial Organization (www.worldcf.org/chotzen.cfm); Children's Craniofacial Association (www.apert.org/apert.htm), and at Craniofacial and Plastic Surgery for Kids, Dallas TX (www.kidsplastsurg.com).

Basis for management recommendations: Derived from complications and American Cleft Palate Association guidelines.

Summary of clinical concerns

General	Learning	Cognitive disability, particularly in those with hydrocephalus
	Behavior	Psychosis (rare)
	Growth	Growth delays, particularly in those with respiratory obstruction
Facial	Face	Shallow orbits, midface hypoplasia, flat forehead, beaked nose
	Eyes	Proptosis with corneal injury, strabismus, lacrimal duct anomalies, ptosis, optic atrophy
	Ears	Otitis media, congenital fixation of the stapedial foot plate (Apert syndrome)
	Nose	Upper respiratory obstruction (deviation of nasal septum, shallow nasal bridge, stenosis or atresia of the posterior choanae)
	Mouth	Mouth breathing, high or cleft palate, dental anomalies (malocclusion, crowded teeth, supernumerary teeth, enamel hypoplasia)
Surface	Skin	Acne vulgaris in Apert, acanthosis nigricans in Crouzon
Skeletal	Cranial	Craniosynostosis of coronal, metopic, lambdoidal sutures, huge fontanel acrocephaly, brachycephaly
	Axial	Cervical vertebral fusion, instability. Cervical spine fusions occur in 68% of patients with Apert syndrome
	Limbs	Syndactyly of digits 2–5 (Apert), syndactyly fingers 2 and 3 with broad thumbs (Saethre–Chotzen), broad thumbs (Pfeiffer), polydactyly (Carpenter), limited joint movement due to synostosis
Internal	Pulmonary	Respiratory obstruction, hypoxemia
	Circulatory	Cardiac anomalies (septal defects, tetralogy of Fallot, transposition of the great arteries)
	Urogenital	Renal anomalies (hydronephrosis, hydroureter), cryptorchidism
Neural	Central	Hydrocephalus, seizures, sleep apnea
	Sensory	Conductive hearing loss, visual deficits
Concerns of frequency >20% are **highlighted**		

Key references

American Cleft Palate-Craniofacial Association (1993). Parameters for evaluation and treatment of patients with cleft lip/palate or other craniofacial anomalies. *Cleft Palate-Craniofacial Journal* 30:S1–8.

Cohen & Kreiborg (1993). Growth pattern in Apert syndrome. *American Journal of Medical Genetics* 47:617–23.

Craniosynostosis syndromes

Preventive medical checklist (0–3 years)

Name _____ Birth date __/__/__ Number _____

Age	Evaluations: key concerns	Management considerations	Notes
New-born ↓ 1 month	Skull exam: sutural ridges, altered shape Skeletal exam: spine, limbs Hearing, vision:[2] proptosis, corneal injury Feeding: cleft palate, dysphagia Respiratory: airway obstruction, apnea Heart: murmur, tachycardia Parental adjustment	❏ Craniofacial team;[1] head imaging ❏ ❏ Skeletal survey;[1] orthopedics[3] ❏ ❏ ABR; ophthalmology[3] ❏ ❏ Feeding specialist; video swallow[3] ❏ ❏ Blood gases; chest X-ray; pulmonology[3] ❏ ❏ Echocardiogram;[3] cardiology[3] ❏ ❏ Family support;[4] genetics ❏	
2 months ↓ 4 months	Growth, development:[5] head size, shape Hearing and vision:[2] otitis, strabismus Feeding: cleft palate, dysphagia Skeletal exam: neck, spine, limbs Neck flexibility;[2] cervical spine fusion Respiratory: airway obstruction, apnea Heart: murmur, tachycardia Other:	❏ Craniofacial team; ECI;[6] family support[4] ❏ ❏ Repeat ABR;[3] ophthalmology;[3] ENT[3] ❏ ❏ Feeding specialist; video swallow[3] ❏ ❏ Orthopedics;[3] neurosurgery[3] ❏ ❏ Cervical spine films; anesthesia precautions ❏ ❏ Blood gases; pulmonology[3] ❏ ❏ Family support;[4] genetics ❏ ❏ ❏	
6 months ↓ 9 months	Growth, development:[5] head size, shape Hearing and vision:[2] otitis, strabismus Skeletal exam: neck, spine, limbs Urogenital: cryptorchidism, renal defects Respiratory: airway obstruction, apnea Other:	❏ Craniofacial team; ECI;[6] family support[4] ❏ ❏ ABR;[3] ophthalmology;[3] ENT[3] ❏ ❏ Orthopedics;[3] neurosurgery[3] ❏ ❏ Urinalysis, BP; renal imaging;[3] urology[3] ❏ ❏ Blood gases; pulmonology[3] ❏ ❏ ❏	
1 year	Growth, development:[5] head size, shape Hearing and vision:[2] otitis, strabismus Skeletal exam: neck, spine, limbs Neck flexibility;[2] cervical spine fusion Respiratory: airway obstruction, apnea Tonsillar herniation: gait, sleep apnea[7] Other:	❏ Craniofacial team; ECI;[6] family support[4] ❏ ❏ ABR;[3] ophthalmology;[3] ENT[3] ❏ ❏ Orthopedics;[3] neurosurgery[3] ❏ ❏ Cervical spine films; anesthesia precautions ❏ ❏ Anesthesia precautions ❏ ❏ Head, foramen magnum MRI;[3] sleep study[3] ❏ ❏ ❏	
15 months ↓ 18 months	Growth, development:[5] head size, shape Hearing and vision:[2] otitis, strabismus Skeletal exam: neck, spine, limbs Respiratory: airway obstruction, apnea	❏ Craniofacial team; ECI;[6] family support[4] ❏ ❏ ABR;[3] ophthalmology;[3] ENT[3] ❏ ❏ Orthopedics;[3] neurosurgery[3] ❏ ❏ Blood gases; pulmonology[3] ❏	
2 years	Growth, development:[5] head size, shape Hearing and vision:[2] otitis, strabismus Skeletal exam: neck, spine, limbs Tonsillar herniation: gait, sleep apnea[7] Neck flexibility[2]	❏ Craniofacial team; ECI;[6] family support[4] ❏ ❏ ABR;[3] ophthalmology;[3] ENT[3] ❏ ❏ Orthopedics;[3] neurosurgery[3] ❏ ❏ Head, foramen magnum MRI;[3] sleep study[3] ❏ ❏ Anesthesia precautions ❏	
3 years	Growth, development:[5] head size, shape Hearing and vision:[2] otitis, strabismus Skeletal exam: neck, spine, limbs Tonsillar herniation: gait, sleep apnea[7] Neck flexibility[2] Heart: murmur, tachycardia Other:	❏ Craniofacial team; ECI;[6] family support[4] ❏ ❏ Audiology; ophthalmology;[3] ENT[3] ❏ ❏ Orthopedics;[3] neurosurgery[3] ❏ ❏ Head, foramen magnum MRI;[3] sleep study[3] ❏ ❏ Anesthesia precautions ❏ ❏ Echocardiogram;[3] cardiology[3] ❏ ❏ ❏	

Craniosynostosis concerns		Other concerns from history	
Craniosynostosis Airway obstruction, sleep apnea Hearing, vision loss Deviated nasal septum Proptosis, optic atrophy Exposure keratitis	Cervical spine fusion Cardiac anomalies Limb, urogenital anomalies Learning differences Hydrocephalus Headaches, seizures	**Family/ history/prenatal** _____ _____ _____ _____	**Social/environmental** _____ _____ _____ _____

Guidelines for the neonatal period should be undertaken *at whatever age* the diagnosis is made; ABR, auditory brainstem evoked response; BP, blood pressure; ECI, early childhood intervention [1]Multidisciplinary assessment and surgical options; distribution of fused sutures and associated anomalies will guide diagnosis and genetic counseling; [2]by practitioner; [3]as dictated by clinical findings; [4]Little People of America for education, medical consultation, and family adaptation; genetic counseling [5]consider developmental pediatrician/ neurologist/genetics clinic according to symptoms and availability; [6]early childhood intervention with occupational therapy for children with significant hypotonia; [7]snoring, pause in breathing, daytime sleepiness, unusual sleep positioning.

Craniosynostosis syndromes

Preventive medical checklist (4–18 years)

Name _____ Birth date __/__/__ Number _____

Age	Evaluations: key concerns		Management considerations		Notes
4 years ↓ 6 years	Growth:[5] head size, shape Development:[2] preschool transition Hearing and vision:[2] otitis, optic atrophy Skeletal exam: neck, spine, limbs Neuro: gait, seizures, sleep apnea[7] Neck flexibility[2] Other:	❏ ❏ ❏ ❏ ❏ ❏ ❏	Craniofacial team[1] Family support;[4] preschool program[5] Audiology; ophthalmology;[3] ENT[3] Orthopedics;[3] neurosurgery[3] Head, foramen magnum MRI;[3] sleep study[3] Anesthesia precautions	❏ ❏ ❏ ❏ ❏ ❏ ❏	
7 years ↓ 9 years	Growth:[5] head size, shape Development:[1] school transition[5] Hearing, vision:[2] nerve compression Skeletal exam: neck, spine, limbs Neuro: gait, seizures, sleep apnea[7] Neck flexibility[2] Other:	❏ ❏ ❏ ❏ ❏ ❏ ❏	Craniofacial team Family support;[4] school progress[6] Audiology;[3] ophthalmology Orthopedics;[3] neurosurgery[3] Head, foramen magnum MRI;[3] sleep study[3] Anesthesia precautions	❏ ❏ ❏ ❏ ❏ ❏ ❏	
10 years ↓ 12 years	Growth, development:[5] head size, shape Hearing, vision:[2] nerve compression Skeletal exam: neck, spine, limbs Neuro: gait, seizures, sleep apnea[7] Other:	❏ ❏ ❏ ❏ ❏	Craniofacial team; school progress[6] Audiology;[3] ophthalmology Orthopedics;[3] neurosurgery[3] ENT;[3] sleep study[3]	❏ ❏ ❏ ❏ ❏	
13 years ↓ 15 years	Growth and development[1] Hearing, vision:[2] nerve compression Skeletal exam: neck, spine, limbs Neuro: gait, seizures, sleep apnea[7] Urogenital: cryptorchidism, renal defects Other:	❏ ❏ ❏ ❏ ❏ ❏	Craniofacial team; school progress[6] Audiology;[3] ophthalmology Orthopedics;[3] neurosurgery[3] Head, foramen magnum MRI;[3] sleep study[3] Urinalysis, BP; renal imaging,[3] urology[3]	❏ ❏ ❏ ❏ ❏ ❏	
16 years ↓ 18 years	Growth and development[1] Hearing, vision:[2] nerve compression Skeletal exam: neck, spine, limbs Neuro: gait, seizures, sleep apnea[7] Other:	❏ ❏ ❏ ❏ ❏	Family support;[4] school progress[6] Audiology; craniofacial team Orthopedics;[3] neurosurgery[3] Head, foramen magnum MRI;[3] sleep study[3]	❏ ❏ ❏ ❏ ❏	
19 years ↓ 23 years	Adult care transition[6] Hearing, vision:[2] nerve compression Skeletal exam: neck, spine, limbs Neuro: gait, seizures, sleep apnea[7] Neck flexibility[2]	❏ ❏ ❏ ❏ ❏	Family support;[4] school progress[6] Audiology; craniofacial team Orthopedics;[3] neurosurgery[3] Head, foramen magnum MRI;[3] sleep study[3] Anesthesia precautions	❏ ❏ ❏ ❏ ❏	
Adult	Adult care transition[6] Hearing, vision:[2] nerve compression Skeletal exam: neck, spine, limbs Neuro: gait, seizures, sleep apnea[7] Neck flexibility[2] Other:	❏ ❏ ❏ ❏ ❏ ❏	Family support[4] Audiology; craniofacial team Orthopedics;[3] neurosurgery[3] Head, foramen magnum MRI;[3] sleep study[3] Anesthesia precautions	❏ ❏ ❏ ❏ ❏ ❏	

Craniosynostosis concerns		Other concerns from history	
Craniosynostosis Hearing, vision loss Deviated nasal septum Proptosis, optic atrophy Exposure keratitis	Cervical spine fusion Cardiac anomalies Limb, urogenital anomalies Learning differences Hydrocephalus, sleep apnea Headaches, seizures	**Family history/prenatal** _____ _____ _____ _____	**Social/environmental** _____ _____ _____ _____

Guidelines for the neonatal period should be undertaken *at whatever age* the diagnosis is made; BP, blood pressure; [1]multidisciplinary assessment and monitoring for progress, surgical complications; consider developmental pediatrician/neurologist/behavior therapist/genetics clinic according to symptoms and availability; [2]by practitioner; [3] as dictated by clinical findings; [4]parent group, family/sib, financial, and behavioral issues with later focus on independent living and employment; [5]preschool program including developmental monitoring and motor/speech therapy; [6]monitor individual education plan, educational testing, balance of special education and inclusion, academic progress, behavioral differences, later vocational planning; [7]snoring, pause in breathing, daytime sleepiness, unusual sleep positioning.

Parent guide to craniosynostosis syndromes

In craniosynostosis, one or more of the gaps in the skull that allow growth (sutures) fuses prematurely and alters head shape. Craniosynostosis can occur as an isolated problem or appear as one of several anomalies in more than 90 craniosynostosis syndromes. Children with fused cranial sutures share many medical and surgical problems, leading to similar strategies of preventive management.

Incidence, causation, and diagnosis

The aggregate frequency of craniosynostosis is about 0.4–0.6 per 1000 live births. The head shape reflects the sutures that are fused. Synostosis of the coronal suture (roughly along a line connecting the ears) produces a "tower" skull (acrocephaly) with a short forehead–occiput distance (brachycephaly). Synostosis of the sagittal suture (from forehead to occiput) produces an elongated head (scaphocephaly, dolichocephaly) with a prominent occiput. Rarely, several sutures are fused to produce the severe anomaly called clover-leaf skull or *Kleebattschädel* anomaly. The pattern of associated malformations will determine the craniosynostosis syndrome diagnosis – Crouzon with facial changes, Apert with fused fingers, Pfeiffer with broad thumbs and toes, Saethre–Chotzen with asymmetry of the digits. Mutations in the fibroblast growth factor receptor-2 (FGFR2) gene cause several craniosynostosis syndromes and DNA diagnosis is available for the more common disorders.

Natural history and complications

Changes in skull shape and restriction of brain and nerve growth produce complications in craniosynostosis disorders. Undergrowth of the midface is common with large fontanelle (soft spot), depressed nasal bridge, deviated nasal septum, stenosis of the nasal passages with airway obstruction, and bulging eyes with corneal injuries from exposure and inadequate tearing. Palatal anomalies (cleft soft palate, highly arched palate) together with flattened cheekbones and protrusion of the jaw cause dental misalignment. A smaller mouth and throat may cause symptoms of obstructive sleep apnea (cessation of breathing during sleep) and heart failure due to inadequate oxygenation (cor pulmonale). Surgical treatment involving resection of the palate, adenotonsillectomy, or even tracheostomy (breathing tube through neck into the windpipe) may be considered for symptomatic patients. Fusions of the neck spine can also occur in these syndromes, mandating cervical (neck) spine X-rays before attempting intubation for general anesthesia. Narrow respiratory structures can impair ear drainage, causing chronic otitis and hearing loss. Hearing deficits and optic nerve problems also occur, along with dental anomalies (extra teeth) and skeletal defects (club foot, fusions of the arm bones, short arms). Mental deficiency and epilepsy have been reported, but mental development is usually normal. Skeletal abnormalities may include fused fingers, asymmetry of the fingers, broad great toes and thumbs, and defects of the cervical (neck) or lumbar (lower back) spine. Anomalies of other systems include short stature, heart defects, kidney anomalies, and cryptorchidism (undescended testes). Occasional patients have had urinary tract or genital anomalies, and inguinal hernias have occurred.

Preventive medical needs

Children with craniosynostosis should be referred to a multidisciplinary craniofacial surgery team that includes input from plastic surgery, ophthalmology, neurosurgery, otolaryngology, and dentistry. Mild asymmetries can be treated with cranial bands to correct their head shape deformity. Brain imaging and skull radiographs, regular evaluation of hearing and vision, Inspection of the eyes for irritation due to protrusion and exposure, and consideration of cervical spine films with anesthesia precautions are useful. Other issues will include the assessment of airway function, the impact on vision and hearing, the distortion of mouth and dental structures, and accessory anomalies of the chest, spine, limbs, and hips. Ultrasound studies of the heart and kidneys may be needed, along with airway assessment and use of oral surgery, tracheostomy, or apnea monitoring. Airway problems can lead to poor nutrition and failure to thrive, so growth of the body as well as the head must be followed closely in children with craniosynostosis syndromes. Surveillance for hydrocephalus (accumulation of fluid in brain cavities), increased intracranial pressure, and cerebellar tonsillar herniation through the foramen magnum is important before and after operations; symptoms may include sleep apnea, altered gait, headaches, or seizures. Regular eye examinations are needed for the detection of optic atrophy or strabismus (wandering eye), and early intervention is important in view of the risks of neurosensory and cognitive problems. The crowded teeth produced by maxillary hypoplasia require early and regular dental care. Periodic urinalyses, blood pressures, and imaging studies of the urinary tract may be considered because of the increased risk of urinary tract anomalies.

Family counseling

Medical counseling should emphasize the excellent surgical outcomes for most patients, with monitoring of development to ensure early intervention services for those with delays. The major syndromes except for Carpenter exhibit autosomal dominant inheritance, so unaffected parents will have a recurrence risk of 2–3% that reflects the possibility of germinal mosaicism (several sperm or eggs in the normal parent with a craniosynostosis mutation). Affected individuals will usually have a 50% recurrence risk with each pregnancy, and DNA diagnosis can be used for prenatal diagnosis of the more common conditions. Carpenter syndrome is autosomal recessive, meaning that parents will have a 25% recurrence risk with each pregnancy. All families should be referred for genetic counseling, which ideally is coupled with the diagnostic evaluation and surgical care as part of a multidisciplinary craniofacial surgery team.

15

Branchial arch and face/limb syndromes

Branchial arch syndromes

Branchial arches are critical for the development of the lower portion of the craniofacies, the muscles of the pharynx and jaw, the cardiac conotruncal region, and the salivary, thymus, and parathyroid glands. In addition, branchial arch mesoderm merges with neural crest cells to form an ectomesenchyme that is important for the development of the cranial nerves. The embryonic derivatives of the branchial arches explain the anomalies seen in children with branchial arch syndromes: craniofacial anomalies of the mandible, maxilla, palate and ears; palatal, salivary gland, and pharyngeal muscle hypoplasias that cause oromotor dysfunction and feeding difficulties; and cranial nerve, optic, otic, and cardiac anomalies that include neurosensory and cognitive deficits. Preventive management is enormously important for children with branchial arch syndromes, since many of their feeding, neurosensory, and learning problems can be anticipated and treated.

Table 15.1 summarizes the clinical manifestations of several branchial arch syndromes. The Goldenhar syndrome-hemifacial microsomia spectrum is the most common, and will be discussed in detail after a review of other branchial arch syndromes.

Branchio-oculo-facial syndrome

Hall first described in 1983 an autosomal-dominant (AD) syndrome consisting of hemangiomatous branchial clefts, eye anomalies, nasolacrimal duct obstruction, and occasion limb or renal anomalies (Jones, 1997, pp. 246–7, Gorlin et al., 2001, pp. 895–7). The branchial clefts may appear as cysts, fistulas, hemangiomas, or cutis aplasia in the lateral neck region, and some patients have had upper lip clefts. Eye anomalies may be severe and include microphthalmia, cataracts, strabismus, colobomata of the irides or retinae, and eyelid anomalies resulting from nasolacrimal duct obstruction and lacrimal gland infection (dacryocystitis). Demirci et al. (2005) noted a lacrimal sac fistula with an orbital dermoid cyst and a hamartoma of the retina and retinal pigment epithelium in one patient. The external ear anomalies may be associated with conductive hearing loss, a risk that is accentuated if

Table 15.1. Branchial arch syndromes

Syndrome	Incidence*	Inheritance	Complications
Branchio-oculo-facial	~20 cases	AD	Branchial cysts, eye a. (strabismus, cataracts, colobomata), ear a., cleft lip/palate, renal a.
Branchio-oculo-renal	1 in 40,000	AD	Ear a., urinary tract a., branchial cysts and fistulas
Goldenhar	1 in 5600	MF	Hemifacial microsomia, cranial asymmetry, eye a. (epibulbar dermoids, lipoepidermoid cysts), micrognathia, cleft lip/palate, cardiac a., limb a., vertebral a., renal a.
Miller	~20 cases	AD	Malar, mandibular, pharyngeal hypoplasia, eye a., hearing loss, post-axial limb a., cardiac and genital a.
Nager	~40 cases	AR, AD	Malar, mandibular, pharyngeal hypoplasia, eye a., hearing loss, thumb and radial a., cardiac and renal a.
Townes–Brocks	~30 cases	AD	External ear a., hearing loss, digital a., imperforate anus
Treacher–Collins	1 in 50,000	AD	Malar, mandibular, pharyngeal hypoplasia, eye a. (colobomata, strabismus, amblyopia), hearing loss, airway obstruction.
Wildervanck	~100 cases	?AD, ?XLR	Klippel–Feil a., abducens palsy with Duane syndrome, hearing loss, facial asymmetry, facial palsy.

Notes:
MF, multifactorial; AD, autosomal dominant; AR, autosomal recessive; XLR, X-linked recessive; a., anomaly.
* Cases or per number of live births.

cleft palate is present. Cystic kidneys and unilateral renal agenesis have been reported, but Lin et al. (2000) demonstrated that branchio-oculo-facial syndrome does not involve mutations in the EYA1 gene and thus is not allelic to the more common branchio-oto-renal (BOR) syndrome.

Preventive management should include early ophthalmology referral with probing, massage, and/or surgery to ensure patency of the nasolacrimal ducts. Audiology screening later in infancy and monitoring of developmental progress are important because some patients have had mental disability. Although renal anomalies have been rare, initial renal ultrasound, periodic screening by urinalysis, and aggressive evaluation after urinary tract infections seems wise.

Branchio-oto-renal syndrome

The BOR syndrome involves anomalies of the external ear including preauricular pits, hearing loss, branchial cysts, and renal anomalies (Jones, 1997, pp. 244–5; Gorlin et al., 2001, pp. 810–13). The condition is AD with an estimated incidence of 1 in 40,000 births. Initial distinctions between a syndrome with branchial findings (BO) and branchial plus renal findings (BOR) have broken down now that both variations were shown to involve mutations in the EYA1 gene at chromosome band 8q13.3, a homolog of the fly developmental gene *eyes absent*. Families that lacked simple point mutations in the EYA1 have suggested another locus is involved, but Chang et al. (2004) and others note that many of these have complex rearrangements of the EYA1 gene that must be documented by different techniques.

Summary of clinical concerns: BOR syndrome management considerations

Craniofacial: The branchial cysts or fistulas occur in 60% of patients, and may present with draining fluid or infection on the lower cervical region.

ENT: Anomalies of the external, middle, and internal ear have been described, with 75% of patients having hearing loss, of which 30% is conductive, 20% sensorineural, and 50% mixed: early auditory evoked response assessment of hearing with imaging of the middle and inner ear if sensorineural hearing loss is documented. Although the hearing loss is not progressive in most instances, periodic audiologic assessment is warranted during childhood and adolescence.

Excretory: Symptomatic urinary tract anomalies occur in about 10% of patients, but some studies revealed 75–100% of patients to have structural anomalies and 33% to have functional anomalies. Renal anomalies may include lethal renal agenesis with Potter sequence and pulmonary hypoplasia: The urinary tract anatomy should be evaluated by an early renal ultrasound, with periodic urinalyses, blood urea nitrogen, and creatinine studies to assess for infection, proteinuria, and evidence of glomerular lesions. Intravenous pyelogram and voiding cystourethrogram studies should be considered in patients with urinary tract infections, since urinary tract anomalies may be subtle.

Parental counseling: BOR syndrome has been confused with related disorders such as hearing loss–ear pit syndromes, renal anomaly–hearing loss, or the Goldenhar spectrum of oculo-auriculo-vertebral anomalies. Recognition of branchial–renal anomaly associations as BOR syndrome, and study of parents to define subtle defects should identify those with a 50% risk for transmission. Limited DNA testing is available to help in suspect cases, and parent or physician information is available at several educational websites including gene reviews at the Gene Clinics site (www.geneclinics.org/profiles/bor/).

Miller syndrome

Patients with Miller syndrome bear facial resemblance to those with Treacher–Collins syndrome and have additional limb defects in the post-axial ray (Jones, 1997, pp. 256–7; Gorlin et al., 2001, pp. 805–7). The face is similar to that in Treacher–Collins or Nager syndrome, but differences include more striking ectropion of the lower lids and more frequent cleft lip/palate with the same small jaw, ear malformations, and hearing loss. Inheritance is AD, and more severe skeletal anomalies such as ulnar hypoplasia, radioulnar synostosis, absent fibula, phocomelia, vertebral anomalies, and cervical ribs assist in differentiation of the Miller, Nager, and Treacher–Collins syndromes (Table 15.1). Some patients have had anomalies of the digestive (midgut volvulus, malrotation) or urinary systems (ureteral reflux, hydronephrosis).

Preventive management involves multidisciplinary craniofacial assessment, evaluation for airway obstruction, screening for vision or hearing loss, and monitoring of nutrition and growth so that feeding problems can be addressed. The presence of cleft palate may require involvement of a cleft palate team. Conical teeth are reported, so dental evaluation is important. Less frequent cardiac (patent ductus arteriosus, ventricular septal defect), intestinal (volvulus, malrotation), urinary (ureteral reflux, hydronephrosis), and genital anomalies (cryptorchidism, micropenis) should also be considered during the initial physical examination to provide appropriate imaging studies and specialty referrals. Initial skeletal examination with appropriate skeletal X-rays (including spine and ribs) is necessary to guide management by orthopedic and hand surgeons. A foundation for Nager and Miller syndromes is available for parent support and information (www.fnms.net/).

Nager syndrome

Nager syndrome consists of abnormal thumbs in addition to mandibulofacial dysostosis reminiscent of that in Treacher–Collins syndrome (Jones, 1997, pp. 258–9; Gorlin et al., 2001, pp. 802–5). Most cases of Nager syndrome exhibit autosomal-recessive (AR) inheritance as supported by consanguinity and consistency of syndrome manifestations; however, some families with AD inheritance may exist provided they are distinct from Treacher–Collins syndrome. Delineation of the two syndromes is complicated, since vertical transmission of thumb anomalies and typical facial dysostosis is evident in some families. Molecular analysis should soon reveal whether thumb anomalies are an occasional manifestation of Treacher–Collins syndrome or whether Nager syndrome exhibits genetic heterogeneity.

Micrognathia is often more severe in Nager syndrome, requiring multidisciplinary craniofacial management as outlined for Treacher–Collins syndrome. Airway obstruction and feeding problems may be more acute than in Treacher–Collins syndrome, and some patients have a Robin sequence with cleft palate or velopalatine insufficiency. The palatal anomalies and frequent laryngeal hypoplasia require even greater attention to speech, with the same annual screening for hearing and vision recommended for Treacher–Collins syndrome (Hunt & Hobar, 2002). Patients with Nager syndrome should have neonatal assessment by a craniofacial surgery team with combined plastic surgery, otolaryngology, dental, pulmonology, and speech therapy services. Early intervention services may be required but intelligence is usually normal. Cardiac and renal anomalies are sufficiently frequent to consider an echocardiogram and renal sonogram as part of the initial diagnostic evaluation. Children with more severe hand defects will need orthopedic and occupational therapy assessments. Radial aplasia, radioulnar synostosis, and limited extension of the elbows may occur.

Accurate genetic counseling requires distinction of Nager from Treacher–Collins syndrome, with provision of a 25% recurrence risk for normal parents of an affected child. A potentially lower risk should be mentioned because of some families with AD inheritance. Parent information can be found at several educational websites and at the Foundation for Nager and Miller syndromes (www.fnms.net/).

Townes–Brocks syndrome

Townes and Brocks in 1972 reported a syndrome consisting of external ear anomalies, limb anomalies, and imperforate anus (Jones, 1997, pp. 260–1; Gorlin et al., 2001, pp. 814–17). Inheritance is AD through mutations in a SALL1 transcription factor on chromosome 16 (Kohlhase, 2000). The ear anomalies range from overturned helices ("lop" ear) to microtia with preauricular tags. Sensorineural hearing loss is common, and the limb anomalies can include triphalangeal or hypoplastic thumbs, abnormal wrist bones, hypoplastic third toes, and cone-shaped epiphyses. Imperforate anus or anal stenosis may be present, and cardiac or urogenital anomalies are sometimes found. Preventive management should include early auditory evoked response and later audiologic monitoring, radiographic skeletal survey with particular attention to the pre-axial regions of the upper limbs, and consideration of renal sonogram to document the urinary tract anatomy. Evaluation of the genitalia is important, since males have had hypospadias and cryptorchidism.

Treacher–Collins syndrome

Treacher–Collins syndrome was recognized in the 1800s but named by the classic description of Treacher–Collins. The disorder is also referred to using the eponyms of Franceschetti and Klein or by the term coined in their article: mandibulofacial dysostosis (Jones, 1997, pp. 250–1; Gorlin et al., 2001, pp. 799–802). It has an incidence of about 1 in 50,000 births, with over 400 cases reported. The syndrome exhibits AD inheritance, with at least 60% representing new mutations; genetic counseling is thus an important aspect of initial management. Mutations in the TCOF1 or treacle gene on chromosome 5 cause the disorder, and at least one mechanism involves decreased transcription of ribosomal RNA (Valdez et al., 2004).

Summary of clinical concerns: Management considerations

Growth and development: Patients with severe micrognathia and Robin sequence may have failure to thrive and developmental delay: Early intervention and neurosensory/developmental assessments.

Craniofacial: Characteristic facial manifestations include flattened cheeks (malar hypoplasia), a notch in the outer third of the lower eyelid (75%), hypoplasia of the supraorbital ridges and zygomatic process, malformed external ears, and down-slanting palpebral fissures: Craniofacial team management with airway assessment and pulmonary function studies for patients with severe micrognathia (Posnick, 1997). Mandibular lengthening may lessen upper airway obstruction, and microsurgical techniques for restoring facial asymmetry may be particularly useful in Treacher–Collins and other branchial arch syndromes (Siebert et al., 1996).

Eye: Visual abnormalities include colobomas of the eyelids and pupils, strabismus (37%), amblyopia (33%), refractive errors (58%), and anisometropia (17%): Neonatal ophthalmology assessment with annual follow-up.

ENT: Hypoplasia of the alae nasae with choanal atresia may contribute to airway obstruction and sleep apnea; hypoplasia of pharyngeal muscles may cause feeding problems; external and middle ear anomalies are common with ear tags, fistulae, malformed ossicles, and conductive hearing loss; the small nasal passages, oral clefts with pharyngeal hypoplasia, and an obtuse cranial base angle may make intubation difficult: Neonatal assessment by otolaryngology if not part of craniofacial surgery team, including initial auditory evoked response and annual hearing assessments; feeding specialists or a cleft palate team may be required to optimize nutrition; anesthesia precautions should be observed and respiration monitored carefully during recovery.

Cardiac: Occasional cardiac defects: Cardiology assessment if symptoms.

Neurologic: Cognitive development is usually normal if hearing loss is anticipated and treated; at least 50% of patients have pure conductive hearing loss as a result of external and middle ear anomalies: School and behavioral assessments with careful monitoring of school progress.

Parental counseling: The normal intellectual potential provides incentive for scrupulous preventive management and an optimistic outlook for parental counseling. AD inheritance implies a 50% recurrence risk for affected individuals and low (1–2%) recurrence for unaffected parents of children with presumed new mutations. Parent and physician information can be found by searching on the syndrome name and at the Treacher–Collins Foundation (http://www. treachercollinsfnd.org/) or at a website organized by an affected individual (www.treachercollins.org/).

Wildervanck syndrome

The Wildervanck syndrome consists of the Klippel–Feil anomaly, hearing loss, and abducens nerve palsy (Gorlin et al., 2001, pp. 813–14; Jones, 1997, pp. 254–5). The abducens palsy produces a Duane syndrome (inability of eye abduction, retraction of the globe and narrowing of the palpebral fissures during eye adduction). Fewer than 100 cases are documented and the majority are female. AD inheritance with sex limitation, X-linked recessive (XLR) inheritance with male lethality, and multifactorial (MF) inheritance mechanisms have been considered. Mental deficiency is rare, and those with significant disability should definitely have chromosome studies.

Eye anomalies include Duane anomaly, epibulbar dermoid cysts and lens subluxation. Anomalies of the external, middle, and/or internal ear can cause sensorineural, conductive, or mixed hearing loss. The Klippel–Feil anomaly may include cervical vertebral fusion with restricted neck mobility; associated basilar impression with brainstem hypoplasia and anomalies of the cervical cord (diastematomyelia) may occur (Balci et al., 2002). Skeletal anomalies can include torticollis, spina bifida occulta, Sprengel deformity, kyphoscoliosis, and rib defects.

Preventive management should include early auditory evoked response studies, ophthalmology assessment, and radiography of the axial skeleton with flexion/ extension views of the cervical spine. Inner ear anomalies may be severe, so cochlear imaging should be considered when there is sensorineural hearing loss. As with other forms of cervical vertebral fusion, periodic radiographic assessment for atlantoaxial instability, basilar impression, and cervical vertebral arthritis should be performed. Some patients may require assessment by the craniofacial surgery team because of facial asymmetry or paralysis, and others will need early intervention services, since mental disability has been described.

Goldenhar syndrome and related defects

Terminology

Goldenhar published in 1952 an influential paper that related eye and ear anomalies to the mandibular hypoplasia that was well known as "hemifacial microsomia" (Jones, 1997, pp. 642–3; Gorlin et al., 2001, pp. 790–8). Unilateral hypoplasia of the jaw with external ear anomalies denoted by the latter term was appreciated in the late 1800s. The publication of Goldenhar initiated a large body of work that delineated a syndrome consisting of craniofacial, ocular, otic, skeletal, cardiac, and renal anomalies. The extreme variability of clinical manifestations has led to several names, including "hemifacial microsomia," "oculo-auriculo-vertebral dysplasia," "facio-auriculo-vertebral spectrum," "first and second branchial arch syndrome," and "Goldenhar complex." From a practical standpoint, it is useful to think of Goldenhar syndrome as a variable spectrum of major anomalies similar to those occurring in associations. Kallen et al. (2004) illustrate the overlap of Goldenhar findings with those of the Coloboma, Heart disease, Atresia choanae, Retarded growth and development, Genital anomalies, and Ear anomalies (CHARGE) or Vertebral, Anorectal, Tracheo-Esophageal, Radial, and Renal defects (VATER) association, an overlap supported by the fact that Goldenhar and VATER manifestations are common in infants of diabetic mothers. The presence of minor anomalies in patients with Goldenhar-like major anomalies should prompt consideration of chromosomal or Mendelian disorders.

Incidence, etiology, and differential diagnosis

The incidence of Goldenhar syndrome will depend on its definition, but including the spectrum from hemifacial microsomia to oculo-auriculo-vertebral defect patterns will yield a figure of at least 1 in 5000 births or more. The disorder exhibits MF inheritance, with rare families showing vertical transmission consistent with AD inheritance. Environmental influences are represented by the ability to induce hemifacial microsomia in the rat arterial disruption or teratogens and the occurrence of Goldenhar anomalies in infants of diabetic mothers. Genetic models include natural or transgenic mouse mutations with branchial arch defects and chromosome abnormalities producing Goldenhar-like patterns (Wilson and Barr, 1983). The variable clinical manifestations of Goldenhar syndrome undoubtedly reflect etiologic heterogeneity, ranging from *in utero* vascular accidents to pure Mendelian disorders. Kallen et al. (2004) suggest these various etiologies act by interfering with early neural crest development.

Differential diagnosis of the branchial arch syndromes can be appreciated by perusing Table 15.1. The most important diagnostic consideration is to exclude Mendelian syndromes such as the BOR or Treacher–Collins syndrome. Trisomy 18 may present with hemifacial microsomia and epibulbar dermoids, but the pattern of other anomalies should allow discrimination from Goldenhar syndrome. The VATER association of vertebral, anorectal, tracheo-esophageal fistula, radial, and renal anomalies has considerable overlap with Goldenhar syndrome, and each disorder is primarily a pattern of major anomalies without a characteristic facies. In most cases, the facial asymmetry and ocular findings of Goldenhar syndrome discriminate it from VATER association. Some patients with Goldenhar syndrome will have the broad nasal region and hypertelorism characteristic of frontonasal dysplasia (Gorlin et al., 2001, pp. 798–9); this conjunction probably reflects the occurrence of cranial malformations in some patients with Goldenhar syndrome (Wilson, 1983).

Diagnostic evaluation and medical counseling

The diagnosis of Goldenhar syndrome should be considered in the presence of unilateral mandibular hypoplasia and ear anomalies, with or without ocular cysts. The initial diagnostic evaluation for children with Goldenhar syndrome depends on the severity and extent of malformation. For children with hemifacial microsomia (unilateral jaw and ear involvement), minimal diagnostic evaluation is needed beyond contact with craniofacial surgery specialists to determine a schedule for repair. Part of the craniofacial evaluation will be auditory evoked response and imaging studies to determine the extent of middle/inner anomalies and hearing loss. For children with hemifacial microsomia and multiple other anomalies that occur with Goldenhar syndrome, an extensive diagnostic evaluation is required. Skeletal radiologic survey for cranial, vertebral, and limb anomalies; echocardiography to evaluate septal defects, transposition, or tetralogy of Fallot; and renal sonography to evaluate the urinary tract anatomy are important. Children with anophthalmia/microphthalmia, frontonasal dysplasia, or severe cranial asymmetry (plagiocephaly) require cranial imaging studies to evaluate brain structure; syringomyelia has been reported. Ophthalmology, otolaryngology, and nutritional evaluations are often needed because of anomalies and/or feeding problems that accompany pharyngeal and salivary gland hypoplasia that is common in Goldenhar syndrome. Airway obstruction may also occur and contribute to poor growth. Chromosomal studies may be considered in patients with severe and extensive anomalies, but a normal result is expected for children with Goldenhar syndrome.

Family and psychosocial counseling

Most families will not have other affected relatives, allowing genetic counseling for a 1–2% recurrence risk appropriate for MF inheritance. A family history is important to rule out unusual instances of AD inheritance. Although an optimistic prognosis for growth and mental development is appropriate for most children, clinicians must consider early feeding problems and the demands of multiple surgeries in providing support for families. Children with anophthalmia, encephaloceles, or severe cranial asymmetry are at risk for mental disability, so the provision of early intervention services and other supportive counseling is needed for their families. The clinical variability of Goldenhar syndrome mandates care in arranging appropriate family contacts. Parent information can be found at various craniofacial surgery sites by searching on the syndrome name, and support groups are available at the Goldenhar Syndrome Support Network (www.goldenharsyndrome.org/).

Natural history and complications

As denoted by the alternative name "first and second branchial arch syndrome," core complications involve the mandibular, maxillary, auditory, and pharyngeal structures. There is facial asymmetry in 20%, mainly reflecting unilateral mandibular aplasia. Malformations of the external ear range from a small and simplified pinna to complete absence of the pinna and ear canal. The pinna may be represented by ear tags, and it is common to find extra cartilaginous tags along a line between the ear and the corner of the mouth. Conductive, sensorineural, or mixed hearing loss is present in at least 15% of cases due to stenosis of the ear canal, malformations of the ossicles, and basilar skull anomalies. These changes also include abnormalities of the temporomandibular joint (Hirschfelder et al., 2004).

The eye and central nervous system are commonly affected, with ocular epibulbar dermoids (milky-white masses with defined edges, 50% of patients), lipoepidermoid cysts (yellowish, diffuse masses, 25% of patients), and anophthalmia/microphthalmia. Ocular motility disorders such as strabismus or Duane syndrome occur in 25% of patients. The implication of microphthalmia/anophthalmia for mental disability fits with an abnormality of neural tissue development in some patients with Goldenhar syndrome: mental retardation (5–15%), microcephaly, encephalocele, lissencephaly, holoprosencephaly, and abnormalities of cranial nerves I-VI and XIII-X have been described.

Oral complications include macrostomia because of lateral clefts, agenesis of the salivary glands (a prominent skin tag near the tragus is predictive of parotid gland agenesis), hypoplasia of the tongue and pharyngeal muscles, delayed development of teeth, and velopalatine insufficiency. Cleft palate with or without cleft lip may occur, and asynchrony of palatal motion may be associated with facial nerve palsies.

Vertebral anomalies are the best known skeletal complications, but anomalous ribs, thumb and radial ray defects, talipes equinovarus, and skull defects have all been noted. Cervical vertebral fusions occur in 20–35% of patients, and these may lead to interference with the articulation of the atlas and basilar skull (basilar impression – Gosain et al., 1994). Visceral anomalies include cardiac defects, pulmonary hypoplasia, renal anomalies, and gastrointestinal defects including imperforate anus.

Goldenhar syndrome preventive medical checklist

As discussed above, the initial evaluation for patients with severe and extensive anomalies of Goldenhar syndrome should include imaging studies of the brain, heart, urinary tract, and skeleton. Careful examination of craniofacial morphology and facial movement is needed, with early referral to craniofacial surgery, otolaryngology, and ophthalmology specialists. Monitoring of head growth (for hydrocephalus, micro-cephaly), of hearing (conductive or sensorineural deficits), and of vision (strabismus, Duane syndrome) is important during infancy and childhood. If renal sonography demonstrates abnormalities of the urinary tract, then periodic urinalyses are needed. Because cervical vertebral fusions are common, cervical spine films are recommended at age 3–5 years when ossification is complete; those with fusions should be followed for symptoms of atlantoaxial instability (neck pain, altered gait, enuresis) or, in adulthood, for cervical osteoarthritis. Gosain et al. (1994) found that posterior inclination of the odontoid relative to the foramen magnum sig-naled a higher risk for basilar impression. These patients require periodic neurol-ogy referral and consideration of CT or MRI scans of the neck.

Later preventive management of Goldenhar syndrome involves the monitoring of hearing, vision, cervical mobility, urinary function, and dentition. Patients with severe cranial asymmetry or brain anomalies will need developmental assessment and possible early intervention/special and inclusive education services. Nutritional problems will usually resolve after the first year as pharyngeal muscles mature, but some patients will require evaluation by nutrition and gastroenterology specialists. Many patients are at risk of airway obstruction, and appropriate precautions should be taken before anesthesia. The occurrence of palatal dysfunction and dental anomalies often requires speech therapy and regular evaluation by dentistry.

Face/limb syndromes

Table 15.2 lists several syndromes that involve altered development of the cranio-facies and limbs. Most are poorly understood, although molecular studies are in progress for many of them. All have a fairly low prevalence, and their preventive management will be summarized briefly.

Acrocallosal syndrome

The acrocallosal syndrome consists of pre- or post-axial polydactyly and absence or hypoplasia of the corpus callosum (Jones, 1997, pp. 226–7; Gorlin et al., 2001, pp. 996–8). It has some similarity to Greig syndrome, and at least one patient has had a mutation in the same GLI3 gene that causes Greig syndrome (Elson et al., 2002). Consanguinity and occurrence in sibs has suggested AR inheritance, but most cases have been isolated. All patients have had mental disability, so early intervention and appropriate family counseling are important for management. An early onset of seizures with hypotonia is predictive of a severe neurologic prog-nosis. Cleft lip/palate has been found in 15%, mandating evaluation for chronic

Table 15.2. Craniofacial–limb anomaly syndromes

Syndrome	Incidence	Inheritance	Complications
Acrocallosal	~25 cases	?AR	DD, agenesis of the corpus callosum, polydactyly, cleft palate
Coffin–Lowry	~100 cases	XLR	DD, coarse face, down-slanting palpebral fissures, broad fingers, soft hands
Coffin–Siris	~30 cases	?AR	DD, coarse face, sparse hair, strabismus, cardiac defects, cleft palate, short fingers, absent nails
Cryptophthalmos (Fraser)	~150 cases	AR	DD, eye a. (cryptophthalmos, microphthalmia), ear a., digital syndactyly, urogenital a.
Fryns	~50 cases	AR	Lethal, coarse face, cleft palate, short fingers, absent nails, diaphragmatic hernia, gastrointestinal a., renal a.
Greig	~50 cases	AD	Frontal bossing, hypertelorism, broad thumbs and great toes, polydactyly
Meckel	~200 cases	AR	Lethal, posterior encephalocele, polydactyly, cystic liver and kidneys
Moebius	~200 cases	Sporadic	DD (15%), facial nerve palsies, mask-like face, digital defects
OFD, Type I	~200 cases	XLD	DD (40%), lobulated tongue, oral frenula, midline cleft lip, cleft palate, syndactyly, brachydactyly, cystic kidneys, hydrocephalus
OFD, Type II	~50 cases	AR	DD, lobulated tongue, midline cleft lip, polydactyly, syndactyly
OFD, Type III	~10 cases	AR	DD, lobulated tongue, dental a., post-axial polydactyly, "see-saw winking"
OFD, Type IV	~20 cases	AR	DD, cleft lip, dental a., polydactyly, syndactyly, tibial dysplasia
OFD, Type V	~20 cases	AR	Median cleft lip, polydactyly
OFD, Type VI	~20 cases	AR	DD (severe), cleft lip, ocular a., polydactyly, cardiac a., cerebellar a.
Otopalatodigital	~200 cases	XLR	DD (mild), frontal bossing, down-slanting palpebral fissures, broad thumbs, great toes
Roberts pseudothalidomide	~100 cases	AR	DD (severe), cleft lip/palate, cataracts, pre-axial limb deficiencies, urogenital a.

Note:

DD, developmental disability; AD, autosomal dominant; AR, autosomal recessive; XLD, X-linked dominant; XLR, X-linked recessive. OFD, oral-facial digital.

otitis and audiology screening in these patients. Occasional brain anomalies include cortical atrophy and cystic lesions, with 75% of patients having seizures.

Coffin–Siris syndrome

Coffin–Siris syndrome is a difficult diagnosis to make because of overlap with conditions such as the fetal hydantoin syndrome. The disorder was described as the combination of coarse facial features, growth failure, and hypoplastic fifth fingers (Gorlin et al., 2001, pp. 1039–40). Affected sibs are among 30 reported cases, but most instances are isolated. Hypoplastic fingernails and the coarse face explain the resemblance to fetal hydantoin syndrome, and one of us (G.N.W.) has seen a patient with suggestive features who was subsequently recognized as having fetal alcohol syndrome. A karyotype should be performed to exclude chromosomal disorders.

Fleck et al. (2001) report a large cohort of patients in whom the most frequent findings were mental deficiency, coarsened facial appearance, feeding difficulties, frequent infections, and hypoplastic fifth fingernails/distal phalanges. Many patients will need follow-up to establish the diagnosis, since growth deficiency, joint laxity, and hypotonia are common manifestations in syndromes, and the sparse scalp hair will require time to become noticeable. Occasional anomalies include cardiac anomalies (30% of patients), cleft palate, strabismus, Dandy–Walker malformation of the brain, and agenesis of the corpus callosum. Once the diagnosis is established – usually by exclusion – ophthalmology, cardiology, neurology, and early intervention referrals should be made. The possibility of AR inheritance should be mentioned, along with psychosocial counseling and planning appropriate for children with severe disabilities. Patients with cleft palate will need monitoring for chronic otitis and hearing loss.

Cryptophthalmos (Fraser) syndrome

Cryptophthalmos syndrome is probably more common than is reflected by the 100 reported cases, since not all affected children have the characteristic eye findings (Jones, 1997, pp. 242–3; Gorlin et al., 2001, pp. 1016–19). The diagnosis is easy when the eyes are hidden by overlying skin, although this can occur as an isolated anomaly. Cryptophthalmos syndrome exhibits AR inheritance, with only 50% of patients surviving infancy. Jadeja et al. (2005) have found mutations in human FRAS1 and FREM2 genes in Fraser syndrome. These genes encode extracellular matrix proteins and in the mouse produce blebs of the spinal cord and skin with renal cysts.

Common manifestations of Fraser syndrome include cryptophthalmos, syndactyly, and abnormal genitalia, with less frequent nasal, external ear, laryngeal, palatal, umbilical, or renal anomalies. Ocular anomalies include colobomata, epibulbar dermoids, and absent lacrimal or meibomian glands in addition to the cryptophthalmos. Nasal hypoplasia with clefts of the alae nasae, pulmonary hypoplasia, cleft lip and palate, dental malocclusion, and auricular anomalies are common, with malformed ear ossicles and conductive hearing loss. Genital anomalies (80%) and unilateral or bilateral renal agenesis (80%) also occur, with 10–15% having anomalies of the urinary tract. A broad range of skeletal anomalies includes cranial asymmetry, parietal foramina, and syndactyly of the digits. Mental deficiency occurs in at least 80% of patients, and 20% have central nervous system anomalies such as encephalocele or Dandy–Walker cyst.

Preventive management for the cryptophthalmos syndrome should include imaging studies of the cranium and brain during the neonatal period, along with renal sonography and skeletal radiographic survey. Most patients will need ophthalmologic evaluation and plastic surgery, and frequent inspection for conjunctivitis, blepharitis, and keratitis is an important aspect of pediatric care. Auditory evoked response and later audiologic monitoring of hearing is recommended, and the occurrence of laryngeal stenosis may require otolaryngologic evaluation for airway obstruction respiratory problems. Examination of the genitalia may suggest urologic referral, and a gonadoblastoma has been documented. Early intervention services are important, particularly in view of the neurosensory and hearing deficits. Supportive counseling for the parents regarding a potentially lethal and handicapping disorder is often needed in the newborn period, and genetic counseling regarding the 25% recurrence risk should be given once the initial shock of diagnosis has subsided.

Fryns syndrome

Fryns syndrome is an AR disorder that consists of facial, limb, ocular, digestive tract, and urogenital anomalies (Jones, 1997, pp. 210–11; Gorlin et al., 2001, pp. 899–902; Slavotinek et al., 2005). Most patients have a diaphragmatic eventration or hernia, with coincident gastrointestinal anomalies such as omphalocele, intestinal atresias, or imperforate anus. The face is typical with coarse features, malformed ears, micrognathia, macrostomia, and a short neck. Corneal clouding and cleft palate are often present. Renal anomalies include renal agenesis, cystic kidney, hydronephrosis, and ureteral cysts; genital anomalies include bicornuate uterus, cryptorchidism, and saddle scrotum. Myoclonic seizures have been reported.

The clinical course is severe, with 60% of affected pregnancies exhibiting polyhydramnios and many cases presenting as stillbirths. Only 14% survive the neonatal period, and brain imaging studies are important for assessment of prognosis since 72% of patients have brain malformations. Recognition of the disorder may avoid unnecessary surgeries and suffering in severely affected patients. Echocardiography and abdominal sonography should be performed in the neonatal period to document anomalies of the heart, diaphragm, and urogenital tracts. Supportive counseling appropriate for infants with a lethal or severe developmental disorder is appropriate, followed by discussion of the 25% recurrence risk; DNA diagnosis is not yet commercially available.

Greig syndrome

Greig syndrome involves broad thumbs and first toes, pre- and/or post-axial polydactyly, and an unusual face with frontal bossing, broad forehead, and hypertelorism (Gorlin et al., 2001, pp. 995–6). It is an AD disorder, and is caused by mutations in the GLI transcription factor gene in chromosome region 7p13. There are few internal anomalies, so preventive management begins with craniofacial surgery and orthopedic evaluations to document anomalies and plan surgical therapy. Inguinal and umbilical hernias have occurred. Rare patients have had mental disability, and brain imaging may be useful in those with delays because agenesis of the corpus callosum and hydrocephalus have been reported.

Meckel syndrome

Meckel syndrome is a lethal, AR disorder that has a broad range of incidence from 1 in 50,000 births up to 1 in 1500 in Finland (Jones, 1997, 184–5; Gorlin et al., 2001, pp. 891–4). Genetic mapping has loci for Meckel syndrome on chromosomes 8, 11, and 17. The presentation is usually striking, with a posterior encephalocele (65–90% of patients), post-axial polydactyly (55–75%), and a distended abdomen due to large, cystic kidneys. Genital anomalies with micropenis and cryptorchidism, cystic changes in the pancreas and liver, and pulmonary hypoplasia are also frequent. The chief preventive measure is to ensure an accurate diagnosis, so that the parents are aware of their 25% recurrence risk. Prenatal diagnosis by ultrasound is very accurate by gestational age 11–14 weeks (Mittermayer et al., 2004).

Moebius syndrome

Moebius syndrome is part of a diverse spectrum of face–limb disorders that involve anomalies of the tongue, mouth, facial nerves, and limbs (Jones, 1997, pp. 646–48; Gorlin et al., 2001, pp. 826–8). The facial paralysis recognized by Moebius can be seen with other oromandibular–limb hypogenesis syndromes that include the hypoglossia–hypodactylia, Hanhart, and Charlie M syndromes. The practical concern for health care professionals is to recognize that facial palsies and feeding problems may occur in children with oromandibular and limb defects, so that appropriate genetic consultation and neurologic/craniofacial evaluation can be arranged.

More than 200 cases of the Moebius syndrome have been reported, and nearly all, like those of other oromandibular–limb syndromes, were sporadic. Cranial nerve palsies are not confined to the seventh nerve, but also may affect nerves III, V, IX, and XII. There is micrognathia with a small mouth and hypoplasia of the tongue. Aplasia of the pectoral muscle (Poland sequence), limb anomalies (clubfoot in 30% of patients), and congenital hip dislocation can also occur.

Preventive management should focus on oromotor function and dental care, since many patients have failure to thrive because of feeding difficulties. Ophthalmologic referral and monitoring should be conducted during childhood because ptosis, nystagmus, and strabismus may occur. Mental deficiency occurs in 10–15%, and early intervention services should be strongly considered in order to monitor neurosensory, facial nerve, and muscular function. Verzijl et al. (2005) conducted detailed cognitive testing on 12 adult patients and found that their incidence of deficits was no greater than that of the normal population. Psychosocial counseling is important for both parents and child, since the mask-like face and inability to smile can cause hardship. Facial function tends to improve with age, and mental deficiency is rarely severe.

Oral-facial-digital syndromes

Like the oromandibular–limb hypogenesis spectrum, the oral-facial-digital (OFD) syndromes are a heterogeneous group of uncommon disorders that are predominantly sporadic in occurrence (Jones, 1997, pp. 262–3; Gorlin et al., 2001, pp. 832–44). Their distinguishing features are clefts and frenula (bands) affecting the tongue, gums, and palate together with polydactyly and/or syndactyly of the digits. As many as nine OFD syndromes have been delineated, of which six are listed in Table 15.2. The X-linked dominant (XLD) OFD syndrome type I is lethal in males, and the OFD1 gene has been identified as an open reading frame (CXORF5 = chromosome X open reading frame 5) within chromosome band Xp22.3. The chief concern for health care professionals should be appropriate genetic, craniofacial, and dental referral so that a diagnostic and preventive care program can be outlined.

The summary of the OFD syndromes in Table 15.2 emphasizes the risk for brain, ocular, oral, lingual, dental, cardiac, renal, and digital anomalies. The initial evaluation should usually include brain imaging, skeletal radiologic survey, and cardiac and/or renal sonography in appropriate patients. Absence of the pituitary gland, and retinal abnormalities have been described. Most patients will need referral to a craniofacial surgery team, with involvement of dental surgeons and orthodontics for oral care. Those patients with cleft palate will need monitoring for chronic otitis and audiologic screening; clinicians should also consider ophthalmologic referral since nystagmus, strabismus, and alternate winking of the eyes ("see-saw winking") have been described in this syndrome group. If the affected patient is male, then the XLD type I OFD syndrome can be excluded; most families will have a 25% recurrence risk befitting AR inheritance. Mental disability is often fairly severe, so early intervention and appropriate psychosocial counseling are important. Monitoring of growth with attention to feeding problems is also needed.

Otopalatodigital syndrome

Taybi first described the otopalatodigital syndrome based on facial changes, short stature, broad thumbs, broad great toes, and irregular digits with broad terminal phalanges. The face is distinctive, with a prominent forehead, down-slanting palpebral fissures, broad nasal root, and down-turned corners of the mouth. The radiographic findings are also quite characteristic, with irregular form and curvature of the fingers and toes, changes in the vertebrae and pelvis, and frontal bossing of the skull (Gorlin et al., 2001, pp. 844–9; Jones, 1997, pp. 270–3). In otopalatodigital syndrome type I, the clinical course is mild and affected males have mild cognitive defects with average IQ in the 75–90 range. A type II otopalatodigital syndrome has been described with more severe skeletal changes and decreased survival; more than 50% of affected patients have died before age 6 months. Both syndromes exhibit XLR inheritance, and they are caused by different alleles of the filamin A gene in chromosome region Xq26–28. The filamin A gene acts to crosslink actin filaments within the microtubular network of cells.

Preventive management of the otopalatodigital syndromes should focus on auditory evoked response and periodic audiology screening for hearing deficits. Preferential speech delays may reflect undetected hearing loss, and early intervention with physical, occupation, and speech therapy is essential for all patients. Cleft palate is a common complication of both otopalatodigital syndromes, providing additional incentive for auditory screening. Apnea secondary to cervical spine anomalies and brainstem compression occurred postoperatively in one patient with otopalatodigital syndrome type II. Genetic counseling for XLR inheritance and a 25% recurrence risk is indicated, with some female carriers exhibiting facial and digital manifestations of the syndrome.

Roberts pseudothalidomide syndrome

The combination of cleft palate and limb reduction defects recognized by Roberts in 1919 was rediscovered by several different observers (Gorlin et al., 2001, pp. 902–5). Hermann used the term "pseudothalidomide syndrome" to emphasize the limb defects, while Opitz, as is his custom, used the family initials S.C. to denote the condition. It is now agreed that pseudothalidomide and SC syndromes share the same spectrum of manifestations with Roberts syndrome. The disorder is AR, and chromosome studies often reveal an unusual phenomenon called premature centromere condensation. This change in chromatin correlates with the causative gene ESCO2, which is the human homolog of a yeast gene that stabilizes sister chromatid pairing (Vega et al., 2005).

Clinical manifestations of Roberts syndrome include microcephaly, cleft lip and palate, cataracts, pre-axial digital defects, flexion contractures, and club feet. Preventive management should include ophthalmologic referral and regular vision screening, craniofacial surgery evaluation for cleft lip and palate, monitoring for chronic otitis and hearing loss, and inspection of the genitalia for cryptorchidism, enlarged penis, or bicornuate uterus. Periodic urinalyses or initial renal sonography should be performed, since horseshoe kidney, polycystic kidneys, and urinary tract anomalies have been reported. Many patients are severely growth retarded and do not survive infancy. Of those who do, 50% have mental disability warranting early intervention referral and appropriate school and legal planning. Occasional cardiac anomalies and thrombocytopenia have also been described.

Preventive management of Goldenhar spectrum

Description: A broad pattern of defects including jaw asymmetry with external ear anomalies (hemifacial microsomia), eye defects such as epibulbar dermoids, and vertebral anomalies; the incidence is about 1 in 5000 live births.

Clinical diagnosis: Pattern of manifestations including mandibular hypoplasia and ear anomalies, often unilateral, with or without ocular cysts. Extreme variability of the craniofacial, ocular, otic, skeletal, cardiac, and renal anomalies led to several names, including "hemifacial microsomia," "oculo-auriculo-vertebral dysplasia," "facio-auriculo-vertebral spectrum," "first and second branchial arch syndrome," and "Goldenhar complex".

Laboratory diagnosis: None available although severely affected patients should have karyotypes because the jaw, ear, and ocular anomalies can occur in chromosomal disorders like cri-du-chat.

Genetics: Multifactorial determination with most cases being sporadic; a 2% recurrence risk was reported for parents of affected children.

Key management issues: Imaging studies of the brain, heart, urinary tract, and skeleton in extensively affected patients, monitoring of head growth (for hydrocephalus, microcephaly), vision (strabismus, Duane syndrome hearing (conductive or sensorineural deficits), tooth development, urinary tract (renal anomalies), early intervention particularly for patients with severe cranial asymmetry or microphthalmia, oromotor and speech therapists for problems due to palatal dysfunction and hypoplastic pharyngeal muscles, cautious anesthesia due to risks for cervical spine fusion and airway obstruction.

Growth charts: No specific charts are available.

Parent information: Parent information can be found at various craniofacial surgery sites by searching on the syndrome name, and support groups are available at the Goldenhar Syndrome Support Network (www.goldenharsyndrome.org/).

Basis for management recommendations: Derived from the complications below as documented by Rollnick et al. (1987); brain imaging studies should be performed on children with severe plagiocephaly or anophthalmia but are not needed in children with mild manifestations.

Summary of clinical concerns

General	Learning	Cognitive disability (5–15%), learning differences, speech problems
	Growth	Low birth weight, failure to thrive
Facial	Eyes	**Strabismus** (25%), **epibulbar dermoids** (50%), **lipoepidermoids** (25%), anophthalmia, microphthalmia
	Ears	**Abnormal pinna** (65%), **preauricular tags** (40%), middle ear anomalies
	Mouth	Dysphagia, decreased salivation, **velopalatal insufficiency** (35%), cleft lip/palate (7–15%), pharyngeal muscle hypoplasia
Skeletal	Cranial	Microcephaly, plagiocephaly, **cranial asymmetry** (20%)
	Axial	**Vertebral anomalies** (30%), **cervical vertebral fusion** (20%), rib anomalies, scoliosis, Klippel–Feil anomaly
	Limbs	Radial anomaly (10%), club feet (20%)
Internal	Pulmonary	Pulmonary hypoplasia, abnormal lung lobation, airway obstruction
	Circulatory	**Cardiac anomalies** (5–58% – ventricular septal defects, tetralogy of Fallot, transposition of the great vessels, dextrocardia)
	Excretory	Renal agenesis, hypoplasia, hydronephrosis, double ureter
Neural	Central	Brain anomalies (encephaloceles, lipomas, teratomas, dermoids, Arnold–Chiari malformation), seizures
	Motor	Cranial nerve anomalies, **facial palsies** (10–20%)
	Sensory	Hearing loss (15%)

Concerns of frequency >20% are **highlighted**

Key references

Gosain et al. (1994). Cervicovertebral anomalies and basilar impression in Goldenhar syndrome. *Plastic and Reconstructive Surgery* 93:498–506.

Kallen et al. (2004). Relation between oculo-auriculo-vertebral (OAV) dysplasia and three other non-random associations of malformations (VATER, CHARGE, and OEIS). *American Journal of Medical Genetics* 127A:26–34.

Wilson GN (1983). Cranial defects in the Goldenhar syndrome. *American Journal of Medical Genetics* 14:435–43.

Goldenhar spectrum

Preventive medical checklist (0–3 Years)

Name _____ Birth date __ / __ / __ Number _____

Age	Evaluations: key concerns	Management considerations		Notes
New-born ↓ 1 month	Morphology exam: external anomalies[2] Morphology exam: internal anomalies[2] Hearing, vision:[2] ear, eye anomalies Feeding: cleft palate, dysphagia Skeletal exam: vertebral, limb defects Parental adjustment[4]	❑ Craniospinal x-rays;[1] ENT;[3] ophthalmology[3] ❑ Cranial, cardiac, GI, renal imaging[1,3] ❑ ABR; ENT;[3] ophthalmology[3] ❑ Feeding specialist; cleft plate team[3] ❑ Skeletal survey;[3] orthopedics[3] ❑ Family support[4]	❑ ❑ ❑ ❑ ❑ ❑	
2 months ↓ 4 months	Growth and development[5] Hearing, vision:[2] ear, eye anomalies Feeding: cleft palate, dysphagia Skeletal exam: vertebral, limb defects Heart, kidneys Respiration: TE fistula, choanal atresia Parental adjustment[4] Other:	❑ ECI;[3,6] family support[4] ❑ ABR;[3] ENT;[3] ophthalmology[3] ❑ Feeding specialist; cleft plate team[3] ❑ Skeletal survey;[3] orthopedics[3] ❑ Sonography;[3] cardiology; urology[3] ❑ Chest X-ray;[3] ENT;[3] pulmonology[3] ❑ Family support[4] ❑	❑ ❑ ❑ ❑ ❑ ❑ ❑ ❑	
6 months ↓ 9 months	Growth and development[5] Hearing, vision:[2] ear, eye anomalies Feeding: dysphagia, small pharynx Neck: cervical spine anomalies Neurologic: brain anomalies, seizures Other:	❑ ECI;[3,6] family support[4] ❑ ABR;[3] ENT;[3] ophthalmology[3] ❑ Feeding specialist, GI[3] ❑ Anesthesia precautions ❑ Neurology;[3] neurosurgery[3] ❑	❑ ❑ ❑ ❑ ❑ ❑	
1 year	Growth and development[5] Hearing, vision:[5] ear, eye anomalies Feeding: dysphagia, small pharynx Respiration: lung agenesis, aspiration Neurologic: brain anomalies, seizures Excretory: renal defects Other:	❑ ECI;[3,6] family support[4] ❑ ABR;[3] ENT;[3] ophthalmology[3] ❑ Feeding specialist, GI[3] ❑ Chest X-ray;[3] ENT;[3] pulmonology[3] ❑ Neurology;[3] neurosurgery[3] ❑ BP, urinalysis; urology[3] ❑	❑ ❑ ❑ ❑ ❑ ❑ ❑	
15 months ↓ 18 months	Growth and development[5] Hearing, vision:[2] ear, eye anomalies Neck: cervical spine anomalies Respiration: lung agenesis, aspiration	❑ ECI;[3,6] family support[4] ❑ ABR;[3] ENT;[3] ophthalmology[3] ❑ Anesthesia precautions ❑ Chest X-ray;[3] ENT;[3] pulmonology[3]	❑ ❑ ❑ ❑	
2 years	Growth and development[5] Hearing, vision:[2] ear, eye anomalies Nutrition: dysphagia, small pharynx Respiration: lung agenesis, aspiration Neurologic: brain anomalies, seizures	❑ ECI;[3,6] family support[4] ❑ ABR;[3] ENT;[3] ophthalmology[3] ❑ Dietician;[3] GI[3] ❑ Orthopedics;[3] neurosurgery[3] ❑ Neurology;[3] neurosurgery[3]	❑ ❑ ❑ ❑ ❑	
3 years	Growth and development[5] Hearing, vision:[2] ear, eye anomalies Nutrition: dysphagia, small pharynx Respiration: lung agenesis, aspiration Neurologic: spine anomalies, AAI Heart, kidneys Other:	❑ ECI;[3,6] family support[4] ❑ Audiology;[3] ENT;[3] ophthalmology[3] ❑ Dietician;[3] GI[3] ❑ Chest X-ray;[3] ENT;[3] pulmonology[3] ❑ Cervical spine flexion–extension radiographs ❑ BP, urinalysis; cardiology;[3] urology[3] ❑	❑ ❑ ❑ ❑ ❑ ❑ ❑	

Goldenhar spectrum concerns		Other concerns from history	
Plagiocephaly Epibulbar dermoids Anophthalmia Ear anomalies, hearing Cardiac anomalies Pulmonary hypoplasia	Renal anomalies Vertebral anomalies enuresis Developmental disability Feeding problems Velopalatal insufficiency Facial nerve palsies	**Family history/prenatal** _____ _____ _____ _____	**Social/environmental** _____ _____ _____ _____

Guidelines for the neonatal period should be undertaken *at whatever age* the diagnosis is made; ABR, auditory brainstem evoked response; BP, blood pressure; GI, gastrointestinal; AAI, atlanto–axial instability; [1] as needed to define internal anomalies and confirm diagnosis; genetic evaluation and chromosome studies should be considered; [2] by practitioner; [3] as dictated by clinical findings; [4] family/sib, financial, and behavioral issues especially if neurologic problems; [5] consider developmental pediatrician/neurologist/behavior therapist/genetics clinic according to symptoms and availability; [6] early childhood intervention including developmental monitoring and motor/speech therapy.

Goldenhar spectrum

Preventive medical checklist (4–18 years)

Name _____ Birth date __ / __ / __ Number _____

Age	Evaluations: key concerns	Management considerations	Notes
4 years ↓ 6 years	Growth: delay if heart, lung disease Development:[2] preschool transition Hearing, vision:[2] ear, eye anomalies Nutrition: dysphagia, small pharynx Respiration: lung agenesis, aspiration Neurologic: spine anomalies, AAI Other:	❏ Growth, developmental monitoring[1] ❏ ❏ Family support;[4] preschool program[5] ❏ ❏ Audiology;[3] ENT;[3] ophthalmology[3] ❏ ❏ Dietician;[3] GI[3] ❏ ❏ Chest X-ray;[3] ENT;[3] pulmonology[3] ❏ ❏ Cervical spine flexion-extension radiographs ❏ ❏ delay if heart, lung disease ❏	
7 years ↓ 9 years	Growth: delay if heart, lung disease Development:[1] school transition[5] Hearing, vision:[2] hearing or vision loss Nutrition: dysphagia, small pharynx Neurologic: brain stem, spine anomalies Heart, kidneys Other:	❏ Growth, developmental monitoring[1] ❏ ❏ Family support;[4] school progress[6] ❏ ❏ Audiology;[3] ENT;[3] ophthalmology[3] ❏ ❏ Dietician;[3] GI[3] ❏ ❏ Neurology;[3] neurosurgery;[3] orthopedics[3] ❏ ❏ BP, urinalysis; cardiology;[3] urology[3] ❏ ❏ ❏	
10 years ↓ 12 years	Growth and development[1] Hearing, vision:[2] hearing or vision loss Nutrition: dysphagia, small pharynx Neurologic: brain stem, spine anomalies Other:	❏ School progress[6] ❏ ❏ Audiology;[3] ENT;[3] ophthalmology[3] ❏ ❏ Dietician;[3] GI[3] ❏ ❏ Neurology;[3] neurosurgery;[3] orthopedics ❏ ❏ ❏	
13 years ↓ 15 years	Growth and development[1] Hearing, vision:[2] hearing or vision loss Nutrition: dysphagia, small pharynx Neurologic: brain stem, spine anomalies Heart, kidneys Other:	❏ School progress[6] ❏ ❏ Audiology;[3] ENT;[3] ophthalmology[3] ❏ ❏ Dietician;[3] GI[3] ❏ ❏ Neurology;[3] neurosurgery;[3] orthopedics[3] ❏ ❏ BP, urinalysis; cardiology;[3] urology[3] ❏ ❏ ❏	
16 years ↓ 18 years	Growth and development[1] Hearing, vision:[2] hearing or vision loss Neurologic: brain stem, spine anomalies Heart, kidneys Other:	❏ Family support;[4] school progress[6] ❏ ❏ Audiology;[3] ENT;[3] ophthalmology[3] ❏ ❏ Neurology;[3] neurosurgery;[3] orthopedics[3] ❏ ❏ BP, urinalysis; cardiology;[3] urology[3] ❏ ❏ ❏	
19 years ↓ 23 years	Adult care transition[6] Hearing, vision:[2] hearing or vision loss Nutrition: dysphagia, small pharynx Neurologic: brain stem, spine anomalies Heart, kidneys Other:	❏ Family support;[4] school progress[6] ❏ ❏ Audiology;[3] ENT;[3] ophthalmology[3] ❏ ❏ Dietician;[3] GI[3] ❏ ❏ Neurology;[3] neurosurgery;[3] orthopedics[3] ❏ ❏ BP, urinalysis; cardiology;[3] urology[3] ❏ ❏ ❏	
Adult	Adult care transition[6] Hearing, vision:[2] hearing or vision loss Nutrition: dysphagia, small pharynx Neurologic: brain stem, spine anomalies Heart, kidneys Other:	❏ Family support[4] ❏ ❏ Audiology;[3] ENT;[3] ophthalmology[3] ❏ ❏ Dietician;[3] GI[3] ❏ ❏ Neurology;[3] neurosurgery;[3] orthopedics[3] ❏ ❏ BP, urinalysis; cardiology;[3] urology[3] ❏ ❏ ❏	

Goldenhar spectrum concerns		Other concerns from history	
Plagiocephaly Epibulbar dermoids Anophthalmia Ear anomalies, hearing Cardiac anomalies Pulmonary hypoplasia	Renal anomalies Vertebral anomalies enuresis Developmental disability Feeding problems Velopalatal insufficiency Facial nerve palsies	**Family history/prenatal** _____ _____ _____ _____	**Social/environmental** _____ _____ _____ _____

Guidelines for the neonatal period should be undertaken *at whatever age* the diagnosis is made; BP, blood pressure; GI, gastrointestinal; AAI, atlanto-axial instability [1] consider developmental pediatrician/neurologist/behavior therapist for children with neurologic dysfunction; [2] by practitioner; [3] as dictated by clinical findings; [4] parent group, family/sib, financial, and behavioral issues with later focus on independent living and employment; [5] preschool program including developmental monitoring and motor/speech therapy; [6] monitor individual education plan – for individuals with disability, include regular educational testing, balance of special education and inclusion, monitor academic progress with screening for behavioral differences and later vocational planning.

Parent guide to Goldenhar spectrum

In 1952, the French physician Goldenhar described patients with extra tissue in the eye (dermoid cysts), asymmetric jaw and ear anomalies (hemifacial microsomia), and vertebral defects. Other names for this variable pattern of anomalies include oculo-auriculo-vertebral dysplasia, facio-auriculo-vertebral spectrum, first and second branchial arch syndrome – Goldenhar spectrum is used here.

Incidence, causation, and diagnosis

The incidence of Goldenhar spectrum is about 1 in 5000 births. The disorder is influenced by genes and the environment (multifactorial determination), and patients with multiple defects and subtle variations in the face, hands, and feet should have chromosome studies. The variable clinical manifestations of Goldenhar spectrum undoubtedly reflect multiple causes, ranging from blood vessel ruptures in the womb to genetic disorders. The diagnosis of Goldenhar spectrum should be considered in the presence of unilateral mandibular hypoplasia and ear anomalies, with or without ocular cysts. The initial diagnostic evaluation depends on the severity and extent of malformation. For children with hemifacial microsomia alone (unilateral jaw and ear involvement), minimal diagnostic evaluation is needed beyond contact with craniofacial surgery specialists to determine a schedule for repair. Part of the craniofacial evaluation will be auditory evoked response and imaging studies to determine the extent of middle/inner anomalies and hearing loss. For children with hemifacial microsomia and multiple other anomalies, skeletal radiography and imaging studies of internal organs is needed to anticipate complications and to differentiate Goldenhar spectrum from similar syndromes that affect the ears and jaw.

Natural history and complications

Complications of Goldenhar spectrum derive from the jaw, cheekbones, ear, and pharyngeal (throat) structures. Facial asymmetry occurs in 20%, particularly involving the jaw. Malformations of the external ear range from a small and simplified pinna (external ear cartilage) to complete absence of the pinna and ear canal. The pinna may be represented by ear tags, and it is common to find extra cartilaginous tags along a line between the ear and the corner of the mouth. Conductive, sensorineural, or mixed hearing loss is present in at least 15% of cases due to narrowing of the ear canal, malformations of the ossicles (internal ear bones), and anomalies of the skull base. The eye is commonly affected, with epibulbar dermoids (milky-white tissue masses with defined edges in the eye – 50% of children), lipoepidermoid cysts (yellowish, diffuse tissue masses – 25% of children), or abnormal eye muscles (strabismus or wandering eye – 25% of children). The presence of anophthalmia/microphthalmia (absent/small eye) increases the chance for brain anomalies and mental disability (5–15%). Oral complications include macrostomia (large mouth) from lateral clefts, agenesis of the salivary glands (a prominent skin tag in front of the ear often signifies parotid salivary gland absence), underdevelopment of the tongue and swallowing muscles, delayed development of teeth, and small pharynx/weak pharyngeal muscles. Cleft palate with or without cleft lip may occur, and asynchrony of palatal motion may correlate with facial weakness. Vertebral (spinal) anomalies are the best known skeletal complications, but anomalous ribs, thumb and wrist defects, club foot, and skull defects have all been noted. Cervical vertebral (neck spine) fusions occur in 20–35% of patients, and these may cause abnormal movement at the base of the skull. Internal anomalies include cardiac defects, small lungs, kidney anomalies, and gastrointestinal defects including imperforate anus (absent anal opening).

Preventive medical needs

The initial evaluation for children with severe and extensive anomalies of Goldenhar syndrome should include imaging studies of the brain, heart, urinary tract, and skeleton. Careful examination of craniofacial morphology and facial movement is needed, with early referral to craniofacial surgery, otolaryngology, and ophthalmology specialists. Monitoring of head growth (for large size suggestive of hydrocephalus or small head, of hearing (conductive or sensorineural deficits), and of vision (deviated eyes or strabismus) is important during infancy and childhood. If abdominal sonograms demonstrate abnormalities of the urinary tract, then periodic urinalyses are needed. Because cervical vertebral (neck spine) fusions are common, cervical spine films are recommended at age 3–5 years when the bones will be visible; those with fusions should be followed for symptoms of atlantoaxial instability (neck pain, altered gait, enuresis) or, in adulthood, for osteoarthritis of the neck bones. Some children with neck spine fusions will need periodic neurology referral and consideration of CT or MRI scans to image the spinal cord. Later preventive management of Goldenhar syndrome involves the monitoring of hearing, vision, cervical mobility, urinary function, and dentition. Patients with severe cranial asymmetry or brain anomalies will need developmental assessment and possible early intervention/special and inclusive education services. Nutritional problems will usually resolve after the first year as pharyngeal (swallowing) muscles mature, but some patients will require evaluation by nutrition and gastroenterology specialists. Many patients are at risk of airway obstruction, and appropriate precautions should be taken before anesthesia. The occurrence of palatal dysfunction and dental anomalies often requires speech therapy and regular evaluation by dentistry.

Family counseling

Most affected children will not have other affected relatives, allowing genetic counseling for a 1–2% recurrence risk in normal parents of an affected child. This same risk will also apply to the affected child when they plan a family. Although an optimistic prognosis for growth and mental development is appropriate for most children, clinicians must consider early feeding problems and the demands of multiple surgeries in providing support for families. The clinical variability of Goldenhar syndrome mandates care in arranging appropriate family contacts.

Part VI

Management of connective tissue and integumentary syndromes

16

Connective tissue disorders

Children with connective tissue weakness and increased joint laxity are at increased risk for a variety of medical problems (Jones, 1997, pp. 472–94; Adib et al., 2005). General manifestations can include increased range of motion and the ability to perform "double-jointed" maneuvers; altered skeletal proportions with elongation of the craniofacies, thorax, and limbs; susceptibility of joints and internal organs to damage during normal function (e.g., joint dislocations, hernias, optic lens dislocations, mitral valve prolapse), and skin fragility manifest by increased bruising, unusual scarring, and stretch marks. Particular syndrome phenotypes depend on the component of connective tissue that is altered and the spectrum of other developmental abnormalities (Table 16.1). Connective tissue dysplasia is a common feature of many different syndromes, but is the primary clinical manifestation for the syndromes discussed in this chapter. The Marfan and Ehlers–Danlos syndromes are prime examples of connective tissue dysplasias, and detailed discussions with checklists are provided. Syndromes with the opposite finding – tight connective tissue that leads to contractures (arthrogryposis) – will be discussed in Chapter 18.

Inspection of Table 16.1 reveals general features of connective tissue dysplasia that can be part of a generalized condition like Down syndrome or homocystinuria or be of primary concern as in the Marfan or Ehlers–Danlos syndromes. The elongated cranium causes a high palate, resulting in tooth crowding and dental problems. Decreased scleral tissue may allow underlying choroid to show through and produce blue/grey sclerae, and increased deformability of the eye or lens can produce myopia with lens trembling or slippage. Mitral valve prolapse is a common sign of heart tissue laxity that in extreme cases may present as the cystic medial necrosis or aortic dilatation of Marfan syndrome. Skeletal changes include a tall and lanky habitus with long digits, increased joint laxity with spontaneous dislocations, pectus, scoliosis, hernias, and flat feet. The skin may be hyperelastic or thin, and is more susceptible to scarring, bruising, and stretch marks.

A clinical dilemma is often to decide whether individuals with these general manifestations of connective tissue laxity are merely expressing family traits or have a

Table 16.1. Syndromes with connective tissue abnormality

Syndrome	Incidence*	Inheritance	Complications
Syndromes with connective tissue abnormality as a primary manifestation			
Beals	~100 cases	AD	Marfanoid habitus, joint contractures, overturned, "crumpled" ears, ectopia lentis, aortic dilatation, septal defects, scoliosis
Cutis laxa	~100 cases	AR, AD	Lax skin, pulmonary emphysema, bronchiectasis, dilated great arteries, hernias, bladder diverticula, gut diverticula
E-D types I–III	1 in 10,000	AD	Joint laxity, elastic skin, "cigarette paper" scars, MVP, scoliosis, hernias, prematurity
E-D type IV	1 in 100,000	AD, AR	Thin skin, arterial ruptures and dissections, bowel ruptures, strokes, hemorrhage
E-D type V	~20 cases	XLR	Joint laxity, kyphosis, hernia, flat feet – rare and possibly not distinct form
E-D type VI	~50 cases	AR	Joint laxity, ocular fragility, elastic skin, scoliosis
E-D type VII	~20 cases	AD	Joint laxity, soft skin, hip dislocation
Homocystinuria	1 in 100,000	AR	Restricted joint mobility, ectopia lentis, myopia, retinal detachment, long and thin limbs, pectus, scoliosis, cognitive disability
Larsen	~200 cases	AD, S	Joint laxity, multiple joint dislocations, cleft palate, laryngeal stenosis, cervical vertebral a.
Marfan	1 in 10,000	AD	Joint laxity, tall stature, ectopia lentis, long and thin limbs, aortic dilatation, pectus, scoliosis, hernias, flat feet
Pseudoxanthoma elasticum	1 in 40,000	AD, AR	Joint laxity, skin thickening, myopia, retinal disease, vascular obstruction and hemorrhage
Stickler syndrome	~200 cases	AD	Joint laxity, Marfanoid habitus, myopia, retinal disease, cleft palate, MVP, hearing loss
Syndromes with connective tissue abnormality as a secondary manifestation			
Down	1 in 800	C	Joint laxity, AAI, high palate, MVP, scoliosis, hernias, extra skin folds
Williams	1 in 25,000	C	Joint laxity, MVP, hernias, scoliosis, bladder diverticuli
Achondroplasia	1 in 16,000	AD	Joint laxity, blue sclerae, scoliosis, prolapsed intervertebral discs
Osteogenesis imperfecta	1 in 20,000	AD	Joint laxity, blue sclerae, MVP, aortic regurgitation, scoliosis, pectus
Homocystinuria	1 in 200,000	AR	Tall stature, ectopia lentis, myopia, high palate, arachnodactyly, pectus, flat feet, scoliosis

Notes:

S, sporadic; AD, autosomal dominant; AAI, atlantoaxial instability; MVP, mitral valve prolapse;
AR, autosomal recessive; XLR, X-linked recessive; E-D, Ehlers–Danlos; C, chromosomal; a., anomalies.
*Reported cases or number per live births.

disease that is life-threatening. Most often this distinction must be clinical, even with the growing knowledge of specific genes responsible for connective tissue disorders. DNA tests are available for fibrillin gene defects in Marfan syndrome and for type I collagen defects in osteogenesis imperfecta, but the large size of these genes and their variable sites of mutation limit sensitivity. Even more complex are the diverse Ehlers–Danlos syndromes where causative genes are known (e.g., type III collagen) but adapted for commercial DNA testing. A reasonable approach is to focus on bottom-line risks, such as cardiac disease, and to be generous with cardiology referral and imaging studies in patients with worrisome signs and symptoms. The preventive strategies outlined here should be generously provided to suspect individuals. Although the lack of definitive diagnosis may be frustrating, education about ophthalmologic, cardiac and orthopedic risks can institute medical monitoring and lifestyle changes that prolong life and preserve function.

Beals syndrome (congenital contractural arachnodactyly)

Thought to be the disorder originally described by Marfan, congenital contractural arachnodactyly was described in 1971 by Beals and Hecht (Jones, 1997, pp. 476–7; Jones et al., 2002). It is an autosomal dominant disorder caused by mutations in the fibrillin-2 gene on chromosome 5. Infants may be suspected of having Marfan syndrome, with long and slender limbs (dolichostenomelia), camptodactyly, ulnar deviation of the fingers, and multiple joint contractures (Jones, 1997, pp. 476–7). Rarely, patients may have ectopia lentis and aortic root dilatation. Other findings include micrognathia, congenital heart defects (septal defects), and "crumpled" ears with overturned and irregular helices. Skeletal deformities include kyphoscoliosis and foot deformities.

Preventive management recommendations can follow the Marfan/General Connective Tissue Checklist, and should include initial ophthalmology and cardiologic evaluation when the diagnosis is considered, periodic examination for skeletal deformities, and physical/occupational therapy for joint contractures. The joint contractures tend to improve, but the kyphoscoliosis may be progressive (Jones et al., 2002).

Cutis laxa syndromes

The defining manifestation of cutis laxa syndromes is very loose skin that hangs in folds and gives affected patients an aged appearance (Gorlin et al., 2001, pp. 502–12). The skin findings link cutis laxa to other Mendelian disorders like and lipoid proteinosis cutis and pseudoxanthoma elasticum, and causative mutations in a membrane transporter in the latter disorder may provide a mechanistic link (Ringpfeil, 2005). Since redundant skin folds are common in disorders such as Down syndrome, De Barsy syndrome, or conditions with accelerated aging (e.g., the gerodermas), one can expect heterogeneity among patients defined by this characteristic. A few patients with autosomal dominant cutis laxa have had mutations in the elastin gene, and one type of recessive cutis laxa was associated with lysyl oxidase deficiency (Ringpfeil, 2005).

Although described as a phenotypic finding in the early 1800s, genetic studies allowed delineation of specific cutis laxa syndromes in the latter part of this century. The autosomal recessive form is most severe, with growth deficiency and respiratory problems producing childhood morbidity and mortality. The skin appears too large for the body, producing skin folds, narrow palpebral fissures (blepharophimosis), and an aged appearance. Abnormal skin fragility or scarring does not occur, but the pulmonary connective tissue seems disproportionately affected with emphysema, pneumonitis, air trapping, respiratory failure, and cor pulmonale. The cardiovascular system is also affected, with tortuous, dilated arteries in the carotid, vertebral, and pulmonary systems. Other complications include diverticulae of the gastrointestinal (pharynx, esophagus, rectum), urinary (bladder), and genital (vagina) tracts. Laxity of the vocal cords may produce a deep voice, and musculoskeletal laxity may produce diaphragmatic, inguinal, or umbilical hernias.

Autosomal dominant cutis laxa is much milder, with presentation as skin laxity in middle to later childhood. The chief complications are cosmetic, with exaggerated skin folds, ptosis, accentuation of nasolabial folds, and an aged appearance. Rarely, the same spectrum of serious problems that complicate the autosomal recessive form are seen: hernias, pulmonary stenosis, mitral valve prolapse, bronchiectasis, and tortuosity of the carotid arteries and aorta. Unlike the recessive disorder, where joint laxity seems minimal, patients with autosomal dominant cutis laxa may have joint dislocations and degenerative arthritis.

Preventive management for the cutis laxa syndromes can follow that outlined in the Ehlers–Danlos/hypermobility syndromes checklist, with surveillance for respiratory problems in the neonatal and infantile periods. Lax pharyngeal tissue poses a risk of obstructive airway disease, and infants may require monitoring for tachypnea as a sign of emphysema or hypoxemia. Imaging studies of the heart and great vessels should be considered in infants with severe cutis laxa, and propensity for pneumonias and bronchiectasis may necessitate therapy to improve pulmonary toilet such as massage or prophylactic antibiotics. The upper airway obstruction, together with hypoxemia, places the affected child at risk of sleep apnea. A history of irregular respirations, stridor, or gasps during sleep plus evidence of growth failure, pectus excavatum, or mouth breathing on examination should prompt sleep studies and referral to otolaryngology. Periodic evaluations for evidence of hernias, bladder or gut diverticulae, and psychosocial needs for cosmetic surgery should be performed.

Homocystinuria

Homocystinuria is a metabolic disorders that produces a syndromic appearance. Homocystinuria is a metabolic finding that can arise in conjunction with several enzyme deficiencies; all except those from nutritional deficiency or defective vitamin B_{12} absorption exhibit autosomal recessive inheritance (Jones et al., 1997, pp. 478–9; Gorlin et al., 2001, pp. 17–161; Mudd et al., 2001). The most common form of homocystinuria is caused by inherited deficiency of cystathionine-β-synthase. Other causes include alterations in folate and vitamin B_{12} metabolism; these disorders are not associated with a Marfanoid phenotype and connective tissue abnormality.

Tall stature, Marfanoid habitus, ectopia lentis, arachnodactyly, scoliosis, and flat feet are frequent findings in patients with homocystinuria, underlying the importance of plasma amino acid levels when the family history cannot discriminate between autosomal recessive homocystinuria and autosomal dominant Marfan syndrome. Osteoporosis is much more common in homocystinuria, as are thromboembolic events that have made homocystinuria carriers of interest in elucidating risk factors for coronary disease. Other differences from Marfan syndrome include downward rather than upward dislocation of the lens, and neurologic manifestations including mental deficiency (median IQ 64 for those not responding to folic acid supplementation), seizures (21%), movement disorders (Arbour et al., 1988; Ekinci et al., 2004), and psychiatric disorders in up to 50% of patients.

Preventive management of homocystinuria begins with a diagnostic evaluation that is best coordinated through metabolic disease specialists at an academic center. Once diagnosis and metabolic monitoring is established, clinical care can follow the recommendations on the Marfan syndrome checklist. It is extremely important to evaluate patients with ectopia lentis for homocystinuria, since there is both treatment and presurgical management that may prevent neurologic catastrophes (e.g., Arbour et al., 1988). Once cystathionine-β-synthase deficiency is confirmed as the cause of homocystinuria, the patient can begin a treatment regimen consisting of dietary methionine restriction; pyridoxine, folate, and betaine; and chronic administration of low-dose aspirin or dipyridamol. The reasons for supplementation are that pyridoxine is a co-factor for cystathionine-β-synthase, folate deficiency can interfere with pyridoxine effect, and betaine helps convert homocystine to methionine. The treatment protocol has shown promising results after long-term follow-up. Patients who respond to low amounts of pyridoxine are particularly benefited, showing higher mean IQ and fewer thrombotic complications. One patient developed diarrhea and pancreatitis that was responsive to betaine. Since dietary methionine levels must be permissive for growth but sufficiently restricted to lower plasma homocystine, regular monitoring through a metabolic disease clinic is recommended. Otherwise, preventive management should include regular ophthalmology, cardiology, and skeletal evaluations as outlined for Marfan syndrome (below). An additional precaution should be anticoagulation, hydration, and oxygenation during surgery so as to lower the risks for thromboembolism (Arbour et al., 1988; Ekinci et al., 2004).

Larsen syndrome

Larsen syndrome consists of increased connective tissue laxity, joint dislocations, club feet, and a flattened face with a shallow nasal bridge (Jones, 1997, 286–7; Gorlin et al., 2001, pp. 888–91). The most striking manifestations affect the skeletal system, with dislocation of the radial head (70%), dislocation of the tibia onto the femur (80%), hip dislocation (80%), and club feet (85%). There may be abnormal segmentation of the carpal and vertebral bones, producing supernumerary bones in the wrist and cervical vertebral anomalies. The latter have been associated with cervical instability and quadriplegia or sudden death. Cardiac anomalies, including septal defects and tortuosity or dilatation of the aorta, have been reported (Baspinar et al., 2005). About 15% of patients have mental deficiency, and sensorineural or mixed hearing loss does occur. Of concern during infancy is laryngotracheomalacia or laryngeal stenosis, which may cause lethal airway obstruction.

Preventive management for Larsen syndrome should include careful orthopedic evaluation and skeletal radiographic survey as soon as the diagnosis is suspected. Evaluation of respiratory function including otolaryngologic assessment of the upper airway is critical, particularly before anesthesia and surgery. Evaluation for signs and symptoms of cardiovascular disease should be conducted periodically, and patients should be counseled to avoid high-impact, collision, or highly competitive sports that are apt to cause joint trauma, dislocation, or degeneration. Audiologic screening is worthwhile in early childhood, and development should be monitored, with referral to early intervention if there is delay. For patients with cleft palate, auditory evoked response studies during infancy, followed by examination and audiology screening for chronic otitis, should be performed. If cervical spine fusions are noted on the initial radiographic survey, then screening for atlantoaxial instability before anesthesia or entry into sports programs or school should be considered. The propensity for joint dislocations in the neck and other regions mandates periodic neurologic evaluations for signs of nerve compression; neurologic and orthopedic referral may be needed in some cases.

Pseudoxanthoma elasticum

Pseudoxanthoma elasticum is a disorder of skin, connective tissue, eyes, heart, and blood vessels that usually presents in the second to third decade of life (Gorlin et al., 2001, pp. 580–4). There are autosomal dominant and autosomal recessive forms of the disease, with an aggregate incidence of about 1 in 40,000 births. Recessive forms are caused by mutations in the ABCC6 membrane transporter gene on chromosome 16.

A characteristic finding is the "peau d'orange," or orange-peel skin, which represents thickening together with yellow papules. The skin becomes leathery and fragile, sometimes perforating over pressure points. Eye findings include myopia and cataracts, with retinal examination revealing typical "angioid streaks" and later hemorrhage or macular degeneration. Abnormal elastin fibers in the blood vessels lead to calcification, obstruction of vascular flow, and hemorrhage. Clinical manifestations of the vasculopathy include intermittent claudication of the limbs, renovascular hypertension, angina of the coronary or celiac arteries, and hemorrhage into the gut, retina, kidney, uterus, bladder, and central nervous system. Intracerebral and subarachnoid hemorrhages may cause neurologic deficits, psychiatric disorders, and seizures during adulthood. Increased joint laxity and vertebral anomalies have been described.

Affected children have been recognized, but usually children are evaluated because a parent or older sib is affected; preventive management should consist of periodic examinations of the eyes, heart, pulses, and skin and testing of the stool for occult blood. Counseling should be given regarding regular medical care as an adult, but women with the disease have lower pregnancy risks than assumed from prior studies (Bercovitch et al., 2005).

Stickler syndrome

Patients with Stickler syndrome may have a Marfanoid habitus (although some have short stature) with vitreoretinal degeneration and detachment, cleft palate, hearing loss, joint laxity, and arthritis (Gorlin et al., 2001, pp. 351–4). There has been controversy about the delineation of Stickler syndrome, in that Marshall, Wagner, and Weissenbacher–Zweymüller all described similar conditions; molecular genetic studies have demonstrated that mutations in the type II collagen alpha 1, the type XI collagen alpha 1, and type XI collagen alpha 2 chain genes (Richards et al., 2000). The original patient described by Weissenbacher and Zweymüller had a mutation in the type XI collagen alpha 2 chain gene, so this disorder along with three or more types of Stickler syndrome can be viewed as a spectrum with overlapping manifestations. More than 200 patients have been reported, and it is estimated the condition accounts for more than 30% of infants with the Robin sequence of micrognathia and cleft soft palate. The various forms are all autosomal dominant, and clinical differences like changes in the retinal vitreous clumping can guide DNA testing strategies that are of value in predicting eye and/or skeletal complications (Richards et al., 2000).

Clinical manifestations of the Stickler syndrome spectrum can include Robin sequence with risks of respiratory obstruction during early infancy, myopia, chorioretinal degeneration with retinal detachment (70%), cataracts, strabismus, flattened midface with cleft palate or velopalatine insufficiency, and multiple skeletal changes. The joint laxity leads to thin, Marfanoid habitus, but at least 25% of patients are short rather than tall. The joints may be enlarged and painful, and there may be flattening of the vertebral bodies with hypoplasia of the pelvis. About 10% of patients develop scoliosis, and many have joint degeneration in later life. Preventive management should include early assessment of the jaw and palate to diagnose Robin sequence; prone positioning during sleep will allow the jaw to descend and prevent obstructive apnea. Early and aggressive ophthalmology evaluation is needed, with close monitoring by retinal specialists. Patients tend to avoid strenuous activity because of joint pain, but they should be counseled about the possibility of high-impact sports augmenting later joint degeneration. Regular evaluations for alignment of the joints and spine are needed.

Generalized joint laxity and the Ehlers–Danlos syndromes

Ehlers–Danlos syndrome is a heterogeneous group of disorders characterized by remarkable joint laxity, elastic skin, and vascular fragility that may compromise internal organs (Jones, 1997, pp. 482–5; Gorlin et al., 2001, pp. 512–28). Table 16.1 lists the more common types of Ehlers–Danlos syndrome, indicating that most exhibit autosomal dominant inheritance. The classical or type I form involves hyperelastic skin, increased joint laxity, and cigarette-paper scars, while type II is similar with less severe features and type III distinguished by joint laxity alone. Type IV is most important to recognize because of its severe vascular complications, and the rare type V is probably not distinct from II (Steinmann et al., 1993). Type VI has ocular complications (ocular fragility, keratoconus), type VII or arthrochalasis multiplex congenita more dislocations of joints, and type VIII has severe periodontal disease; because all of these manifestations may occur in classical types I–II, their distinctness is established only in those type VI patients that have mutations in the lysyl hydroxylase gene. The former type IX (occipital horn disease) is now separated from the Ehlers–Danlos group and classified as an X-linked from of cutis laxa that involves altered copper metabolism.

Molecular analysis has demonstrated type V collagen mutations in about one-half of patients with classical or type I Ehlers–Danlos syndrome (Malfait et al., 2005), while type III collagen is mutated in some cases with type IV. Type VII patients have had type I collagen mutations, but these were excluded in the classical form (Malfait et al., 2005). The lysyl hydroxylase gene mutations in type VI undoubtedly foreshadow other genes affecting fibrillar structure/metabolism that will be mutated in the Ehlers–Danlos spectrum. With the present limited ability for clinical and molecular delineation, about 90% of individuals diagnosed with Ehlers–Danlos syndrome will be affected with types I–III, about 4% with the severe type IV, and another 6% with other types. These numbers are obviously dependent on how many individuals with increased joint laxity are classified as Ehlers–Danlos syndrome. The less common types of Ehlers–Danlos syndrome will now be discussed before outlining preventive measures for the more prevalent group with types I–III.

Ehlers–Danlos syndrome type IV

The ecchymotic or arterial form of Ehlers–Danlos syndrome (type IV) is the most severe of these disorders. It is an autosomal dominant disorder caused by mutations in type III collagen. Mortality is significant, with 40% of affected patients dying before age 40 (Gorlin et al., 2001, pp. 519–21). The skin is not elastic but is thin and translucent with visible venous patterns. There is a subtle facial resemblance among patients, with a thin nose and prominent eyes producing an aged appearance. The weakened vascular tissue is evidenced superficially by varicose veins and internally by aneurysms, dissections, and hemorrhages that may damage a variety of organs. Intestinal ruptures may present as abdominal pain, and bleeding into limbs may produce compartment syndromes. Myocardial infarction and cerebrovascular hemorrhage and strokes may occur in younger individuals with type IV Ehlers–Danlos syndrome.

Preventive management of Ehlers–Danlos syndrome type IV consists of attempts to minimize strain that might provoke bleeding episodes since no curative treatment is available (Steinmann et al., 1993). Strenuous exercise and collision sports should be prohibited, and cough or constipation should be treated with antitussives and laxatives. Anticoagulant therapy and aspirin therapy should be avoided (Steinmann et al., 1993). Early response to bleeding is important, since surgery and angiography have high rates of complications. Vascular fragility can be significant, so medical procedures should avoid intramuscular injections or indwelling catheters. Because recurrence of colon perforation is so common, colectomy is recommended after the first episode (Steinmann et al., 1993). Pregnancy is highly dangerous, with a 20% mortality rate per pregnancy in one review of 26 patients (Lurie et al., 1998). Early termination before 16 weeks is recommended, with careful monitoring, restricted activity and elective cesarean section delivery (after steroid therapy to aid fetal lung development) for those who continue pregnancy (Lurie et al., 1998).

Ehlers–Danlos syndrome type VI

Type VI Ehlers–Danlos syndrome is also called the "ocular-scoliotic" type because of ruptured globes, retinal detachment, and severe kyphoscoliosis. It is an autosomal recessive disorder, but the responsible gene has not been characterized. Thoracic cage deformity and hypotonia may cause pulmonary restrictions and episodes of pneumonia during infancy. Early death has been reported. Preventive management consists of frequent musculoskeletal evaluation, regular ophthalmologic referral, and medical counseling to avoid strenuous exercise or collision sports. Infants should be watched for signs of pulmonary compromise or pneumonia, and orthopedic monitoring will often be necessary for progressive scoliosis.

Ehlers–Danlos syndrome type VII

Patients with Ehlers–Danlos syndrome type VII (arthrochalasis multiplex congenita) are most striking for joint hypermobility, multiple subluxations or dislocations, and tearing of ligaments. The disorder is autosomal dominant, and is caused by mutations in type I collagen (different regions of the gene from those causing osteogenesis imperfecta). Infants may have congenital hip dislocation and hypotonia. Motor development is often delayed, and many patients have severe scoliosis. Preventive management consists of avoidance of strenuous activity, with appropriate orthopedic monitoring for dislocations and subluxations.

Ehlers–Danlos syndrome types I–III

Terminology

Ehlers described patients with lax joints and elastic skin in 1901, while Danlos reported unusual scarring and skin fragility in 1908 (Gorlin et al., 2001, pp. 512–28). Subsequent work has defined many types of Ehlers–Danlos syndrome, as described above and summarized in Table 16.1. Types I–III are very similar, with types II being milder and type III being "benign" joint hypermobility without skin fragility and "cigarette-paper" scarring. However, patients with increased joint laxity can have numerous complications, and the checklist accompanying this discussion is intended for all types of Ehlers–Danlos syndrome including any patient with dramatic joint hypermobility (Adib et al., 2005).

Incidence, etiology, and differential diagnosis

The overall incidence of Ehlers–Danlos syndromes is estimated to be 1 in 5000 births, with types I–III comprising the majority of cases (Steinmann et al., 1993). All three disorders are autosomal dominant and mutations in collagen V genes can be demonstrated in about one-half of the cases (Malfait et al., 2005). DNA testing is neither routinely available nor very sensitive, so clinical distinction between classical and rare forms of Ehlers–Danlos syndrome must be made, being particularly alert for patients with type IV (greater risks of hemorrhage and vascular disruption) or type VI (greater risks of globe rupture or retinal detachment (Table 16.1)). The normal elasticity of skin in type IV and the lack of typical scarring in types IV and VI should aid in differentiating the disorders. As mentioned above, the large number of syndromes with connective tissue laxity and the difficulty in distinguishing patients with simple hypermobility are clinically challenging. Physicians would be wise to consider any patient with dramatic joint laxity as a candidate for the Ehlers–Danlos group, and use the accompanying checklist as a reminder of potential complications.

Two clinical signs that are helpful in recognizing Ehlers–Danlos syndromes are the Meténier sign (easy eversion of the upper eyelids) and the Gorlin sign (ability to touch the nose with the tongue (Gorlin et al., 2001, pp. 512–28). Signs of joint hypermobility include passive bending of the wrist and thumb to touch the forearm and the ability to wrap one arm behind the back and reach the umbilicus.

Diagnostic evaluation and medical counseling

Most children with types I–III Ehlers–Danlos syndrome present in early childhood because of motor delay from joint laxity and hypotonia. Patients with type I may also present because of increased bruisability, skin fragility, or unusual scarring. Several commercial laboratories offer DNA testing for collagen V mutations in types I–III Ehlers–Danlos syndrome, collagen III mutations in type IV, lysyl oxidase gene mutations in type VI, or collagen I mutations in type VII (see www.genetests. org). These tests have low sensitivity except in clear-cut cases of type IV. Other evaluations should include ophthalmologic examination as a baseline and to exclude more severe forms of Ehlers–Danlos syndrome. Echocardiography is also warranted after the diagnosis is made so that mitral valve prolapse and congenital heart defects (pulmonic stenosis, septal defects) can be ruled out. The tendencies for bruising and scarring bring some children with Ehlers–Danlos syndrome type I to attention because of suspected child abuse.

Family and psychosocial counseling

Patients with Ehlers–Danlos syndrome types I–III have a 50% risk to transmit the condition, and couples should be counseled regarding the risks for prematurity, and bladder or rectal prolapse during pregnancy and delivery (Steinmann, 1993). The normal lifespan and intelligence in these disorders warrants optimistic counseling with emphasis on periodic evaluation of the eyes and heart. However, Lumley et al. (1994) reported significant psychosocial problems among 41 adults and seven children with Ehlers–Danlos syndrome. They noted anxiety, depression, anger, sexual difficulties, reproductive concerns, and frustration with the medical care system (Lumley et al., 1994). Psychological intervention was recommended for some families. Parent information and support can be found at the Ehlers–Danlos Syndrome Foundation (www.ednf.org/), the Ehlers–Danlos Support Group (www.ehlers–danlos.org/), and at various educational sites by searching on the syndrome name.

Natural history and complications

The complications of Ehlers–Danlos syndrome types I–III include prematurity, since the extra-embryonic membranes are fetal in origin and may exhibit fragility. Mothers face an increased risk for postpartum hemorrhage and prolapse of the uterus or bladder. Neonates have increased joint mobility but few other complications; infants often come to attention because of developmental delay due to joint laxity and easy bruisability.

As children grow older, their chief complications affect the eyes, heart, skin, and skeleton. The face may be unusual, with occasional blue sclerae and epicanthal folds. Eye anomalies include microcornea, strabismus, angioid streaks, and detachment of the retina. The teeth may have abnormal enamel and dentin formation, with altered tooth morphology. The gums are fragile, and periodontal disease can occur at an early age. Subluxation of the temporomandibular joint may occur. Skin findings include hyperelasticity, gaping wounds from minor trauma, and formation of finely wrinkled, pigmented scars that are likened to cigarette paper. There may be nodules under the skin (pseudotumors), and calcified cysts occur in about 30% of patients. Thinning of the skin makes acrocyanosis more prominent in children and varicosities more prominent in adults. Skeletal anomalies include flat feet, genu recurvatum, club feet, and kyphoscoliosis. Inguinal or umbilical hernias are more common. Occasional features include reflux nephropathy and peripheral neuropathy.

Ehlers–Danlos syndrome types I–III preventive medical checklist

Knowledge of Ehlers–Danlos syndrome types I–III during pregnancy allows planning for the possibility of maternal hemorrhage, bleeding from episiotomy wounds or lacerations, and observation for bladder or rectal prolapse. There will be a 50% risk of the infant being affected, with a higher risk for prematurity . After birth, the infant should be evaluated for signs of joint laxity and skin elasticity, with ophthalmologic and cardiologic consultation in suspect patients. For children without a family history, ophthalmologic and cardiologic evaluations should be performed once the diagnosis is considered. Fragility of the gums and mild hypotonia may lead to feeding problems, so nutrition and growth, eyes, heart, skin, and joints should be assessed during each pediatric visit. Dental referral should be performed once the child has teeth. Because scoliosis and joint dislocations are common, a baseline orthopedic evaluation may be worthwhile once the child begins walking.

In the adolescent and adult years, surveillance of the eyes, skin, and joints should continue with auscultation for signs of mitral or tricuspid valve prolapse. Patients who have had an earlier echocardiogram to rule out congenital heart lesions can probably be followed symptomatically, but changing auscultatory or clinical signs warrant repeat echocardiography. Counseling to avoid high-impact or collision sports and minimize joint/skin trauma is worthwhile. Bracing and fusions seem to be the most common methods for orthopedic treatment of injured joints including spinal fusions for severe scoliosis.

Marfan syndrome

Terminology

Marfan syndrome, like other connective tissue dysplasias, may present with increased joint laxity and consequent skeletal changes. Like type IV Ehlers–Danlos syndrome, it is associated with more severe cardiovascular anomalies such as aortic dilatation and cardiac valvular disease. Marfan described the clinical pattern of elongated body proportions, tall stature, ocular changes such as myopia or ectopia lentis, and cardiac changes, although his original patient is now thought to have been affected with Beals syndrome (Jones, 1997, pp. 472–3; Gorlin et al., 2001, pp. 327–34). Affected patients have long, narrow, and hyperextensible fingers ("arachnodactyly") and limbs ("dolichostenomelia"). A degenerative process affecting the aorta and other blood vessels in Marfan syndrome is termed "cystic medial necrosis." Like other findings of the disorder, cystic medial necrosis of the aorta by itself is suggestive but not diagnostic of Marfan syndrome.

Incidence, etiology, and differential diagnosis

The incidence of Marfan syndrome is estimated to be as high as 1 in 10,000 births, and occurs in many ethnic groups. The disorder exhibits autosomal dominant inheritance with 15% of patients representing new mutations. Marfan syndrome is caused by mutations at the fibrillin-1 locus on chromosome 15; the large size of the gene and the diverse nature of the mutations had so far not allowed routine DNA diagnostic testing. Isolated ectopia lentis has also been related to a fibrillin-1 mutation, and Beals syndrome is caused by mutations in fibrillin-2 on chromosome 5. The differential diagnosis includes other connective tissue dysplasias such as homocystinuria or Beals syndrome; it would have given comfort to Dr. Marfan to realize the many patients reported as having Beals syndrome are thought now to have Marfan syndrome (Pyeritz, 1993). The ear anomalies seen in Beals syndrome or the demonstration of normal homocysteine levels should differentiate these conditions from Marfan syndrome.

Interpretation of autopsy or surgical specimens may be difficult because cystic medial necrosis can occur as an isolated finding or in congenital syphilis. Furthermore, ectopia lentis can occur as an isolated abnormality with autosomal dominant inheritance, and mitral valve prolapse occurs in otherwise normal people as well as in several connective tissue disorders and conditions such as fragile X syndrome. Diagnostic criteria have been published that require at least one major manifestation in patients with an affected first-degree relative and two major manifestations in patients with an unremarkable family history. The two major criteria are most often aortic dilatation by echocardiography and lens laxity/dislocation by ophthalmologic slit lamp examination; skeletal X-rays to demonstrate acetabular protrusion or head/spinal MRI studies to demonstrate dural ectasia offer additional signs (Gorlin et al., 2001, p. 327). Pyeritz (1993) has emphasized the arbitrary and age-sensitive nature of these criteria, asserting that Marfan syndrome is one end of a continuum of connective tissue abnormality that is a challenge for molecular diagnosis and clinical delineation to resolve.

Although molecular testing could help delineate this spectrum, DNA testing is still insensitive in that the fibrillin gene is large and most families have unique mutations (see www.genetests.org for the several laboratories offering DNA testing). Another problem with testing is variable expressivity, in that relatives with identical fibrillin gene mutations may span the range from virtually no symptoms to multiple complications and early death (Buoni et al., 2004).

Diagnostic evaluation and medical counseling

Many patients with Marfan syndrome will not present in the newborn period. Some show signs in later childhood and still others are identified as asymptomatic adults who have an affected relative. Once the diagnosis is suspected, all patients should have an ophthalmologic examination and echocardiography by a cardiologist who is experienced with the condition. The aortic root diameter can be plotted against norms for the patient's age and size, allowing recognition of subclinical dilatation. Optic lens dislocation may not be obvious, and slit lamp exam with a fully dilated pupil may be needed to detect lens hyperkinesia due to laxity of the ciliary ligament (Pyeritz, 1993). Many patients with Marfan syndrome will not have either of these major findings, making decisions about preventive management difficult. If the physician judges the patient is at risk of Marfan syndrome, medical counseling should include prohibition of collision or highly competitive sports, and of isometric exercises that adversely strain cardiac output (Pyeritz, 1993). Emotional stress should also be avoided where possible. Such advice is better accepted after the tragic death of certain athletes, but difficult to enforce in asymptomatic adolescents. Pregnancy is thought to be of higher risk in Marfan syndrome, but Meijboom et al. (2005) reported minimal complications in women whose aortic root was less than 40 mm in width.

Family and psychosocial counseling

Genetic counseling for Marfan syndrome is straightforward numerically but complicated in terms of medical recommendations and patient self-image. All at-risk patients should be referred to a genetic specialist and probably to an experienced cardiologist for detection of subtle manifestations. Affected individuals will have a 50% risk of transmitting the condition, and severely affected females should be informed of higher complication rates during pregnancy (Meijboom et al., 2005). Fetal diagnosis by ultrasound can sometimes be made in the third trimester of pregnancy, allowing parental adjustment and perinatal planning.

In counseling adults with the Marfan syndrome, clinicians must mention the possibility of aortic aneurysm and sudden death to encourage compliance with preventive measures, but it is also important to emphasize that many patients are asymptomatic throughout life. Improvement in the lifespan of patients with Marfan syndrome has been described, with expected survival of 72 years in the 1990s compared to 48 years in the 1970s. Examination of at-risk adults for suggestive skeletal features is recommended but may elicit disagreements from patients who do not wish to consider the diagnosis. Echocardiography is a useful arbiter, since the results lead directly to a management plan of caution and surveillance (when negative) or of discussion of beta-blocker or angiotensin-converting enzyme inhibitor therapy when positive (Kim et al., 2005; Yetman et al., 2005). When the diagnostic criteria are fulfilled, initiation of therapy can be started even in the absence of aortic dilatation. Parent support groups include the National Marfan Syndrome Foundation (www.marfan.org/) and the Canadian Marfan Syndrome Association (www.marfan.ca/).

Natural history and complications

When signs of Marfan syndrome are recognized during infancy or childhood, the outcome is often poor. Infants frequently have serious cardiac abnormalities (83%), and these may be lethal in early childhood (10–20%). Affected infants often have congenital hand contractures and megalocornea. For more typical patients presenting in adolescence to young adulthood, complications affect the eye (ectopia lentis in 70%, myopia in 60%), heart (abnormal echocardiogram in 96%, aortic root enlargement in 84%, and mitral valve prolapse in 58%), and skeleton (kyphoscoliosis in 44%, pectus deformity in 68%, and flat feet in 44%). Other clinical findings include strabismus (90%), a mid-systolic click typical of mitral valve prolapse (30%), murmur suggestive of aortic regurgitation (10%), or a murmur suggestive of mitral regurgitation (6%). Most are tall (56% greater than 95th centile for age), most had arachnodactyly (88%), and some had obvious stretch marks (24%). Since most studies concern older adolescents or adults, these frequencies of complications can be viewed as maxima for children.

The cardiac symptoms of adolescents and adults with Marfan syndrome include palpitations, dyspnea, and light-headedness associated with mitral valve prolapse (not with arrhythmias), and chest pain related to pneumothorax or aortic dissection. Recurrence of aortic dissection after surgical repair emphasizes that Marfan syndrome is a disease of the entire aorta. It is clear that life-long monitoring of cardiac status is needed in Marfan syndrome, since some complications occur after cardiac surgery. Thoracic surgical management of children may require different approaches (Tsang et al., 1994).

Besides the cardinal ocular, cardiac, and skeletal manifestations, other complications of Marfan syndrome can include a high palate with dental crowding, severe scoliosis with restrictive pulmonary disease and cor pulmonale, unusual lens shape (microspherophlakia) with later predisposition to cataracts, retinal lattice degeneration with rare detachment, increased bruisability but normal healing of skin, and ectasia of the spinal dura with occasional nerve root pain in the neck and pelvic pain due to anterior meningocele (Pyeritz, 1993; Foran et al., 2005). Locomotor symptoms including spinal pain, arthralgia, ligament injury, and fracture are frequent in adults with Marfan syndrome but rare in children. Spondylolisthesis occurs in 6% of older individuals, and some affected women may have severe osteoporosis (Gorlin et al., 2001, p. 329).

Marfan syndrome preventive medical checklist

In neonates with skeletal changes suggestive of Marfan syndrome (elongated limbs and fingers, hand contractures, hernias, pectus), echocardiography and ophthalmologic evaluation should be performed (Committee on Genetics, 1996). These same evaluations should be performed on older patients at the time of diagnosis or when affected relatives bring them to attention, providing they have suggestive clinical findings. Regular evaluations of the eyes, heart, and skeletal system then constitute the core of management, including dental and optometric assessments when children are old enough. Because of the risk of scoliosis, adolescents may require evaluation by orthopedics at the time surrounding puberty.

Several studies have documented the better outlook for patients afforded by long-term beta-adrenergic blockade (propranolol, atenolol) or angiotensin-converting enzyme inhibitors (enalopril – Kim et al., 2005; Yetman et al., 2005). A longer experience with beta-adrenergic blockade has demonstrated that it slows the progression of aortic dilatation, and beta-blocker therapy should be considered once the diagnosis of Marfan syndrome is made. Severely affected children should definitely receive therapy, while others can have activity restrictions with regular monitoring of aortic root size in patients with mild dilation. The varying experience and indications for thoracic surgery in Marfan syndrome (e.g., Pyeritz, 1993; Kim et al., 2005) emphasize the need for patients to be followed by cardiologists and cardiovascular surgeons who are experienced with the disorder.

Preventive management of Marfan syndrome

Description: Clinical pattern caused by mutations in the fibrillin-1 gene in 50% of cases; incidence is 1 in 1000–2500 affecting both males and females.

Clinical diagnosis: Manifestations include ectopia lentis and dilatation or aneurysm of the aorta in individuals with generalized connective tissue laxity, producing a tall and thin body build ("Marfanoid habitus"), long fingers ("arachnodactyly") and limbs ("dolichostenomelia"), skin striae and easy bruising, concave chest (pectus excavatum), scoliosis, hernias, and flat feet. Major objective criteria for diagnosis include aortic dilatation relative to age/size via echocardiogram and lens laxity or dislocation by slit lamp exam; minor objective criteria include acetabular protrusion on hip X-ray and dural ectasia by spinal/head MRI. Minor subjective criteria include the skeletal or skin manifestations of lax connective tissue as listed above. Two objective criteria plus subjective findings are required for diagnosis.

Laboratory diagnosis: Mutations in the fibrillin gene on chromosome 15 cause Marfan syndrome, but DNA diagnosis is not very sensitive because the fibrillin gene is large and many families have unique mutations.

Genetics: The disorder exhibits autosomal dominant inheritance with 15% of patients representing new mutations. Affected individuals have a 50% risk for transmission to offspring.

Key management issues: Echocardiography and ophthalmologic evaluation at the time of diagnosis; subsequent monitoring of the eyes, heart, and skeletal system, including regular ophthalmology, cardiology, dentistry, dental, and orthopedic evaluations; consideration of β-adrenergic blocking drugs such as propranolol to treat aortic dilation.

Growth charts: Specific charts available in Pyeritz et al. (1985).

Parent information and support: National Marfan Syndrome Foundation (www.marfan.org/) and the Canadian Marfan Syndrome Association (www.marfan.ca/).

Basis for management recommendations: Guidelines formulated by the Committee on Genetics, American Academy of Pediatrics (1996).

Summary of clinical concerns

General	Learning	Verbal-performance discrepancy (rare), occasional problems with visual attention
	Behavior	Hyperactivity (rare)
	Growth	**Tall stature** (58%), **low upper/lower segment ratio** (77%), asthenic habitus
Facial	Eyes	**Ocular anomalies** (70%) – ectopia lentis (60%), myopia (34%), retinal detachment (6.4%); lens dislocation
	Mouth	**High palate** (40–60%), cleft palate, dental malocclusion, mandibular prognathism, temporomandibular joint disease
Surface	Neck/trunk	**Pectus excavatum** (68%), **inguinal hernia** (22%)
	Epidermal	Alopecia
Skeletal	Cranial	Dolichocephaly, prominent supraorbital ridges, mandibular prominence, temporomandibular joint disease
	Axial	**Scoliosis** (44%), spondylolisthesis (6%)
	Limbs	**Arachnodactyly** (88%), **flat feet** (44%), joint laxity, recurrent dislocations of fingers and patellae, limited elbow flexion, later arthritis
Internal	Digestive	Biliary tract anomalies
	Circulatory	**Cardiac dysfunction** (98%), **aortic enlargement** (84%), **mitral valve dysfunction** (69%), **abnormal echocardiogram** (87%), **mitral prolapse** (67–100%), **cardiac arrythmias** (33%), aneurysms of descending aorta or pulmonary artery, risk for bacterial endocarditis
	Pulmonary	Reduced vital capacity, spontaneous pneumothorax (4.4%), emphysema, reduced vital capacity with increased anesthesia risks
	RES	Clotting tendencies
	Excretory	Renal vein thrombosis, nephrotic syndrome
	Genital	Primary hypogonadism
Neural	Central	Sacral meningocele, dural ectasia, sleep apnea
	Motor	Muscle weakness, decreased skeletal muscle mass
	Sensory	**Visual deficits** (20%)

RES, reticuloendothelial system; **concerns** of frequency >20% are **highlighted**

Key references

Committee on Genetics, AAP (1996). Health supervision for children with Marfan syndrome. *Pediatrics* 98:978–82.

Meijboom, et al. (2005). Pregnancy and aortic root growth in the Marfan syndrome. *European Heart Journal* 26:914–20.

Pyeritz (1993). Marfan syndrome. In: *Connective Tissue and Its Heritable Disorders*, eds P. M. Royce & B. Steinmann, pp. 437–68. New York: Wiley-Liss.

Pyeritz, et al. (1985). Growth and anthropometrics in the Marfan syndrome. In: *Endocrine Genetics and the Genetics of Growth*, eds C. J. Papadatos & C. S. Bartsocas, pp. 355–66. New York: Alan R. Liss.

Marfan syndrome

Preventive medical checklist (0–3 years)

Name _____ Birth date __ / __ / __ Number _____

Age	Evaluations: key concerns	Management considerations		Notes
New-born ↓ 1 month	Dysmorphology: anomalies Hearing, vision:[2] eye examination Feeding: cleft palate, poor intake Heart: murmur, dilation Urogenital: renal, genital defects Skeletal: pectus, lung restriction, hernias Parental adjustment	☐ Genetic evaluation[1] ☐ ABR; ophthalmology[3] ☐ Feeding specialist, video swallow[3] ☐ Echocardiogram; cardiology ☐ Abdominal sonogram; urology[3] ☐ Orthopedics;[3] pulmonology[3] ☐ Family support[4]	☐ ☐ ☐ ☐ ☐ ☐ ☐	Patients with neonatal manifestations often have severe disease
2 months ↓ 4 months	Growth, development:[5] motor weakness Hearing, vision:[2] strabismus, lens laxity Feeding: cleft palate, poor intake Heart: murmur, dilation Urogenital: renal, genital defects Skeletal: neck laxity, lung restriction Parental adjustment Other:	☐ Marfan growth charts; ECI[6] ☐ Ophthalmology[3] ☐ Feeding specialist; video swallow[3] ☐ Echocardiogram;[3] cardiology[3] ☐ Urinalysis, BP; urology[3] ☐ Pulmonology;[3] anesthesia precautions ☐ Family support[4] ☐	☐ ☐ ☐ ☐ ☐ ☐ ☐ ☐	
6 months ↓ 9 months	Growth, development:[5] motor weakness Hearing, vision:[2] strabismus, lens laxity Heart: murmur, dilation Urogenital: renal, genital defects Skeletal: pectus, joint laxity Other:	☐ ECI[6] ☐ Ophthalmology[3] ☐ Echocardiogram;[3] cardiology[3] ☐ Urinalysis, BP; urology[3] ☐ Orthopedics;[3] anesthesia precautions ☐	☐ ☐ ☐ ☐ ☐ ☐	
1 year	Growth, development:[5] motor weakness Hearing, vision:[2] strabismus, lens laxity Heart: murmur, dilation Urogenital: renal, genital defects Skeletal: neck laxity, lung restriction Dural ectasia: nerve root, pelvic pain Other:	☐ ECI[6] ☐ Ophthalmology[3] ☐ Echocardiogram;[3] cardiology[3] ☐ Urinalysis, BP; urology[3] ☐ Pulmonology;[3] anesthesia precautions ☐ Head, spine MRI[3] ☐	☐ ☐ ☐ ☐ ☐ ☐ ☐	
15 months ↓ 18 months	Growth, development:[5] motor weakness Hearing, vision:[2] strabismus, lens laxity Heart: murmur, dilation Skeletal: joint laxity, lung restriction	☐ ECI[6] ☐ Ophthalmology[3] ☐ Echocardiogram;[3] cardiology[3] ☐ Orthopedics;[3] anesthesia precautions	☐ ☐ ☐ ☐	
2 years	Growth, development:[5] motor weakness Vision, teeth:[2] myopia, lens, malocclusion Heart: murmur, dilation Dural ectasia: nerve root, pelvic pain Skeletal: joint laxity, lung restriction	☐ ECI[6] ☐ Ophthalmology, dentistry ☐ Echocardiogram;[3] cardiology[3] ☐ Head, spine MRI[3] ☐ Orthopedics;[3] anesthesia precautions	☐ ☐ ☐ ☐ ☐	
3 years	Growth, development:[5] motor weakness Vision, teeth:[2] myopia, lens, malocclusion Heart: murmur, dilation Dural ectasia: nerve root, pelvic pain Urogenital: renal, genital defects Skeletal: joint laxity, lung restriction Other:	☐ Marfan growth charts; ECI;[6] family support[4] ☐ ☐ Ophthalmology, dentistry ☐ Echocardiogram;[3] cardiology[3] ☐ Head, spine MRI[3] ☐ Urinalysis, BP; urology[3] ☐ Orthopedics;[3] anesthesia precautions ☐	☐ ☐ ☐ ☐ ☐ ☐	

Marfan syndrome concerns

		Other concerns from history	
Myopia, lens dislocation Retinal detachment Cleft palate, feeding problems Dental malocclusion Mitral, aortic valve dysfunction Arterial dilation, aneurysms	Ventricular arrhythmias Renal thrombosis, hypogonadism Umbilical, inguinal hernia Joint laxity, dislocations Meningocele, dural ectasia	**Family history/prenatal** _____ _____ _____ _____	**Social/environmental** _____ _____ _____ _____

Guidelines for the neonatal period should be undertaken *at whatever age* the diagnosis is made; ABR, auditory brainstem evoked response; BP, blood pressure; [1]clinical genetic and subspecialty evaluations are crucial for correct diagnosis and counseling – should include retinal examination, echocardiogram, pelvic X-rays, and possibly head/spine MRI; [2]by practitioner; [3]as dictated by clinical findings; [4]parent group, family/sib, financial, and behavioral issues for severely affected children; [5]consider developmental pediatric or genetics clinic according to symptoms and availability; [6]early childhood intervention if muscle weakness, feeding problems.

Marfan syndrome

Preventive medical checklist (4–18 years)

Name _____ Birth date __/__/__ Number _____

Age	Evaluations: key concerns	Management considerations	Notes
4 years ↓ 6 years	Growth:[1] tall stature Development:[2] preschool transition Vision, teeth:[2] myopia, lens, malocclusion Heart: valvular disease, aneurysms Dural ectasia, sleep apnea Skeletal: joint laxity, lung restriction Other:	❏ Marfan syndrome charts[1] ❏ ❏ Family support;[4] preschool program[5] ❏ ❏ Ophthalmology; dentistry ❏ ❏ Cardiology; activity restrictions; beta-blockers[3] ❏ ❏ Head, spine MRI;[3] sleep study[3] ❏ ❏ Orthopedics;[3] anesthesia precautions ❏ ❏ ❏	
7 years ↓ 9 years	Growth:[1] tall stature Development:[1] school transition[5] Vision, teeth:[2] myopia, lens, malocclusion Heart: valvular disease, aneurysms Urogenital: renal, genital defects Skeletal: joint laxity, lung restriction Other:	❏ Marfan syndrome charts[1] ❏ ❏ Family support;[4] school progress[6] ❏ ❏ Ophthalmology; dentistry ❏ ❏ Cardiology; activity restrictions; beta-blockers[3] ❏ ❏ Urinalysis, BP; urology[3] ❏ ❏ Orthopedics;[3] anesthesia precautions ❏ ❏ ❏	
10 years ↓ 12 years	Growth and development[1] Vision, teeth:[2] myopia, lens, malocclusion Heart: valvular disease, aneurysms Skeletal: pectus, scoliosis, hernias Other:	❏ School progress[6] ❏ ❏ Ophthalmology; dentistry ❏ ❏ Cardiology; activity restrictions; beta-blockers[3] ❏ ❏ Orthopedics;[3] anesthesia precautions ❏ ❏ ❏	
13 years ↓ 15 years	Growth and development[1] Vision, teeth:[2] myopia, lens, malocclusion Heart: valvular disease, aneurysms Dural ectasia, sleep apnea Urogenital: renal, genital defects Other:	❏ Marfan charts;[1] school progress[6] ❏ ❏ Ophthalmology; dentistry ❏ ❏ Cardiology; activity restrictions; beta-blockers[3] ❏ ❏ Head, spine MRI;[3] sleep study[3] ❏ ❏ Urinalysis, BP; urology[3] ❏ ❏ ❏	
16 years ↓ 18 years	Growth and development[1] Vision, teeth:[2] myopia, lens malocclusion Heart: valvular disease, aneurysms Skeletal: pectus, scoliosis, hernias Other:	❏ Family support;[4] school progress[6] ❏ ❏ Ophthalmology; dentistry ❏ ❏ Cardiology; activity restrictions; beta-blockers[3] ❏ ❏ Orthopedics;[3] anesthesia precautions ❏ ❏ ❏	
19 years ↓ 23 years	Adult transition: body image, activity Vision, teeth:[2] myopia, lens, malocclusion Heart: valvular disease, aneurysms Skeletal: joint laxity, contractures Renal, pulmonary abnormalities	❏ Physical therapy/trainer;[3] cosmetic surgery[3] ❏ ❏ Ophthalmology; dentistry ❏ ❏ Cardiology; activity restrictions; beta-blockers[3] ❏ ❏ Head, spine MRI;[3] sleep study[3] ❏ ❏ Urinalysis, BP; urology[3] pulmonology[3] ❏	
Adult	Body image, activity guidance Vision, teeth:[2] myopia, lens, malocclusion Heart: valvular disease, aneurysms Skeletal: arthritis, scoliosis, flat feet Renal, pulmonary abnormalities Dural ectasia, sleep apnea Other:	❏ Physical therapy/trainer;[3] cosmetic surgery[3] ❏ ❏ Audiology;[3] ENT;[3] ophthalmology;[3] ❏ ❏ Cardiology; activity restrictions; beta-blockers[3] ❏ ❏ Orthopedics;[3] anesthesia precautions ❏ ❏ Urinalysis, BP; urology[3] pulmonology[3] ❏ ❏ Head, spine MRI;[3] sleep study[3] ❏ ❏ ❏	Fertile women have risks for aortic aneurysm during pregnancy and for chromosome anomalies in offspring.

Marfan syndrome concerns		Other concerns from history	
Tall stature Myopia, lens dislocation Retinal detachment, cataracts Dental malocclusion, TMJ disease Mitral, aortic valve dysfunction Arterial aneurysms, arrythmias	Scoliosis, pulmonary restriction Joint laxity, hernias, fractures Ligament tears, arthritis Dural ectasia, sleep apnea Learning differences	**Family history/prenatal** _____ _____ _____ _____	**Social/environmental** _____ _____ _____ _____

Guidelines for the neonatal period should be undertaken *at whatever age* the diagnosis is made; BP, blood pressure; TMJ, temporomandibular joint; [1]consider developmental pediatric or genetics clinic according to symptoms and availability; [2]by practitioner; [3]as dictated by clinical findings; [4]parent group, family/sib, financial, and behavioral issues for rare patients with learning differences, debilitating illness; [5]preschool program including developmental monitoring and motor therapy if needed; [6]monitor for learning differences, avoid high intensity/collision sports, monitor for depression due to body habitus, activity restrictions.

Parent guide to Marfan syndrome

Marfan syndrome is a clinical pattern consisting of elongated body proportions, tall stature, ectopia lentis (slipped lens), skeletal abnormalities including pectus (concave chest), scoliosis (curved spine), and, of most concern, progressive dilation of the aorta (large artery near heart) and heart valves.

Incidence, causation, and diagnosis

Marfan syndrome has an incidence of 1 in 10,000 births and occurs in many ethnic groups. The disorder exhibits autosomal dominant inheritance with 15% of patients representing new genetic changes (mutations). Marfan syndrome is caused by mutations in the fibrillin-1 gene on chromosome 15; DNA testing is available but not very sensitive because of the large size of the gene and the diverse nature of the mutations have so far not allowed routine DNA diagnostic testing. The differential diagnosis includes other connective tissue dysplasias such as homocystinuria or Beals syndrome; abnormal blood amino acids in the former and ear anomalies in the latter disorder allow differentiation. Clinical diagnosis requires two objective manifestations (cardiovascular, eye, hip joint, or stretching of the craniospinal lining – dural ectasia) demonstrated by specialty studies plus suggestive skeletal signs – long face, high palate, long fingers (arachnodactyly), joint laxity, pectus, scoliosis, hernias, flat feet.

Natural history and complications

Newborns with signs of Marfan syndrome have a severe outlook with heart disease in over 80% and risks for early death. For the more typical patients who present in mid-childhood to adolescence, complications include eye problems (ectopia lentis, myopia); heart problems (abnormal echocardiogram, aortic root enlargement, floppy mitral valve), and skeletal problems (spinal curvature or scoliosis, chest concavity, flat feet). On clinical examination, 30% will have a click typical of mitral valve prolapse (floppy mitral valve), 10% a murmur suggestive of a dilated aortic valve, and 6% a murmur suggestive of a dilated mitral valve. Most are tall with a long face, high palate causing dental problems, long fingers, joint laxity, hernias, and fragile skin with obvious stretch marks. The cardiac symptoms of adolescents and adults with Marfan syndrome include palpitations, shortness of breath, light-headedness associated with mitral valve prolapse, and chest pain related to pneumothorax (ruptured lung) or aortic dissection (tearing of the aortic artery). Other complications can include severe spinal curvature with restrictive lung disease and heart failure; cataracts or retinal problems with detachment; increased bruisability but normal healing of skin; and stretching of the spinal cord lining (dura) with neck or abdominal pain. Spinal pain, arthralgia, ligament injury, and fracture occur in most adults with Marfan syndrome, but not in children. Women with Marfan syndrome have more severe osteoporosis (bone softening) and risks for aortic artery dissection during pregnancy.

Preventive medical needs

All patients should have an ophthalmologic examination and echocardiography by a cardiologist who is experienced with the condition when the diagnosis is made. The aortic root diameter can be plotted against norms for the patient's age and size, allowing recognition of early aortic dilation. Consultation with cardiology and cardiothoracic surgery should occur initially and annually to consider timing of beta-blocker therapy and aortic patch surgery. Optic lens dislocation may not be obvious, and slit lamp exam with a fully dilated pupil may be needed to detect increased lens motion due to laxity of its suspensory ligament. Newborns with signs of Marfan syndrome should be carefully monitored for cardiopulmonary changes, and infants watched for palatal problems and referred to early childhood intervention for likely motor delays due to muscle weakness. The likely heart defects and joint laxity require care during anesthesia. Regular evaluations of the eyes, heart, and skeletal system are the core of management, with attention to pectus, scoliosis, and flat feet in adolescence. Severe skeletal defects can cause pulmonary restriction and cosmetic problems for teenagers/young adults. Restriction of high-intensity or collision sports is necessary because of risks for eye injury, joint fatigue, and sudden cardiac death. An activity program with monitoring for withdrawal or depression may be needed for individuals with severe stigmata. The varying experience and indications for thoracic surgery in Marfan syndrome emphasize the need for patients to be followed by cardiologists and cardiovascular surgeons who are experienced with the disorder.

Family counseling

Genetic counseling for Marfan syndrome is straightforward numerically but complicated in terms of medical recommendations and patient self-image. All at-risk patients should be referred to a genetic specialist and probably to an experienced cardiologist for detection of subtle manifestations. Affected individuals will have a 50% risk of transmitting the condition, but 15% are new mutations that imply minimal recurrence risks for parents. Fibrillin-1 DNA testing is available but not yet sensitive enough for routine use. Fetal diagnosis by ultrasound can sometimes be made in the third trimester of pregnancy, allowing parental adjustment and perinatal planning. Medical counseling should include prohibition of collision or highly competitive sports, and of isometric exercises that place strain on the heart. Emotional stress should also be avoided where possible. Such advice is better accepted after a tragic death in the family, but difficult to enforce in asymptomatic adolescents. Teenagers and young adults may have poor self image due to severe pectus or frail body habitus, and physical trainers/guided activity programs or cosmetic surgeries may be helpful. Pregnancy is thought to be of higher risk in Marfan syndrome, but one study reported minimal complications in women whose aortic root diameter was less than 40 mm in width. Improved management has enhanced the average lifespan of patients with Marfan syndrome from 48 years in the 1970s to 72 years in the 1990s.

Preventive management of Ehlers–Danlos/hypermobility syndromes

Description: The Ehlers–Danlos (E-D) disorders comprise a broad range of conditions with connective tissue weakness. Their most characteristic signs are joint hypermobility and skin fragility with scarring, but some forms have risks for cardiovascular changes. Incidence of the entire category is 1 in 5000 live births, 90% with E-D types (I–III) where skin and joint changes predominate.

Clinical diagnosis: E-D types I–III and V are characterized by changes in the eyes (myopia, strabismus), skin (enhanced elasticity and fragility, poor wound closure, "cigarette paper" scarring), trunk (inguinal and umbilical hernias), and skeleton (increased joint laxity, joint dislocations, pectus, scoliosis, flat feet, ligament tears, arthritis). It may be difficult to distinguish patients with familial joint laxity/hypermobility from those with E-D syndrome, and any individual with dramatic joint laxity deserves consideration of the specified preventive management strategies. E-D type IV is a more severe disorder with risks for arterial aneurysms and dissections, particularly during pregnancy.

Laboratory diagnosis: DNA diagnosis is available for type V collagen gene mutations that account for 50% of patients with E-D types I–III disease, for type III collagen mutations in E-D type IV, and for lysyl oxidase gene mutations in E-D type VII. The number of different syndromes and as yet uncharacterized genes limit the sensitivity of DNA diagnosis.

Genetics: Autosomal-dominant inheritance for most E-D types with a 50% risk for affected individuals to transmit the disease. Type IV and other disorders with severe joint laxity may exhibit autosomal recessive inheritance. Pregnancy risks for E-D types I–III include premature delivery for affected infants and bladder or rectal prolapse for affected mothers; those for type IV are sufficiently severe to warrant early termination or planned premature delivery.

Key management issues: Ophthalmologic and cardiologic evaluation in suspect cases, monitoring of the skin, eyes, teeth, and joints with auscultation for signs of valvular prolapse or insufficiency, counseling to avoid high-impact or collision sports, bracing and fusions for injured joints or severe scoliosis, counseling and monitoring for pregnancy risks.

Growth charts: Growth is usually normal, allowing the use of standard growth charts.

Parent information: The Ehlers–Danlos Syndrome Foundation (www.ednf.org/), the Ehlers–Danlos Support Group (www.ehlers-danlos.org/), and various educational sites accessed by searching on the syndrome name.

Basis for management recommendations: Derived from the complications listed below.

Summary of clinical concerns

General	General	Fragile fetal membranes, prematurity, decreased life span and high pregnancy risks in type IV
	Behavior	Higher rates of psychiatric problems
Facial	Eyes	**Epicanthal folds** (25%), microcornea, strabismus, myopia, blue sclerae, retinal detachment, keratoconus, easy eversion of eyelids (Menetrier sign), glaucoma (E-D type VI)
	Ears	Overturned helices
	Mouth	Tooth enamel hypoplasia, deformed teeth, periodontal disease, fragile oral mucosa, absent frenula, temporomandibular joint subluxation
Surface	Neck/trunk	**Inguinal hernias** (10–20%), umbilical hernias
	Epidermal	Hyperelastic skin, pigmented "cigarette-paper" scares, enhanced scarring, enhanced skin fragility with gaping wounds after trauma, molluscoid pseudotumors or spheroids (calcified cysts over bony prominences), easy bruising, varicose veins, ecchymoses with type IV
Skeletal	Axial	**Kyphoscoliosis** (15–20%), thoracic asymmetry, atlantoaxial subluxation (type IV)
	Limbs	Joint laxity, flat feet, **genu recurvatum** (25%), club feet (5%), congenital hip dislocation, joint effusions and dislocations, osteoarthritis (20–60%), acrocyanosis
Internal	Digestive	Gastrointestinal diverticula, rectal prolapse, constipation
	Circulatory	Cardiac septal defects, bicuspid aortic valve, mitral valve prolapse, tricuspid valve prolapse, dilation of aortic root, high rate of **arterial dissection/aneurysm** (80%) presenting as stroke, abdominal pain, flank pain due to bowel rupture in E-D type IV
	Pulmonary	Spontaneous pneumothorax, cavitary lesions (E-D type IV)
	RES	Hematomas, bleeding after surgeries
	Excretory	Bladder prolapse
	Genital	Uterine prolapse
	Motor	Peripheral neuropathy with brachial plexus palsy, lumbosacral plexopathy
	Sensory	Vision loss

RES, reticuloendothelial system; **concerns** of frequency >20% are **highlighted**

Key references

Lumley, et al. (1994). Psychosocial functioning in the Ehlers–Danlos syndrome. *American Journal of Medical Genetics* 53:149–52.

Lurie, et al. (1998). The threat of type IV Ehlers–Danlos syndrome on maternal well-being during pregnancy: early delivery may make the difference. *Journal of Obstetrics and Gynaecology* 18:245–8.

Steinmann, et al. (1993). The Ehlers–Danlos syndrome. In: *Connective Tissue and Its Heritable Disorders*, eds P. M. Royce & B. Steinmann, pp. 351–407. New York: Wiley-Liss.

Ehlers–Danlos/hypermobility

Preventive medical checklist (0–3 years)

Name _____ Birth date __/__/____ Number _____

Age	Evaluations: key concerns	Management considerations	Notes
New-born ↓ 1 month	Skeletal: dislocations, hernias Hearing, vision:[2] eye examination Heart: murmur, dilation GI: constipation, rectal prolapse Parental adjustment	❑ Genetic evaluation;[1] orthopedics[3] ❑ ❑ ABR; ophthalmology[3] ❑ ❑ Echocardiogram;[3] cardiology[3] ❑ ❑ GI specialist[3] ❑ ❑ Family support[4] ❑	
2 months ↓ 4 months	Growth, development:[5] muscles, feeding Hearing, vision:[2] strabismus Skeletal: dislocations, hernias, AAI Heart: murmur, dilation GI: constipation, rectal prolapse Skin: scarring, bruising Other:	❑ ECI[6] ❑ ❑ Ophthalmology[3] ❑ ❑ Orthopedics;[3] anesthesia precautions ❑ ❑ Echocardiogram;[3] cardiology[3] ❑ ❑ GI specialist[3] ❑ ❑ Family support[4] ❑ ❑ ❑	
6 months ↓ 9 months	Growth, development:[5] muscles, feeding Hearing, vision:[2] strabismus Skeletal: dislocations, hernias, AAI Heart: murmur, dilation GI: constipation, rectal prolapse Other:	❑ ECI[6] ❑ ❑ Ophthalmology[3] ❑ ❑ Orthopedics;[3] anesthesia precautions ❑ ❑ Echocardiogram;[3] cardiology[3] ❑ ❑ GI specialist[3] ❑ ❑ ❑	
1 year	Growth, development:[5] muscles, feeding Hearing, vision:[2] strabismus Skeletal: dislocations, hernias, AAI Heart: murmur, dilation Skin: scarring, bruising Other:	❑ ECI[6] ❑ ❑ Ophthalmology[3] ❑ ❑ Orthopedics;[3] anesthesia precautions ❑ ❑ Echocardiogram;[3] cardiology[3] ❑ ❑ Family support[4] ❑ ❑ ❑	
15 months ↓ 18 months	Growth, development:[5] muscles, feeding Hearing, vision:[2] strabismus Skeletal: dislocations, hernias, AAI Heart: murmur, dilation	❑ ECI[6] ❑ ❑ Ophthalmology[3] ❑ ❑ Orthopedics;[3] anesthesia precautions ❑ ❑ Echocardiogram;[3] cardiology[3]	
2 years	Growth, development:[5] muscles, feeding Hearing, vision:[2] strabismus Skeletal: walking, alignment, AAI Heart: murmur, dilation Skin, gums: bruising, fragility	❑ ECI[6] ❑ ❑ Ophthalmology[3] ❑ ❑ Orthopedics;[3] anesthesia precautions ❑ ❑ Echocardiogram;[3] cardiology[3] ❑ ❑ Dentistry; family support[4] ❑	
3 years	Growth, development:[5] motor weakness Hearing, vision:[2] strabismus Skeletal: walking, alignment, AAI Heart: murmur, dilation Skin, gums: bruising, fragility GI: constipation, rectal prolapse Other:	❑ ECI[6] ❑ ❑ Ophthalmology[3] ❑ ❑ Orthopedics;[3] cervical spine X-rays[3] ❑ ❑ Echocardiogram;[3] cardiology[3] ❑ ❑ Dentistry; family support[4] ❑ ❑ GI specialist[3] ❑ ❑ ❑	

Ehlers–Danlos concerns		Other concerns from history	
Myopia, blue sclerae Retinal detachment Fragile gums, periodontitis Mitral, aortic valve dysfunction Arterial dilation, aneurysms	Rectal, bladder prolapse Umbilical, inguinal hernia Joint laxity, dislocations Skin bruising, scarring	**Family history/prenatal** _____ _____ _____ _____	**Social/environmental** _____ _____ _____ _____

Guidelines for the neonatal period should be undertaken *at whatever age* the diagnosis is made; ABR, auditory brainstem evoked response; AAI, atlantoaxial instability; GI, gastrointestinal; [1]clinical genetic and subspecialty evaluations are crucial for correct diagnosis and counseling – should include ophthalmology examination and skeletal X-rays as dictated by symptoms; [2] by practitioner; [3]as dictated by clinical findings; [4]parent and health care education, avoid erroneous reports of child abuse; [5]consider genetics clinic according to symptoms and availability; [6]early childhood intervention if muscle weakness, dislocations.

Ehlers–Danlos/hypermobility

Preventive medical checklist (4–18 years)

Name _____ **Birth date** __/__/____ **Number** _____

Age	Evaluations: key concerns	Management considerations		Notes
4 years ↓ **6 years**	Growth, development: motor weakness Vision:[2] myopia, retinal changes Skeletal: scoliosis, joints, AAI Heart: murmur, dilation Skin, gums: bruising, fragility GI: rectal prolapse, intestinal bleeding Other:	❑ Preschool program[5] ❑ Ophthalmology[3] ❑ Orthopedics;[3] anesthesia precautions ❑ Cardiology;[3] activity restrictions ❑ Dentistry; dermatology;[3] family support[4] ❑ GI specialist[3] ❑	❑ ❑ ❑ ❑ ❑ ❑ ❑	
7 years ↓ **9 years**	Growth and development[1] Vision:[2] myopia, globe trauma Skeletal: dislocations, hernias, AAI Arteries, lungs: aneurysms, ectasias Skin, gums: bruising, fragility GI: rectal prolapse, intestinal bleeding Other:	❑ School transition[6] ❑ Ophthalmology[3] ❑ Orthopedics;[3] anesthesia precautions ❑ Cardiology;[3] pulmonology;[3] activity restrictions ❑ Dentistry; dermatology;[3] family support[4] ❑ GI specialist[3] ❑	❑ ❑ ❑ ❑ ❑ ❑ ❑	
10 years ↓ **12 years**	Growth and development[1] Vision:[2] myopia, retinal changes Skeletal: scoliosis, joints, AAI Arteries, lungs: aneurysms, ectasias Other:	❑ School progress[6] ❑ Ophthalmology[3] ❑ Cardiology;[3] activity restrictions ❑ Echocardiogram[3]; Cardiology[3] ❑	❑ ❑ ❑ ❑ ❑	
13 years ↓ **15 years**	Growth and development[1] Vision:[2] myopia, globe trauma Skeletal: dislocations, hernias, AAI Arteries, lungs: aneurysms, ectasias GI: rectal prolapse, intestinal bleeding Other:	❑ School progress[6] ❑ Ophthalmology[3] ❑ Orthopedics;[3] cervical spine X-rays[3] ❑ Cardiology;[3] activity restrictions ❑ GI specialist[3] ❑	❑ ❑ ❑ ❑ ❑ ❑	
16 years ↓ **18 years**	Growth and development[1] Vision:[2] myopia, retinal changes Skeletal: scoliosis, joints, AAI Skin, gums: bruising, fragility Other:	❑ Family support;[4] school progress[6] ❑ Ophthalmology[3] ❑ Orthopedics;[3] anesthesia precautions ❑ Dentistry; dermatology;[3] family support[4] ❑	❑ ❑ ❑ ❑ ❑	
19 years ↓ **23 years**	Adult transition: body image, activity[6] Vision:[2] myopia, globe trauma Skeletal: dislocations, hernias, AAI Arteries, lungs: aneurysms, ectasias Skin: scarring, bruising	❑ Physical therapy/trainer;[3] cosmetic surgery[3] ❑ Ophthalmology[3] ❑ Orthopedics;[3] anesthesia precautions ❑ Cardiology;[3] activity restrictions ❑ Dermatology;[3] family support[4]	❑ ❑ ❑ ❑ ❑	
Adult	Body image, activity guidance[6] Vision:[2] myopia, trauma, retina Skeletal: tendons, joints, AAI Arteries, lungs: aneurysms, ectasias Skin, gums: bruising, fragility GI: rectal prolapse, intestinal bleeding Other:	❑ Physical therapy/trainer;[3] cosmetic surgery[3] ❑ Ophthalmology[3] ❑ Orthopedics;[3] cervical spine X-rays[3] ❑ Cardiology;[3] activity restrictions ❑ Dentistry; dermatology[3] ❑ GI specialist[3] ❑	❑ ❑ ❑ ❑ ❑ ❑ ❑	Pregnancy risks for premature rupture of membranes, high mortality with E-D type IV.

Ehlers–Danlos concerns		Other concerns from history	
Myopia, blue sclerae Retinal detachment Fragile gums, periodontitis Mitral, aortic valve dysfunction Arterial dilation, aneurysms	Rectal, bladder prolapse Umbilical, inguinal hernia Joint laxity, dislocations Joint tears, arthritis Skin bruising, scarring	**Family history/prenatal** _____ _____ _____ _____	**Social/environmental** _____ _____ _____ _____

Guidelines for the neonatal period should be undertaken *at whatever age* the diagnosis is made; AAI, atlantoaxial instability; GI, gastrointestinal; [1]consider genetics clinic according to symptoms and availability; [2]by practitioner; [3]as dictated by clinical findings; [4]parent and provider education, avoid erroneous reports of child abuse; [5]for those with motor weakness, severe complications or handicaps; [6]avoid high intensity or collision sports, guidance for alternative activities, counseling regarding pregnancy risks, and alertness for psychosocial problems including anxiety, depression, reproductive concerns, and frustration with the medical care system.

Parent guide to Ehlers–Danlos/hypermobility syndromes

Ehlers described patients with lax joints and elastic skin in 1901, while Danlos reported unusual scarring and skin fragility in 1908. Subsequent work has defined many types of Ehlers–Danlos (E-D) syndrome, most involving the eyes, skin, and joints. Types I–III are very similar, with type II being a mild form of type I and type III consisting of joint hypermobility that merges with that seen in otherwise normal individuals. Other types of Ehlers–Danlos syndrome are rare, including the type IV with disease of the blood vessels.

Incidence, causation, and diagnosis

The overall incidence of Ehlers–Danlos syndromes is estimated to be 1 in 5000 live births, with types I–III comprising over 90% of cases. The majority are autosomal dominant, with some cases of type IV exhibiting autosomal recessive inheritance. Collagen gene mutations (collagen gene V in E-D types I–III, collagen gene III in E-D type IV) and mutations in genes modifying collagen or elastin filaments have been identified for some disorders, but clinical rather than DNA diagnosis is required for most patients. It is important to differentiate the more common E-D types from rarer disorders like E-D type IV (with greater risks of blood vessel breakdown and bleeding) or VI (with greater risks of eye rupture or retinal detachment). It is important to recognize that a large number of syndromes involve increased laxity of connective tissue and that normal families may display increased joint laxity – recent information suggests that any individual with dramatic joint hypermobility should be followed for eye and skeletal complications with guidance towards activities that minimize joint wear and injury. The Meténier sign (easy eversion of the upper eyelids) and Gorlin sign (ability to touch the nose with the tongue) are helpful signs of connective tissue weakness, and signs of joint hypermobility include passive bending of the wrist and thumb to touch the forearm and to wrap one arm behind the back and reach the umbilicus.

Natural history and complications

The complications of Ehlers–Danlos syndrome types I–III include prematurity, since the extra-embryonic membranes are fetal in origin and may exhibit fragility. Mothers face an increased risk for postpartum hemorrhage and prolapse of the uterus or bladder. Neonates have increased joint mobility but few other complications; infants may come to attention because of motor delay due to joint laxity or with severe bruising/gaping lacerations that are sometimes interpreted as child abuse. As children grow older, their chief complications affect the eyes, heart, skin, and skeleton. The face may be unusual, with occasional blue sclerae (whites of the eyes and epicanthal folds (folds at the corner of the eye). Eye anomalies include small cornea, strabismus (deviated gaze), and retinal changes such as orange streaks or detachment. The teeth may have abnormal enamel and dentin formation, with altered tooth morphology. The gums are fragile, and periodontal disease can occur at an early age. Locking of the temporomandibular (temple-jaw) joint may occur. Skin findings include marked looseness, gaping wounds from minor trauma, and formation of finely wrinkled, pigmented scars that are likened to cigarette paper. There may be nodules under the skin (spheroids or calcified cysts) in 30% of patients. Thinning of the skin makes blue discoloration with cold (acrocyanosis) more prominent in children and varicose veins more prominent in adults. Skeletal anomalies include curved spine, bowed legs, flat feet, or club feet. Inguinal or umbilical hernias are more common. Occasional features include urinary tract infections due to bladder reflux or loss of sensation in the extremities (peripheral nephropathy).

Preventive medical needs

Knowledge that a pregnant woman is affected with E-D syndromes types I–III allows planning for the possibility of maternal bleeding from episiotomy wounds or lacerations, and observation for bladder or rectal prolapse. There will be a 50% risk of the infant being affected, with a higher risk for rupture of membranes and prematurity. After birth, the infant should be evaluated for signs of joint laxity and skin elasticity, with ophthalmologic and cardiologic consultation in suspect patients. For the majority of patients with joint hypermobility with or without skin changes, counseling to limit high intensity/collision sports and monitoring of joint and skeletal status will then be sufficient. However, the potential for serious cardiovascular complications should be borne in mind, with ready referral to cardiology or gastroenterologists for cardiopulmonary symptoms or intestinal/abdominal complaints. If E-D type IV is suspected based on severe early bruising and/or heart findings, then early and annual cardiology assessments are essential. Dental care is even more important in these children, and the potential for scoliosis (spinal curvature) and joint dislocations make a baseline orthopedic evaluation worth considering once the child begins walking. In the adolescent and adult years, surveillance of the eyes, skin, and joints should continue with auscultation for signs of heart disease. Patients who have had an earlier echocardiogram to rule out congenital heart lesions can probably be followed symptomatically, but changing auscultatory or clinical signs warrant repeat echocardiography. Bracing and fusions seem to be the most common methods for orthopedic treatment of injured joints, including spinal fusions for severe curvatures. Cosmetic surgery and/or physical therapy/trainer consultation regarding alternative activities may be worthwhile for adolescents and young adults to promote a healthy lifestyle and body image.

Family counseling

Patients with Ehlers–Danlos syndrome types I–III have a 50% risk to transmit the condition, and couples should be counseled regarding the risks for prematurity, and bladder or rectal prolapse during pregnancy and delivery. The normal life span and intelligence in these disorders warrants optimistic counseling with emphasis on periodic evaluation of the eyes and heart. However, psychosocial problems such as anxiety, depression, anger, sexual difficulties, reproductive concerns, and frustration with the medical care system are frequently reported in patients with Ehlers–Danlos syndrome. Psychological intervention is therefore beneficial for some families. Parent support groups are available (see p. 1).

17

Integumentary syndromes

Syndromes with primary manifestations affecting the integument comprise a diverse group of relatively rare conditions (Table 17.1). In this chapter, they are categorized as ectodermal dysplasias, albinism, other pigmentary disorders,

Table 17.1. Integumentary syndromes

Syndrome or disease	Incidence*	Inheritance	Complications
Ectodermal dysplasias			
Hypohidrotic ectodermal dysplasia	1 in 100,000	XLR	Sparse hair, dry and hypohidrotic skin, keratitis, sinusitis, absent teeth, conical teeth, high fevers
Ectrodactyly–ectodermal dysplasia-cleft palate (EEC) syndrome	~100 cases	AD	Sparse hair, hypohidrotic skin, photophobia, keratitis, cleft lip/palate, absent teeth, ectrodactyly
Albinism			
Oculocutaneous albinism, type 1	1 in 20,000	AR	Ocular a. (foveal hypoplasia, strabismus, nystagmus), white skin, no tanning
Oculocutaneous albinism, type 2	1 in 20,000	AR	Ocular a. (foveal hypoplasia, strabismus, nystagmus), white skin, no tanning
Ocular albinism	1 in 100,000	XLR, AR	Ocular a. (foveal hypoplasia, strabismus, nystagmus)
Other pigmentary disorders			
Goltz–Gorlin syndrome	~200 cases	XLR	Hyper- or hypo-pigmented linear streaks on the skin, eye a. (colobomata, strabismus), syndactyly, brachydactyly, urogenital a., cognitive disability
Hypomelanosis of Ito	~50 cases	C	Hypopigmented macules and streaks on the skin, microcephaly, seizures, cognitive disability

(*cont.*)

Table 17.1. (*cont.*)

Syndrome or disease	Incidence*	Inheritance	Complications
Incontinentia pigmenti	~200 cases	XLR	Sparse hair, vesicular or pigmented skin, absent teeth, conical teeth, microcephaly, hydrocephalus, seizures, cognitive disability
LEOPARD syndrome	~100 cases	AD	Lentigines, ptosis, hypertelorism, cardiac a., scoliosis, genital a., short stature, cognitive disability
Waardenburg syndrome	~1400 cases	AD	White forelock, dystopia canthorum, heterochromia of the irides, strabismus, sensorineural deafness, Hirschsprung a.
Hemangioma syndromes			
Ataxia–telangiectasia	1 in 100,000	AR	Ataxia, facial and conjunctival telangiectasias, frequent infections, early graying, predisposition to cancer, immune deficiency
Bloom syndrome	~200 cases	AR	Short stature, microcephaly, facial erythema and telangiectasias, hypogonadism, predisposition to cancer, immune deficiency
Osler–Rendu–Weber syndrome	1 in 100,000	AD	Multiple hemorrhagic telangiectasias, pulmonary arteriovenous fistulas, urinary tract bleeding, gastrointestinal bleeding, intracranial bleeding
Rothmund–Thomson syndrome	~150 cases	AR	Short stature, photosensitivity, sparse hair, facial erythema, cataracts, strabismus, dental a., hyper- and hypo-pigmentation of skin (poikiloderma), hypogonadism, predisposition to sarcomas
Disorders with radiation sensitivity and/or rapid aging			
Cockayne syndrome	~75 cases	AR	Short stature, photosensitivity, sparse hair, retinitis, accelerated aging, early death
Progeria	~75 cases	Sporadic	Short stature, photosensitivity, sparse hair, joint degeneration, atherosclerosis, accelerated aging
Xeroderma pigmentosum	1 in 200,000	AR	Short stature, skin pigmentation, squamous and basal cell carcinomas, early death

Notes:

AR, autosomal recessive; AD, autosomal dominant; XLR, X-linked recessive; C, chromosomal; a., anomalies.

*Cases or per number of live births.

hemangiomatous disorders, and disorders of radiation sensitivity/accelerated aging. Each disorder will receive a fairly brief description, as only albinism is sufficiently common to be encountered frequently by health professionals.

Ectodermal dysplasias

Hypohidrotic ectodermal dysplasia

Described in the mid-1800s, including mention by Charles Darwin, hypohidrotic ectodermal dysplasia is prototypic of more than 100 disorders that exhibit abnormalities in the hair, teeth, nails, and integumentary glands (Jones, 1997, pp. 540–2; Gorlin et al., 2001, pp. 540–5). The incidence is 1 in 100,000 births, with the majority of families exhibiting X-linked recessive inheritance and having mutations in the ectodysplasin-A gene at chromosome band Xq13. Because many disorders have manifestations of ectodermal dysplasia associated with other defects, differential diagnosis is substantial and complex. Referral to genetic, dentistry, and dermatology specialists is therefore essential for diagnosis and counseling. Decreased numbers of sweat pores can be assessed by a variety of methods, including hypohidrosis by standard sweat testing as performed for diagnosis of cystic fibrosis or by applying starch–iodine mixtures to skin surfaces and noting the distribution and numbers of sweat pores.

Clinical manifestations include a typical face in affected males, with sparse hair, absent or missing eyelashes, frontal bossing with depressed nasal bridge, absence of many permanent teeth, conical maxillary and canine teeth, and protuberant, full lips due to maxillary and dental hypoplasia. The skin is soft and dry, due to the absence of sebaceous glands, and there is scanty body hair. The nails grow slowly and are fragile or spoonshaped. The breasts are hypoplastic, and may be entirely absent in female carriers. Abnormal nasal mucosa and salivary gland function may lead to allergies, sinusitis, and dryness of the mouth. Of most concern in children, the hypohidrosis may lead to elevated temperatures during exertion or illness; all families should be counseled about antipyretics and bathing strategies to lower body temperature during these episodes.

Preventive management for hypohidrotic ectodermal dysplasia and related conditions should include early referral to ophthalmology to assess lacrimal gland function and to monitor possible complications such as glaucoma or keratitis. Regular dental evaluation is also important, and reconstruction strategies are needed in those with significant anodontia (Martin J. W. et al., 2005), and otolaryngologic referral may be needed for the management of atrophic rhinitis, sinusitis, or dysphonia due to atrophy of laryngeal mucosa. Cosmetic approaches become important in later childhood and adolescence, with possible need for false teeth or a wig.

Parental counseling must distinguish among other ectodysplasia syndromes and rare cases with autosomal dominant or recessive inheritance. Affected females will have a 25% recurrence risk for severely affected males due to X-linked recessive inheritance and a 50% risk for mildly affected daughters with hair and teeth changes or even amastia. Isolated cases may represent new mutations (1/3 chance) or offspring of asymptomatic female carriers (2/3 chance), and DNA testing is available (see www.genetests.org). Parent information and support is available at the National Foundation for Ectodermal Dysplasias (www.nfed.org/) or the Ectodermal Dysplasia Society (www.ectodermaldysplasia.org/).

Ectrodactyly–Ectodermal dysplasia-clefting (EEC) syndrome

Ectrodactyly, also called "split hand" or "lobster-claw deformity," can occur as an isolated anomaly that exhibits autosomal-dominant inheritance. Ectrodactyly, together with ectodermal dysplasia and clefts of the lip and palate, constitutes a rare, autosomal-dominant condition with approximately 100 reported cases in the literature (Jones, 1997, pp. 294–5; Gorlin et al., 2001, pp. 878–82). The Hay–Wells syndrome, with ankyloblepharon (adhesions binding together the lateral palpebral fissures), cleft palate and ectodermal dysplasia, is a closely related disorder that also exhibits autosomal-dominant inheritance (Jones, 1997, pp. 296–7). The Rapp–Hodgkin syndrome, also autosomal dominant, consists of ectodermal dysplasia, cleft lip/palate, and genital anomalies (Jones, 1997, pp. 543–4).

Summary of clinical concerns: EEC/Hay–Wells/Rapp–Hodgkin syndrome management considerations

Growth and development: Some patients will have mental disability, and scores have been devised to correlate surgical and rehabilitative approaches with outcomes in social functioning (Diano et al., 2003): Monitoring of development with referral of those with delays to early intervention and preschool programs. Particular attention should be given to hearing screens and speech development.

Eyes: Eye anomalies include absent lacrimal glands with tearing, photophobia, and keratitis: Ophthalmology assessment upon diagnosis and regular care including lubricants.

ENT: Problems can include cleft lip/palate with chronic otitis, conductive hearing loss, abnormal voice, dry vocal cords, dental anomalies including absent, conical, or hypoplastic teeth: Care is best coordinated by craniofacial and orthopedic surgery teams that will include ophthalmologic and otolaryngologic assessment of lacrimal gland and hearing function; cleft palate team for feeding, surgical, and respiratory concerns; and maxillofacial surgery assessment of dental anomalies.

Surface-skin: Sparse hair and eyelashes with decreased sweating. In Caucasian patients, the skin and hair are hypopigmented, and there are hypoplastic sebaceous and sweat glands: Surveillance for and warnings about hyperpyrexia in childhood is necessary.

Urogenital: Genitourinary defects include renal duplication, renal aplasia, hydronephrosis, and cryptorchidism: Initial genital examination and renal sonogram
with monitoring of urinalysis, blood pressure, and appropriate urology consultation to manage the urogential anomalies.

Parental counseling: The ECC, Hay–Wells, and Rapp–Hodgkin syndromes are results
of mutations in a TP63 signal transduction pathway that is homologous to the
p53 tumor suppressor gene (Ray et al., 2004); TP63 mutations are responsible
for type I EEC syndrome and for some patients with Hay–Wells and
Rapp–Hodgkin syndromes. These disorders can be viewed as variations on a
genetic theme, and their complications and preventive management will be
similar. Parental counseling is best performed after genetics and dermatology
evaluation to ensure correct diagnosis. A 50% recurrence risk for affected
patients and a low recurrence for unaffected parents of *de novo* cases are usual,
but parents with minimal signs may have the gene with incomplete penetrance.
Limited DNA testing is available for unclear cases or recurrence risks (see
www.genetests.org), and parent information can be found at the ectodermal
dyplasia organizations listed above or by searching on the syndrome names.

Albinism

Many conditions involve alterations in the production or distribution of melanin,
producing light-colored hair, eyes, and/or skin (Sethi et al., 1996; Orlow, 1997; Carden
et al., 1998). Tyrosinase deficiency accounts for the classical and most common
albinism phenotype, but many other gene products interact to influence melanocyte
maturation and distribution (King et al., 1995). Many melanin-regulating genes
have been characterized and related to homologous genes in mice [skin (King
et al., 2001; Tomita and Suzuki, 2004)]. Often useful in the differential diagnosis of
albinism disorders is the presence of ocular abnormalities such as foveal hypoplasia,
strabismus, and nystagmus; these changes reflect the role of melanin in ocular
development (King et al., 1995).

Primary albinism can be divided into two categories: oculocutaneous albinism
(which affects the hair, skin, and eyes) and ocular albinism (which affects only the
eyes). The differences relate to separate derivation of melanocytes in the hair and
skin (neural crest origin) and those in the retinal pigmentary epithelium (neurectoderm of the developing optic cup).

Oculocutaneous albinism type 1

Oculocutaneous albinism type 1 includes four sub-types with autosomal-recessive
inheritance. Diagnostic assays are available using the classic hair-bulb assay (incu-
bation with tyrosine to produce brown coloration) or molecular analysis that characterizes mutations in the tyrosinase gene (King et al., 2001). Because these assays

are not widely used, specific frequencies for the many sub-types of albinism are not known. The general prevalence for albinism ranges from 1 in 10,000 to 1 in 50,000; it is found in all ethnic groups and in all regions of the world.

Heterogeneity of oculocutaneous albinism type 1 includes patients who are tyrosinase-negative and have virtually no pigment throughout their life, patients with residual tyrosinase activity who develop some pigment including distinctive yellow hair, and patients with temperature-sensitive tyrosinase who develop pigment in their distal extremities because these have lower temperature. The latter individuals are analogous to the distal pigment in Siamese cats or Himalayan mice.

Clinical manifestations of oculocutaneous albinism type 1 are generic, albeit milder, for other types of albinism. Melanin within the retinal epithelium and choroid plays an important role in the development of the visual system. As a result, patients with oculocutaneous albinism type 1 have a hypoplastic fovea with reduced visual acuity that cannot be corrected with glasses. There is also misrouting of optic fibers at the chiasm, resulting in alternating strabismus that usually does not develop into amblyopia. Also resulting from the decreased visual acuity and/or developmental abnormalities is nystagmus, which is present from birth in the majority of patients with severe albinism. Absence of melanin pigment in the inner ear also produces changes in the auditory evoked response and enhances patients' susceptibility to noise or drug-induced hearing loss. Occasional patients develop malignant melanoma.

Tyrosinase-negative oculocutaneous albinism type 1 is distinguished by the absence of pigmentation at birth. Tyrosinase-negative individuals are born with white hair, white skin, and light blue irides that appear pink in certain lights. The hypopigmentation phenotype is constant for all ethnic groups and changes little with age. Exposure to sun usually produces erythema, burning, and little tanning, although patients with residual pigment can tan. As mentioned above, forms of oculocutaneous albinism type 1 that retain partial or temperature-sensitive tyrosinase activity can develop some skin pigment and hair color.

Preventive management of oculocutaneous albinism type 1 includes an early diagnostic evaluation and later protective care. Ocular abnormalities are essential for the diagnosis, and may be documented by visual evoked response testing if foveal hypoplasia and nystagmus are not obvious by clinical inspection. The finding of tyrosinase on hair-bulb assay is helpful for medical counseling in that later acquisition of pigment and less stigmatization can be anticipated. Ophthalmologic examination is essential throughout life, and school arrangements must include provision for large-type texts, appropriate seating, and use of high-contrast visual materials (King et al., 2001). Auditory evoked response studies are not indicated in oculocutaneous albinism unless one of the rare syndromes involving albinism and deafness is suspected.

Parents should be counseled about the damaging effects of loud noise, and told to warn health care professionals about the risks of ototoxic antibiotics in their child. The most important protective measures will be to minimize exposure to sun, using sunglasses, long-sleeved clothing, hats, and sunscreens (sun protection factor above 25). Counseling should include practical advice about the occurrence of damaging high-intensity ultraviolet in late morning/early afternoon and its reflections from sandy beaches or clouds should be provided. Parents will have a 25% recurrence risk consistent with an autosomal-recessive disorder, and DNA testing is available for confirmation of diagnoses (see www.genetests.org). Parent information for various types of albinism is available at NOAH– National Organization for Albinism and Hypopigmentation disorders (www.albinism.org/), Albinism Fellowship UK (www.albinism.org.uk/).

Oculocutaneous albinism type 2

Formerly distinguished as tyrosinase-positive, "partial," "imperfect," or "incomplete" albinism, oculocutaneous albinism type 2 is caused by a mutation in the P gene, the human homologue of the *pink* gene causing a form of murine albinism (King et al., 2001; Tomita and Suzuki, 2004). This gene is found within the chromosome 15 region that is deleted or abnormally imprinted in the Prader–Willi and Angelman syndromes. Alterations of the P gene explain why some patients with the Prader–Willi and Angelman syndromes have albinoid characteristics such as optic abnormalities, light hair, blue eyes, and pale skin.

Depending on their geographic area, Caucasian individuals with oculocutaneous albinism type 2 vary from minimal (e.g., Scandinavian origin) to moderate (e.g., Mediterranean origin) pigment at birth. The milder patients are hard to distinguish from normal individuals of European descent, who change from blond hair, white skin, and blue eyes as children to darker shades as adults. Most affected individuals of African origin have yellow or yellow-red hair at birth, with blue eyes and white skin (King et al., 2001). In both blacks and whites, affected individuals acquire some pigment with age, including pigmented nevi and freckles with minimal tanning of the skin. Preventive management will be as outlined for oculocutaneous albinism type 1, with ophthalmologic monitoring, provision for visual assistance at school, and protection from sun. Genetic counseling and parent resources are also the same, with parent information available at NOAH–National Organization for Albinism and Hypopigmentation disorders (www.albinism.org/), Albinism Fellowship UK (www.albinism.org.uk/).

Ocular albinism

Two major types of ocular albinism have been described, one exhibiting X-linked recessive and the other autosomal-recessive inheritance. In each disorder, the distinguishing characteristic is hypopigmentation that is limited to the eye. King et al. (2001) emphasized that subclinical cutaneous hypopigmentation is present in individuals with ocular albinism, and that African–American individuals with X-linked ocular albinism may have hypopigmented macules on the skin. The clinical manifestations of ocular albinism are foveal hypoplasia, hypopigmented retina, decreased visual acuity, and nystagmus. The irides are translucent and light blue to brown, with a more normal brown color in African–Americans. Patches of retinal hypopigmentation and iris translucency are found in 80% of female carriers of the X-linked form of ocular albinism, but these females rarely have ocular symptoms. Preventive management of individuals with ocular albinism consists of the same ophthalmologic monitoring and school measures mentioned above for oculocutaneous albinism, with alertness for sensorineural deafness that is occasionally associated (King et al., 2001). Genetic counseling requires distinction between the X-linked and autosomal-recessive forms – both with a 25% recurrence risk except with isolated male cases: these have a 1/3 chance to be new mutations if it is the X-linked form. DNA testing can help with this distinction (see www.genetests.org) and parent information is available at NOAH – National Organization for Albinism and Hypopigmentation disorders (www.albinism.org/), Albinism Fellowship UK (www.albinism.org.uk/).

Other pigmentary disorders

Recent progress has been made in understanding complex patterns of lesions produced by certain genetic skin disorders (Paller, 2004). Many of these disorders are caused by genes with severe effects on cell growth/development, so that patients surviving to be born often exhibit somatic mosaicism (mixtures of normal and mutant, or of single-mutant and double-mutant cells). Effects of the mutation on skin, when they are manifest during embryogenesis, may occur in segments of the body or trace the migration of the earliest ectodermal precursors – the lines of Blaschko. Linear patterns of light and dark, inflammation or tumor can result, depending on the onset and degree of mosaicism Segmental café-au-lait spots or neurofibromata in patients mosaic for neurofibromatosis-1 (autosomal-dominant mosaicism) is an example, as are the patterned lesions of hypomelanosis of Ito (chromosomal mosaicism), and Goltz syndrome or incontinentia pigmenti (X-linked mosaicism) discussed below. Mosaicism can be straightforward as mutant/non-mutant cells (type 1) or complex with a primary mutation causing mild skin changes of wide distribution and a secondary loss of heterozygosity (removing the normal allele) causing exacerbation along lines of Blaschko [type 2 mosaicism (Paller, 2004)]. These types of mosaicism have been confirmed by molecular analysis of affected/normal or severe/mild skin regions, and Paller (2004) points out that future studies may allow correlation of skin patterns with mutant percentages in germ cells, allowing precise risks for transmission to be assigned.

Focal dermal hypoplasia (Goltz–Gorlin syndrome)

More than 200 cases of focal dermal hypoplasia have been reported after the initial descriptions of Goltz in 1962 and Gorlin in 1963 (Jones, 1997, pp. 532–3; Gorlin et al., 2001, pp. 571–6). Over 90% of affected patients are female, raising the possibility of X-linked dominant inheritance with male lethality.

Summary of clinical concerns: Goltz–Gorlin syndrome management considerations

Growth and development: Short stature (25%).

Eye: Eye anomalies (40% of patients) include colobomata of the iris or retina, microphthalmia, strabismus, ectopia lentis, and nystagmus: Initial and regular ophthalmology evaluations.

ENT: Mixed hearing loss is fairly common, with cleft palate and dental problems (hypoplastic enamel, missing teeth, abnormal dental roots) being frequent (Balmer et al., 2005): Early auditory evoked response and audiology assessment, regular dental care, cleft palate team when appropriate.

Surface-skin: Skin findings are distinctive in Goltz–Gorlin syndrome, with linear or reticular hyperpigmented lesions and telangiectases. Supernumerary nipples, asymmetry of the breasts, and subcutaneous nodules are also common, and the finger and toenails are often hypoplastic or malformed.

Skeletal: Skeletal changes include fused or short fingers, absent or extra fingers, scoliosis, congenital hip dislocation, and rib anomalies: Regular skeletal examinations screening for congenital dislocated hip and later scoliosis.

Gastrointenstinal: Omphalocele, diaphragmatic hernia, umbilical hernia: Neonatal evaluations with appropriate surgical referral.

Urogenital: Urogenital defects include hydronephrosis, horseshoe kidney, labial hypoplasia, and cryptorchidism: Renal sonogram when diagnosis is made, monitoring for urinary tract infections, referral to urology when anomalies are detected.

Neurologic: Only 15% have mild mental disability, but brain anomalies including hydrocephalus, Arnold–Chiari malformation, or spina bifida have been reported: Consider neurology referral and head magnetic resonance imaging (MRI) in those with rapid head growth or other symptoms.

Parental counseling: Balmer et al. (2004) support the mechanism of X-linked dominant inheritance of Goltz syndrome by demonstrating the tooth enamel hypoplasia and root changes show the patchy pattern expected from Lyonization effects (random inactivation of the mutated versus normal X chromosome during embryogenesis). Recurrence risks could theoretically be up to 50% for affected females, depending on whether they transmit their normal or mutated X chromosome. Mothers of new cases should be examined carefully for manifestations, but in general should have very low recurrence risks for future children. Parent information is available at several medical education sites by searching on the syndrome name.

Hypomelanosis of Ito syndrome

Originally recognized by Ito in 1952, the combination of depigmented whorls and macules together with neurologic problems has been called hypomelanosis of Ito syndrome or incontinentia pigmenti achromians (Jones, 1977, pp. 504–5). The latter name reflects the idea that the hypomelanosis resembles a negative image of the pigmented lesions in incontinentia pigmenti. Hypomelanosis of Ito is clearly a heterogeneous phenotype with one cause being chromosomal mosaicism (Sybert, 1994). In these patients, cell lines of different chromosome constitution are differently pigmented and produce linear markings along the lines of Blaschko as described for type I mosaicism above (Paller, 2004). Several different chromosomes have been involved. Skin biopsy and fibroblast culture may be required to demonstrate the mosaicism, since some patients have normal peripheral blood karyotyping.

In other patients with hypomelanosis of Ito syndrome, the presence of macrocephaly and limb asymmetry suggests a hamartosis or overgrowth syndrome analogous to neurofibromatosis. Neurologic problems include micro- or macrocephaly, seizures, and mental disability, which may be more severe than predicted by the degree of mosaicism. Some patients have ocular anomalies (microphthalmia, strabismus, nystagmus, the latter two suggestive of ocular albinism).

Preventive management of hypomelanosis of Ito should initially focus on the presence of neurologic abnormalities, for these will establish the need for early intervention and neurosensory evaluations. Cranial sonography and neurology evaluation should be performed on children with small head circumference or with neurologic symptoms. Subsequent management will include regular ophthalmologic assessment, monitoring of growth for asymmetry and of development for learning problems, and skeletal evaluation for limb length discrepancies and scoliosis. The skin lesions may be more apparent by Wood's light examination, and it is important to note that they are not preceded by vesicular or verrucous rashes of the type seen in incontinentia pigmenti.

Parents will typically have low recurrence risks and not require chromosome studies; information is available at several medical education sites by searching on the syndrome name.

Incontinentia pigmenti

While vesicular and pigmentary skin lesions are most characteristic of incontinentia pigmenti, more than 50% of patients have manifestations outside of the integument (Jones, 1997, pp. 502–3; Gorlin et al., 2001, pp. 551–4). The disorder was best defined by the work of Bloch, Sulzberger, and others in the 1920s, and it is sometimes referred to as Bloch–Sulzberger syndrome. Incontinentia pigmenti exhibits X-linked dominant inheritance with high lethality in males that results in over 97% of patients being female. Genetic mutations in the NF-kappaB essential modulator

(NEMO) cause incontinentia pigmenti, and less severe mutations in this gene cause ectodermal dysplasia with immunodeficiency in males (Bruckner, 2004).

There are four phases in the clinical course of incontinentia pigmenti, inflammatory, verrucous, hyperpigmented, and atrophic. The first occurs in infancy, often presenting as an eczematoid rash with eosinophilia that may reach as high as 70–80% of the peripheral white blood cell count. The rash is typically vesicular, with clustered or linear lesions that change to papules after the first month of life. Coincident with or shortly after the vesicular phase is the second phase of hyperkeratosis, consisting of warty lesions over the dorsal surfaces of the digits, joints, and limbs. Finally, the third and most characteristic phase appears, with linear or reticular patches of brown/gray pigment. There may be prominent whorls of pigmented and depigmented areas that usually fade in early childhood; remnants of these pigmentary changes can often be found in adults. The pigmentary findings may be confused with the hypomelanosis of Ito spectrum, which includes chromosomal mosaicism as an etiology, or the rare Naegeli syndrome, which exhibits autosomal-dominant inheritance. Referral to dermatology and a diagnostic skin biopsy should thus be part of the initial diagnostic evaluation for incontinentia pigmenti.

Other complications are reminiscent of ectodermal dysplasia with sparse hair and conical or absent teeth. The eye anomalies are more severe, with optic atrophy, strabismus, cataract, and retinal detachment. Correlating with optic atrophy are numerous central nervous system abnormalities in 35–40% of patients. Mental disability, microcephaly, hydrocephalus, and seizures may occur. Several patients with incontinentia pigmenti have suffered from frequent and unusually severe infections, but no specific defect in immunity has been characterized.

Preventive management for incontinentia pigmenti should include dermatologic and genetic referral during the initial diagnostic evaluation, ophthalmologic referral and monitoring to evaluate strabismus and/or retinal changes, and dental referral to evaluate and treat tooth anomalies. Some children with microcephaly and pigmentary changes will need chromosome studies on peripheral blood and skin fibroblasts to exclude somatic chromosomal mosaicism that is found in hypomelanosis of Ito (see above). Early intervention and psychosocial counseling services should be provided for children with incontinentia pigmenti until mental development is ascertained to be normal. Head circumference should be closely monitored during the first 2 years of life, since children are at risk for microcephaly or hydrocephalus. CT or MRI scanning of the head should be considered in children with abnormal head circumference or severe developmental delay.

Parent information is available at the Incontinentia Pigmenti International Foundation (imgen.bcm.tmc.edu/IPIF/), and there is an overview of information and experience from a parent of an affected daughter (mom_2_three_ip.tripod.com/).

LEOPARD syndrome

"LEOPARD" is an acronym coined by Gorlin and colleagues in 1971 as a mnemonic to describe an autosomal-dominant syndrome: *L*entigines, *E*lectrocardiographic conduction abnormalities, *O*cular hypertelorism, *P*ulmonary stenosis, *A*bnormalities of the Genitalia, *R*etardation of growth, and *D*eafness (Jones, 1997, pp. 531–2; Gorlin et al., 2001, pp. 555–8). Most cases of the disorder are caused by mutations in the same protein-tyrosine phosphatase non-receptor-11 (PTPN11) gene that is altered in Noonan syndrome, explaining their sharing of facial, cardiac, and genital abnormalities.

The cognate black–brown spots are usually distributed over the entire body, and may coalesce to form large patches (café-noir spots) in LEOPARD syndrome. Electrocardiographic changes include a superiorly oriented QRS axis with occasional bundle branch or complete heart block. Atrial septal defects in addition to valvular pulmonic stenosis (40% of patients) can occur, along with hypertrophic cardiomyopathy. These same cardiac findings occur in Noonan syndrome, as do the facial characteristics (hypertelorism, epicanthal folds, ptosis), short stature, genital anomalies (hypospadias, cryptorchidism), skeletal anomalies (pectus excavatum, cubitus valgus, scoliosis), and mild mental retardation seen in LEOPARD syndrome. Other complications can include renal agenesis, brain anomalies, and delayed puberty.

Preventive management for LEOPARD syndrome is identical to that for Noonan syndrome outlined in Chapter 10. In fact, the Noonan syndrome preventive management checklist could be used for children with LEOPARD syndrome. Essentials of prevention include early and regular hearing assessment, echo- and electrocardiography, periodic cardiologic assessment, evaluation of the genitalia and follow-up for micropenis, evaluation for pectus and scoliosis, and referral to early intervention with provision for inclusive education to help children with disabilities. Parent counseling is dependent on examination of parents to look for mild features – affected individuals will have a 50% transmission risk, while normal parents of affected children will have low recurrence risks. DNA testing of the PTPN11 gene is available, and parent information can be found at several medical education sites by using the syndrome name.

Waardenburg syndrome

Waardenburg syndrome is an autosomal-dominant disorder that involves hypertelorism, ventromedial hypopigmentation, and sensorineural deafness (Jones, 1997, pp. 234–5; Gorlin et al., 2001, pp. 561–6). Clinical manifestations also can include poliosis (white forelock), early graying of the hair, dystopia canthorum (lateral displacement of the inner canthi to produce a broad nasal bridge), eye anomalies such as cataracts, strabismus, or hypoplasia of the irides, and facial hirsutism with prominent eyebrows. Other pigmentary findings may include heterochromia of the irides (differently colored eyes) and vitiligo.

Several types of Waardenburg syndrome have been delineated based on clinical manifestations and molecular studies. Type I has dystopia canthorum and is caused by mutations in the PAX 3 gene, a homologue of the fruit fly *paired* gene that is important in early development. Type II does not have dystopia canthorum and is now separated into four subtypes (A–D) based on different causative mutations (a transcription factor identified in mice with microphthalmia on chromosome 3 accounts for type IIA). Type III is associated with upper limb defects (also called Klein–Waardenburg syndrome), and type IV with Hirschsprung disease (Waardenburg–Shah syndrome). The prevalence is estimated at 2–3 per million, with type II being 20 times more common than I and III/IV being very rare.

Complications of Waardenburg syndrome include increased susceptibility to dacryocystitis and bilateral congenital sensorineural hearing loss in 20% of type I patients, 50% of type II patients. Other abnormalities have included Hirschsprung disease, anal atresia, Sprengel deformity, sacral dimple, spina bifida, and limb defects with elbow and digital contractures. Cleft lip/palate also occurs, and homozygous patients with severe manifestations have been reported.

Preventive management of Waardenburg syndrome should include early hearing assessment with auditory evoked response, then audiology screening, regular ophthalmologic examinations, monitoring of feeding and bowel function to rule out intestinal atresias or Hirschsprung disease, and examination of the skeleton. Patients with thoracic or limb anomalies should have a complete skeletal radiographic survey to identify more subtle defects, and physical therapy may be required to maximize mobility. Family counseling should include contact with advocates for the deaf in appropriate cases, and explanation of 50% transmission risks in affected patients. Germ-line mosaicism has been reported, so normal parents of affected children may have risks above zero; the lack of facial characteristics in some forms emphasizes the importance of hearing testing to ensure parents are normal. Numerous medical information sites can be found by searching on the syndrome name.

Disorders with telangiectasias

Ataxia–telangiectasia

The combination of ataxia with telangiectasias of the ears, conjunctiva, and cheeks is an autosomal-recessive disorder with an incidence of about 1 in 100,000 births. The ataxia derives from cerebellar anomalies that include atropy and diminished numbers of Purkinje cells. There are other ocular anomalies such as strabismus, photophobia, and nystagmus, and the face becomes rigid with a staring expression and fixation nystagmus (Gorlin et al., 1990, pp. 469–71). Sinopulmonary infections are recurrent in 75–80% of patients, often with decreased amounts of serum immunoglobulin A. Ataxia–telangiectasia could also be categorized as an accelerated aging/neoplasia syndrome, since there is early graying, scleroderma of the skin with poikiloderma (mixed streaks of hypo- and hyperpigmentation), and a predisposition to lymphomas, Hodgkin disease, leukemias, and carcinomas (stomach, skin, liver, ovary, breast; Lynch et al., 1994). Telangiectasias may also affect the oral and nasal mucosa, producing epistaxis.

Preventive management of ataxia–telangiectasia should include regular ophthalmologic examinations, initial neurologic evaluation with consideration of cerebellar imaging, and regular pediatric follow-up with alertness for upper respiratory infections, sinusitis, and lymphoid or solid tumors. Serum immunoglobulin electrophoresis may be useful in deciding whether gamma-globulin therapy may be tried; many patients also have thymic hypoplasia and diminished cellular immunity.

Osler–Rendu–Weber syndrome (Hereditary hemorrhagic telangiectasia)

Hereditary hemorrhagic telangiectasia is an autosomal-dominant disorder with symptomatology that depends on which organs are afflicted with angiodysplasias. The prevalence of the disorder is about 1 in 100,000 individuals, with accounts of more than 1500 persons in the literature. Infants are rarely affected, and pediatric management will usually concern older children or adolescents. Superficial telangiectasias often occur on the cheeks, ears, and nasal mucosa, with 95% of patients experiencing severe epistaxis (Gorlin et al., 1990, pp. 476–8; Jones, 1997, p. 524). The lips, tongue, and gingiva are also frequent sites of telangiectasias, and bleeding from the mouth can be a serious complication. Pulmonary arteriovenous fistulas (15–25% of patients), gastrointestinal lesions (20–45%), urinary tract lesions, and cerebral lesions leading to intracranial hemorrhage and cerebral abscess are other abnormalities that can cause death. As expected for a disorder with multiple telangiectasias, platelet trapping and thrombocytopenia can occur.

Preventive management for Rendu–Weber–Osler syndrome requires careful initial examination for superficial telangiectasias and subsequent monitoring for evidence of internal lesions. Minor traumas such as tooth brushing may elicit superficial bleeding, so counseling regarding gentle grooming techniques and initial management of nose/mouth bleeding with ice and compresses should be provided. Regular urinalysis and stool guaiac screening are useful for the detection of internal bleeding, and regular blood pressure/cardiac assessments should be made for evidence of arteriovenous fistulas. Complaints of chest pain or headache require thorough evaluation to exclude pulmonary or intracranial bleeding.

Rothmund–Thomson syndrome

Rothmund–Thomson syndrome is an autosomal-recessive disorder that involves short stature, mixed hyper- and hypopigmentation of the skin (poikiloderma), photosensitivity, eye anomalies, and hypogonadism (Jones, 1997, pp. 148–9).

The eye anomalies include cataracts, strabismus, and microcornea. The teeth are also abnormal, with microdontia, supernumerary teeth, and absent teeth (Gorlin et al., 1990, pp. 489–91). Most patients have short stature with thin hair and dysplastic nails. Skeletal anomalies (thumb or radial aplasia), genital anomalies (micropenis in males, scanty menstruation with infertility in females), and predisposition to sarcomas (squamous cell, osteosarcomas) have been described.

Preventive management of Rothmund–Thomson syndrome should include monitoring of growth and genital development, with consideration of endocrinologic evaluation for growth hormone deficiency/supplementation. Dermatologic evaluation of the skin and regular ophthalmologic examinations are important, and cosmetic options may be needed for the sparse hair, eyebrows, and eyelashes. Cystic lesions and fragility of the bones together with acquired flexion contractures mandate periodic physical therapy and orthopedic evaluation. Patients should avoid exposure to sun and observe the same precautions of long-sleeved clothing and sunscreen recommended for patients with albinism.

Disorders with radiation sensitivity and/or rapid aging

Cockayne syndrome

Cockayne syndrome is now known to denote a group of disorders that share autosomal-recessive inheritance, growth failure, and accelerated aging. (Jones, 1997, pp. 144–5; Gorlin et al., 2001, pp. 596–600, 767–9). The cerebro-oculo-facial syndrome, also known as Pena–Shokeir type II, belongs in this category while other conditions with microcephaly and eye changes (e.g., MICRO syndrome, congenital infections) do not (Graham et al., 2004). Skin fibroblasts from patients in the Cockayne syndrome group exhibit enhanced death rates when exposed to ultraviolet light due to a defect in nucleotide excision repair. By co-cultivating cell lines from different Cockayne patients, specific sub-types of the disease can be recognized since mutations in different DNA repair genes will complement each other and restore normal ultraviolet light sensitivity. Several complementation groups have been identified for classical Cockayne patients with normal infancies and later accelerated aging, while others have been identified in patients with the cerebro-oculo-facial syndrome presentation that exhibits microcephaly and severe problems at birth. Some of the responsible genes have been isolated, including the DNA excision repair genes Cockayne syndrome A (CSA), CSB, or excision repair complementation 6 (ERCC6). These genes are highly conserved in evolution and have homologues that mediate radiation sensitivity in yeast. This conservation testifies to their essential role in DNA repair, their severe human phenotypes, and their extreme effects may give insight into natural aging processes.

Clinical manifestations of the Cockayne syndrome group will vary in presentation from infancy to mid-childhood. They include a characteristic face with sunken eyes and a prominent nose, growth delay beginning in the second to third year of life, photosensitivity with erythematous dermatitis appearing on sun-exposed areas, retinitis pigmentosa, and progressive mental disability with microcephaly, ataxia, and demyelination. As the patient reaches mid- to later childhood, the full complement of aging-related disabilities can occur, including diabetes mellitus, hypertension, osteoporosis, and cachexia. The transition from normal infancy to childhood elder is one of the most striking in medicine, as the affected teenager lays helpless, contracted, senile, and feeble, with sparse hair, wrinkled skin, and cataracts that reminds one of a nursing home patient. Death is inevitable in the severe form, but some of the complementation groups are associated with a milder course.

Preventive management for Cockayne syndrome will include an initial diagnostic evaluation to document retinitis (ophthalmologic evaluation), demyelination (MRI or CT head scan), and skeletal radiographic survey to document thickening of the skull bones, platyspondyly, and osteoporosis. Subsequent management will be chiefly palliative, with maintenance of calories (gastrostomy is often required), avoidance of sunlight, and screening for glycosuria, hypertension, and bony deformities secondary to osteoporosis. Regular ophthalmologic examinations may be helpful in preserving some vision.

Parental counseling should emphasize early intervention/preschool services for early presentations, providing therapy and support for families. The Share and Care Cockayne syndrome Support Group (www.cockayne-syndrome.org/) has international affiliations with parent and professional information, and several medical information sites can be accessed by searching on the syndrome name. Many states have programs for medically dependent children that can help with nursing care; these applications should be initiated when significant disabilities first appear, as there may be long waiting periods. The nursing assistance should transition to hospice services once the child is severely affected and bed ridden. Genetic counseling will emphasize the 25% recurrence risk for autosomal-recessive disease regardless of classical or infantile presentation; fibroblast sensitivity to ultraviolet light can be quantified as an assay for diagnosis and prenatal diagnosis, now supplemented by DNA testing for mutations in the CSA and CSB genes offered by a few laboratories (see www.genetests.org). Mutations in these genes account for 80% of affected patients.

Xeroderma pigmentosum

Patients with xeroderma pigmentosum also exhibit photosensitivity and damage from sunlight, with progressive freckling and hemangiomatosis. Like Cockayne syndrome, the disorder is autosomal recessive and exhibits a degenerative course with loss of scalp hair, loss of subcutaneous fat, and progressive mental disability (Jones, 1997, pp. 552–3; Gorlin et al., 2001, pp. 600–606). Also like Cockayne, studies in cultured fibroblasts have defined many complementation groups and defined mutations in non-excision DNA repair genes. Many of the genes responsible for xeroderma pigmentosum participate in a non-excision repair complex with those affected in Cockayne syndrome, are related through highly conserved evolutionary motifs, and are denoted by similar names [e.g., Xeroderma Pigmentosum A-XPA, ERCC3, etc. (Hengge, 2005)].

The usual presentation in xeroderma pigmentosum is marked sensitivity to sunlight manifest in early childhood. Sun-exposed areas develop freckles that enlarge and are interspersed with light spots to produce a "salt and pepper" appearance. Skin atropy, lipodystrophy, hair loss, and telangiectasias produce an aged appearance, and scarring may interfere with eye or mouth opening. The most severe problem concerns predisposition to keratosis and skin neoplasms such as basal cell carcinomas, squamous cell carcinomas, and melanomas – these may appear as early as age 2 years. Oral complications include pigmented macules on the lip and tongue that may degenerate into squamous cell carcinomas. Ocular complications (40%) include photophobia, conjunctivitis, and persistent lacrimation, and neurologic complications (20%) include spasticity, hyporeflexia, and movement disorders with athetosis and ataxia. Sensorineural deafness and mental retardation occur more often in the Sanctis–DeCacchione sub-type, and the more severe forms have progressive microcephaly with cortical atrophy.

Preventive management consists first of sunlight avoidance and protection, then of facial, dental, and eye care to minimize the effects of scarring, photophobia and conjunctivitis. Patients must be monitored closely for neoplasm of the skin and mouth, and early intervention/developmental assessments will be needed in those with severe skin manifestations, for they are most likely to have neurologic problems. Early developmental pediatric and neurology referral to manage motor delays, speech apraxias, spasticity, peripheral neuropathy, incoordination, and movement disorders are needed in such patients.

Parental counseling will involve the same medical assistance and hospice programs as discussed for Cockayne syndrome for those with severely affected patients, and parent information is available from the Xeroderma Pigmentosum Society (www.xps.org/). An exciting development is the initiation of clinical trials of gene therapy directed at the skin (Hengge, 2005), and parents should be made aware of such trials through the support group with options for referral to appropriate centers. Such options emphasize the importance of genetic counseling for the 25% recurrence risk and of skin fibroblast studies or DNA testing to confirm the sub-type and allow prenatal diagnosis (see www.genetests.org).

Progeria (Hutchinson–Gilford syndrome)

Hair loss and accelerated aging are the most dramatic signs of the Hutchinson–Gilford progeria syndrome, but growth failure, hearing loss, dental crowding, joint contractures, joint degeneration, and atherosclerotic cardiovascular disease are additional features (Jones, 1997, pp. 138–41; Gorlin et al., 2001, pp. 584–5). Recently, the disorder has been traced to mutations in the lamin A gene that encodes a constituent of the nuclear matrix (Pollex and Hegele, 2004). Similarities of progeria to the later-onset Werner syndrome of accelerated aging are indicated by the fact that some patients classified as Werner were found to have lamin A mutations and reclassified as progeria. Complications of progeria can be further correlated with other phenotypes caused by lamin A mutations – cardiomyopathy with conduction defects, Emery–Dreifuss and limb-girdle muscular dystrophy, lipodystrophy, mandibuloacral dysplasia aging syndrome, and even one form of Charcot–Marie–Tooth syndrome. The demonstration of heterozygous lamin A mutations indicates that progeria is an autosomal-dominant disorder, with most affected patients having mutations and rare affected siblings due to germinal mosaicism.

Children with progeria begin with normal growth that plateaus after the first year and remains at the 3-year-old level. Hair and eyebrow loss begins in the second year, and the face becomes distinctive with a prominent cranium, absent eyebrows and lashes, small ears, beaked nose, and micrognathia. Intelligence is normal with occasional sensorineural hearing loss. There is progressive thinning of the skin with lipoatrophy and an aged appearance. Skeletal changes include osteolysis of the terminal phalanges and hip joints, which provide diagnostic clues on skeletal radiographs. Cardiac changes include murmurs and cardiomyopathy, with severe atherosclerosis, myocardial infarctions, and strokes that limit life span to an average of 13–14 years.

Preventive management of progeria should include early hearing assessment, maintenance of nutrition, regular dental care, and surveillance of joint movement so that contractures and degeneration can be ameliorated with splinting and/or physical therapy. Cardiovascular symptoms can appear as early as 5 years of age, so cholesterol screening and treatment with resins, drugs, or lipophoresis should be carried out from birth. Family support is important, and information can be found at the Hutchinson–Gilford Progeria syndrome Network (www.hgps.net/), the Progeria Research Foundation (www.progeriaresearch.org/), and the Progeria Project Foundation (www.progeriaproject.com/). Most parents will have a low but not negligible recurrence risk of 1–2% because of possible germinal mosaicism.

Part VII

The management of neurologic and neurodegenerative syndromes

Although many malformation syndromes affect the nervous system, some are more distinctive for unusual neurologic or neurodegenerative manifestations. Chapter 18 will discuss syndromes that involve unusual neuromuscular symptoms, such as the arthrogryposes, and Chapter 19 will discuss some chronic metabolic disorders that are associated with neurodegeneration. Selected metabolic disorders with acute presentations are discussed in Chapter 20. The classic reference of Scriver et al. (2001) provides an encyclopedic and detailed description of inborn errors of metabolism, and this reference should be consulted for detailed therapeutic management.

18

Neurologic syndromes including the arthrogryposes

Abnormalities of development have a disproportionate impact on the more complex body structures, illustrated by the nervous and cardiovascular systems. Most malformation syndromes involve neurologic abnormalities, but this chapter focuses on those notable for pain insensitivity, brain anomalies, or congenital contractures (Table 18.1).

Table 18.1. Syndromes with brain anomalies and/or arthrogryposis

Syndrome	Incidence*	Inheritance	Complications
Syndromes with neuropathy and/or self-mutilation			
Riley–Day	1 in 10,000 (J)	AR	Hypotonia, fixed facial expression, keratitis, scoliosis, dysarthric speech, Charcot joints
HSAN I	~50 cases	AD	Sensory neuropathy (feet), foot ulcers, shooting leg pains, deafness, peroneal atrophy
HSAN II	~50 cases	AR	Sensory neuropathy (digits), acroosteolysis, digital mutilation, hyperhidrosis, Charcot joints
HSAN III Riley–Day	1 in 10,000 (J)	AR	Sensorimotor and autonomic neuropathy, hypotonia, fixed facial expression, keratitis, scoliosis, dysarthric speech, Charcot joints
HSAN IV	~25 cases	AR	Sensorimotor/autonomic neuropathy, hyperpyrexia, hypohidrosis, orodigital mutilation
Lesch–Nyhan	~150 cases	XLR	Dystonia, choreoathetosis, hyperuricemia, neurodegeneration, orodigital mutilation
Syndromes with brain anomalies			
Aicardi	~25 cases	XLD	Agenesis of the corpus callosum, lacunar retinal defects, costovertebral a.
FG	~50 cases	XLR	Frontal hair whorl, ptosis, imperforate anus
Walker–Warburg	~50 cases	AR	Lissencephaly, retinal detachment, muscular dystrophy

(cont.)

Table 18.1. (*cont.*)

Syndrome	Incidence*	Inheritance	Complications
Syndromes with contractures (arthrogryposis)			
Amyoplasia	1 in 10,000	Sporadic	Limb contractures, micrognathia, muscle atrophy, "policeman's tip" position of hands
Marden–Walker	~50 cases	AR	Limb contractures, immobile facies, blepharophimosis, scoliosis, FTT, DD
Multiple pterygium	~60 cases	AR	Limb and digital contractures, pterygia of neck and limbs, cleft palate, scoliosis, genital a.
Pena–Shokeir I	1 in 10,000	AR	Camptodactyly, club feet, hypertelorism, pulmonary hypoplasia, urogenital a., cardiac a.
Pena–Shokeir II	~25 cases	AR	Hip and knee ankyloses, microcephaly, brain a., cataracts, degenerative course, DD
Popliteal pterygium	~80 cases	AD	Limb and digital contractures, popliteal pterygia, cleft palate, genital a.
Schwartz–Jampel	~50 case	AR	Limb contractures, puckered facies, blepharophimosis, scoliosis, FTT, DD
Whistling face (Freeman–Sheldon)	~65 cases	AD, AR	Distal limb contractures, microstomia and "whistling face," facial immobility, deviated ("windvane") fingers

Notes:

J, Jewish population; HSAN, hereditary sensory and autonomic neuropathy; AD, autosomal dominant; AR, autosomal recessive, XLR, X-linked dominant; XLD, X-linked dominant; DD, developmental disability; FTT, failure to thrive.

* Cases or per number of live births.

Pain insensitivity syndromes

Familial dysautonomia (Riley–Day syndrome) and the hereditary sensory neuropathies

Riley–Day syndrome has an incidence of 1 in 10–20,000 births in Ashkenazic Jews and is 100-fold more rare in non-Jewish populations (Gorlin et al., 2001, pp. 733–6). It is an autosomal-recessive syndrome involving generalized dysfunction of the peripheral nervous system. Many of the clinical manifestations of Riley–Day syndrome overlap with other genetic disorders that are grouped together as hereditary sensory and autonomic neuropathies (HSAN). Four types of HSAN have been delineated (Table 18.1), and other types undoubtedly occur. In contrast to patients with Riley–Day syndrome, those with other types of HSAN may exhibit self-mutilation of the lips and hands (Table 18.1).

Familial dysautonomia is caused by mutations in the IkappaB kinase complex-associated protein gene, with a specific splicing mutation responsible for 95% of affected patients of Ashkenazi Jewish origin (Casella et al., 2005). The disorder was formerly diagnosed by a lack of axon flare after intracutaneous injection of 0.01 ml of 1:10,000 histamine solution or miosis of the pupil after exposure to 0.0625% pilocarpine eyedrops; now DNA diagnosis is available and very sensitive for families of Jewish background.

Neonatal manifestations of Riley–Day syndrome include breech presentation (30%), premature rupture of membranes (30%), and neonatal hypotonia and feeding problems with a poor suck (60%). In childhood, there is growth delay, diminished deep-tendon reflexes, fixed or frightened facial expression, absent tears, absent tongue papillae, and hypersalivation. There is also indifference to pain but hypersensitivity to touch (dysesthesia), episodic appearance of erythematous macules over the trunk and limbs, and progressive scoliosis appearing around age 8–9 years. Intelligence is normal, but speech is often monotonous or slurred. Other manifestations of neuropathy include sleep apnea (insensitivity to carbon dioxide), Charcot joints (insensitivity to pain), keratitis and corneal ulceration (absent corneal reflex and tears), recurrent aspiration and drooling (diminished gag reflex and dysphagia), and cold hands and feet with poor tolerance of exercise (diminished epinephrine response). Additional complications of the HSAN group include scarring of the lips and fingers, risks of osteomyelitis and fractures, severe dental decay with self-extraction of teeth, and occasional intestinal perforation.

Preventive management for Riley–Day syndrome and related sensory neuropathies should include early and regular ophthalmologic evaluations to protect against corneal abrasions and vision loss. Feeding and nutrition should be watched closely, with regular chest radiographs to assess chronic aspiration and pneumonia. Sleep studies should be performed in later childhood and adolescence, and regular dental care is needed for malocclusion and crowding in Riley–Day syndrome, or for dental caries in the HSAN group. Anesthesia is accompanied by risks of hypotension and cardiac arrest. Orthopedic referral should be considered in early adolescence because of scoliosis and joint damage from pain insensitivity. Early intervention may be needed because of motor delays, and psychosocial counseling should be facilitated for adolescents because of their somatic and behavioral differences.

Lesch–Nyhan syndrome

Lesch–Nyhan syndrome is an X-linked recessive disorder that causes severe self-mutilation and mental deficiency in affected males (Gorlin et al., 2001, pp. 736–8; Jinnah & Friedmann, 2001). The original description of the disease was followed shortly by the demonstration of hypoxanthine-guanine phosphoribosyl transferase deficiency as the basic defect. Molecular analysis is now available, which allows the recognition of female carriers who have a 25% risk of having affected sons (see www. genetests.org). More than 150 cases have been reported.

Clinical manifestations of Lesch–Nyhan syndrome include a normal neonatal period with onset of hypertonia and motor delay by age 6 months. The neurologic features usually lead to the diagnosis, with opisthotonic posturing, dystonia, and choreoathetosis in most patients. The onset of self-mutilation occurs between ages 4 months and 4 years, involving the lips, fingers, and shoulders. Mental deficiency is often severe, with dysarthric speech and occasional normal intelligence. Hyperuricemia can cause orange "sand" or "crystals" in the diaper, with later nephrolithiasis and obstructive uropathy. Subcutaneous or auricular tophi are common, but gouty arthritis is not. Interestingly, patients with partial enzyme deficiencies have hyperuricemia and gouty arthritis without neurologic problems (Rossiter & Caskey, 1995). Other clinical manifestations include propensity for infection, megaloblastic anemia because of folate deficiency, and testicular atrophy.

Preventive management for Lesch–Nyhan syndrome consists of pharmacologic therapy for hyperuricemia, hydration to prevent urinary tract stones or damage, and restraints to minimize the injuries from self-mutilation. Early neurologic evaluation and early intervention services are important, although no effective medication for the dystonia or choreoathetosis has been found. Periodic urinalyses, blood urea nitrogen and creatinine, and complete blood counts should be performed to screen for renal or hematologic problems. Hyman (1996) reviewed the behavioral modification, pharmacologic, and physical restraints that have been employed for patients with self-mutilation. Behavior enhancement through positive reinforcement of alternative activities (e.g., crafts rather than hand in mouth), together with elbow restraints that allow freedom of the hands, offer the best options for patients with Lesch–Nyhan syndrome (Hyman, 1996). The anticonvulsants, antidepressants, and neuroleptics that have been tried in other disorders with self-mutilation have not been effective in Lesch–Nyhan syndrome. Parent and physician-oriented information can be found at numerous medical education sites by searching on the syndrome name.

Syndromes with brain anomalies

Aicardi syndrome

Aicardi and colleagues characterized a syndrome involving myoclonic epilepsy, brain anomalies including agenesis of the corpus callosum, and chorioretinal defects or "lacunae" in 1969 (Aicardi, 2005; Jones, 1997, pp. 534–5). The disorder usually affects females, and is thought to follow X-linked dominant inheritance with male lethality. Two severely affected males have been reported, supporting this hypothesis. Several patients have had chromosome anomalies centering on the Xp22.3 region, providing a candidate location for the responsible gene that has not yet been characterized.

With their microcephaly and retinal defects, infants with Aicardi syndrome must first be distinguished from those with congenital infections. Clinical manifestations include persistent hyperplastic primary vitreous, costovertebral defects with absent or malformed ribs, scoliosis, hemivertebrae, and various benign or malignant tumors. Mental disability is usually severe, but survival can be prolonged. Menezes et al. (1994) reported 76% survival at age 6 years and 40% survival at age 15 years, with 21% of the patients being able to walk or crawl and 29% having some language ability.

Preventive management of Aicardi syndrome will require an initial evaluation including cranial MRI scan, skeletal radiographic survey, and ophthalmologic examinations. Patients with seizures should have neurologic evaluations, and typical electroencephalographic findings have been reported. Anticonvulsant therapy, attention to nutrition with tube feeding or gastrostomy, and early intervention referrals will be needed. Parents will have an extremely low recurrence risk, and parent information is available at the Aicardi Syndrome Foundation (www.aicardisyndrome.org/) or at several medical education websites.

Walker–Warburg syndrome

Walker–Warburg syndrome is one of a group of disorders with muscle-eye-brain disease that includes Fukayama congenital muscular dystrophy (Gorlin et al., 2001, pp. 731–3). It was first delineated using the acronym "HARD-E," where the letters stood for Hydrocephalus, Agyria, Retinal Dysplasia, and Encephalocele (Jones, 1997, pp. 192–3). Walker and Warburg published descriptions of affected patients, and the agyria places Walker–Warburg syndrome in the group of lissencephalies that includes the Miller–Dieker syndrome with submicroscopic chromosome 17 deletions (see Chapter 9). Some patients with the condition have had mutations in the protein O-mannosyltransferase (POMT1) gene that contributes to glycosylation of alpha-dystroglycan – the dual role of dystroglycans in cortical development and muscle structure explains why some patients with Walker–Warburg syndrome have muscle changes (sometimes called Norman–Roberts syndrome) and why patients with mutations in other POMT1 gene regions have limb-girdle or Fukayama muscular dystrophy with no cerebral anomalies (Balci et al., 2005).

Summary of clinical concerns: Walker–Warburg syndrome management considerations

General: The disorder is lethal when there are severe brain anomalies, with 65% dying in the first 3 months: Early head MRI scan can guide palliative care.

Growth and Development: Monitoring of head growth to detect enlargement and hydrocephalus, and evaluation of feeding with consideration of nasogastric tube or gastrostomy for those with severe muscle weakness.

Eye: Eye anomalies include microphthalmia, iris hypoplasia, cataracts, retinal hypoplasia with detachment, and optic nerve hypoplasia: Early ophthalomology assessment and follow-up depending on the prognosis.

Urogenital: Hydronephrosis and cryptorchidism have been described: Neonatal genital examination and monitoring of urinalyses; consider renal sonogram and urology referral with signs or symptoms.

Neurologic: Walker–Warburg patients have lissencephaly, hydrocephalus and other brain anomalies including arrhinencephaly, absent corpus callosum, or Dandy–Walker malformation. As mentioned above, some patients have a peculiar type of muscular dystrophy: The initial evaluation should include a cranial MRI scan and ophthalmologic examination, and many patients will require neurosurgical evaluation.

Parental counseling: Parents should receive genetic counseling for autosomal-recessive inheritance and a 25% recurrence risk; prenatal diagnosis has been accomplished by cerebral findings on ultrasound, but its sensitivity has not been defined. Psychosocial counseling with assistance for medically compromised children and transition to hospice care should be provided.

Syndromes with congenital contractures (Arthrogryposis syndromes)

Many different disorders have been grouped under the term "arthrogryposis multiplex congenita," which encompasses any newborn with multiple contractures (Jones, 1997, pp. 170–83, 214–25; Gorlin et al., 2001, pp. 765–89). Hall (1997, 1998) demonstrated that arthogryposis multiplex congenita is not a specific autosomal-recessive disorder but a group of specific syndromes with varying inheritance and accessory manifestations. Many arthrogyposis conditions reflect constraint *in utero* (deformation), and exhibit improvement that is enhanced by multidisciplinary management (Staheli et al., 1998).

Contractures of the limbs and digits form a spectrum from mildly decreased range of motion, to obvious deformity with webbing across the joint, to severe ankylosis with fixation. The severity of joint limitation and deformity will reflect the degree and duration of fetal immobility, since the rule for fetal limb and lung development is "use it or lose it" (Hall, 1997). Joint contractures have many genetic and environmental causes, including maternal myasthenia gravis, experimental curare paralysis, agenesis of spinal motor ganglia (e.g., severe Werdnig–Hoffman disease), myopathies presenting in fetal life, and constraint of fetal movement by uterine anomalies or amniotic bands. The webs, joint contractures, muscle atrophy, and pulmonary problems are thus variations on a theme of fetal immotility that occur in several arthrogryposis syndromes (Table 18.1). Several specific conditions will now be discussed, followed by a section that outlines general preventive management for these various disorders.

Amyoplasia

Children with amyoplasia have decreased skeletal muscle mass with specific changes in limb positioning (Jones, 1997, pp. 170–1). The cause of the disorder is unknown, but trunk and limb muscles are replaced by fibrous tissue and fat with predilection for the upper shoulder girdle (Sells et al., 1996; Bernstein, 2002). It is usually a sporadic condition, and in pure form is conceived as a disruption of muscle development rather than as a malformation syndrome. Intellectual potential is normal, and functional outcomes depend on the distribution of muscle aplasia and on the aggressiveness of physical therapy and surgical treatment (Bernstein, 2002).

The face may be round, with glabellar hemangiomas and micrognathia. The hands are held in the typical "policeman's tip" configuration with the shoulders internally rotated, the wrists flexed, and the palms extended backward. The knees may be flexed or extended and the hips are flexed. Club feet, scoliosis, dimpling over the affected joints, and atrophic muscles are characteristic. Amyoplasia occurs more commonly in twins, where it is usually discordant. The diagnostic evaluation is clinical; muscle biopsies are non-specific with decreased numbers of muscle fibers (Jones, 1997, pp. 170–1; Hall, 1998).

Preventive management of amyoplasia can follow the general arthrogryposis checklist (see below). Hall (1998) and Sells et al. (1996) place particular emphasis on physical therapy to preserve what little muscle is present. However, it is important for an experienced therapist to be involved, since fractures can occur (Staheli et al., 1998). The normal intelligence and frequent improvement in patients with amyoplasia warrant optimistic medical counseling, since 85% of patients are ambulatory and achieve independent function (Sells et al., 1996). Parental counseling should emphasize the low recurrence risk and hopeful outlook, and information is available at several medical education sites and from parents of an affected child (www.forabby.com/).

Marden–Walker and Schwartz–Jampel syndromes

Marden–Walker and Schwartz–Jampel syndromes exhibit similar manifestations of joint contractures, feeding problems, failure to thrive, abnormalities of the facial muscles, and eye anomalies (Gorlin et al., 2001, pp. 779–83). Schwartz–Jampel syndrome (also known as chondrodystrophic myotonia) involves increased tone of the facial muscles, with a characteristic puckering of the lips and grimace that is present in the neonatal period. Marden–Walker syndrome involves decreased tone of the facial muscles, with decreased mobility of the mouth and sagging cheeks. Marden–Walker syndrome also involves earlier onset of contractures and more severe developmental delay than does Schwartz–Jampel syndrome, and the latter condition involves a chondrodysplasia with bowed long bones, acetabular dysplasia, and metaphyseal widening.

Both conditions exhibit autosomal-recessive inheritance, and prenatal diagnosis may be approached through ultrasonography. Schwartz–Jampel syndrome is heterogenous with mutations documented in the HSPG2 gene (a heparan sulfate proteoglycan within the basement membrane of cells also called perlecan) or the leukemia inhibitory factor receptor (LIFR or gp190 chain) gene (Dagoneau et al., 2004). Gene(s) responsible for Marden–Walker syndrome have not been characterized.

Preventive management of Schwartz–Jampel and Marden–Walker syndromes can follow the general arthrogryposis checklist with attention to certain special concerns. Both conditions will require attention to feeding and nutrition, and specialists in oromotor function may be helpful (Staheli, 1998). Anesthesia must be performed by experienced personnel because of potential mobility constraints, pulmonary hypoplasia, or kyphoscoliosis. Ophthalmologic assessment and follow-up is important because of ptosis, blepharospasm, and/or myopia in Schwarz–Jampel syndrome and ptosis, blepharophimosis, and/or strabismus in Marden–Walker syndrome. Renal cysts have been observed, and may be a clue for prenatal ultrasound diagnosis. Orthopedic and physical therapy evaluations are emphasized because both syndromes have multiple skeletal changes in addition to joint contractures, including pectus and scoliosis. Mental deficiency occurs in 25% of patients with Schwartz–Jampel syndrome and nearly all cases of Marden–Walker syndrome, indicating the importance of early intervention services and developmental assessments. Alertness for aspiration and pneumonias should be maintained, with immunoglobulin A deficiency being reported in Schwartz–Jampel syndrome. Carbamezapine has been beneficial in treating the myotonia of Schwartz–Jampel syndrome. Marden–Walker syndrome was first reported as a connective tissue dysplasia, so periodic evaluation for hernias, easy bruising, stretch marks, and mitral valve prolapse should be performed as with the disorders discussed in Chapter 16.

Schwartz–Jampel and Marden–Walker syndromes are proven autosomal recessives with 25% recurrence risks for parents of affected children. Pediatric genetic referral is essential for accurate diagnosis of these complex disorders that overlap with other arthrogryposis syndromes. Parent information on the syndromes is available at medical education sites and there is a support network for Marden–Walker syndrome listed on WebMD: (my.webmd.com/hw/health_guide_atoz/shc29maw.asp).

Multiple pterygium, popliteal pterygium, and Bartsocas–Papas syndromes

An overlapping group of disorders is characterized by arthrogyposis and *in utero* immobility that produces webs (pterygia) over the affected joints (Jones, 1997, pp. 304–7; Gorlin et al., 2001, pp. 771–9). These disorders may be confused with those involving a webbed neck (e.g., Noonan syndrome, Turner syndrome) or with other forms of arthrogryposis, since any condition with prenatal onset of limb immobility may produce webbing. Multiple pterygium syndrome is distinguished by having pterygia of the neck with cervical vertebral anomalies and frequent kyphoscoliosis (Table 18.1). Popliteal webs, kyphoscoliosis, club feet, and digital syndactyly can occur in all three conditions, but digital defects, ectrodactyly, and unusual bands between jaw and neck occur in popliteal pterygium syndrome. Bartsocas–Papas syndrome has hypoplastic/absent thumbs with more severe popliteal pterygia.

Complications include low birth weight with significant neonatal mortality in Bartsocas–Papas syndrome. Occasional choanal atresia or cleft palate can produce respiratory and feeding problems with aspiration, and conductive or sensorineural deafness is reported. Upper airway problems can join with severe kyphoscoliosis and pulmonary restriction to produce recurrent pulmonary infections and hypoxia. Limb contractures can involve the fingers and larger joints, producing camptodactyly, club feet, and webs that must be dissected carefully to avoid nerve damage during surgical correction. Frequent syndactyly and digital defects are signified by a characteristic finding in popliteal pterygium syndrome, where a triangle of skin extends over the dorsum of the great toenail (Gorlin et al., 2001, p. 775). Webs in the genital region can produce cryptorchidism and scrotal abnormalities.

Preventive management of the multiple and popliteal pterygium syndromes can follow the recommendations in the arthrogryposis checklist with more aggressive orthopedic and plastic surgical management to mobilize joints and remove webs (Staheli et al., 1998). Pulmonary complications and cervical vertebral fusion in multiple pterygium syndrome mandate careful evaluations before anesthesia. Urologic evaluation of the genital anomalies may also be needed. Recurrent pneumonias due to severe kyphoscoliosis may lead to early death in multiple pterygium syndrome, but the normal intelligence in patients with these conditions supports an optimistic and aggressive medical outlook.

Inheritance is autosomal dominant for most cases of multiple pterygium syndrome and autosomal recessive for popliteal pterygium or Bartsocas–Papas syndromes. Parents of infants with multiple pterygium syndrome will have a negligible recurrence risk consistent with new mutations, while those of infants with popliteal pterygium or Bartocas–Papas syndromes will have 25% recurrence risks. Causative genes have not been defined for these disorders, so the diagnosis remains clinical. Several lethal syndromes with pterygia have been reported, and pediatric genetic evaluation is essential for correct diagnosis, prognosis, and counseling.

Pena–Shokeir syndrome types I and II

In 1974, Pena and Shokeir wrote a seminal description of children with congenital contractures that gave rise to two different eponymic syndromes with autosomal-recessive inheritance (Jones, 1997, 174–7; Gorlin et al., 2001, pp. 765–9). Pena–Shokeir type I syndrome is now considered a non-specific phenotype or sequence with limb contractures, facial changes (hypertelorism, high nasal bridge, malformed ears, micrognathia), and pulmonary hypoplasia. Pena–Shokeir type II syndrome is a more specific syndrome with limb contractures, microcephaly, unusual facies (enophthalmos, microphthalmia), and brain anomalies (agenesis of the corpus callosum, cerebellar hypoplasia). The type II disorder has also been called cerebro-oculo-facial syndrome (COFS); it has a degenerative course resembling that of Cockayne syndrome, and shares cellular sensitivity to UV light and mutations with that disorder (discussed in Chapter 17).

Pena–Shokeir type I syndrome has a rather high incidence of 1 in 10,000 births, reflecting its phenotypic heterogeneity. A variety of neurologic or muscular injuries that render the fetus immobile can cause the Pena–Shokeir type I phenotype. Some prefer the term "fetal akinesia sequence" to indicate that immobility of the fetal limbs results in contractures (arthrogryposis, ankylosis) and that decreased fetal respiratory excursions result in pulmonary hypoplasia. In support of this view is the similar phenotype obtained when rodent fetuses are paralyzed *in utero*.

Additional manifestations of Pena–Shokeir type I syndrome include webbing of the neck, small chest, and contractures that can involve any of the limb joints or digits. There are also cardiac anomalies (25%), urinary tract anomalies (30%), and genital anomalies such as cryptorchidism (virtually 100%), hypospadias (20%), or labial hypoplasia (15%). Pena–Shokeir type II patients can have cataracts, dislocation or contracture of limb joints, scoliosis, and a degenerative course with wasting of subcutaneous tissue.

Preventive management of the Pena–Shokeir syndrome type I can utilize the arthrogryposis checklist, with the different palliative management for type II discussed in Chapter 17. Genetic counseling regarding the possibility of a 25% recurrence risk for normal parents with affected children should be mentioned, but many cases have been sporadic. Prenatal diagnosis by sonography is possible for severe cases through detection of fetal hydrops or other anomalies, but second trimester detection cannot be guaranteed. Antibodies against acetylcholine receptors in some patients and affliction of offspring of mothers with myasthenia gravis provide clues for gene characterization in Pena–Shokeir type I, and there will undoubtedly be several genes and environmental factors that cause the phenotype. Parent information and updates on research progress is available at several medical education websites.

Whistling face (Freeman–Sheldon) syndrome

The puckered lips and immobile face of the Freeman–Sheldon syndrome are so distinctive that the "whistling face" description should be retained. Not surprisingly, the syndrome was recognized some time ago and has been separated from other forms of "distal" arthrogryposis (Jones, 1997, pp. 214–5; Gorlin et al., 2001, pp. 783–6). Most families show vertical transmission consistent with autosomal-dominant inheritance, but some pedigrees involve consanguinity typical of autosomal-recessive inheritance.

Complications of whistling face syndrome include enopthalmos, hypertelorism or strabismus, microstomia with an "H"-like cleft on the chin, puckered lips, micrognathia, facial immobility, small nasal alae, ulnarly deviated ("windvane") fingers, and congenital contractures of the hips and knees including club feet and kyphoscoliosis. There are early feeding problems and failure to thrive (30%), and a few patients have had mental disability.

Preventive management of whistling face syndrome should follow the recommendations of the arthryogyposis checklist with emphasis on evaluation of early nutrition and respiratory function. Some children have suffered aspiration and death, and anesthesia requires considerable evaluation and expertise. There are variants of the condition with severe micrognathia and Pierre Robin sequence that accentuate these respiratory problems. The improvement in joint function seen with many forms of arthrogryposis can be particularly evident in Freeman–Sheldon syndrome, so medical management should be aggressive and optimistic (Staheli et al., 1998).

The sporadic occurrence of most cases implies a low recurrence risk for parents, but consanguinity has been reported and some variants are clearly recessive with a 25% recurrence risk. Pediatric genetic evaluation is again essential for accurate diagnosis. Parent information is available at a Freeman–Sheldon Parent Support Group (www.fspsg.org/), a site organized by a parent of an affected daughter (www.heartofanangel.com/LeahRose/fss1.html) and at various medical education websites.

Arthrogryposis syndromes

Terminology

Arthrogryposis multiplex congenita is a phenotype that has now been separated into many different syndromes. A conglomerate of signs and symptoms including deformity or fixation of the joints (limb contractures or ankylosis), dimpling over the joints, pterygia (webbing) across the joints, bony deformities (kyphoscoliosis) are seen in various arthrogryposis syndromes, and it may be difficult to classify individual patients (see checklist; Hall, 1981; Jones, 1997, pp. 170–83, 214–25; Staheli et al., 1998). Joint contractures and pulmonary hypoplasia may occur as a "fetal akinesia sequence" that is caused by fetal nerve or muscle dysfunction as well as maternal constraint (uterine anomaly, twin pregnancy).

Incidence, etiology, and differential diagnosis

The overall incidence of arthrogryposis is about 1 in 10,000 births (Hall, 1981), with some individual syndromes being quite rare (Table 18.1). As discussed above, any abnormality of the fetal genotype, the maternal metabolism, or the *in utero* environment that decreases fetal movement can produce congenital contractures. Severe fetal Werdnig–Hoffman disease or myopathy, maternal myasthenia gravis, and uterine constraints (twin pregnancy, bicornuate uterus) are all causes of arthrogryposis. Because several syndromes with arthrogryposis as a component exhibit autosomal-recessive inheritance, the older, all-inclusive name "arthrogryposis multiplex congenita" was often described as an autosomal-recessive disease. One of the more common forms of arthrogryposis (amyoplasia) is not genetic.

The differential diagnosis of children with congenital contractures is extensive, including many neuromuscular disorders in addition to the syndromes listed in Table 18.1. Chromosomal disorders (e.g., trisomy 18 that can be confused with Pena–Shokeir type I syndrome) and metabolic diseases (e.g., Zellweger syndrome with club feet) may include congenital contractures as a presenting symptom. Distinctive clinical findings include the "policeman's tip" positioning in amyoplasia, the pulmonary hypoplasia in Pena–Shokeir type I syndrome, the deeply set eyes in Pena–Shokeir type II syndrome, the puckered lips of Schwartz–Jampel or whistling face syndrome, and the webbing extending over the great toes in popliteal pterygium syndrome.

Diagnostic evaluation and medical counseling

A thorough physical examination is the cornerstone of diagnostic evaluation for the arthrogryposis syndromes. Webs, dimples, and positioning should be noted and the range of motion of each limb segment noted for future reference. Inspection for associated anomalies of the facies, eyes, mouth, trunk, and genitalia should then be conducted; children with a small thorax should be watched for evidence of respiratory insufficiency. Additional investigations may include cranial MRI scans in children with microcephaly, and a skeletal radiographic survey for the detection of osteopenia, fractures, cervical spine fusions, sacral fusions, etc. If there are minor anomalies of the craniofacies and limbs, then chromosomal studies should be performed. Ophthalmologic evaluations for cataracts, strabismus, or ptosis are important as a prelude to regular vision checks. Medical counseling will usually be optimistic unless there is severe pulmonary hypoplasia or evidence of microcephaly and facial dysmorphology. Many children with severe joint contractures make remarkable progress in motor rehabilitation.

Family and psychosocial counseling

Table 18.1 illustrates that syndromes with congenital contractures may be inherited as autosomal-dominant or autosomal-recessive diseases. If one includes severe presentations of neuropathies or myopathies, the X-linked recessive inheritance may also occur. The most likely inheritance mechanism will be autosomal recessive with a 25% recurrence risk, but amyoplasia (sporadic occurrence) or whistling face syndrome (autosomal dominant in some cases) may be associated with a minimal recurrence risk. Psychosocial counseling is needed for parents when severe developmental disabilities or major rehabilitative efforts are needed. Parent information is available from AVENUES: A National Support Group for Arthrogryposis Multiplex Congenita, (www.sonnet.com/avenues/); the Arthrogryposis Group (TAG: http://www.tagonline.org.uk/), a patient story (hometown.aol.com/arthrogryposisc/), and from numerous medical information sites by searching on the term "arthrogryposis."

Natural history and complications

Although many children with congenital contractures have an excellent prognosis, those with involvement of the central nervous system have increased morbidity and mortality. The complications of arthrogryposis mainly concern the bones and joints, but the syndromes listed in Table 18.1 illustrate numerous other problems that may occur. The arthrogryposis checklist, part 1, lists many of the more common complications of the arthrogryposis syndromes, including feeding and nutrition, ocular anomalies, high or cleft palate, micrognathia, hernias, kyphoscoliosis, limb contractures with or without webs, gastrointestinal anomalies, pulmonary hypoplasia and/or chronic pneumonitis, cardiac anomalies, urogenital anomalies, brain anomalies, and neurosensory deficits. After treatment of the contractures, later complications can include dental crowding, hernias, restrictive lung disease, degenerative arthritis, and motor disabilities.

Arthrogryposis syndromes preventive medical checklist

Once the initial assessment of cranial, skeletal, pulmonary, and urogenital development is completed, the clinician should initiate aggressive orthopedic and physical therapy to preserve muscle function and mobilize joints (Staheli et al., 1998). Therapists must be cautioned to avoid forcing movement when there is ankylosis or osteopenia, and a skeletal radiographic survey is helpful to point out fragile areas. Ophthalmologic evaluations should be performed initially to document anomalies and serially to monitor vision. Feeding may be compromised by a high or cleft palate, by micrognathia, or by a small mouth with constricted lips; feeding evaluation and education are therefore essential. Observation of stool and urinary patterns is also important to rule out intestinal or genitourinary anomalies.

Later management (see checklist) will consist of monitoring skeletal growth and symmetry, continued neurosensory testing including audiometric and ophthalmologic evaluations, orthopedic and physical medicine assessments to provide appliances or therapies for motor limitations, and dental evaluations to exclude tooth crowding or malocclusion (Staheli, 1998). Patients with neurologic symptoms may require school evaluations and family counseling appropriate for children with severe disabilities.

Preventive management of arthrogryposis syndromes

Description: Clinical pattern of joint restriction caused by fetal immobility; the various syndromes have an overall incidence of about 1 in 10,000 live births. Various disorders with an:

Clinical diagnosis: Abnormal brain, peripheral nerve, or muscle function during embryofetal development produces deformity or fixation of the joints (limb contractures or ankylosis), dimpling over the joints, pterygia (webbing) across the joints, and bony deformities (kyphoscoliosis, club feet). Abnormalities may be confined to the musculoskeletal system in disorders such as amyoplasia, but other arthrogryposis syndromes include a broader spectrum of brain, heart, and kidney defects.

Laboratory diagnosis: Some chromosomal disorders will include arthrogyposis, so chromosome studies may be performed to exclude other conditions. A few syndromes have characterized mutations (like the DNA repair defect in Pena–Shokeir type II), but lack of commercial DNA testing necessitates a clinical diagnosis for most arthrogryposis disorders.

Genetics: Autosomal recessive inheritance applies for many disorders involving arthrogyposis, but amyoplasia (sporadic occurrence) or Freeman–Sheldon(autosomal dominant in some cases) may imply a minimal recurrence risk for normal parents having an affected child.

Key management issues: Aggressive orthopedic and physical therapy to preserve muscle function and mobilize joints, avoiding forced positioning in the presence of ankylosis or osteopenia; evaluation of feeding, stool, and urinary patterns to rule out anomalies; dental evaluations to exclude tooth crowding or malocclusion; monitoring of hearing, vision, growth, and skeletal development; early intervention and family support for patients with microcephaly and severe disabilities.

Growth charts: The dependence of stature on the degree of limb deformity and its variation among syndromes precludes the use of specific charts; regular charts should be used to monitor head growth and weight gain.

Parent information: AVENUES: A National Support Group for Arthrogryposis Multiplex Congenita, (www.sonnet.com/avenues/); The Arthrogryposis Group (TAG: http://www.tagonline.org.uk/), and a patient story (hometown.aol.com/arthrogryposisc/).

Basis for management recommendations: Multidisciplinary management outlined in detail by Staheli et al. (1998), complications below as documented by Hall (1997); Hall et al. (1998).

Summary of clinical concerns

General	Learning	**Cognitive disability**, learning differences for patients with microcephaly, drooling, poor speech
	Growth	**Failure to thrive**, short stature, **oromotor dysfunction**
Facial	Facies	Epicanthal folds, large or malformed ears, hemangiomas, micrognathia
	Eyes	**Ptosis**, microphthalmia, corneal opacities, strabismus
	Nose	**Broad nasal root**, choanal atresia
	Mouth	Dysphagia, small mouth, restricted mouth opening, cleft or high palate, dental crowding, microstomia, lower lip pits
Surface	Neck/trunk	Torticollis, short, webbed, or immobile neck; umbilical hernias, inguinal hernias
	Epidermal	Extensible skin, widely spaced nipples, single palmar creases, decreased scalp hair
Skeletal	Cranial	Macrocephaly, **microcephaly**, cranial asymmetry, craniosynostosis
	Axial	**Kyphosis, scoliosis**, fusion of cervical vertebrae, spina bifida occulta
	Limbs	**Pterygia, ankyloses**, synostoses, **contractures** of large joints; camptodactyly of digits, **dislocated hips**, **club feet**, syndactyly, ectrodactyly, osteoporosis, degenerative arthritis
Internal	Digestive	Gastroschisis, intestinal atresias
	Circulatory	**Cardiac anomalies** (as high as 25%), cardiomyopathies
	Pulmonary	Pulmonary hypoplasia, restrictive lung disease, respiratory obstruction, laryngeal stenosis
	RES	Thymus hypoplasia
	Excretory	**Renal anomalies**, hydronephrosis, urinary tract infections
	Genital	**Cryptorchidism, hypospadias**, micropenis, labial hypoplasia
Neural	Central	**Microcephaly**, brain anomalies, seizures, intracranial calcifications
	Motor	**Muscle weakness, decreased skeletal muscle mass**, decreased movements, motor delays, myotonia, malignant hyperthermia during anesthesia
	Sensory	Hearing and vision deficits

RES, reticuloendothelial system; **concerns** of frequency >20% are **highlighted**

Key references

Bernstein, R. M. (2002). Arthrogryposis and amyoplasia. *Journal of the American Academy of Orthopaedic Surgery* 10:417–24.

Hall, J. (1997). Arthrogryposis multiplex congenita: etiology, genetics, classification, diagnostic approach, and general aspects. *Journal of Pediatric Orthopaedics* 6:159–66.

Hall, J. G. (1998). Overview of arthrogryposis. In *Arthrogryposis: A Text Atlas*, eds L. T. Staheli et al., pp. 1–26. Cambridge UK: Cambridge University Press.

Arthrogryposis syndromes

Preventive medical checklist (0–3 years)

Name _____ Birth date __/__/__ Number _____

Age	Evaluations: key concerns	Management considerations		Notes
New-born ↓ 1 month	Dysmorphology: anomalies	❏ Genetic evaluation[1]	❏	
	Hearing, vision: eye exam[2]	❏ ABR; ophthalmology[3]	❏	
	Feeding: cleft palate, poor intake	❏ Feeding specialist; video swallow[3]	❏	
	Heart: murmur	❏ Echocardiogram;[3] cardiology[3]	❏	
	Urogenital: renal, genital defects	❏ Abdominal sonogram, urology[3]	❏	
	Skeletal: joints, lung, restriction, hernias	❏ Orthopedics;[3] pulmonology[3]	❏	
	Parental adjustment	❏ Family support[4]	❏	
2 months ↓ 4 months	Growth, development:[5] motor weakness	❏ ECI[6]	❏	
	Hearing, vision[2]	❏ Ophthalmology[3]	❏	
	Feeding: cleft palate, poor intake	❏ Feeding specialist; video swallow[3]	❏	
	Heart: murmur	❏ Echocardiogram;[3] cardiology[3]	❏	
	Urogenital: renal, genital defects	❏ Urinalysis, BP; urology[3]	❏	
	Skeletal: neck, lungs, joints, limbs	❏ Pulmonology;[3] anesthesia precautions	❏	
	Parental adjustment	❏ Family support[4]	❏	
	Other:	❏	❏	
6 months ↓ 9 months	Growth, development:[5] motor, feeding	❏ ECI[6]	❏	
	Hearing, vision:[2] strabismus	❏ Ophthalmology[3]	❏	
	Heart: murmur	❏ Echocardiogram;[3] cardiology[3]	❏	
	Urogenital: renal, genital defects	❏ Urinalysis, BP; urology[3]	❏	
	Skeletal: neck, lungs, joints, limbs	❏ Orthopedics;[3] anesthesia precautions	❏	
	Other:	❏	❏	
1 year	Growth, development:[5] motor, feeding	❏ ECI[6]	❏	
	Hearing, vision:[2] strabismus	❏ Ophthalmology	❏	
	Heart: murmur	❏ Echocardiogram;[3] cardiology[3]	❏	
	Urogenital: renal, genital defects	❏ Urinalysis, BP; urology[3]	❏	
	Skeletal: neck, lungs, joints, limbs	❏ Pulmonology;[3] anesthesia precautions	❏	
	Dural ectasia: nerve root, pelvic pain	❏ Head, spine MRI[3]	❏	
	Other:	❏	❏	
15 months ↓ 18 months	Growth, development:[5] motor, feeding	❏ ECI[6]	❏	
	Hearing, vision:[2] strabismus	❏ Ophthalmology[3]	❏	
	Heart: murmur	❏ Echocardiogram;[3] cardiology[3]	❏	
	Skeletal: neck, lungs, joints, limbs	❏ Orthopedics;[3] anesthesia precautions	❏	
2 years	Growth, development:[5] motor, feeding	❏ ECI[6]	❏	
	Hearing, vision:[2] strabismus	❏ Ophthalmology, dentistry	❏	
	Heart: murmur	❏ Echocardiogram;[3] cardiology[3]	❏	
	Urogenital: renal, genital defects	❏ Urinalysis, BP; urology[3]	❏	
	Skeletal: neck, lungs, joints, limbs	❏ Orthopedics;[3] anesthesia precautions	❏	
3 years	Growth, development:[5] motor, feeding	❏ ECI;[6] family support[4]	❏	
	Hearing, vision:[2] strabismus	❏ Ophthalmology, dentistry	❏	
	Heart: murmur	❏ Echocardiogram;[3] cardiology[3]	❏	
	Urogenital: renal, genital defects	❏ Urinalysis, BP; urology[3]	❏	
	Skeletal: neck, lungs, joints, limbs	❏ Orthopedics;[3] anesthesia precautions	❏	
	Other:	❏	❏	

Arthrogryposis concerns		Other concerns from history	
Craniosynostosis	Cardiac anomalies	**Family history/prenatal**	**Social/environmental**
Microphthalmia, cataracts	Joint contractures, pterygia	_____	_____
Strabismus	Club feet, hip dislocation	_____	_____
Small mouth, dysphagia	Urogenital anomalies	_____	_____
High, cleft palate	Microcephaly, seizures	_____	_____
Pulmonary hypoplasia	Inguinal, umbilical hernias	_____	_____

Guidelines for the neonatal period should be undertaken *at whatever age* the diagnosis is made; ABR, auditory brainstem evoked response; BP, blood pressure; [1]clinical genetic and subspecialty evaluations are crucial for correct diagnosis and counseling – should include surface and skeletal examination, skeletal X-rays, and head/spine MRI with cranial/neck changes; [2]by practitioner; [3]as dictated by clinical findings; [4]parent group, family/sib, financial, and behavioral issues for severely affected children; [5]consider development pediatric or genetics clinic according to symptoms and availability; [6]early childhood intervention with motor/speech therapy.

Arthrogryposis syndromes

Preventive medical checklist (4–18 years)

Name _____ Birth date __ / __ / ____ Number _____

Age	Evaluations: key concerns	Management considerations		Notes
4 years ↓ 6 years	Growth: head size, short stature Development:[2] preschool transition Hearing, vision, teeth[2] Heart: murmur Urogenital: renal, genital defects Skeletal: neck, lungs, joints, limbs Other:	❑ ❑ ❑ ❑ ❑ ❑ ❑	Specialty clinics;[1] endocrinology[3] Family support;[4] preschool program[5] Ophthalmology; dentistry Echocardiogram;[3] cardiology[3] Urinalysis, BP; urology[3] Orthopedics;[3] anesthesia precautions ❑	
7 years ↓ 9 years	Growth: head size, short stature Development:[1] school transition[5] Hearing, vision, teeth[2] Heart: murmur Urogenital: renal, genital defects Skeletal: neck, lungs, joints, limbs Other:	❑ ❑ ❑ ❑ ❑ ❑ ❑	Specialty clinics;[1] endocrinology[3] Family support;[4] school progress[6] Ophthalmology; dentistry Echocardiogram;[3] cardiology[3] Urinalysis, BP; urology[3] Orthopedics;[3] anesthesia precautions ❑	
10 years ↓ 12 years	Growth: head size, short stature Hearing, vision, teeth[2] Urogenital: renal, genital defects Skeletal: neck, lungs, joints, limbs Other:	❑ ❑ ❑ ❑ ❑	Specialty clinics;[1] school progress[6] Ophthalmology; dentistry Urinalysis, BP; urology[3] Orthopedics;[3] anesthesia precautions ❑	
13 years ↓ 15 years	Growth: head size, short stature Hearing, vision, teeth[2] Heart: murmur Urogenital: renal, genital defects Skeletal: neck, lungs, joints, limbs Other:	❑ ❑ ❑ ❑ ❑ ❑	Specialty clinics;[1] school progress[6] Ophthalmology; dentistry Echocardiogram;[3] cardiology[3] Urinalysis, BP; urology[3] Orthopedics;[3] anesthesia precautions ❑	
16 years ↓ 18 years	Growth: head size, short stature Hearing, vision, teeth[2] Urogenital: renal, genital defects Skeletal: neck, lungs, joints, limbs Other:	❑ ❑ ❑ ❑ ❑	Family support;[4] school progress[6] Ophthalmology; dentistry Urinalysis, BP; urology[3] Orthopedics;[3] anesthesia precautions ❑	
19 years ↓ 23 years	Adult transition: body image, activity Hearing, vision, teeth[2] Heart: murmur Urogenital: renal, genital defects Skeletal: neck, lungs, joints, limbs	❑ ❑ ❑ ❑ ❑	Physical therapy/trainer;[3] cosmetic surgery[3] Ophthalmology; dentistry Echocardiogram;[3] cardiology[3] Urinalysis, BP; urology[3] Orthopedics;[3] anesthesia precautions	
Adult	Body image, activity guidance Hearing, vision, teeth[2] Heart: murmur Urogenital: renal, genital defects Skeletal: neck, lungs, joints, limbs Skeletal: arthritis, osteoporosis Other:	❑ ❑ ❑ ❑ ❑ ❑ ❑	Physical therapy/trainer;[3] cosmetic surgery[3] Audiology;[3] ophthalmology;[3] dentistry Echocardiogram;[3] cardiology[3] Urinalysis, BP; urology[3] Orthopedics;[3] anesthesia precautions Rheumatology[3] ❑	Fertile women have risks for aortic aneurysm during pregnancy and for chromosome anomalies in offspring.

Arthrogryposis concerns		Other concerns from history	
Craniosynostosis Microphthalmia, cataracts Strabismus Small mouth, dental crowding High, cleft palate Pulmonary hypoplasia	Cardiac anomalies Joint contractures, pterygia Arthritis, osteoporosis Urogenital anomalies Microcephaly, seizures Inguinal, umbilical hernias	**Family history/prenatal** _____ _____ _____ _____	**Social/environmental** _____ _____ _____ _____

Guidelines for the neonatal period should be undertaken *at whatever age* the diagnosis is made; BP, blood pressure; [1]consider developmental pediatric, neurology, or genetics clinic according to symptoms and availability; [2]by practitioner; [3]as dictated by clinical findings; [4]parent group, family/sib, financial, and behavioral issues for rare patients with learning differences, debilitating illness; [5]preschool program including developmental monitoring and motor/speech therapy; [6]monitor individual education plan, educational testing, balance of special education and inclusion, academic progress, behavioral differences, later vocational planning.

Parent guide to arthrogryposis syndromes

The words "arthro" (joint) and "gryposis" (curved), combined as the term "arthrogryposis multiplex congenital," are now known to denote findings in many different disorders. Fetal immobility can lead to fixation of joints (contractures) with webbing across the joint and ankylosis. Arthrogryposis can result from maternal myasthenia gravis, brain anomalies with central denervation, agenesis of spinal nerves (e.g., severe Werdnig–Hoffman disease), muscle diseases presenting in fetal life, or constraint of fetal movement by uterine anomalies or amniotic bands. Joint contractures and pulmonary hypoplasia may occur as a "fetal akinesia sequence."

Incidence, causation, and diagnosis

The overall incidence of arthrogryposis is about 1 in 10,000 births, with many individual syndromes being quite rare. Because several syndromes with arthrogryposis as a component exhibit autosomal recessive inheritance, the older, all-inclusive name "arthrogryposis multiplex congenita" was often described as an autosomal recessive disease. It is now recognized that many forms of arthrogryposis, like the common disorder amyoplasia, are not inherited. The differential diagnosis of children with congenital contractures is extensive, including many neuromuscular or chromosomal disorders. Sometimes a specific genetic condition like Werdnig–Hoffman disease can be recognized, or a chromosome study can reveal a diagnosis like trisomy 18. In most cases the diagnosis is clinical, requiring careful examination and follow-up to define a characteristic pattern of anomalies. Distinctive clinical findings include the "policeman's tip" positioning in amyoplasia, the small and dysfunctional lungs in Pena–Shokeir type I syndrome, the deeply set eyes in Pena–Shokeir type II syndrome, the puckered lips of Schwartz–Jampel or whistling face syndrome, and the webbing extending over the great toes in popliteal pterygium syndrome. A thorough physical examination is the cornerstone of diagnostic evaluation for the arthrogryposis syndromes. Webs, dimples, and positioning should be noted and the range of motion of each limb segment noted for future reference. Inspection for associated anomalies of the facies, eyes, mouth, trunk, and genitalia should then be conducted; children with a small thorax should be watched for evidence of respiratory problems. Additional investigations may include cranial MRI scans in children with small heads or skeletal X-rays for the detection of thin, soft bones, fractures, cervical (neck) spine fusions, etc. In many cases, chromosomal studies should be performed for exclusion. Ophthalmologic evaluations for cataracts, strabismus (deviated gaze), or ptosis (hooded lids) are important as a prelude to regular vision checks.

Natural history and complications

Although many children with congenital contractures have an excellent prognosis, those with involvement of the central nervous system or lungs may have increased morbidity and mortality. The complications of arthrogryposis mainly concern the bones and joints, but other problems may occur. Common complications of the arthrogryposis syndromes involve feeding and nutrition, ocular anomalies, high or cleft palate, small jaw and dental problems, hernias, spinal curvatures, limb contractures with or without webs, gastrointestinal anomalies, small lungs with or without chronic pneumonias, heart defects, kidney and genital anomalies, brain anomalies, and hearing and/or vision problems. After treatment of the contractures, later complications can include dental crowding, hernias, lung disease, degenerative arthritis, and motor disabilities.

Preventive medical needs

Once the initial assessment of cranial, skeletal, pulmonary, and urogenital development is completed, aggressive orthopedic and physical therapy should be initiated to preserve muscle function and mobilize joints. Therapists must be cautioned to avoid forcing movement when there are fixed joints or thin bones, and skeletal X-rays are helpful for highlighting fragile areas. Ophthalmologic evaluations should be performed initially to document anomalies and serially to monitor vision. Feeding may be compromised by a high or cleft palate, by a small jaw, or by a small mouth with constricted lips; feeding evaluation and education are therefore essential. Observation of stool and urinary patterns is also important to rule out intestinal or genitourinary anomalies. Later management will include monitoring of skeletal growth, audiometric and ophthalmologic evaluations, orthopedic and physical medicine assessments to provide appliances or therapies for motor limitations, and dental evaluations to exclude tooth crowding or misalignment. Patients with neurologic symptoms may require early intervention, school evaluation, and family counseling appropriate for children with severe disabilities.

Family counseling

Medical counseling will usually be optimistic unless there is severe pulmonary hypoplasia or evidence of microcephaly and facial dysmorphology. Many children with severe joint contractures make remarkable progress in motor rehabilitation. Syndromes with congenital contractures may be inherited as autosomal dominant or autosomal recessive diseases. If one includes severe presentations of nerve or muscle diseases, then X-linked recessive inheritance may also occur. The most likely inheritance mechanism will be autosomal recessive with a 25% recurrence risk for normal parents with an affected child. However, many mild forms are either autosomal dominant or not inherited, so unaffected parents may have a low recurrence risk. One distinctive pattern that is quite common is amyoplasia (literally, no growth of muscles). These children have decreased musculature in their upper shoulder girdle and hands that curve in the "policeman's tip" position such that their thumbs are bent back against their arm with their palms opened upward. The legs may be similarly involved, but other anomalies are uncommon. Children with amyoplasia have an excellent prognosis for functional improvement and for normal intelligence; their parents have a minimal recurrence risk. Families can benefit from psychosocial counseling when severe developmental disabilities are present or major rehabilitative efforts are needed.

Part VIII

Management of neurodegenerative metabolic disorders

With several hundred diseases and an aggregate frequency of 1 in 600 births, a complete discussion of metabolic disorders is beyond the scope of this book. The classic reference of Scriver et al. (2001) provides an encyclopedic and detailed description of inborn errors of metabolism. Selected here are several of the more common diseases that illustrate the role of generalists in the care of patients with metabolic disorders. Since the focus of this book is congenital malformations, emphasis is given to disorders that produce alterations in appearance and/or morphogenesis. From the standpoint of morphogenesis, these are metabolic dysplasias in the sense that they cause altered histiogenesis (see Chapter 1). Examples include the glycogen-storage diseases ("cherubic" facies and hepatomegaly), the mucopolysaccharidoses (coarsened face with dysostosis multiplex), and a variety of neuromuscular diseases with hypotonic facies (bitemporal hollowing, down-turned corners of the mouth) with other malformations (e.g., brain anomalies, limb defects, hepatorenal disease, and contractures that can occur in the Smith–Lemli–Opitz or Zellweger syndromes).

Most patients with inborn errors of metabolism will require consistent input from metabolic specialists for monitoring of injurious metabolites, dietary counseling, and prognostication. Ideally, the primary physician would coordinate general health care issues including growth, development, and school issues, leaving metabolic management to the specialist. In practice, the sweep of managed care may force many primary physicians to coordinate more of the dietary and metabolic management of patients with inborn errors of metabolism. Disorders that are unresponsive to dietary treatment, discussed in Chapter 19, are more similar to malformation syndromes in requiring chronic preventive management to realize an optimal quality of life. Despite their known or suspected metabolic etiology, these metabolic dysplasia syndromes are like other chronic disorders in needing informed primary care physicians to ensure optimal preventive care after the initial diagnostic evaluation.

19

Organellar and miscellaneous neurodegenerative disorders

Partitioning of the cell into organellar compartments offers the advantage and vulnerability of specialized function. Genetic mutations that alter the structure or targeting of organellar proteins may disrupt the entire organelle and produce multiple metabolic abnormalities. Examples of generalized organellar dysfunction include alterations of the mannose-6-phosphate targeting in lysosomes (e.g., I-cell disease), deletions of mitochondrial DNA (e.g., Kearns–Sayre syndrome), and mutations in peroxisomal membrane proteins (e.g., Zellweger syndrome). Other genetic mutations affect only one organellar protein, producing a more limited and specific phenotype (e.g., Fabry disease, Leber hereditary optic neuropathy, or adrenoleukodystrophy).

The dietary manipulations that are effective for the "small"-molecule disorders have limited use for organellar disorders. Deficiencies of lysosomal enzymes often lead to "storage" diseases, with the accumulation of "large" molecules that are internally synthesized and independent of dietary sources. Other lysosomal diseases, as well as disorders affecting the structure of mitochondria or peroxisomes, may involve an excess or deficiency of molecules within cellular compartments; these molecules are less accessible to manipulation by diet.

Many organellar disorders are progressive, involving a phase of normal development until the accumulation of metabolites interferes with organ function. Often several organs are affected, particularly the brain, eye, heart, liver, and skeleton. Most of the disorders exhibit insidious loss of previously acquired developmental milestones, followed by neurodegeneration and death. The age at which the deceleration of development occurs and the rate of progression vary widely. In a few diseases, and in some variants within a disease category, the nervous system is spared. Selected disorders affecting lysosomal, mitochondrial, or peroxisomal function are described in this chapter, with an emphasis on those causing syndromal disease. A miscellaneous category of metabolic dysplasias is also discussed, based on similarities in clinical presentation and natural history.

Lysosomal enzyme deficiencies

Lysosomes are one of several cytoplasmic organelles that form a network of protein transport between the plasma membrane and the Golgi apparatus (Sabatini & Adesnik, 2001). Endosomes from the Golgi may fuse with coated vesicles from the cell surface, acquire mannose-6-phosphate receptors that lead to the import of hydrolytic enzymes (multivesicular bodies), and shed these receptors to become a mature lysosome. External or internal cellular macromolecules can be transferred to the Golgi or to lysosomes via the multivesicular bodies, and those routed to mature lysosomes are degraded for the recycling of components. Deficiency of a single lysosomal hydrolase leads to abnormal accumulation of its substrate, causing lysosomal engorgement and disruption of other lysosomal hydrolases. Several types of macromolecules can then build up in susceptible organs. As outlined in this chapter, lysosomal enzyme deficiencies can be classified as lipidoses, mucolipidoses (oligosaccharidoses), or mucopolysaccharidoses according to the predominant type of macromolecule that is stored (Table 19.1).

Table 19.1. Selected lysosomal enzyme deficiencies

Disease or syndrome	Incidence*	Deficient enzyme	Complications
Neurolipidoses			
Krabbe disease	1 in 200,000	Galactosyl-ceramidase	ND, blindness, deafness
Metachromatic leukodystrophy	1 in 50,000	Arylsulfatase A	ND, altered gait, incontinence, seizures, quadriparesis
Niemann–Pick diseases	1 in 40,000 (J)	Sphingomyelinase	ND, visceromegaly,
Tay–Sachs, Sandhoff disease (G_{M2} gangliosidoses)	1 in 4000 (J) 1 in 100,000	Hexaminidase A,B	ND, cherry red spot
Other lipidoses			
Fabry disease	1 in 40,000	α-galactosidase	Angiokeratoma, band cataract, vascular disease, nerve pain, renal failure, hypohydrosis
Gaucher disease type I	1 in 1000 1 in 100,000	Glucocerebrosidase	ND (types 2,3), visceromegaly, bleeding, bone crises, joint disease, pulmonary disease
Gaucher disease types II, III			
Oligosaccharidoses			
G_{M1} gangliosidosis	~50 cases	β-Galactosidase	ND, Hurler-like, cherry red spots

(cont.)

Table 19.1 (*cont.*)

Disease or syndrome	Incidence*	Deficient enzyme	Complications
I-cell disease	~50 cases	Phosphotransferase	ND, Hurler-like
Pseudo–Hurler syndrome	~50 cases	Phosphotransferase	ND, Hurler-like
Multiple sulfatase deficiency	~50 cases	Sulfatases	ND, Hurler-like, cherry red spot, ichthyosis
Mannosidosis	~50 cases	α-Mannosidase	ND, Hurler-like, seizures, cataracts
Mannosidosis	~50 cases	β-Mannosidase	ND, Hurler-like, hearing loss, infections
Fucosidosis	~100 cases	α-Fucosidase	ND, Hurler-like, angiokeratomas, hypohidrosis
Sialidosis	~50 cases	Sialidase	ND, Hurler-like, cherry red spot, angiokeratomas
Aspartylglucosaminuria	~100 cases	Aspartyl hydrolase	ND, Hurler-like, cataracts
Mucopolysaccharidoses			
Hurler syndrome (type IH)	1 in 100,000	α-Iduronidase	ND, coarse face and skin, viscous mucous, pectus, gibbus, dysostosis, visceromegaly
Scheie syndrome (type IS)	1 in 500,000	α-Iduronidase	
Hunter syndrome (type II)	1 in 65,000	Iduronate sulfatase	ND, Hurler-like
San Filippo syndrome (type III)	1 in 24,000	Heparan sulfatase	ND, Hurler-like (later onset)
Morquio syndrome (type IV)	1 in 40,000	β-Galactosidase	Dysostosis, short neck and trunk
Maroteaux–Lamy (type VI)	1 in 100,000	Arylsulfatase B	Hurler-like
Sly syndrome (type VII)	~20 cases	β-Glucuronidase	ND, Hurler-like

Notes:
(J), Jewish population; ND, neurodegeneration.
*Cases or per number of live births.

Lysosomal diseases: Lipidoses and mucolipidoses (oligosaccharidoses)

The storage of lipid material is a common feature of several lysosomal enzyme deficiencies. Many, like Tay–Sachs disease, Sandhoff disease, Niemann–Pick disease, metachromatic leukodystrophy, G_{M2} gangliosidosis, or Krabbe disease, are predominantly neurodegenerative disorders that will not be discussed here. Preventive management of the neurolipidoses will involve regular neurologic, audiologic, and ophthalmologic evaluations that attend to neurosensory deficits, seizures, and progressive neurodevastation. Most neurolipidoses are lethal, autosomal-recessive diseases requiring genetic counseling, extensive psychosocial support, physical/occupational therapy, and hospice services.

Other lipidoses affect many other structures besides the brain and eyes. Some of these involve the storage of both lipids and oligosaccharides, leading to a phenotype that resembles the mucopolysaccharidoses. These disorders have been called mucolipidoses or, because there is not a true "mucolipid" substance, oligosaccharidoses. Disorders of glycoprotein degradation including the mannosidoses, fucosidosis, and sialidoses could also be classified as oligosaccharidoses. Selected lipidoses and oligosaccharidoses are summarized in Table 19.1.

Disorders of glycoprotein degradation

Mannosidoses, fucosidosis, sialidoses, and aspartylglucosaminuria are autosomal-recessive disorders caused by well-characterized enzyme deficiencies that allow prenatal diagnosis (Thomas, 2001). Inspection of a blood smear for vacuolated lymphocytes and urine screening for mannose, fucose, sialyl, or aspartylglucosamine oligosaccharides allow suspicion of the diagnoses, followed by demonstration of the appropriate enzyme deficiency in leucocytes. Recent advances have characterized the genes for most of these deficiencies, allowing direct DNA diagnosis in many cases (Gururaj et al., 2005). Enzyme therapy trials are underway for these more severe lysosomal deficiencies, although penetration through the blood–brain barrier is still problematic.

Each of the glycoprotein degradation diseases may be associated with a Hurler-like syndrome reminiscent of the mucopolysaccharidoses. Other clinical manifestations include moderate to severe mental retardation and seizures, cataracts and corneal opacities (α-mannosidosis, aspartylglucosaminuria), cherry red spots (sialidosis), hearing loss (β-mannosidosis), recurrent infections (β-mannosidosis), sweat abnormalities with hypohidrosis (fucosidosis), and angiokeratomas of the skin (fucosidosis, β-mannosidosis, sialidosis; Thomas, 2001). There are subtypes within these disorders that vary in their onset and progression. Adult survival is common in certain types of sialidosis and in aspartylglucosaminuria.

Preventive management should be similar to that outlined for the mucopolysaccharidoses, with focus on neurologic, ophthalmologic, and orthopedic evaluations (Thomas, 2001). Audiologic monitoring is particularly important for patients with mannosidosis and fucosidosis, and visual deterioration is noted in patients with sialidosis. Patients with aspartylglucosaminuria are susceptible to pulmonary infections and cardiac valvular disease in adulthood. The early intervention and psychosocial services emphasized for patients with mucopolysaccharidoses are certainly needed for severely affected patients with mannosidoses, fucosidosis, sialidoses, and aspartylglucosaminuria.

Fabry disease

Fabry disease was described in 1898 and initially named angiokeratoma corporis diffusum universale because of its characteristic skin lesions (Gorlin et al., 2001, pp. 154–7; Desnick et al., 2001). It is an X-linked disorder caused by a deficiency of α-galactosidase, encoded by a locus in chromosome region Xq22. There is progressive deposition of glycolipids into the endothelium of blood vessels, accounting for most of the clinical manifestations. On the skin, glycolipid deposition produces dark-red to blue telangiectasias that cluster over the umbilicus, thorax, thighs, buttocks, and knees. There is also ectodermal dysplasia with sparse body and facial hair together with hypohidrosis. Blood vessel changes in many other organs produce retinal and conjunctival aneurysms with cloudiness of the cornea and a whitish band in the lens called "Fabry cataract". Proteinuria with azotemia and renal failure, myocardial infarction, and cerebrovascular disease causes increased morbidity and mortality, with a mean survival of 41 years for untransplanted patients. Chronic pain from paresthesias begins in childhood, and these episodic crises of burning pain may drive patients to attempt suicide. Growth retardation, delayed puberty, abdominal pain, lymphedema of the limbs, and avascular necrosis of the femoral head are less common findings.

Preventive management for Fabry disease should include regular ophthalmologic evaluations, dermatologic monitoring of the skin lesions with possible cosmetic treatments, and periodic monitoring of blood pressure, renal functions, heart, and urinary sediment. Growth and development should be followed in early childhood, with possible referral for early intervention services if there are delays. Pain management is important, and clinicians should consider referring severely affected patients to pain specialists. Diphenylhydantion and carbamazapine have been helpful in suppressing painful crises. The α-galactosidase is a lysosomal enzyme that is taken up by deficient cells, so renal transplantation and enzyme therapies have had some success (Desnick et al., 2001).

Gaucher disease

Gaucher disease was described in 1882 based on a patient with massive splenomegaly (Beutler & Grabowski, 2001). Three types of the disease have been recognized, with types 2 and 3 being much rarer and having severe to moderate neurologic involvement. All three types are autosomal recessive, and involve accumulation of glucocerebroside due to deficiency of β-glucosidase. The incidence is about 1 in 1000 births for the Ashkenazic Jewish population and 1 in 100,000 in non-Jewish populations.

Clinical manifestions of type 1 Gaucher disease include neurologic (spinal cord compression due to collapse of vertebrae), pulmonary (infiltrative disease with clubbing), gastoenterologic (hepatomegaly and occasional liver failure), hematologic (thrombocytopenia, splenic infarction or rupture), and skeletal (painful "bone crises," fractures) abnormalities. Type 2 (acute neuronopathic) Gaucher disease may present as hydrops fetalis or infantile oculomotor abnormalities (e.g., strabismus). Severe neurologic features (hypertonia, choreoathetosis, seizures) and visceromegaly are present during infancy, and death usually occurs by age 2 years. Type 3 Gaucher disease resembles type 2 in presenting with oculomotor changes and visceromegaly. The usual onset is between infancy and age 14 years, with survival to the third or fourth decade.

The diagnostic evaluation may include a bone marrow to demonstrate the foam-laden Gaucher cells, but should rest on the demonstration of β-glucosidase deficiency in leucocytes. DNA analysis for β-glucosidase gene mutations is also available, and is preferred when a mutation has been demonstrated in affected relatives.

Preventive management for Gaucher disease is outlined by Beutler & Grabowski (2001). After diagnosis, the first consideration is splenectomy for patients with massive splenomegaly or severe thrombocytopenia (platelet count less than 40,000). The need for penicillin prophylaxis of overwhelming infection may be mitigated by performing a partial splenectomy. With the advent of enzyme therapy, splenectomy is less commonly performed. Skeletal abnormalities may be severe, and periodic orthopedic evaluations should be performed. Patients should be counseled to avoid high-intensity exercise; swimming is a good choice for minimizing joint deterioration. Hip, knee, and shoulder joint replacements have been helpful in alleviating pain and restoring mobility, but surgeons should be experienced in dealing with bone thinning and pseudofractures. Phosphonates have shown anecdotal but not controlled benefits in treating bone disease.

Although the ability to target exogenous enzymes to lysosomes has made this category an attractive candidate for enzyme therapy, Gaucher disease is one of the few disorders where this has been achieved. Modified enzyme from human placenta (Ceredase or alglucerase) and reombinant enzymes produced in bacteria are available, as are substrate reduction therapies (Jmoudiak & Futerman, 2005). Though expensive, these treatments are effective in reducing hematologic and skeletal complications in patients with Gaucher disease. Some manifestations (e.g., pulmonary disease) are less responsive to therapy, mandating continued monitoring for hematologic, orthopedic, and pulmonary problems in Gaucher patients. Bone marrow transplant is also effective, but has the usual disadvantage of a 10–15% mortality rate.

G$_{M1}$ gangliosidosis, I-Cell disease, and pseudo-Hurler polydystrophy

Children with early and severe features of Hurler syndrome but with minimal urine mucopolysaccharide excretion were initially designated as having pseudo-Hurler syndrome. Since some children with these clinical features (e.g., those with

G_{M1} gangliosidosis) had cherry red spots reminiscent of neurolipidosis, the term "mucolipidosis" was coined to designate the combined findings. Methods for detecting urine oligosaccharides by thin-layer chromatography replaced this name with the chemically accurate designation of oligosaccharidoses (Jones, 1997, pp. 450–71; Gorlin et al., 2001, pp. 139–54; Thomas, 2001). The severe, aggregate manifestations of oligosaccharidoses relate in part to the many varieties of accumulated polysaccharides. Deficiency of a multisubstrate enzyme (β-galactosidase in G_{M1} gangliosidosis) or deficiency of multiple enzymes due to a disruption of the mannose-6-phosphate targeting system (I-cell disease, pseudo-Hurler polydystrophy) accounts for the accumulation of these complex oligosaccharides. Inclusions may be seen in leucocytes and fibroblasts, explaining the term "inclusion-cell disease." Multiple sulfatase deficiency also has a severe, multienzyme deficiency phenotype that combines features of lipidosis and mucopolysaccharidosis (see below).

G_{M1} gangliosidosis, I-cell disease, and pseudo-Hurler polydystrophy all have an onset of Hurler-like features at birth or during infancy. A cherry red spot is often seen in G_{M1} gangliosidosis, with corneal clouding more common in I-cell disease and pseudo-Hurler polydystrophy. All can exhibit rapid progression of neurologic symptoms and Hurler-like somatic manifestations. As with other lysosomal storage disorders, there are milder clinical variants within these categories. Preventive management is essentially the same as detailed below for the mucopolysaccharidoses. An emphasis on preserving neurosensory, joint, and respiratory functions is important for patients with milder disease; survival is often limited to early childhood in the severe forms.

Multiple sulfatidosis

Most forms of sulfatide lipidosis (metachromatic leukodystrophies) cause neurodegeneration and death without an unusual appearance. However, children with multiple sulfatase deficiency lack not only the arylsulfatases responsible for metachromatic leukodystrophy but also the mucopolysaccharide sulfatases that are deficient in disorders such as Hunter syndrome. These children have features resembling the mucopolysaccharidoses, and the disorder has been Austin syndrome.

Clinical manifestations include a loss of milestones in the second year, with progressive development of hearing loss, blindness, and seizures. Features of mucopolysaccharidosis may appear simultaneously with the neurologic deterioration, or may appear later. They include subtle coarse facies, visceromegaly, joint contractures, pectus, and gibbus. Ichthyosis and cherry red spots may occur in multiple sulfatase deficiency as distinguishing features from the mucopolysaccharidoses. Preventive management should be as outlined for the mucopolysaccharidoses, with the additional provision of skin lotions for the treatment of ichthyosis. Some amelioration of symptoms has been produced by bone marrow transplantation, but the procedure has worsened the clinical course of patients who are already deteriorating (Hopwood & Ballabio, 2001).

Lysosomal diseases: Mucopolysaccharidoses

The mucopolysaccharidoses are a group of neurodegenerative disorders that exhibit somatic changes of the face and skeleton (Table 19.1). They are lysosomal storage diseases, caused by a deficiency of enzymes that sculpt complex chains of carbohydrate and protein (glycosaminoglycans). Glycosaminoglycans are a prominent component of the extracellular matrix, explaining the thickened secretions and subcutaneous tissues in children with mucopolysaccharidosis (Jones, 1997, pp. 450–71; Gorlin et al., 2001, pp. 139–54; Neufeld Muenzer, 2001). The typical somatic changes embodied by Hurler syndrome are also seen in certain lipidoses or oligosaccharidoses (Table 19.1) distinguished from the mucopolysaccharidoses by their lower amounts of urinary glycosaminoglycans. The mucopolysaccharide-storage disorders offer a compelling strategy for enzyme or gene therapy that is derived from the classic experiments of Neufeld and colleagues: the deficient enzymes often contain a mannose-6-phosphate "tag" that targets them to lysosomes of the appropriate cells and allows a restoration of degradative function (Neufeld & Muenzer, 2001).

In contrast to neurolipidoses such as Tay–Sachs or Krabbe diseases, the mucopolysaccharide/oligosaccharide-storage diseases develop a Hurler-like syndrome that extends beyond the neurodegeneration of the retina and brain (Table 19.1). At times that vary from birth to later adolescence, depending on the disease and/or severity, the patients develop insidious symptoms. These include coarsening of the facial features, thickening of the skin and hair, thickened secretions that cause chronic rhinorrea or communicating hydrocephalus, joint contractures, and skeletal deformities. The Hurler-like appearance becomes manifest during late fetal development in the infantile form of G_{M1} gangliosidosis, during early childhood in the Hurler and Hunter syndromes, and during adolescence in the milder forms of San Filippo or Maroteaux–Lamy syndromes (Table 19.1).

The degree of mental disability versus connective tissue or skeletal involvement varies among the different mucopolysaccharide-storage disorders and among different patients with the same disorder. Patients with San Filippo syndrome have severe mental disability with milder somatic features, while those Morquio or Maroteaux–Lamy syndromes have normal mentality with severe somatic features. Despite these variations, a common set of strategies for diagnosis and preventive management are required for the mucopolysaccharidoses and oligosaccharidoses. The descriptions below are directed toward patients with mucopolysaccharidoses I (Hurler), II (Hunter), VI (Maroteaux–Lamy) and VII (Sly) syndromes, but can be modified for relevance to other conditions listed in Table 19.1. These modifications are outlined briefly in the sections devoted to complications and management.

Terminology

The mucopolysaccharidoses were first identified by the classical reports of Hurler and Hunter in the early 1900s. Distinctive clinical manifestations and subsequent characterization of enzyme deficiencies led to the delineation of seven types, each bearing the eponym of its discoverer (Table 19.1). Scheie disease was initially designated as type V until it was realized that both Scheie and Hurler syndromes involve a deficiency of α-iduronidase. Although descriptive of their high content in mucus and their core polysaccharide chain, the substances designated as "mucopolysaccharides" are more properly termed "glycosaminoglycans." Many forms of glycosaminoglycans exist, and the relative proportions of keratan sulfate, dermatan sulfate, or heparan sulfate excreted in the urine can give preliminary insight into the type of mucopolysaccharidosis.

Incidence, etiology, and differential diagnosis

The incidence of disorders with the syndrome of coarse facies and dysostosis multiplex is estimated at 1 in 10,000–20,000 births, depending on the age of ascertainment. Individual disorders, exemplified by Hurler (1 in 100,000 births), Scheie (1 in 500,000 births), or Hunter (1 in 65,000 births) syndromes, are much more rare. The etiology of these disorders is a deficiency of lysosomal proteins that incorporate or degrade complex glycosaminoglycans within lysosomes. Specific enzyme deficiencies have been characterized for all of the clinically delineated mucopolysaccharide and oligosaccharide syndromes, and antibodies to the affected proteins have led to the cloning and characterization of the responsible genes. Following the rule for other enzymes involved in the same metabolic pathway or process, the genes responsible for mucopolysaccharide accumulation are distributed widely across the genome. All are autosomal-recessive disorders, with the exception of Hunter syndrome which is X-linked recessive. Proper biochemical and molecular diagnosis of affected children allows prenatal diagnosis in subsequent pregnancies. Neonatal screening can be highly sensitive for certain of these disorders, but a simple, effective strategy for detecting the entire category is not yet available (Meikle et al., 2004). Early detection would have advantages for prevention of complications, and will become more important as enzyme and gene therapies are perfected.

The differential diagnosis is chiefly concerned with distinguishing among the members of the mucopolysaccharidosis/mucolipidosis category. Disorders with later-onset of the characteristic facial and skeletal changes, such as San Filippo syndrome, may be confused with other causes of mental retardation and bony deformities.

Chromosomal disorders and syndromes with contractures may be confused until the appropriate biochemical studies are performed.

Diagnostic evaluation and medical counseling

The presenting complaints of children with mucopolysaccharidoses will usually be developmental delay with or without unusual facial or skeletal findings. The more severe disorders may present with hydrops fetalis, infantile hydrocephalus, or even multiple fractures suggestive of osteogenesis imperfecta. For mildly stigmatized patients, an ophthalmologic examination for corneal clouding, skeletal radiographic survey for evidence of dysostosis, and a urine mucopolysaccharide screen are often obtained as evidence that the patient fits into the mucopolysaccharidosis category. Chromosomal studies may be considered for exclusion, and cranial imaging or liver biopsy may be obtained if there is macrocephaly or hepatosplenomegaly. It should be emphasized that random urine samples may give false negative results for mucopolysaccharides if they are too dilute, or false positive results if they are stored at room temperature and contaminated by bacteria. Nonspecific indicators of altered mucopolysaccharide metabolism, such as the measurement of radioactive sulfate accumulation in fibroblasts, may also give anomalous results. Patients with suggestive clinical findings should have serum, leucocyte, or fibroblast enzyme assays performed for the disorders in question; several academic centers offer panels of relevant leucocyte and serum assays. Serum levels of lysosomal enzymes are elevated in disorders such as mucolipidosis II (I-cell disease) where defective lysosomal transport allows the egress of multiple degradative enzymes.

Medical counseling must be tailored to the particular type of mucopolysaccharidosis or oligosaccharidosis. Many of these disorders are uniformly fatal, with the lifespan depending on complications and the dedication of the family to chronic care. Contact with centers doing enzyme therapy should be initiated when the diagnosis is confirmed, because benefits for visceral function are established even though neurodegenerative problems remain (Wraith et al., 2005). Patients with G_{M1} gangliosidosis or I-cell disease will usually die in early childhood; those with Hurler or Hunter syndromes, in later childhood or adolescence. Complicating predictions are the varying phenotypes caused by similar enzyme deficiencies; the iduronidase deficiencies in Hurler and Scheie disease cause early death in the former disorder but allow a virtually normal life in the latter. Mild variants have also been described having the same iduronate sulfatase deficiency found in Hunter syndrome. In general, children with stigmata manifest in early childhood face a terminal illness with severe neurodevastation that renders them bedridden and dependent on gastrostomy feedings. Attention to the type of enzyme deficiency is also important, with the Morquio or Maroteaux–Lamy syndromes exhibiting normal intelligence despite severe somatic changes. Emphasis on minimizing pain and maximizing the quality of life is recommended, without attempting to predict the exact timing of disability and death.

Family and psychosocial counseling

Because all of the mucopolysaccharidoses and oligosaccharidoses are autosomal or X-linked recessive, a 25% recurrence risk can be predicted for subsequent children. In the X-linked Hunter syndrome, only males will have phenotypic expression unless carrier females experience deletion of their normal X chromosome locus due to chromosome rearrangement. Prenatal diagnosis is available through chorionic villus biopsy or amniocentesis, although overlap of heterozygote and affected homozygote enzyme levels have caused errors in some instances. In some of the disorders, common molecular mutations have been characterized that allow DNA diagnosis.

Psychosocial counseling is extremely important in the more severe mucopolysaccharidoses because of the terrible burden of these diseases. Not only must parents learn that their apparently normal child will experience degeneration and death, but also they must witness the progressive coarsening and deformity of their child. Many patients also have severe behavioral changes that disrupt family life, with aggression, biting, hyperactivity, and inability to sleep. The large size and aggressiveness of some children warrant special measures for confinement, including a secured area to put the child and allow respite during selected family activities and sleep. Contacts with psychosocial and pastoral counseling services should be facilitated for all families with severely affected children, and parent information/support is available at The National Mucopolysaccharidosis (MPS) society (www.mpssociety.org/index.html) or numerous medical education sites. Clinical trials of bone marrow or umbilical cord transplantation are also underway, and can be accessed at the National Institute of Health (NIH) clinical trials website (www.clinicaltrials.gov/).

Natural history and complications

The majority of patients with mucopolysaccharidoses exhibit macrocephaly and early increase of growth until medical complications accumulate (see checklist). In Hurler syndrome, the accelerated growth falls off between 1 and 2 years of age, in Hunter syndrome, between 3 and 6 years. Behavioral changes often accompanying the plateauing of development, with poor attention span, aggressive behavior, and temper tantrums. Hydrocephalus may be present. Chronic rhinorrhea and otitis are common, and the thick mucus together with a large tongue places patients at risk of airway obstruction or sleep apnea. Corneal clouding is prominent in the Hurler and Maroteaux–Lamy syndromes, but absent in Hunter syndrome. The skeletal changes include progressive contractures of the extremities and deformity of the chest and spine (pectus, gibbus scoliosis). Inguinal and umbilical hernias as well as congenital hip dislocation may attest to the general affliction of connective tissue. Deformities of the thoracic cage, together with thickened alveolar secretions, often produce restrictive lung disease and interstitial pneumonitis. Odontoid hypoplasia and platyspondyly may cause cervical spinal cord compression, adding another source of unacknowledged pain or apnea.

As the disease progresses, the cardiac valves may become infiltrated and lead to congestive heart failure. Dental cysts and thin enamel may compromise oral hygiene and interfere with feeding, and infiltration of the intestine can produce chronic diarrhea. Joint fixations and neurosensory deficits lead to a withdrawn, bedridden patient with cardiorespiratory compromise. Pneumonias are a frequent cause of death. Distinctive findings among the mucopolysaccharidoses include more severe hearing loss in Hunter syndrome and the appearance of somatic features in later childhood or adolescence in Scheie syndrome. There are milder somatic features despite severe neurodegeneration in the four subtypes of San Filippo syndrome, thoracic dysplasia suggestive of a skeletal dysplasia in Morquio syndrome, and more severe cardiovascular infiltration in Maroteaux–Lamy syndrome. Hearing loss is prominent in both Morquio and Maroteaux–Lamy syndromes, and both usually have normal intellectual potential if not compromised by neurosensory deficits and medical problems. Sly syndrome exhibits striking variability, with some patients presenting as hydrops fetalis and others having only mild mental disability.

The mucopolysaccharidoses preventive medical checklist

If not part of the initial diagnostic evaluation, then a cranial MRI scan, ophthalmologic examination, audiologic assessment, and skeletal radiographic survey should be performed as soon as a specific enzymatic diagnosis is made. Neurosensory evaluation is extremely important, and regular audiometric, and ophthalmologic evaluations are essential. Periodic examination of the skeleton is also important, with referral to orthopedics for the treatment of congenital hip dislocation, joint contractures, or scoliosis. Physical and occupational therapy are needed to maintain joint mobility, and these should be initiated through early intervention services. Radiologic evaluation of the cervical spine should be performed routinely, and patients with stridor, upper airway obstruction, gasping respirations, or apnea need sleep studies and otolaryngologic evaluation. Patients with Morquio syndrome are at particular risk for quadriparesis due to atlantoaxial instability. Hydrocephalus and cervical spinal cord compression may be sources of pain that the patient cannot describe, so a high index of suspicion is necessary with consideration of craniospinal MRI scans. Undetected pain, including discomfort from upper respiratory congestion and serous otitis, may exacerbate difficult behavior. Careful medical surveillance is an important adjunct to psychosocial and pastoral supports, which should be facilitated for all families.

Depending on the type of mucopolysaccharidosis, later changes in the cardiac valves, joints, and teeth may occur in midchildhood (Hurler syndrome) up to the third or fourth decade (Scheie syndrome). Regular cardiac and skeletal evaluations are needed, with good histories and range-of-motion examinations to detect joint problems such as carpal tunnel syndrome. Formal cardiology referral with echocardiography should be performed during the initial phase of disease progression as judged by somatic and skeletal features. Because corneal clouding and hearing loss may progress during adulthood in the Scheie, Morquio, and Maroteaux–Lamy syndromes, ophthalmologic and audiometric assessments should be performed throughout life. Bone marrow transplant has been tried in several types of mucopolysaccharide disease with promising results. Younger children with minimal brain and visceral dysfunction are the best candidates.

Organellar disorders: Mitochondrial and peroxisomal diseases

The mitochondria and peroxisomes have key roles in lipid metabolism, and their pathology has significant consequences for lipid-rich structures – brain, nerves, retina, and skin. Each organelle is separated from the cell matrix by membranes, and each has an organized interior structure that can be disrupted by alterations in key proteins. Single gene mutations can cause multiple deficient enzymes and overlapping metabolic changes, complicating the diagnosis and classification of these organellar disorders. Mitochondria also have their own genome, present in some 1000 copies per cell, with additional complexity due to interaction of nuclear-encoded and mitochondrial-encoded products and to mixtures of normal and mutant mitochondrial genomes (heteroplasmy). Diagnosis of mitochondrial and peroxisomal disorders requires collaboration of dysmorphology, metabolism, and pathology subspecialists, and often ends up with a categorical (e.g., complex I deficiency, generalized peroxisomal import disorder) rather than specific diagnosis. Management will focus on the nervous system, with imaging developmental, and neurosensory assessments.

Mitochondrial disorders encoded by nuclear DNA

Mitochondria contain a large complement of proteins that contribute to the two mitochondrial membranes and mediate import of peptides and other metabolites into the organelle (Robinson, 2001; Shofner & Wallace, 2001; Wallace et al., 2001). Mitochondria contain unique ribosomes and protein synthesis mechanisms, and serve in respiratory and oxidation pathways that supply energy for the cell. Many mitochondrial proteins are encoded by nuclear DNA and imported into the organelle, exemplified by most components of the respiratory chain. Metabolic disorders caused by the alteration of nuclear-encoded mitochondrial proteins will exhibit Mendelian inheritance: usually autosomal recessive but occasionally X-linked recessive inheritance (Table 19.2). Other mitochondrial proteins are synthesized by the 16-kilobase mitochondrial genome, which is transmitted to embryonic cells in the maternal oocyte cytoplasm. Genetic disorders involving mitochondrial genome-encoded proteins often exhibit maternal inheritance, meaning that all offspring of

Table 19.2. Mitochondrial, peroxisomal, and miscellaneous metabolic dysplasias

Disease or syndrome	Incidence*	Inheritance	Complications
Mitochondrial diseases caused by nuclear genes			
Glutaric aciduria II	~50 cases	AR	ND, acidosis, hypotonia, abnormal facies, demyelination, renal cysts, genital a.
Leigh disease, lactic acidemias	?	AR, XLR	ND, lactic acidosis, hypotonia, brain a., optic atrophy, ophthalmoplegia
Mitochondrial diseases caused by mitochondrial genes			
Kearn–Sayre disease	~300 cases	Maternal, AD, AR	Ptosis, ophthalmoplegia, retinitis, hearing loss, diabetes, hypoparathyroidism, myopathy, lactic acidosis
Peroxisomal diseases			
Adrenoleukodystrophy	1 in 50,000	XLR	ND, visual loss, adrenal insufficiency
Infantile Refsum disease	~50 cases	AR	ND, hypotonia, unusual facies, liver disease, hearing loss, retinitis, ichthyosis
Neonatal adrenoleukodystrophy	~200 cases	AR	ND, hypotonia, unusual facies, seizures, demyelination, brain a.,
Zellweger syndrome	1 in 50,000	AR	ND, hypotonia, unusual facies, demyelination, brain a., liver disease, renal cysts, stippled epiphyses
Miscellaneous metabolic dysplasias			
Carbohydrate-deficient glycoprotein syndrome	~50 cases	AR	ND, liver disease, ataxia, retinitis, strabismus, abnormal fat, coagulopathy
Smith–Lemli–Opitz syndrome	~150 cases	AR	ND, hypotonia, abnormal facies, polydactyly, renal cysts, genital a.

Notes:

AR, autosomal recessive; XLR, X-linked recessive; ND, neurodegeneration; a., anomalies AD auto somal dominant,

*Cases or per number of live births.

affected mothers but no offspring of affected fathers exhibit the trait. In practice, the 1000 mitochondria in each cell may become heterogeneous in their genomic and/or protein structure, a phenomenon termed heteroplasmy. Clinical manifestations of mitochondrial genome-encoded disorders may thus change with time, representing the proportion of abnormal genomes within cells of susceptible tissues. Maternal inheritance may therefore be obscured by absent manifestations in mothers or offspring that have small proportions of abnormal mitochondria in the cells of susceptible tissues. Direct analysis of mitochondrial DNA is now available to distinguish between nuclear and mitochondrial-encoded disorders, and to measure the degree of heteroplasmy.

An underlying theme in the pathogenesis of mitochondrial DNA mutations is a diminished cellular energy supply. Any given mitochondrial DNA phenotype probably depends on the degree to which mitochondrial respiratory function is disrupted, the energy requirements of particular tissues and developmental stages, and the proportions of altered mitochondria. The most common manifestation of decreased energy supply is lactic acidemia. If the lactic acidemia is pronounced during the neonatal period, infants may have a slightly unusual facies. Other disorders with acidosis and severe hypotonia, such as glutaric acidemia type II, will have more extensive dysmorphology reminiscent of Zellweger syndrome (see below).

Glutaric acidemia type II

Accumulation of glutaric acid, a five-carbon dicarboxylic acid, occurs in two very different disorders. Type I glutaric acidemia is a defect in lysine metabolism associated with macrocephaly, hypotonia, dystonia, and Reyelike episodes with vomiting, hepatomegaly, and encephalopathy (Frerman & Goodman, 2001). Death often occurs in the first decade. Type II glutaric acidemia is caused by an abnormality of the electron transfer flavoprotein (ETF) that is part of the mitochondrial respiratory chain (Frerman & Goodman, 2001). Similar disorders are caused by deficiencies of ETF or its dehydrogenase, and both exhibit autosomal-recessive inheritance consistent with their encoding by the nuclear genome.

Clinical manifestations of glutaric acidemia type II are of three types: neonatal onset with malformations, neonatal onset without malformations, and onset in later childhood (Frerman & Goodman, 2001). Major and minor anomalies include macrocephaly, a large anterior fontanel, high forehead, broad nasal root, telecanthus, rocker bottom feet, renal cysts, hypospadias, and chordee (Wilson et al., 1989). The neonatal presentation usually includes hypotonia and hepatomegaly associated with severe hypoglycemia and metabolic acidosis. Most patients with neonatal onset die in early infancy, often with hypertrophic cardiomyopathy. Later-onset patients have presented in early to later childhood with vomiting, hypoglycemia, and acidosis. The initial diagnostic evaluation should include: urine organic acid and ketone determination – potentially revealing glutaric, ethylmalonic, and adipic acids but no ketones; serum glucose, electrolyte, hepatic transaminase, and carnitine levels – potentially revealing hypoglycemia, acidosis, and liver disease; cranial MRI scan – potentially revealing demyelination; and abdominal CT scan – potentially showing renal cysts. A definitive diagnosis can be made by demonstrating deficiency of ETF or its dehydrogenase in cultured fibroblasts or liver.

Preventive management for glutaric acidemia II will be limited in neonatal onset patients, but should include chest radiography to monitor heart size, frequent electrolyte studies to monitor acidosis, and periodic urinalyses to monitor aminoaciduria and renal disease. Therapy with oral riboflavin (100–300 mg/day) and oral carnitine (100 mg/kg/day) have had some benefit in later-onset patients but not with neonates (Frerman & Goodman, 2001). A low fat and protein diet may also be helpful. Genetic and psychosocial counseling are important for parents, and later-onset patients should have early intervention services.

Leigh disease and lactic acidemias

Leigh disease, also known as subacute necrotizing encephalomyelopathy, is a phenotype that is produced by a variety of defects in the mitochondrial respiratory chain. The presentation has onset from early infancy to middle childhood, and includes hypotonia, developmental delay with regression, optic atrophy, strabismus, nystagmus, irregularities in breathing, muscle weakness, and lactic acidosis. Later neurologic symptoms may include ataxia and spasticity. The cranial MRI scan shows demyelination and/or hyperintense areas near the thalamus and basal ganglia. Occasional patients have retinitis or hypertrophic cardiomyopathy, and some have the ragged red fibers visualized on muscle biopsy specimens that are characteristic of mitochondrial disease (Shofner, 2001).

The diagnosis of Leigh disease involves an analysis of respiratory chain components in muscle or leucocytes. Alterations in cytochrome c (respiratory complex IV) are most common, but abnormalities of NADH dehydrogenase (respiratory complex I) or pyruvate dehydrogenase have also been reported. DNA analysis is the preferred diagnostic method, since several common mutations have been described. While most mutations causing Leigh disease have been in nuclear-encoded genes, a few examples with maternal inheritance have been demonstrated. It is important to realize that the phenotype is extremely variable and heterogeneous, overlapping with other mitochondrial diseases such as pigmentary retinopathy with degeneration or mitochondrial myopathy (Shofner, 2001).

Also overlapping with the Leigh disease phenotype are numerous disorders of the mitochondrial respiratory chain that produce chronic lactic acidemia. The most common of this group is deficiency of the pyruvate dehydrogenase complex. Pyruvate dehydrogenase deficiency can cause severe neonatal lactic acidemia and death, more moderate lactic acidemia with severe developmental retardation, or intermittent lactic acidemia with ataxia after a carbohydrate load (Robinson, 2001). Clinical variability is probably related to the presence of multiple subunits in the pyruvate dehydrogenase complex, one of which is encoded on the X chromosome. Other causes include deficiency of enzymes in the glycolytic pathway (phosphenolpyruvate carboxykinase, pyruvate carboxylase). Lactic acidemias can exhibit autosomal recessive or X-linked recessive inheritance.

The initial diagnostic evaluation for children with Leigh disease or lactic acidemias should be performed in conjunction with metabolic disease specialists and include serum glucose, hepatic transaminase, electrolyte, lactate, and pyruvate levels. A high pyruvate and a high lactate (normal lactate/pyruvate ratio) would suggest defects in pyruvate dehydrogenase or other diseases such as glycogen-storage disease or defects in fatty acid oxidation. A high lactate/pyruvate ratio suggests a respiratory defect typical of Leigh disease and other mitochondrial disorders. A cranial MRI scan, ophthalmologic examination, and muscle biopsy should then reveal the typical basal ganglia demyelination, retinitis, or ragged red fibers of Leigh/respiratory chain disease, or demonstrate the more limited phenotype of lactic acidemia and neurodegeneration. Analysis for common mutations associated with Leigh disease or assay of pyruvate dehydrogenase and pyruvate carboxylase can then proceed as appropriate. The category of lactic acidemias is still expanding, and specific enzyme or DNA alterations may not be identified in many patients. Preventive management is limited to periodic neurologic and ophthalmologic evaluations, control of lactic acidosis, monitoring of growth and nutrition, and referral for early intervention services.

Several therapies have been tried for respiratory chain disorders and lactic acidemias, but disease heterogeneity has complicated the interpretation of results (Shofner, 2001; Robinson, 2001). A low-carbohydrate, ketogenic diet may be helpful for children with pyruvate dehydrogenase deficiency. Dichloroacetate at levels of 15–200 mg/kg/day often reduces lactate levels by 20% and has few side effects. Menadione (vitamin K_3) at 1.1–1.5 mg/kg/day and ascorbic acid at 50 mg/kg/day have been tried as electron donors to cytochrome c. Coenzyme Q (4.3 mg/kg/day), thiamine (100 mg/day), and riboflavin (300 mg/day as mentioned above) have also been tried. None of these treatments has produced a dramatic reversal of neurologic deterioration.

Mitochondrial disorders encoded by mitochondrial DNA

Mutations in the mitochondrial genome produce an overlapping group of disease findings that depend on the location and extent of altered DNA. Single nucleotide mutations may produce a limited phenotype such Leber hereditary optic neuropathy (LHON) or maternally inherited sensorineural deafness (Shofner & Wallace, 2001). Large mitochondrial DNA deletions often affect several organ systems, exemplified by Kearns–Sayre syndrome. The findings in Kearns–Sayre syndrome are quite variable, and overlap with those of other mitochondrial DNA mutations. Among these are Pearson syndrome (bone marrow failure, pancreatic dysfunction with diabetes mellitus, ataxia, myopathy), diabetes mellitus with deafness, mitochondrial encephalopathy with ragged red fibers (MERRF), mitochondrial encephalopathy with lactic acidemia and strokes (MELAS), and myoneuro-gastrointestinal disorder (encephalopathy, diarrhea, malabsorption, weight loss, external ophthalmoplegia, and peripheral neuropathy (Wallace et al., 2001)).

Kearns–Sayre syndrome

Patients with Kearns–Sayre syndrome show manifestations before age 20 that include ophthalmoplegia, retinitis pigmentosa, generalized myopathy, and occasional cardiac conduction defects (Wallace et al., 2001). If the onset of symptoms occurs after age 20, the patients are classified as having chronic progressive external ophthalmoplegia with or without other manifestations. Both diseases are associated with mitochondrial DNA deletions that occur during embryogenesis and increase their proportions with age, causing progressive disease. Another closely related condition is Pearson syndrome, with bone marrow failure, pancreatic insufficiency, and similar neurologic problems. Associated clinical manifestations in this spectrum of disorders include lactic acidemia, seizures, dementia, ataxia, optic atrophy, hearing loss, cardiac arrhythmias, diabetes mellitus, hypoparathyroidism, gastrointestinal dysmotility, renal failure with glomerulosclerosis, and neuropathies (Shofner and Wallace, 2001). Some patients have had renal tubular acidosis and others severe atrophy of the choroid and sclera which resembles choroidemia. Diagnosis is made by analysis of mitochondrial DNA for deletions and, more rarely, duplications. Preventive management for patients with Kearns–Sayre syndrome, chronic progressive external ophthalmoplegia, and overlapping conditions will include regular ophthalmologic, neurologic, and audiometric assessments; serum glucose, calcium, electrolyte, blood urea nitrogen, creatinine, and lactate monitoring; periodic electrocardiography; and, depending on the age of onset, referral for early intervention, special education, or job training services. Trial of coenzyme Q, vitamin K, and/or ascorbate therapy as mentioned above may be considered.

Peroxisomal diseases: Categories and specific disorders

Peroxisomes are single-membraned organelles that contain over 40 proteins, many with a prominent role in lipid metabolism. They were first observed by electron microscopy and called "microbodies," then named peroxisomes based on their content of catalase and peroxidases (Wilson et al., 1988; Gould et al., 2001). Clinical interest in peroxisomes was intensified when their absence from the liver of patients with Zellweger syndrome was discovered). A spectrum of diseases was soon defined, each involving abnormal peroxisomal structure or deficiencies of peroxisomal enzymes. Several peroxisomal diseases are summarized in Table 19.2.

A major distinction among peroxisomal diseases is whether they cause severe disruption of peroxisome structure, with multiple enzyme deficiencies, or whether they involve deficiency of a single enzyme that is located within peroxisomes (Gould et al., 2001). Acatalasemia, X-linked adrenoleukodystrophy, and rhizomelic chondrodysplasia punctata are disorders that may be caused by deficiency of a single peroxisomal enzyme deficiency (catalase, ALDP protein, and dihydroxyacetone phosphate acyltransferase enzyme respectively), and their phenotypes (mouth ulcers, neurodegenerative disease, skeletal dysplasia) are strikingly different. Peroxisomal diseases that involve multiple enzyme deficiencies have overlapping clinical manifestations that often involve the central nervous system; many of these patients have a syndrome of hypotonia and facial features that is most dramatic in Zellweger syndrome (Wilson et al., 1988). Patients with multiple deficiencies of peroxisomal enzymes also have a common metabolic profile with elevated very-long-chain fatty acids, elevated pipecolic and phytanic acids, and deficient plasmalogens. In a few cases, these multiple enzyme deficiency diseases have been shown to involve alterations in proteins within the peroxisomal membrane. It is therefore logical that mutations that disrupt the entire peroxisomal structure would cause a severe and multifaceted phenotype due to multiple enzymic deficiencies, while those that affect a single peroxisomal enzyme have a more limited and specific phenotype (Wilson et al., 1988; Gould et al., 2001).

Zellweger and colleagues reported the first patients with Zellweger syndrome in 1964, although two of their patients proved to have a separate disorder. The Refsum syndrome of ataxia, retinitis, and ichthyosis was described in 1946, and in 1974, severely affected patients with similar features were described as infantile Refsum syndrome (Wilson et al., 1988). The neurologic and adrenal changes of adrenoleukodystrophy, recognized initially as an X-linked disorder in 1923, were described as an autosomal recessive, neonatal variety in 1978 (Table 19.2). Grouping of these apparently separate diseases as a peroxisomal disease category was made possible when biochemical markers of peroxisome dysfunction were characterized: elevated very-long-chain fatty acids and deficient plasmalogens. Soon it was realized that patients presenting as Zellweger syndrome, neonatal adrenoleukodystrophy, or infantile Refsum syndrome had alterations in the metabolism of very-long-chain fatty acid and plasmalogens. Unlike adult adrenoleukodystrophy or Refsum syndrome, these early-onset disorders had similar phenotypes due to generalized peroxisomal dysfunction (Wilson et al., 1988).

As with other multifaceted disorders, observers have seized upon component manifestations of Zellweger syndrome and reported affected patients as having separate conditions. Some patients described as having "chondrodysplasia punctata," "hyperpipecolatemia," or infantile Refsum disease undoubtedly are part of the spectrum of Zellweger syndrome, and it will require further biochemical and molecular characterization to achieve a precise delineation of the generalized peroxisomal disease category (Wilson, 1986). Rhizomelic chondrodysplasia punctata is discussed in more detail in Chapter 11. Detection of reduced red cell plasmalogens is particularly useful in this condition.

Although population surveys have estimated incidences for Zellweger syndrome as low as 1 in 100,000 births, the aggregate incidence of generalized peroxisomal disorders is thought to be 1 in 25,000–50,000 births (Gorlin et al., 2001, pp. 168–74). The generalized peroxisomal disorders exhibit autosomal-recessive inheritance, and selected patients with Zellweger syndrome have had mutations in the 70- or 35-kDa peroxisomal membrane proteins. Alterations in very-long-chain fatty acid degradation, plasmalogen synthesis, or numerous other pathways presumably account for the effects on embryogenesis and neural development. There is little understanding of the pathogenesis of peroxisomal disorders, but the ability to increase peroxisome density by administering oral agents offers some promise for pre- and postnatal therapy.

The differential diagnosis includes many other disorders with hypotonia, neurologic dysfunction, and congenital contractures (Wilson et al., 1988). Congenital myopathies, disorders producing stippling of the epiphyses (chondrodysplasia punctatas), and even Down syndrome have been confused. It may be difficult to separate Zellweger syndrome from other generalized peroxisomal disorders because of the similar profile of enzymic deficiencies and metabolic alterations. Even the classical Zellweger phenotype is heterogeneous, since studies investigating the correction of cells in culture have suggested that mutations at thirteen different genetic loci can cause this phenotype. Several of these loci have been characterized, and encode peroxisomal membrane proteins.

Peroxisomal disorders: Diagnostic evaluation and management

Children with generalized peroxisomal disorders often come to medical attention because of infantile hypotonia, and frequently have cranial MRI scans that may show demyelination. Additional diagnostic findings include retinitis pigmentosa detected by ophthalmologic examination, stippled epiphyses detected by radiographic survey, and periportal fibrosis with iron storage on liver biopsy performed for hepatomegaly. The diagnosis is confirmed by a demonstration of altered metabolites, particularly the sensitive and specific assay for serum very-long-chain fatty acids developed by Moser and colleagues (Gould et al., 2001). Additional metabolic testing includes assay of erythrocyte plasmalogens and serum phytanic acid; leucocyte or fibroblast enzyme assay to demonstrate deficiencies of dihydroxyacetone phosphate acyltransferase (Wilson et al., 1986), phytanic oxidase, or sedimented catalase may also be employed (Gould et al., 2001). All of these measures are usually

abnormal in patients with severe Zellweger syndrome, while more selective elevations of very-long-chain fatty acids (neonatal adrenoleukodystrophy) or phytanic
acid (infantile Refsum disease) may point toward other disorders.

Most important for medical counseling is the age of presentation and the severity of neurologic features. Severely hypotonic neonates with brain anomalies by
MRI have a severe prognosis, with likely death during infancy. It should be remembered that hepatic disease in Zellweger syndrome may be fulminant in the first few
months and subside, so prognosis should be based on neurologic manifestations.
Even milder patients with a Zellweger syndrome phenotype will have significant
neurosensory deficits and mental disability. Parents should be prepared for a
potentially lethal and handicapping disorder.

All of the generalized peroxisomal disorders are autosomal recessive, implying a
25% recurrence risk for future pregnancies. Prenatal diagnosis is reliable by measuring elevated metabolites or enzyme deficiencies in chorionic villi or amniocytes.
Psychosocial and pastoral support appropriate for a potentially lethal disorder
should be facilitated. Parent information can be found at a site by parents of a child
with infantile Refsum disease (www.pacifier.com/~mstephe/) and at various medical
education sites by searching on "peroxisomal disorders."

The natural history of peroxisomal disorders varies from a turbulent and lethal
neonatal course to a chronic debilitating condition with survival into adulthood.
Patients with Zellweger syndrome have facial features that derive from the hypotonia
and dysostosis. Patients with milder Zellweger syndrome, neonatal adrenoleukodystrophy, or infantile Refsum disease have similar but less dramatic craniofacial findings. The anterior fontanel is large, the forehead is prominent, and there is a broad
nasal root with down-turned corners of the mouth and micrognathia. Single palmar
creases, a high palate, and club feet are residua of *in utero* hypotonia, and there may
be Brushfield spots and epicanthal folds reminiscent of Down syndrome. Additional
clinical manifestations include congenital heart defects, liver disease with hepatitis
and cirrhosis, renal cysts, genital anomalies such as hypospadias and cryptorchidism,
and intestinal anomalies (pyloric stenosis, malrotation). Patients with infantile
Refsum syndrome are more likely to have ichthyosis.

The clinical course is dominated by neurologic abnormalities including seizures,
sensorineural deafness, blindness, and severe mental disability. Neuropathologic
analysis has been performed on 46 patients with Zellweger syndrome, showing
pachymicrogyria (67%), heterotopias or migration defects (48%), gliosis (35%),
demyelination (22%), and agenesis of the corpus callosum (20%) or olfactory lobes
(7%; Wilson et al., 1986). Poor nutrition and failure to thrive are usual, with most
patients requiring gastrostomy feedings. The high palate leads to dental crowding,
and proteinuria or urinary tract abnormalities (horseshoe kidney, renal agenesis)
may occur.

After or during the initial diagnostic evaluation, a cranial MRI or CT scan, skeletal survey, renal sonogram, auditory evoked response study, electroretinogram, and screening of liver functions should be performed. Ophthalmologic and neurologic assessments will usually be indicated to evaluate lens opacities, retinal pigmentation, seizure activity, and hypotonia. Feeding and nutrition should be followed carefully, since many patients will require high-calorie formulas, and nasogastric or gastrostomy feedings. Coagulation profiles and precautions against bleeding may be required if there is liver disease, and some patients have had esophageal varices. Occasional patients have presented with hypothyroidism, so monitoring of thyroid, hearing, vision, and nutrition is important in early childhood. Early intervention and psychosocial counseling appropriate for children with severe disabilities is appropriate.

Long-term survivors will need monitoring of developmental progress, hearing and vision. Speech therapy and dental evaluations for tooth crowding are also important. Periodic urinalyses are advised to evaluate aminoaciduria and potential infections; children with abnormal genitalia should have urologic assessment and monitoring during puberty. Adrenal function may be compromised in the peroxisomal disorders, so steroid supplementation may be considered during acute illnesses. A corticin stimulation test can be performed to confirm subtle adrenal insufficiency. Cataracts and ichthyosis can be late complications, so regular skin and eye examinations are needed.

Dietary therapy has been attempted in the peroxisomal disorders by minimizing dietary oleic acid and dairy products containing phytanic acid (Gould et al., 2001). Dietary supplementation of ether lipids produced increases in erythrocyte plasmalogens, but no long-term clinical improvements (Wilson et al., 1986). Martinez et al. (2000) have reported docosahexaenoic acid deficiency in those with generalized and more restricted peroxisomal phenotypes, and have shown improved cerebral myelination and biochemical functions in patients given oral docosahexaenoic acid.

Miscellaneous metabolic disorders

Carbohydrate-deficient glycoprotein syndrome

A wide variety of signs and symptoms can occur in the carbohydrate-deficient glycoprotein syndrome, including mental disability, growth failure, ataxia, seizures, strokes, strabismus, retinal degeneration, cardiomyopathy with pericardial effusions, elevated hepatic enzymes, renal microcysts, and unusual distribution of body fat (Gorlin et al., 2001, pp. 174–6). More than 150 patients have been reported, and the inheritance is autosomal recessive. The initial symptoms are often hypotonia and developmental delay, with peau d'orange appearance of the skin and lipodystrophy being the most distinctive features. Multiple glycoproteins have abnormal carbohydrate moieties, causing deficiencies of the coagulation proteins S and C, antithrombin III, and factor IX, with abnormal transferrin being used as a diagnostic marker from serum. There is as yet no mapping data or knowledge of the gene responsible for carbohydrate-deficient glycoprotein syndrome.

Preventive management should consist of an initial diagnostic evaluation including a cranial MRI scan, screening of serum coagulation factors as well as transferrin, cardiologic evaluation to screen for cardiomyopathy or pericardial effusion, and ophthalmologic evaluation to screen for strabismus or retinal changes. Hematologic referral to consider anticoagulant therapy should be considered in patients with low levels of protein S, C, and antithrombin III; hyperreflexia, ataxia, and muscle atrophy in children have been attributed to strokelike episodes. Variants exist with mild mental disability, but most families should be referred for early intervention and psychosocial services.

Smith–Lemli–Opitz syndrome

Many years after the description of Smith–Lemli–Opitz syndrome of microcephaly, growth delay, and facial and genital abnormalities, a defect in cholesterol metabolism has been recognized in these patients (Jones, 1997, pp.112–5; Gorlin et al., 2001, pp. 1147–51). The original patients had a very distinctive phenotype with a low birth weight, microcephaly, a broad nasal root, micrognathia, genital anomalies including cryptorchidism and hypospadias, and syndactyly of toes 2 and 3. A more severe, type II disorder has been suggested, with more severe prenatal growth retardation and genital anomalies. Both disorders exhibit autosomal-recessive inheritance and elevations of the metabolite 7-dehydrocholesterol, and they are allelic conditions deriving from the 7-dehydrocholesterol reductase gene on chromosome 11. Smith–Lemli–Opitz syndrome can now be viewed as one of several morphologic disorders with defective cholesterol synthesis, including X-linked dominant chondrodysplasia punctata type 2, congenital hemidysplasia with ichthyosiform erythroderma and limb defects (CHILD syndrome), a lethal bone dysplasia with hydrops (HEM dysplasia), and some cases of Antley–Bixler syndrome (Porter, 2003).

Summary of clinical concerns: Smith–Lemli–Opitz syndrome management considerations

General: The many potential affected systems mandage comprehensive initial evaluation to screen for anomalies of brain, heart, skeleton, urinary tract and internal genitalia. The timing of cranial, cardiac, skeletal, abdominal, and pelvic imaging studies should be coordinated with the severity of illness and the probability of neonatal survival.

Growth and development: Early feeding and nutrition is important to monitor because of hypotonia (50% of infants) or hypertonia (30% of older children): All patients will need early intervention assessment, and those with significant disabilities will require preschool, rehabilitative, and psychosocial counseling services.

Facial: Distinctive appearance with the ptosis (85%), broad nasal root, anteverted nares (75%), and small jaw.

Eye: Cataracts, strabismus (40%): Early and regular ophthalmologic evaluations.

ENT: Cleft palate (40%) or broad lateral palatine ridges that give the appearance of a high palate (60%), chronic otitis, frequent infections: The debilitated condition and infectious susceptibility of these patients, together with palatal anomalies require surveillance for infections including chronic otitis. Regular audiologic assessments are needed.

Skeletal: Postaxial polydactyly (25%), congenital hip dislocation, and deformations like scoliosis may require orthopedic evaluation.

Cardiac: Congenital heart lesions (20%) include septal defects, tetralogy of Fallot, and aberrant subclavian artery: Echocardiography and cardiology evaluation with symptoms.

Gastrointestinal: Pyloric stenosis, gastointestinal reflux, Hirschsprung disease (in more severe patients): Imaging studies and gastroenterology evaluation with symptoms.

Urogenital: Genital anomalies include hypospadias (50%), cryptorchidism (50%), and genital ambiguity with internal testes and Mullerian duct remnants in some males. Renal anomalies (45%) include cystic or hypoplastic kidneys: Neonates with ambiguous genitalia require multidisciplinary assessment from urology, endocrinology, and genetics to determine sex assignment, and early renal sonogram plus monitoring for hypertension or urinary tract infections should be performed on all patients.

Neurologic: Brain abnormalities include hydrocephalus, seizures, agenesis of corpus callosum, and hypoplasia of cerebellar vermis: Neurologic evaluation if behavior suggests seizures or if there is severe hypertonicity that interferes with feeding.

Parental counseling: Many patients, particularly with the type II Smith–Lemli–Opitz syndrome, have a lethal disorder that merits palliative management sufficient for diagnosis and genetic counseling. However, milder forms of the disorder have been described, and occasional patients survive to adulthood. Blood for the measurement of elevated 7-dehydrocholesterol levels should be obtained in all suspect patients, since a positive result provides the option for prenatal diagnosis in subsequent pregnancies. Chromosomal studies will be indicated in most patients with Smith–Lemli–Opitz syndrome to exclude other diagnoses. One study suggests a higher rate of suicidal behavior in carrier parents, correlating with their potential deficiency in cholesterol metabolism (Lalovic et al., 2004), but separation of parenting stressors and correlation with cholesterol metabolite levels remains to be done. Initial hopes that cholesterol supplementation might improve neurologic functions have not been realized, but there may be some benefit in monitoring 7-dehydrocholesterol levels so as to minimize reported liver toxicity (Sikora et al., 2004). There is an advocacy and exchange site for the disorder (members.aol.com/slo97/), and many educational sites can be accessed by searching on the syndrome name.

Preventive management of the mucopolysaccharidoses

Description: Clinical pattern produced by storage of mucopolysaccharides in tissues, including progressive changes in the face, skeleton, heart, and brain. The aggregate incidence of all types is 1 in 10,000–20,000 births.

Clinical diagnosis: Variable, progressive pattern of manifestations that includes a coarse facial appearance, thickened skin and hair, chronic rhinorrhea, thickened gums, skeletal changes in the cranium, thorax and limbs, and mental deterioration. The progression is insidious with timing in early childhood for Hunter and Hurler syndromes, later childhood in Maroteaux–Lamy and San Filippo syndromes. Morquio syndrome resembles a skeletal dysplasia.

Laboratory diagnosis: Deficiency of specific lysosomal enzyme in leucocytes or fibroblasts.

Genetics: All types exhibit recessive inheritance with Hunter syndrome being X-linked recessive.

Key management issues: Cranial MRI, ophthalmology, audiology, skeletal survey at the time of diagnosis; monitoring of hearing, vision, respiratory status, and sleep, periodic examination for congenital hip dislocation, joint contractures, or scoliosis; radiographic evaluation for cervical spinal cord compression or hydrocephalus with irritability or respiratory problems, monitoring of the cardiac valves, joints, and teeth as the disease progresses. Enzyme therapy is available for some disorders (Wraith et al., 2005).

Growth charts: Early overgrowth, later short stature in most types, no specific charts are available.

Parent information: National Mucopolysaccharidosis Society (MPS – www.mpssociety.org/index.html).

Basis for management recommendations: Derived from complications cited in the references below as cited in Gorlin et al. (2001), Neufeld & Meunzer (2001). Clinical judgement should guide the use of imaging studies that require anesthesia, but the subtle manifestations of hydrocephalus or spinal cord compression should be realized.

Summary of clinical concerns

General	Learning	Cognitive disability, neurodegeneration
	Behavior	Poor attention span, outbursts, aggression
	Growth	Early tall stature, later short stature
Facial	Facies	Coarse appearance, chronic rhinitis, chronic otitis
	Eyes	Strabismus, corneal clouding, retinal degeneration, ptosis
	Nose	Chronic rhinorrea, thick mucus, upper respiratory infections
	Mouth	Large tongue, dental cysts, large alveolar ridges, gingivitis, abnormal tooth positions, thin enamel, large adenoids, sleep apnea, limited temporo-mandibular joint motion
Surface	Neck/trunk	Short neck, umbilical hernias, inguinal hernias, pectus
	Epidermal	Hirsutism, coarse hair and skin, skin nodules
Skeletal	Cranial	Macrocephaly, microcephaly, J-shaped sella, craniosynostosis
	Axial	Platyspondyly, odontoid hypoplasia, and kyphoscoliosis (particularly in Morquio); spinal cord compression and cervical myelopathy (particularly in Maroteaux–Lamy), widened ribs
	Limbs	Carpal tunnel syndrome, congenital hip dislocation, joint contractures, camptodactyly or claw-deformities of fingers
Internal	Digestive	Chronic diarrhea, hepatosplenomegaly
	Circulatory	Aortic insufficiency and cardiac valvular lesions (adults), mitral valve prolapse
	Pulmonary	Interstitial pneumonitis, airway obstruction
Neural	Central	Hydrocephalus, headaches, seizures, neurodegeneration
	Motor	Motor delays
	Sensory	Optic and otic nerve dysfunction, hearing and vision loss

Concerns of frequency >20% are **highlighted**

Key references

Gorlin, et al. (2001). *Syndromes of the Head and Neck*. New York: Oxford. pp. 119–39.

Neufeld & Muenzer (2001). The mucopolysaccharidoses. In: *The Metabolic and Molecular Bases of Inherited Disease*, 8th edn, ed. Scriver et al., pp. 3421–52. New York: McGraw-Hill, Inc.

Wraith, et al. (2005). Laronidase treatment of mucopolysaccharidosis I. *BioDrugs* 19:1–7.

Mucopolysaccharidosis

Preventive medical checklist (0–3 years)

Name _____ Birth date __ / __ / ____ Number _____

Age	Evaluations: key concerns	Management considerations		Notes
New born ↓ **1 month**	Dysmorphology: anomalies Hearing, vision: eye examination[2] Feeding: macroglossia, dysphagia Skeletal: neck, joints, hernias Neurologic: hydrocephalus Parental adjustment	☐ Genetic/metabolic evaluation[1] ☐ ABR; ophthalmology ☐ Feeding specialist; video swallow[3] ☐ Skeletal X-rays;[3] orthopedics[3] ☐ Neurology;[3] head/neck MRI[3] ☐ Family support[4]	☐ ☐ ☐ ☐ ☐ ☐	
2 months ↓ **4 months**	Growth, development:[5] head size Hearing, vision: otitis, corneae[2] Feeding: macroglossia, dysphagia Skeletal: neck, joints, hernias Neurologic: hydrocephalus Heart: murmur Parental adjustment Other:	☐ ECI[6] ☐ ABR;[3] ophthalmology;[3] ENT[3] ☐ Feeding specialist; video swallow[3] ☐ Skeletal X-rays;[3] orthopedics[3] ☐ Neurology;[3] head/neck MRI[3] ☐ Echocardiogram;[3] cardiology[3] ☐ Family support[4] ☐	☐ ☐ ☐ ☐ ☐ ☐ ☐ ☐	
6 months ↓ **9 months**	Growth, development:[5] head size Hearing, vision: otitis, corneae[2] Feeding: macroglossia, dysphagia Skeletal: neck, joints, hernias Neurologic: hydrocephalus, AAI, sleep[7] Other:	☐ ECI[6] ☐ ABR;[3] ophthalmology;[3] ENT[3] ☐ Feeding specialist; video swallow[3] ☐ Skeletal X-rays;[3] orthopedics[3] ☐ Neurology;[3] head/neck MRI;[3] sleep study[3] ☐	☐ ☐ ☐ ☐ ☐ ☐	
1 year	Growth, development:[5] head size Hearing, vision: otitis corneae[2] Airway, heart, lungs, feeding, gums Skeletal: neck, spine, joints, hernias Neurologic: hydrocephalus, AAI, sleep[7] Other:	☐ ECI[6] ☐ ABR;[3] ophthalmology;[3] ENT[3] ☐ Diet;[3] cardiology;[3] pulmonology;[3] dentistry ☐ Orthopedics;[3] anesthesia precautions ☐ Neurology;[3] head/neck MRI;[3] sleep study[3] ☐	☐ ☐ ☐ ☐ ☐ ☐	
15 months ↓ **18 months**	Growth, development:[5] head size Hearing, vision: otitis corneae[2] Skeletal: neck, spine, joints, hernias Neurologic: hydrocephalus, AAI, sleep[7]	☐ ECI[6] ☐ ABR;[3] ophthalmology;[3] ENT[3] ☐ Orthopedics;[3] anesthesia precautions ☐ Neurology;[3] head/neck MRI;[3] sleep study[3]	☐ ☐ ☐ ☐	
2 years	Growth, development:[5] head size Hearing vision: otitis corneae[2] Airway, heart, lungs, feeding, gums Skeletal: neck, spine, joints, hernias Neurologic: hydrocephalus, AAI, sleep[7]	☐ ECI[6] ☐ Audiology/ABR;[3] ophthalmology;[3] ENT[3] ☐ Diet;[3] cardiology;[3] pulmonology;[3] dentistry ☐ Orthopedics;[3] anesthesia precautions ☐ Neurology;[3] head/neck MRI;[3] sleep study[3]	☐ ☐ ☐ ☐ ☐	
3 years	Growth, development:[5] head size Hearing, vision: otitis, corneae[2] Airway, heart, lungs, feeding, gums Skeletal: neck, spine, joints, hernias Neurologic: hydrocephalus, AAI, sleep[7] Other:	☐ ECI;[6] family support[4] ☐ Audiology; ophthalmology;[3] ENT[3] ☐ Diet;[3] cardiology;[3] pulmonology;[3] dentistry ☐ Orthopedics;[3] anesthesia precautions ☐ C-spine films; neurology;[3] sleep study[3] ☐	☐ ☐ ☐ ☐ ☐ ☐	

Mucopolysaccharidosis concerns		Other concerns from history	
Hydrocephalus, craniosynostosis Corneal clouding, glaucoma Chronic otitis, hearing loss Large tongue, dysphagia Frequent infections Infiltrative pulmonary disease	Cardiac valve disease Hip dislocation, kyphosis Inguinal, umbilical hernias Motor, speech delays Microcephaly, seizures AAI, sleep apnea	**Family history/prenatal** _____ _____ _____ _____	**Social/environmental** _____ _____ _____ _____

Guidelines for the neonatal period should be undertaken *at whatever age* the diagnosis is made; ABR, auditory brainstem evoked response; AAI, atlantoaxial instability; [1]subspecialty evaluations crucial for diagnosis and counseling – should include surface and skeletal examination, skeletal X-rays, head/spine MRI if cranial/neck changes, enzyme/DNA studies, and consideration of enzyme/transplant therapy; [2]by practitioner; [3]as dictated by clinical findings; [4]parent group, family/sib, financial, and behavioral issues; [5]consider developmental pediatric, neurology, or genetics clinic according to symptoms and availability; [6]early childhood intervention if muscle weakness, feeding problems; [7]snoring, pause in breathing, daytime sleepiness, unusual sleep positioning.

Mucopolysaccharidosis

Preventive medical checklist (4–18 years)

Name _____ Birth date__/__/____ Number _____

Age	Evaluations: key concerns	Management considerations		Notes
4 years ↓ **6 years**	Growth: head size, short stature Development:[2] preschool transition Hearing, vision:[2] corneae, otitis Airway, heart, lungs, gums, teeth Skeletal: neck, spine, joints, hernias Neurologic: hydrocephalus, AAI, sleep[7] Other:	❑ Specialty clinics[1] ❑ Family support;[4] preschool program[5] ❑ Audiology; ophthalmology;[3] ENT[3] ❑ Cardiology;[3] pulmonology;[3] dentistry ❑ Orthopedics;[3] anesthesia precautions ❑ Neurology;[3] head/neck MRI;[3] sleep study[3] ❑	❑ ❑ ❑ ❑ ❑ ❑ ❑	
7 years ↓ **9 years**	Growth: head size, short stature Development:[1] school transition[5] Hearing, vision:[2] corneae, strabismus Airway, heart, lungs, gums, teeth Skeletal: neck, spine, joints, hernias Neurologic: hydrocephalus, AAI, sleep[7] Other:	❑ Specialty clinics;[1] endocrinology[3] ❑ Family support;[4] school progress[6] ❑ Audiology; ophthalmology[3] ❑ Cardiology;[3] pulmonology;[3] ENT;[3] dentistry ❑ Orthopedics;[3] anesthesia precautions ❑ Neurology;[3] head/neck MRI;[3] sleep study[3] ❑	❑ ❑ ❑ ❑ ❑ ❑ ❑	
10 years ↓ **12 years**	Growth: head size, short stature Hearing, vision:[2] corneae, strabismus Airway, heart, lungs, gums, teeth Skeletal: neck, spine, joints, hernias Other:	❑ Specialty clinics;[1] school progress[6] ❑ Audiology; ophthalmology[3] ❑ Cardiology;[3] pulmonology;[3] ENT;[3] dentistry ❑ Orthopedics;[3] anesthesia precautions ❑	❑ ❑ ❑ ❑ ❑	
13 years ↓ **15 years**	Growth: head size, short stature Hearing, vision:[2] corneae, strabismus Airway, heart, lungs, gums, teeth Skeletal: neck, spine, joints, hernias Neurologic: AAI, regression, sleep[7] Other:	❑ Specialty clinics;[1] school progress[6] ❑ Audiology; ophthalmology[3] ❑ Cardiology;[3] pulmonology;[3] ENT;[3] dentistry ❑ Orthopedics;[3] anesthesia precautions ❑ C-spine films; neurology;[3] sleep study[3] ❑	❑ ❑ ❑ ❑ ❑ ❑	
16 years ↓ **18 years**	Growth: head size, short stature Hearing, vision:[2] corneae, strabismus Airway, heart, lungs, gums, teeth Skeletal: neck, spine, joints, hernias Other:	❑ Family support;[4] school progress;[6] ❑ Audiology; ophthalmology[3] ❑ Cardiology;[3] pulmonology;[3] ENT;[3] dentistry ❑ Orthopedics;[3] anesthesia precautions ❑	❑ ❑ ❑ ❑ ❑	
19 years ↓ **23 years**	Adult transition: nutrition, activity[6] Hearing, vision:[2] strabismus Airway, heart, lungs, gums, teeth Skeletal: neck, spine, joints, hernias Neurologic: AAI, regression, sleep[7]	❑ Dietician;[3] physical therapy/trainer[3] ❑ Audiology; ophthalmology[3] ❑ Cardiology;[3] pulmonology;[3] ENT;[3] dentistry ❑ Orthopedics;[3] anesthesia precautions ❑ Neurology;[3] head/neck MRI;[3] sleep study[3]	❑ ❑ ❑ ❑ ❑	
Adult	Nutrition, activity guidance Hearing, vision:[2] strabismus Airway, lungs, gums, teeth Heart: valve dysplasia, aneurysms Skeletal: neck, spine, joints, hernias Neurologic: AAI, regression, sleep[7] Other:	❑ Dietician;[3] physical therapy/trainer[3] ❑ Ophthalmology, dentistry ❑ Pulmonology;[3] ENT;[3] dentistry ❑ Cardiology; echocardiogram ❑ Orthopedics;[3] anesthesia precautions ❑ Neurology;[3] head/neck MRI;[3] sleep study[3] ❑	❑ ❑ ❑ ❑ ❑ ❑ ❑	

Mucopolysaccharidosis concerns		Other concerns from history	
Corneal clouding, glaucoma Dental anomalies, gingivitis Large tongue, poor airway Frequent infections Infiltrative pulmonary disease	Cardiac valve disease Kyphoscoliosis Inguinal, umbilical hernias AAI, sleep apnea Hydrocephalus, seizures Neurodegenerative disease	**Family history/prenatal** _____ _____ _____ _____	**Social/environmental** _____ _____ _____ _____

Guidelines for the neonatal period should be undertaken *at whatever age* the diagnosis is made; AAI, atlantoaxial instability; [1]consider developmental pediatric, neurology, or genetics clinic according to symptoms and availability; [2]by practitioner; [3]as dictated by clinical findings; [4]parent group, family/sib, financial, and behavioral issues; [5]preschool program including developmental monitoring and motor/speech therapy; [6]monitor individual education plan, educational testing, balance of special education and inclusion, academic progress, behavioral differences, later vocational planning.

Parent guide to the mucopolysaccharidosis

The mucopolysaccharidoses (MPS) are a group of disorders that may affect the brain, eyes, face, and skeleton. They are lysosomal storage diseases in which complex chemicals accumulate in cells and disrupt function, producing neurodegeneration, eye, and skeletal changes that vary according to the specific enzyme deficiency.

Incidence, causation, and diagnosis

The aggregate incidence is 1 in 10,000–20,000 births with individual disorders like Hurler (1 in 100,000 births), Scheie (1 in 500,000 births), or Hunter syndromes (1 in 65,000 births) being more rare. A useful but not completely reliable screening test for the MPS disorders is to test for elevated mucopolysaccharides (GAGs) in the urine. The urine screen must then be supplemented with enzyme assays or DNA analysis to define the specific enzyme deficiency and type of MPS. The degree of mental disability versus connective tissue or skeletal involvement varies among the different MPS storage disorders and among different patients with the same disorder. The mucolipidoses or oligosaccharidoses are a class of disorders with similar clinical findings but negative urine MPS screen. Children with suggestive findings must have thorough clinical imaging studies and enzyme studies even when urine MPS screening is negative. The more severe MPS and oligosaccharidosis disorders may present with hydrops fetalis (swelling of the fetus), infantile hydrocephalus (fluid accumulation in brain cavities), or multiple fractures/thin bones reminiscent of brittle bone diseases. It should be emphasized that random urine samples may give false negative results for GAGs if they are too dilute, or false positive results if they are stored at room temperature and contaminated by bacteria.

Natural history and complications

Patients with MPS have a similar clinical course that varies degree, age of onset, and extent of neurologic versus skeletal complications. Most will exhibit increased head size and increased growth until medical complications accumulate. Behavioral changes often accompany the plateau in development, with poor attention span, aggressive behavior, and temper tantrums. Hydrocephalus (accumulation of fluid in brain cavities), chronic runny nose and ear infections, large tongue and thick mucous with airway obstruction, large adenoids with sleep apnea (cessation of breathing), corneal clouding, contractures of the extremities, deformities of the chest (pectus) or spine (gibbus, scoliosis), inguinal or umbilical hernias, and congenital hip dislocation may occur depending on type. Restrictive lung disease, pneumonias, cardiac valvular disease (in adulthood), and spinal compression (causing neck pain or tilt, sleep apnea, sleep problems) may occur, Dental cysts and thin enamel may compromise oral hygiene and interfere with feeding, and infiltration of the intestine can produce chronic diarrhea. Joint fixations and neurosensory deficits lead to a withdrawn, bedridden patient with cardiorespiratory compromise in the more severe forms.

Preventive medical needs

Cranial MRI scan, ophthalmologic examination, audiologic assessment, and skeletal X-rays should be performed as soon as a specific enzymatic diagnosis is made. Neurosensory evaluation is extremely important, and regular audiometric and ophthalmologic evaluations are essential. Periodic skeletal examinations are needed for congenital hip dislocation, joint contractures, or scoliosis (spinal curvature). Physical and occupational therapy are needed to maintain joint mobility, and these should be initiated through early intervention services. Evaluation of the cervical spine and upper airway should be performed before anesthesia, with sleep and otolaryngologic studies as needed. Patients with Morquio syndrome are at particular risk for spinal nerve damage and leg weakness due to neck spine instability, and most types have risks for hydrocephalus or cervical cord compression that can hasten degeneration. Later changes in the eyes, cardiac valves, joints, and teeth require appropriate assessments during adulthood. Enzyme therapy, bone marrow, or umbilical cord transplants provide a source of normal enzyme and should be considered when the diagnosis is made.

Family counseling

Medical counseling must be tailored to the particular type of MPS or oligosaccharidosis, with appropriate palliative care after neurodegeneration becomes severe. Many of these disorders are uniformly fatal, with the life span depending on complications and the dedication of the family to chronic care. Because the MPS/oligosaccharidoses are autosomal or X-linked recessive, a 25% recurrence risk can be predicted for subsequent children. In the X-linked Hunter syndrome, only males will have disease. Pre-implantation diagnosis (when DNA mutations are known) and routine prenatal diagnosis (for enzyme deficiencies) are options. Psychosocial counseling is extremely important for parents of severely affected children, who must face deterioration and behavior changes that can disrupt family life. Large and aggressive children may require a secured room for protection and family respite. Contacts with psychosocial and pastoral counseling services should be facilitated for all families with severely affected children.

20

Metabolic dysplasias susceptible to dietary treatment

The provision of dietary treatment is a powerful strategy for preventive management that is available for selected inborn errors of metabolism. Newborn screening programs allow recognition of certain of these disorders (e.g., phenylketonuria, galactosemia), while clinical acumen must be utilized for others (e.g., glycogen storage diseases).

An algorithm for approaching patients with suspected inborn errors of metabolism is presented in Chapter 1. The approach emphasizes the differences between abnormalities in "small" molecule metabolism (acute presentations with seizures, coma, hypoglycemia, acidosis, hyperammonemia, sepsis, or organ failure) and abnormalities in "large" metabolism (facial changes, visceromegaly, or neurodegeneration). While there is overlap between these simplified categories, the "small" molecule disorders are often diagnosed by amino acid and organic acid screening, while the "large" molecule disorders are recognized by neurologic, ophthalmologic, and tissue biopsy studies. In this chapter, the "small" molecule diseases are represented by galactosemia and phenylketonuria, while the "large" molecule diseases are represented by the glycogen storage diseases.

The definitive diagnosis for any inborn error of metabolism is to characterize a primary defect in the responsible gene (by DNA diagnosis) or its protein product (by enzyme assay). Often the demonstration of abnormal metabolites in plasma, urine, or affected tissues allows categorization of the disease and guides selection of the gene or enzyme to be tested. Participation of a metabolic disease specialist in the initial diagnostic evaluation is strongly recommended for interpretation of complex laboratory results (e.g., urine organic acid profiles). After the diagnosis is confirmed, the primary physician assumes the more important role in management, either as a partner in ensuring dietary compliance or as a director of the preventive management program.

This chapter will discuss treatable metabolic diseases according to four categories: disorders of carbohydrate, amino acid, organic acid, and fatty acid metabolism. Among these disorders, only the glycogen storage diseases have sufficient population incidence and diversity of preventive measures to warrant presentation of a detailed checklist.

Disorders of carbohydrate metabolism

The provision of glucose to cells is important for energy production in highly active tissues such as liver, skeletal muscle, and heart. Numerous steps in the provision of glucose to cells can be interrupted, including dietary intake, digestion into small molecules, absorption into the blood stream, conversion of other carbohydrates into glucose, maintenance of serum glucose levels, intake of glucose into cells, and storage of materials for gluconeogenesis during fasting. Hypoglycemia is the prototypic symptom of inborn errors of carbohydrate metabolism such as galactosemia or glycogen storage diseases. Dietary deprivation, intestinal malabsorption, or inaccessibility of glucose to cells (e.g., diabetes mellitus) represent other alterations of carbohydrate metabolism that are better discussed in nutrition, gastroenterology, or endocrinology texts (Table 20.1).

Galactosemia

The most common cause of galactosemia is deficiency of the enzyme galactose-1-phosphate uridyl transferase (GALT). The incidence ranges from 1 in 35,000 to 1 in 190,000 births, with an average figure of 1 in 62,000 births (Holton et al., 2001; Zaffanello et al., 2005). The diagnosis is often suspected from clinical manifestations of vomiting, diarrhea, and jaundice after breast or formula feeding in the newborn period, and a urine clinitest will be positive for reducing substances (sugars such as glucose or galactose and other metabolites with aldehyde groups). In the 38 states with newborn screening programs, report of an elevated serum galactose should be returned within 1–2 weeks, but this may occur after serious complications have occurred. Timely collection of neonatal blood spots and follow-up of infants for feeding problems and jaundice may also challenge health care professionals in this era of early discharge from the nursery. A change to lactose-free formula should be instituted immediately once galactosemia is considered, until referral to metabolic specialists and assay of blood for GALT enzyme deficiency can confirm or exclude the diagnosis.

Clinical manifestations of galactosemia most commonly include cataracts, vomiting, diarrhea, and indirect hyperbilirubinemia in the neonatal period. The jaundice may occur after the usual physiologic elevation of bilirubin, and there may be associated hemolysis, which masks the disease. Cataracts may be visible only on slit-lamp examination. Less commonly, infants are acutely ill with the lethargy, hypotonia, hepatic disease, and cerebral edema that will usually occur if lactose is not removed from the diet. There is predisposition to *E. coli* sepsis, and it is recommended that

Table 20.1. Disorders of carbohydrate metabolism

Disease	Incidence*	Deficient enzyme, locus	Clinical manifestations
Fructose-1,6-diphosphatase deficiency	Unknown	Fructose-1, 6-diphosphatase	Hypoglycemia, lactic acidosis
Galactosemia, severe	1 in 50,000	GALT, 9p13, 4 kb gene, 11 exons, Q188R mutation in 70%	Neonatal liver disease, sepsis, later MR if untreated, ovarian failure with certain mutations
Galactosemia, mild	Unknown	Galactokinase 17q21	Cataracts
GSD type Ia (von Gierke)	1 in 100,000	G-6-Pase, 17p	Hypoglycemia, hyperuricemia, lactic acidemia, hepatomegaly
GSD type Ib	1 in 200,000	Abnormal microsomal transport G-6-Pase	Type Ia plus neutopenia
GSD type II (Pompe)	1 in 100,000	α-Glucosidase	Cardiac disease, early death
GSD types III and IV	1 in 100,000	Debrancher (1p21) or brancher (3p12) enzyme	Mild type Ia (III) or fatal cirrhosis (type IV)
GSD types VI and VIII	1 in 200,000	Phosphorylase kinase (unknown or Xp22)	Mild type Ia

Note:

GSD, glycogen storage disease; GALT, galactose-1-phosphate uridyl transferase; G-6-P, glucose-6-phosphate; 9p17, band 17 on the short arm of chromosome 9.

* per number of live births.

infants with *E. coli* infections be screened for GALT enzyme deficiency. Later manifestations include more chronic presentation in later infancy or childhood with failure to thrive, cataracts, hepatomegaly, and developmental delay. Even with dietary treatment, there is a significant incidence of speech problems (62% of sibs recognized and treated as newborns), decreased IQ, poor school performance, and psychological problems such as lack of motivation and withdrawal. Females may have streak or hypoplastic ovaries, hypergonadotropic hypogonadism (75%), amenorrhea, premature menarche, and infertility.

Preventive management of galactosemia begins with removal of breast milk or formula from the diet, followed by dietary counseling through experienced nutritionists at a metabolic disease center. Failure to remove lactose from the diet produces liver failure with cirrhosis, renal tubular dysfunction with aminoaciduria, cataracts, and death. Soybean formula (e.g., Isomil) or Nutramigen are recommended formulas, although the former has galactose-containing sugars such as raffinose and the latter is derived from cow's milk. The dangers of lactose in fruit and vegetables have been emphasized by some, but others feel that this lactose is not available for absorption and metabolism (Holton et al., 2001). Since galactose is not an essential nutrient, complete omission is the goal of dietary therapy. Assay of erythrocyte galactose-1-phosphate levels may be performed to monitor dietary compliance, but there is imperfect and controversial correlation between these levels and galactose intake. Milk avoidance should certainly be maintained throughout life, but other foods (e.g., cakes and bread) may be permitted in adolescence and adulthood. Better intellectual outcomes have been demonstrated in sibs having dietary restriction from birth as compared to their older sibs who required several weeks to over 1 year to make the diagnosis.

Because intellectual and ovarian dysfunction can occur even in well-controlled patients, developmental and speech assessments should be performed on children with galactosemia. Speech apraxias are particularly common, and older children have had cerebellar ataxias and tremors reminiscent of neurodegenerative disease. Since these changes may relate to kernicterus or other neonatal complications, galactosemics with turbulent neonatal histories should probably receive early intervention and preschool services. Monitoring of females for menstrual irregularities is also important, and pelvic sonography may be indicated when there is concern about puberty or fertility. Quarterly visits to the metabolic clinic are recommended for young children, with annual visits being sufficient for older and more stable patients.

Hereditary fructose intolerance and fructose 1,6-bisphosphatase deficiency

Hereditary fructose intolerance is a self-limiting disease that exerts its most severe effects during infancy (Steinmann et al., 2001; Santer et al., 2005). It is an autosomal-recessive disorder that leads to deficiency of aldolase and accumulation of fructose-1-phosphate in tissues. Infants and young children may present with severe vomiting, failure to thrive, hypoglycemia, jaundice, diarrhea, hepatic and renal disease. Reducing substances may be found in the urine, but definitive diagnosis may require a fructose challenge. Even small amounts of sucrose, fructose, or sorbitol may be lethal for some patients, although most survive and become normal when they are able to control their diet and avoid fructose-rich foods. Nutritional counseling is still needed once the diagnosis is suspected, since even the small amounts of fructose allowed by self-selection may cause hepatomegaly and growth failure. Monitoring of growth, development, and yearly assessment in the metabolic/nutrition clinic is appropriate preventive management for patients with hereditary fructose intolerance. Families and older patients should carry emergency treatment cards that emphasize the dangers of intravenous fluids containing sucrose, fructose, or sorbitol.

Fructose 1,6-bisphosphatase (FDPase) deficiency is a more severe disorder than hereditary fructose intolerance. More than 85 patients with this autosomal-recessive disorder have been reported, and it can be diagnosed by assaying the cognate enzyme in liver. FDPase deficiency usually presents in the newborn period, with severe hypoglycemia, acidosis, hyperventilation, hypotonia and coma. Unlike hereditary fructose intolerance, the patients rarely have hepatic or renal disease and there is no aversion to eating sweets or fruits containing fructose. Usually there are episodic attacks of inanition, vomiting, convulsions, hypoglycemia, and acidosis before the diagnosis is recognized. These attacks are provoked by febrile illnesses and fasting. The clinical course is benign once fructose and sucrose are excluded from the diet, but high-carbohydrate diet, frequent feeding, and treatment of intercurrent episodes with glucose and intravenous fluids may be required. Preventive management consists of nutritional counseling and early pediatric evaluation for intercurrent infections, watching for vomiting, diarrhea, and acidosis. Families should be counseled regarding the danger of sucrose-containing intravenous fluids, and emergency treatment cards stipulating this prohibition should be carried by affected patients. For patients who are doing well, yearly visits to the metabolic clinic are sufficient.

Glycogen storage diseases

Terminology

Glycogen storage diseases are a group of genetic disorders that produce alterations in the amount or structure of glycogen. Since storage of glycogen occurs mainly in liver and muscle, the diseases were first classified based on the spectrum of hepatic and muscular disease (Chen, 2001). Type I glycogen storage disease was described as "hepato-nephromegalia glycogenica" by von Gierke in 1929, and the disease is still known by that eponym. Types III (Cori or Forbes disease), IV (Anderson disease) and VI (Hers disease) are also hepatic glycogenoses, while type II (Pompe disease with cardiac manifestations) and types V and VII (McArdle and Tarui diseases with muscle cramping) are muscle glycogenoses. Type II (Pompe) glycogen storage disease is a lysosomal storage disease that is quite different from other glycogenoses, and it emphasizes that glycogen storage is one cause of cardiomyopathy (Arad et al., 2005).

Incidence, etiology, and differential diagnosis

The incidence of all types of glycogen storage diseases is about 1 in 20–25,000 births, with types I–IV accounting for over 90% of patients. Most follow the general rule for metabolic diseases and exhibit autosomal-recessive inheritance; the exceptions are the group of heterogenous disorders that comprise the X-linked recessive type VI category. Enzymes that regulate glucose/glycogen interconversion are responsible for the glycogen storage diseases, including type I (glucose-6-phosphatase), type II (lysosomal α-glucosidase), type III (debranching enzyme), type IV (branching enzyme), type V (muscle phosphorylase), type VI (phosphorylase and phosphorylase kinase), and type VII (phosphofructokinase). Differential diagnosis for the hepatic disorders will include other causes of hypoglycemia and acidosis: galactosemia, fructose bisphosphatase deficiency, fatty acid oxidation disorders or even infectious hepatitis may be considered until the typical metabolic profile and excess hepatic glycogen are demonstrated. Pompe disease can simulate endocardial fibroelastosis and other cardiomyopathies until the characteristic shortened P–R interval is demonstrated by electrocardiography. The muscle cramping of types V and VII can be confused with other disorders that interfere with muscle energy metabolism (i.e., hexokinase deficiency) until exercise testing, phosphorus magnetic resonance imaging, and muscle enzyme assays are employed.

Diagnostic evaluation and medical counseling

Although a variety of intravenous tolerance tests and associated imaging studies can be performed, the primary technique for diagnosis of glycogen storage diseases should involve biopsy of the appropriate organ followed by histologic and enzymatic study of the hepatic or muscle tissue. The exception is Pompe disease, where the abnormal lysosomal enzyme (α-glucosidase) is best assayed in fibroblasts grown from skin biopsy. The enzyme can be assayed in leucocytes prepared from whole blood, but α-glucosidase isozymes may contribute residual activities that are more difficult to interpret. Medical counseling can be optimistic for glycogen storage diseases other than types II and IV. Although patients with types I and III disease may have short stature and protuberant abdomens, improvements in management and natural amelioration after puberty allows normal adult function for many affected individuals. Emphasis on adherence to treatment regimens is important, since treatment is clearly related to the degree of short stature and adult complications. Families of patients with type II or type IV disease require psychosocial, pastoral, and hospice support appropriate for the early lethality of these disorders.

Family and psychosocial counseling

The recurrence risk for parents of children with glycogen storage disease will be 25%, with type VI families having the risk for affected sons rather than daughters. Carrier mothers do not have manifestations of type VI glycogen storage disease, so that enzyme assay of maternal tissues is required to determine if index patients with type VI disease represent new mutations. Molecular analysis is now possible for most types of glycogen storage disease since gene mutations responsible for their respective enzyme deficiencies have been characterized (see www.genetests.org).

Family counseling for patients with hepatic glycogenoses I and III should emphasize the importance of maintaining adequate carbohydrate supplies so that growth failure, abnormal body build, and medical complications can be minimized. Similar counseling regarding avoidance of high-intensity exercise should be given to patients with muscle glycogenoses types V and VII. Parent information and support is available at the Association for Glycogen Storage Disease in the United States (www.agsdus.org/) and United Kingdom (www.agsd.org.uk/home/), as well as several medical education sites accessed by searching on "glycogen storage disease" or particular syndrome names.

Natural history and complications

The key derangement in patients with hepatic glycogenoses is the inability to mobilize hepatic glycogen into circulating glucose. Abnormal amounts or structures of glycogen accumulate and produce hepatomegaly, while the block in glucose liberation causes hypoglycemia, lactic acidosis, hyperuricemia, and hyperlipidemia. Lipids also accumulate in the liver and contribute to the hepatomegaly. The types of hepatic glycogenoses present variations on this theme of glycogen accumulation and glucose scarcity. In type I, shunting of glucose-6-phosphate through glycolysis causes increased lactate and acidosis. The lactate competes with renal urate excretion, and joins with increased nucleotide turnover to cause hyperuricemia. The exaggerated glycolysis also increases pools of NADH/NADPH and glycerol, favoring triglyceride synthesis and fatty liver. Types III and VI involve the same pathogenetic mechanisms as in type I, but to lesser degrees. In type IV, the accumulating glycogen is hepatotoxic and leads to early death from liver failure. The cause of toxicity is not known (Chen, 2001).

As a result of these metabolic alterations, patients with hepatic glycogenoses exhibit early clinical manifestations of hypoglycemia, seizures, and lactic acidosis. In later childhood, they may have short stature, cherubic or "doll-like" facies with increased adiposity, protuberant abdomen with hepatomegaly, and skin xanthomas. Ocular changes may include atrophy of the retinal pigment epithelium. After puberty, which is often delayed, there is short stature, pancreatitis secondary to hyperlipidemia, gouty tophi, and arthritis secondary to hyperuricemia, and renal disease with proteinuria, Fanconi syndrome, hypertension, hyperfiltration, or renal failure. Osteoporosis and pulmonary hypertension have also been reported, but increased atherosclerosis from hyperlipidemia has not been demonstrated. Most patients with type I glycogen storage disease develop hepatic adenomas in their second to third decade of life, and these are subject to hemorrhage or malignant transformation. The hepatic adenomas and hepatocellular carcinomas may reflect increased amounts of long-chain, dicarboxylic fatty acids that are associated with peroxisome proliferators and liver cancers in rodents.

Glycogenoses other than type I exhibit either milder or different clinical manifestations. Biochemical analysis of glucose-6-phosphatase compartmentalization in the cell has revealed a sub-type of glycogen storage disease type I that has been designated type Ib. In addition to the clinical problems detailed above, these patients have neutropenia with recurrent bacterial infections, mouth ulcers, and intestinal lesions that present as inflammatory bowel disease. Type III patients have more frequent cirrhosis, particularly if they are Japanese, and later-onset muscular weakness and wasting. Type III patients may also develop arrythmias (Arad et al., 2005). Type VI patients may have growth delay, motor delay, mild hepatitis, hepatomegaly, and hyperlipidemia in childhood, but show improvement with age to become virtually asymptomatic in adulthood. The severe cirrhosis in type IV, the cardiomyopathy in type II, and the intermittent muscle cramping in types V and VII have already been mentioned as exceptions to the clinical manifestations summarized for types I, III, and VIII.

Hepatic glycogen storage disease preventive medical checklist

The initial management concern in children with hepatic glycogenoses is to restore glucose homeostasis and prevent hypoglycemic seizures, lactic acidosis, hyperuricemia, and hyperlipidemia (Chen, 2001). Enzymic or DNA diagnosis is required to distinguish milder type III and VI patients who may not require therapy. Two dietary treatment methods are efficacious in preventing hypoglycemia and its secondary complications. The first involves placement of a nasogastric tube for administration of nocturnal glucose drip feedings. The rate is 8–10 mg/kg/min in an infant and 5–7 mg/kg/min in older children. During the day, a high-carbohydrate diet is administered to comprise a total load of 65–70% carbohydrate, 10–15% lipid, and 20–25% fat with about 33% of total intake administered as the nocturnal infusion. The first oral feeding must follow cessation of the infusion by no more than 30 min, and precautions to ensure pump and tube function are important since interruptions have been associated with sudden hypoglycemia and death. The second dietary treatment involves oral administration of uncooked cornstarch at 1.6 g/kg every 4 h for infants younger than 2 years, changing to 1.75–2.5 g/kg every 6 h. The cornstarch provides a slow-release form of glucose and is supplemented to provide a diet with similar composition to that mentioned for nocturnal infusion.

Once dietary therapy is instituted, monitoring of growth and development, glucose levels, liver size, liver function tests, and tongue size is important. Patients with glycogen storage disease type Ib will require complete blood counts to monitor neutropenia, and inspection for mouth ulcers. Patients with type Ib disease who develop inflammatory bowel disease have been treated with colony-stimulating factors. Periodic assessments by an experienced dietician and metabolic specialist is recommended, and the option of liver transplantation should be considered in severe cases. Allopurinol should be given for children with hyperuricemia, maintaining the serum urate concentration below 6.4 mg/mL. A bleeding time should be obtained prior to any surgery, and abnormal values corrected by intravenous glucose administration. In general, 10% dextrose solutions should be used for intravenous therapy rather than Ringer's lactate. Fructose and galactose should also be limited in the diet of type I patients since these sugars cannot be converted to glucose.

Management of older children with hepatic glycogen storage disease should include monitoring of glucose, liver function, uric acid, renal function, and liver size. The occurrence of hepatomas should be monitored by abdominal examination and periodic abdominal ultrasound, with periodic α-fetoprotein measurements to check for transformation to hepatocarcinoma. If there is poor growth, referral to endocrinology may be considered, and women should be counseled about worsening symptoms that occur with pregnancy. The presence of malignant hepatic tumors would constitute an immediate indication for liver transplant, and some patients have required renal transplant because of chronic renal failure. Many patients with long-term dietary treatment are now reaching adulthood, and the outlook for normal stature and regression of hepatic adenomas seems good.

Disorders of amino acid metabolism

Disorders of amino acid metabolism may be present acutely in the newborn period (hyperglycinemia, urea cycle disorders) or gradually with developmental delay and seizures. The usual diagnostic procedures are a serum ammonia, plasma amino acids, and urine organic acids. Newborn screening is an important method for recognizing aminoacidopathies such as phenylketonuria, since dietary treatment can prevent mental retardation. Few of the amino acid disorders are associated with an abnormal facies or congenital malformations (Table 20.2). Homocystinuria does involve an altered body habitus and is discussed in Chapter 16.

Phenylketonuria

Elevated plasma concentration of phenylalanine is associated with three categories of disease (Scriver & Kaufman, 2001). The most frequent is classical phenylketonuria (PKU), due to deficiency of phenylalanine hydroxylase enzyme. Patients with PKU require diets low in phenylalanine to have normal mental development. Milder deficiencies of phenylalanine hydroxylase produce hyperphenylalaninemia, a benign variant which rarely requires dietary treatment. A third category involves deficiency of biopterin, the cofactor for phenylalanine hydroxylase, and is more refractory to dietary management. Another disease occurs in infants of mothers

Table 20.2. Disorders of amino acid metabolism

Disease	Incidence*	Deficient enzyme, locus	Clinical manifestations
Phenylketonuria	1 in 10,000	<1% PAH, 12q22, 90 kb gene with 13 exons, >100 diverse mutations	MD, mousy odor, seizures if untreated
Hyperphenylalaninemia	1 in 20,000	>1% PAH, 12q22, subset of mutations	None – benign phenotype
Hyperphenylalaninemia	1 in 1,000,000	Dihydropteridine reductase, 4p15	Severe MD, seizures
Tyrosinemia type I	unknown	Fumarylacetoacetate hydrolase, 15q23	Liver disease, cirrhosis
Oculocutaneous albinism	1 in 30,000	Tyrosinase, 11q14	Pale skin, eyes, sun sensitivity, nystagmus
Alkaptonuria	1 in 100,000	Homogentisic acid oxidase, 3q2	Dark urine, pigmented cartilage, arthritis
Homocystinuria	1 in 350,000	Cystathionine-β-synthase deficiency, 21q21	Marfanoid habitus, vascular thromboses
Maple syrup urine disease	1 in 180,000	Branched chain keto-acid dehydrogenase subunits, 1p31, 6p21, 7q31, 19q13	MD, ketoacidosis; lactic acidosis with E3 subunit deficiency

* per number of live births.

with uncontrolled PKU during pregnancy; these infants have congenital anomalies and developmental delay reminiscent of fetal alcohol syndrome.

PKU, like hyperphenylalaninemia and the biopterin deficiencies, is an autosomal-recessive disorder. The incidence of PKU is 1 in 10,000 births in caucasian populations, while hyperphenylalaninemia is four- or five-fold lower and the biopterin deficiencies 100-fold lower. Children with PKU are often lightly pigmented, presumably because of tyrosine deficiency (tyrosine is the product of phenylalanine hydroxylase) and decreased melanin synthesis. Developmental delay, seizures, scleroderma-like changes, and skin rashes may occur. Demyelination of the brain may be demonstrated on cranial MRI scan if dietary control is inadequate. Untreated patients with PKU will have severe mental retardation, while adolescents terminating treatment may have depression, distractibility, anxiety, and agoraphobia.

Preventive management for PKU begins with accurate diagnosis. Health care providers must be vigilant to ensure that newborn screening is performed in an era of early neonatal discharge. Elevated phenylalanine in blood spots is often reported within 10–14 days and a repeat sample is requested. Children with confirmed elevations should be referred to a metabolic disease center for quantitative blood phenylalanine and tyrosine determinations and biopterin testing. Once the diagnosis of PKU is confirmed, forceful medical and dietary counseling of the parents is essential to ensure compliance with a diet low in phenylalanine. Parents should also be cautioned about aspartame, the artificial sweetener that contains phenylalanine. Genetic counseling regarding the 25% recurrence risk and the feasibility of prenatal diagnosis by DNA analysis should be mentioned. Some patients, particularly those with biopterin deficiencies, have some mental disability despite good dietary compliance.

After the initial diagnostic evaluation and counseling, management consists of monitoring of nutrition and development. Many states have guidelines for management of children with PKU. Follow-up is best coordinated with a metabolic center and a nutritionist knowledgable about phenylalanine-free foods and formulae. Parents should be encouraged to compile 3-day diet records when the child is 6 months, 1 year, 2 years, and 3 years old to assess knowledge and compliance. Most programs recommend monitoring of blood phenylalanine and tyrosine levels at least every 6 months and more often if compliance is in question. A variety of child behavior and developmental testing should also be performed. Termination of the diet has been tried at age 6 years, but most centers recommend lifelong restriction. Teenagers are often aware of decreased concentration and school abilities when their intake of phenylalanine increases. Women with PKU must be counseled regarding the risks of pregnancy, since they must have good dietary control before and during the embryonic period. Many of these women have difficulty resuming a stringent diet, particularly when they have mental disability. Infants born to poorly controlled mothers may have microcephaly, growth failure, congenital heart disease, ocular, and orthopedic anomalies. Preventive management of these infants can utilize the checklist for fetal alcohol syndrome that is presented in Chapter 5.

Maple syrup urine disease

Maple syrup urine disease involves accumulation of branched chain amino and organic acids, producing acidosis, and neurologic symptoms (Chuang & Shih, 2001). It is an autosomal-recessive disorder with a frequency of about 1 in 185,000 births. The primary defects involve alteration of the branched chain α-keto-acid dehydrogenase, a complex of at least five proteins and a thiamine cofactor. In the most severe variety, neonates become lethargic at age 4–7 days, then progress to hypotonia, dystonic posturing, ketosis, and acidosis. Subtle dysmorphic features that may accompany acidosis in patients with maple syrup urine disease, pyruvate dehydrogenase deficiency, and related disorders. Seizures, coma, and a bulging fontanelle and a maple syrup odor may be noted. The diagnosis is made by blood amino acid and urine organic acid profiles, which show the branched chain amino acids and keto acids (valine, leucine, isoleucine). Several milder forms of the disease have been described and discriminated by molecular analysis; one of these responds to thiamine.

Preventive management relies on a sufficiently early diagnosis to avoid severe neurologic lesions. The initial diagnosis and dietary counseling is best made at a metabolic center, where the specialized testing and dietary management is available. Once the diagnosis is suspected, thiamine at 50–300 mg/day should be given for at least 3 weeks. Special formulas lacking in branched chain amino acids should be administered, and blood branched chain amino acid levels followed weekly for 6 months. Once the levels are stable, determinations can occur at 6–12 month intervals, but regular evaluations for skin and mouth lesions should occur. Intercurrent infections and/or dehydration can be lethal to these patients, and parents should be warned to contact their physician early for symptoms of illness, loss of appetite, or behavioral changes. Exchange transfusion and parenteral nutrition may be required during acute episodes (Chuang & Shih, 2001). Many patients sustain some neurologic damage, so early intervention and other services appropriate for children with disabilities are needed.

Disorders of organic and fatty acid metabolism

The prominent symptom of organic acidemias is metabolic acidosis. In disorders of fatty acid oxidation, acute decompensation may occur after a normal early childhood, often related to fasting and an intercurrent illness. Several organic acidemias and fatty acid oxidation disorders are accompanied by hypoglycemia and absence of the usual ketones. More than eight disorders of fatty acid oxidation have been described, epitomized by medium chain coenzyme A dehydrogenase deficiency. Affected patients have episodic hypoglycemia, acidosis, and carnitine deficiency, sometimes with cardiomyopathy and skeletal myopathy. They do not have an unusual appearance or congenital malformations. The pediatrician must be alert for disorders of fatty acid oxidation, since children may have lethargy and acidosis only in concert with routine infections; a blood acylcarnitine profile should be obtained in those with several such episodes, or who seem to become extraordinarily sick from a routine illness. Supplemental newborn screening, which is essentially an acylcarnitine profile on the neonatal blood spot, is becoming more widely used and will allow presymptomatic detection of fatty acid oxidation disorders. Once recognized, the shorter and medium chain disorders can be treated successfully with low fat diets, frequent feeding, and carnitine supplementation.

While many fatty acid disorders and organic acidemias exhibit demyelination, seizures, and other neurologic problems, they are not typically associated with dysmorphology. An exception is biotinidase or multiple carboxylase deficiency, where patients may have ocular problems, deafness, and alopecia.

Biotinidase and holocarboxylase synthetase deficiencies

Biotin is a vitamin cofactor for several carboxylase enzymes including proprionyl coenzyme A carboxylase and pyruvate carboxylase. These mitochondrial carboxylases

Table 20.3. Organic acidemias and fatty acid oxidation disorders

Disease	Incidence*	Deficient enzyme, locus	Clinical manifestations
Propionic acidemia	Unknown	Propionyl-CoA carboxylase subunits, 3q13, 13q22	MD, acidosis, hypoglycemia, hyperammonemia, neutropenia
Methylmalonic acidemia	1 in 20,000	Methylmalonyl-CoA mutase, 6p12	Same as propionic
Methylmalonic acidemia plus homocystinuria	Unknown	Methylcobalamin (vit. B12) synthesis	MD, milder acidosis, neutropenia
Multiple carboxylase deficiency	1 in 25,000	Biotinidase	Sparse hair, rashes, acidosis, anion gap
Multiple carboxylase deficiency	Unknown	Holocarboxylase synthetase deficiency	Sparse hair, rashes, acidosis, anion gap
LCHAD deficiency	Unknown	Long-chain hydroxyacyl CoA dehydrogenase	Liver disease, cardiomyopathy
MCAD deficiency	1 in 20,000	Medium chain acyl-CoA dehydrogenase, 1p31	Nonketotic hypoglycemia, acidosis, sudden death
SCAD deficiency	Unknown	Short chain acyl-CoA dehydrogenase	MD, lethargy, vomiting, hypotonia

* Per number of live births.

are important for fatty acid synthesis and amino acid catabolism, and their combined deficiency produces elevations of lactate, propionate, ammonia, alanine, and ketone bodies (Fenton et al., 2001). Biotin is chemically attached to these carboxylases (biotinylation), and must be recycled through action of the enzyme biotinidase. Defective biotinylation (holocarboxylase synthetase deficiency) or defective biotin recycling (biotinidase deficiency) are two disorders that produce similar clinical results: organic aciduria, acidosis, variable neurologic problems, skin rashes, and alopecia. These disorders are important to recognize because they can be partially or completely cured by administration of biotin (Table 20.3).

Holocarboxylase synthetase deficiency has been described in less than 20 patients, producing lactic acidosis, ketosis, organic aciduria including propionic and lactic acids, hyperammonemia, skin rashes, poor feeding, lethargy, seizures, ataxia, and hair loss. More than 100 patients have been described with biotinidase deficiency, a later-onset disorder with similar clinical symptoms. Children with either disorder have increased susceptibility to bacterial and fungal infections, and patients have died with disseminated sepsis before treatment can be given. Most children with holocarboxylase synthetase deficiency present before 3 months, while that age is the median age of presentation for patients with biotinidase deficiency.

The initial diagnostic evaluation for children with biotin deficiencies should include urine organic acids, blood amino acids, blood ammonia, glucose, electrolytes, neurology, and ophthalmology examinations. The definitive diagnosis is established by enzyme assay of component carboxylases and biotinidase in serum, leucocytes, or fibroblasts. Preventive management for disorders of biotin metabolism begins with administration of 60–80 mg/day of oral biotin when the diagnosis is suspected. Biotin therapy is curative if begun before severe infection or neurologic devastation. Prenatal diagnosis is also available for these autosomal-recessive disorders, and administration of 10 mg/day of oral biotin to mothers during the last trimester, followed by treatment of the infant, has resulted in normal children with demonstrable enzyme deficiencies. It is not clear if prenatal in addition to postnatal therapy is necessary for these normal outcomes. Once treatment is begun, the child should have regular assessments of hearing, vision, and development. Audiometry and ophthalmology evaluations are particularly important, since hearing loss and optic atrophy respond more slowly to therapy (Fenton et al., 2001). Feeding and nutrition should also be carefully monitored in early childhood. Baseline neurologic and dermatologic examinations may be useful to detect motor weakness, ataxia, and rashes that may persist despite successful biotin therapy. Early intervention services should be considered in children with prominent neurologic symptoms or developmental delays; speech problems have been recognized in less than 10% of treated patients with biotinidase deficiency.

Preventive management of glycogen storage diseases

Description: Clinical patterns caused by deficiency of enzymes for glycogen degradation, resulting in liver and muscle disease. Their overall incidence is 1 in 20–25,000 births.

Clinical diagnosis: Pattern of manifestations including short stature, cherubic face, prominent abdomen with enlarged liver, and liver disease with recurrent hypoglycemia, hypercholesterolemia, hyperuricemia, and acidosis. Type I is the classic hepatic disease with type Ib having neutropenia; types III and VI are milder versions of type I while type IV has lethal cirrhosis; type II lethal cardiac, and types V, VII skeletal muscle disease.

Laboratory diagnosis: Liver biopsy to document glycogen storage, specific enzyme assays in liver biopsy tissue.

Genetics: Autosomal recessive with a 25% recurrence risk after the first affected child; type VI is X-linked recessive.

Key management issues: Dietary therapy with complex carbohydrates coordinated by a metabolic disease center, monitoring of growth, development, glucose levels, liver size, liver function tests, and tongue size; assessment of blood counts and inspection for mouth ulcers in type Ib; allopurinol therapy for hyperuricemia; screening for hepatic tumors by abdominal examination, periodic abdominal ultrasound, and α-fetoprotein measurements; bleeding times prior to surgery; endocrine referrals for poor growth; options for liver transplantation in severe cases; counseling women about worsening disease during pregnancy.

Growth Charts: Short stature is common, but no specific charts are available.

Parent information: Available at the Association for Glycogen Storage Disease in the United States (www.agsdus.org/) and United Kingdom (www.agsd.org.uk/home/).

Basis for management recommendations: Complications as summarized by Chen (2001).

Summary of clinical concerns

General	Behavior	Rebellious because of abnormal appearance, short stature
	Growth	**Short stature**, failure to thrive (types II, IV)
	Tumors	**Hepatic adenomas** (decades 2–3), hepatocarcinoma
Facial	Eyes	Retinal lesions (hyperlipidemia)
	Mouth	Oral ulcers (type Ib)
Surface	Neck/trunk	**Protuberant abdomen**
	Epidermal	Skin xanthomas
Skeletal	Limbs	Gouty arthritis (postpubertal), osteoporosis
Internal	Digestive	**Hepatomegaly**, intermittent diarrhea, pancreatitis, inflammatory bowel disease (type Ib), lethal cirrhosis (Type IV)
	Pulmonary	Pulmonary hypertension
	Circulatory	Congestive heart failure (type I), severe cardiomyopathy and short P–R interval (type II), later cardiomyopathy (type III)
	Endocrine	Delayed puberty, normal fertility
	Metabolic	Hypoglycemia, lactic academia, hyperuricemia, hyperlipidemia
	RES	Easy bruising, epistaxis, prolonged bleeding time (impaired platelet adhesion due to hypoglycemia), neutropenia in type Ib
	Excretory	Enlarged kidneys; proteinuria, glomerular disease, hypertension, nephrocalcinosis, renal failure in adulthood, myoglobinuria and acute renal failure (types V, VII)
	Genital	Polycystic ovaries in females without acne/hirsutism
Neural	Central	Seizures (hypoglycemia), hypotonia (type IV)
	Motor	Muscle atrophy, severe myopathy (type IV), later myopathy (types III, V, VII), cramps (types V, VII)

RES, reticuloendothelial system; **concerns** of frequency >20% are **highlighted**

Key references

Arad, et al. (2005). Glycogen storage diseases presenting as hypertrophic cardiomyopathy. *New England Journal of Medicine* 352: 362–72.

Chen (2001). Glycogen storage diseases. In *The Metabolic and Molecular Bases of Inherited Disease*, 8th edn, eds C. R. Scriver et al., pp. 1521–2. New York: McGraw-Hill, Inc.

Glycogen storage diseases

Preventive medical checklist (0–3 years)

Name _____ Birth date __ / __ / ____ Number _____

Age	Evaluations: key concerns	Management considerations	Notes
Newborn ↓ 1 month	Initial examination: hepatomegaly, hypotonia Hearing, vision[2] Metabolic, blood counts, coagulation Heart: cardiomyopathy[3] Neuromuscular: myopathy[3] Diagnostic evaluation Parental adjustment	❑ Metabolic evaluation; genetic counseling[1] ❑ ❑ ABR ❑ ❑ CBC/diff; coagulation studies; liver panel ❑ ❑ EKG;[3] echocardiogram;[3] cardiology[3] ❑ ❑ Neurology[3] ❑ ❑ Liver, muscle or skin biopsy; enzyme studies ❑ ❑ Family support[4] ❑	
2 months ↓ 4 months	Growth, development, hearing, vision[2] Nutrition: macroglossia;[3] hypoglycemia[3] Metabolic: glucose, lytes, urate Blood counts, coagulation, hepatorenal Heart: cardiomyopathy[3] Neuromuscular: myopathy[3] Parental adjustment Other:	❑ ECI;[6] ABR[3] ❑ ❑ Feeding specialist;[3] night feeding;[3] GI[3] ❑ ❑ Serum metabolic panel ❑ ❑ CBC/diff; clotting factors; BUN; liver enzymes ❑ ❑ EKG;[3] echocardiogram;[3] cardiology[3] ❑ ❑ Neurology[3] ❑ ❑ Family support[4] ❑ ❑ ❑	
6 months ↓ 9 months	Growth, development, hearing, vision[2] Nutrition: macroglossia;[3] hypoglycemia[3] Metabolic: glucose, lytes, urate Blood counts, coagulation, hepatorenal Heart: cardiomyopathy[3] Other:	❑ ECI[6] ❑ ❑ Feeding specialist;[3] night feeding;[3] GI[3] ❑ ❑ Serum metabolic panel ❑ ❑ CBC/diff; clotting factors; BUN; liver enzymes ❑ ❑ EKG;[3] echocardiogram;[3] cardiology[3] ❑ ❑ ❑	
1 year	Growth, development, hearing, vision[2] Nutrition: macroglossia;[3] hypoglycemia[3] Metabolic: glucose, lytes, urate Blood counts, coagulation, hepatorenal Heart: cardiomyopathy[3] Neuromuscular: myopathy[3] Other:	❑ ECI;[3,6] family support[3,4] ❑ ❑ Feeding specialist;[3] night feeding;[3] GI[3] ❑ ❑ Serum metabolic panel ❑ ❑ CBC/diff; clotting factors; BUN; liver enzymes ❑ ❑ EKG;[3] echocardiogram;[3] cardiology[3] ❑ ❑ Neurology[3] ❑ ❑ ❑	
15 months ↓ 18 months	Growth, development, hearing, vision[2] Nutrition: macroglossia;[3] hypoglycemia[3] Metabolic: glucose, pH, lytes, urate Blood counts, coagulation, hepatorenal	❑ ECI[6] ❑ ❑ Feeding specialist;[3] night feeding;[3] GI[3] ❑ ❑ Serum metabolic panel ❑ ❑ CBC/diff; clotting factors; BUN; liver enzymes ❑	
2 years	Growth, development, hearing, vision[2] Nutrition: macroglossia;[3] hypoglycemia[3] Metabolic: glucose, lytes, urate Blood counts, coagulation, hepatorenal Heart: cardiomyopathy[3]	❑ ECI;[3,6] family support[3,4] ❑ ❑ Feeding specialist;[3] night feeding;[3] GI[3] ❑ ❑ Serum metabolic panel ❑ ❑ CBC/diff; clotting factors; BUN; liver enzymes ❑ ❑ EKG;[3] echocardiogram;[3] cardiology[3] ❑	
3 years	Growth, development, hearing, vision[2] Nutrition: macroglossia;[3] hypoglycemia[3] Metabolic: glucose, lytes, urate Blood counts, coagulation, hepatorenal Heart: cardiomyopathy[3] Neuromuscular: myopathy[3] Other:	❑ ECI;[3,6] family support[3,4] ❑ ❑ Feeding specialist;[3] night feeding;[3] GI[3] ❑ ❑ Serum metabolic panel ❑ ❑ CBC/diff; clotting factors, BUN, liver enzymes ❑ ❑ EKG;[3] echocardiogram;[3] cardiology[3] ❑ ❑ Neurology[3] ❑ ❑ ❑	

Glycogen storage concerns		Other concerns from history	
Hypoglycemia, acidosis High urate, lipids Epistaxis Prolonged bleeding time Proteinuria	Cardiomyopathy Hepatomegaly Hepatic adenomas Neutropenia, infections[5] Hypotonia, motor delay	**Family history/prenatal** _____ _____ _____ _____	**Social/environmental** _____ _____ _____ _____

Guidelines for the neonatal period should be undertaken *at whatever age* the diagnosis is made; ABR, auditory brainstem evoked response; CBC/diff, blood count and differential; lytes, electrolytes; GI, gastrointestinal; BUN, blood urea nitrogen; [1]metabolic and enzyme studies essential for correct diagnosis; [2]by practitioner; [3]as dictated by clinical findings–GI studies for types I, III–IV, VI, VIII; cardiac studies for types II, IV; muscular studies for types V, VII; feeding and early intervention for severe types II, IV; [4]parent group, family/sib, financial, and behavioral issues for those with types II, IV; [5]consider developmental pediatrics–genetics–neurology–gastroenterology according to symptoms and availability; [6]early childhood intervention including developmental monitoring and motor/speech therapy for myopathies and severe types.

Glycogen storage diseases

Preventive medical checklist (4–18 years)

Name _____ Birth date __/__/____ Number _____

Age	Evaluations: key concerns	Management considerations	Notes
4 years ↓ **6 years**	Growth, preschool transition[1,5] Nutrition: hypoglycemia[3] Metabolic: glucose, lytes, urate, lipids Blood counts, coagulation, hepatorenal Heart;[3] kidneys;[3] liver mass[3] Neuromuscular;[3] skeletal[3] Other:	❑ Family support;[4] preschool program[5] ❑ ❑ Dietician;[3] night feeding;[3] GI[3] ❑ ❑ Serum metabolic, lipid panel ❑ ❑ CBC/diff; clotting factors; BUN; liver enzymes ❑ ❑ Cardiology;[3] BP;[3] urinalysis;[3] liver sonogram[3] ❑ ❑ Neurology;[3] skeletal X-rays;[3] orthopedics[3] ❑ ❑ ❑	
7 years ↓ **9 years**	Growth, school transition[1,5] Nutrition: hypoglycemia[3] Metabolic: glucose, lytes, urate, lipids Blood counts, coagulation, hepatorenal Heart;[3] kidneys;[3] liver mass[3] Neuromuscular;[3] skeletal[3] Other:	❑ Family support;[4] endocrinology[3] ❑ ❑ Dietician;[3] night feeding;[3] GI[3] ❑ ❑ Serum metabolic, lipid panel ❑ ❑ CBC/diff; clotting factors; BUN; liver enzymes ❑ ❑ Cardiology;[3] BP;[3] urinalysis;[3] liver sonogram[3] ❑ ❑ Neurology;[3] skeletal X-rays;[3] orthopedics[3] ❑ ❑ ❑	
10 years ↓ **12 years**	Growth and development:[1,5] short stature Nutrition: hypoglycemia[3] Metabolic: glucose, lytes, urate, lipids Blood counts, coagulation, hepatorenal Other:	❑ Family support;[4] endocrinology[3] ❑ ❑ Dietician;[3] night feeding;[3] GI[3] ❑ ❑ Serum metabolic, lipid panel ❑ ❑ CBC/diff; clotting factors; BUN; liver enzymes ❑ ❑ ❑	
13 years ↓ **15 years**	Growth and development:[1,5] short stature Nutrition: hypoglycemia[3] Metabolic: glucose, lytes, urate, lipids Blood counts, coagulation, hepatorenal Heart;[3] kidneys;[3] liver mass[3] Other:	❑ Family support;[4] endocrinology[3] ❑ ❑ Dietician;[3] night feeding;[3] GI[3] ❑ ❑ Serum metabolic, lipid panel ❑ ❑ CBC/diff; clotting factors; BUN; liver enzymes ❑ ❑ Cardiology;[3] BP;[3] urinalysis;[3] liver sonogram[3] ❑ ❑ ❑	
16 years ↓ **18 years**	Growth and development:[1,5] short stature Nutrition: hypoglycemia;[3] obesity[3] Metabolic: glucose, lytes, urate, lipids Blood counts, coagulation, hepatorenal Other:	❑ Family support;[4] school progress[6] ❑ ❑ Dietician;[3] night feeding;[3] GI[3] ❑ ❑ Serum metabolic, lipid panel ❑ ❑ CBC/diff; clotting factors; BUN; liver enzymes ❑ ❑ ❑	
19 years ↓ **23 years**	Adult care transition[1,6] Nutrition: hypoglycemia[3] Metabolic: glucose, lytes, urate, lipids Blood counts, coagulation, hepatorenal Heart;[3] kidneys;[3] liver mass[3]	❑ Family support;[4] school progress[6] ❑ ❑ Dietician;[3] night feeding;[3] GI[3] ❑ ❑ Serum metabolic, lipid panel ❑ ❑ CBC/diff; clotting factors; BUN; liver enzymes ❑ ❑ Cardiology;[3] BP;[3] urinalysis;[3] liver sonogram[3] ❑	
Adult	Adult care transition[6] Nutrition: hypoglycemia[3] Metabolic: glucose, lytes, urate, lipids Blood counts, coagulation, hepatorenal Heart;[3] kidneys;[3] liver mass[3] Neuromuscular;[3] skeletal[3] Other:	❑ Family support[4] ❑ ❑ Dietician;[3] night feeding;[3] GI[3] ❑ ❑ Serum metabolic, lipid panel ❑ ❑ CBC/diff; clotting factors; BUN; liver enzymes ❑ ❑ Cardiology;[3] BP;[3] urinalysis;[3] liver sonogram[3] ❑ ❑ Neurology;[3] skeletal X-rays;[3] orthopedics[3] ❑ ❑ ❑	

Glycogen storage concerns		Other concerns from history	
Short stature Hypoglycemia, acidosis High urate, lipids Epistaxis, coagulopathy Proteinuria	Cardiomyopathy Hepatomegaly, hepatic tumors Neutropenia, infections[5] Renal failure Osteopenia, lumbar lordosis	**Family history/prenatal** _____ _____ _____ _____	**Social/environmental** _____ _____ _____ _____

Guidelines for the neonatal period should be undertaken *at whatever age* the diagnosis is made; ABR, auditory brainstem evoked response; CBC/diff, blood count and differential; lytes, electrolytes; GI, gastrointestinal; BP, blood pressure; BUN, blood urea nitrogen; [1]metabolic and enzyme studies essential for correct diagnosis; [2]by practitioner; [3]as dictated by clinical findings – GI studies for types I, III–IV, VI, VIII; cardiac studies for types II, IV; muscular studies for types V, VII; consider transplants for severely affected individuals; [4]parent group, family/sib, financial, and behavioral issues for those with types II, IV; [5]consider developmental pediatrics/genetics/neurology/gastroenterology according to symptoms and availability; preschool program including developmental monitoring and motor/speech therapy for those with disabilities; [6]monitor individual education plan, educational testing, academic progress, problems socialization due to short stature and prominent abdomen, behavioral differences, later vocational planning.

Parent guide to glycogen storage diseases

Glycogen storage diseases are a group of genetic disorders that produce alterations in the amount or structure of glycogen. Glycogen is a complex sugar that is released slowly by the body, providing energy between meals. Storage of glycogen occurs mainly in liver and muscle, and the diseases can be classified according to which of these organs they affect. Type I (von Gierke), III (Cori or Forbes), IV (Anderson) and VI (Hers) are mainly diseases of the liver, while type II (Pompe), V (McArdle), and VII (Tarui) are muscle diseases with cramping). Type IV can have heart disease with lethal cirrhosis, while type II has lethal heart disease and myopathy.

Incidence, causation, and diagnosis

The incidence of all types of glycogen storage diseases is about 1 in 20–25,000 births, with types I–IV accounting for over 90% of patients. Most exhibit autosomal recessive inheritance except for X-linked recessive type VI category. Enzymes that regulate glucose/glycogen interconversion are responsible for the glycogen storage diseases including type I (glucose-6-phosphatase), type II (lysosomal α-glucosidase), type III (debranching enzyme), type IV (branching enzyme), type V (muscle phosphorylase), type VI (phosphorylase and phosphorylase kinase), and type VII (phosphofructokinase). Differential diagnosis for the liver disorders will include other causes of hypoglycemia (low blood sugar) and acidosis: galactosemia, fructose bisphosphatase deficiency, fatty acid oxidation disorders or even infectious hepatitis may be considered. Pompe disease can simulate other cardiomyopathies (heart muscle diseases) until the characteristic shortened P–R interval is demonstrated by electrocardiography. The muscle cramping of types V and VII can be confused with other disorders that interfere with muscle energy metabolism (i.e., hexokinase deficiency) until exercise testing, phosphorus MRI imaging, and muscle enzyme assays are employed. The primary technique for diagnosis of glycogen storage diseases should involve biopsy of the appropriate organ followed by pathologic study and enzyme testing of liver, skin, or muscle tissue.

Natural history and complications

The key derangement in patients with liver glycogen storage diseases is the inability to mobilize liver glycogen into circulating glucose. Abnormal amounts or structures of glycogen accumulate and produce hepatomegaly, while the block in glucose liberation causes metabolic abnormalities such as low-blood sugar, high lactic acid and acidosis, increased uric acid, and increased serum lipids. Type IV may lead to early death due to liver toxicity of the accumulating glycogen. Patients with hepatic glycogenoses exhibit early clinical manifestations of hypoglycemia, seizures and acidosis with later short stature, cherubic or "doll-like" facies, protuberant abdomen with large liver, and skin xanthomas (fatty deposits). After puberty, which is often delayed, there is short stature, pancreatitis because of high blood lipids, gouty arthritis due to the high uric acid, and kidney disease with protein in the urine. The kidney disease can lead to high blood pressure and kidney failure. Osteoporosis (soft bones) and lung damage from high blood pressure have also been reported, but hardening of the arteries from high blood lipids has not been demonstrated. Most patients with type I glycogen storage disease develop hepatic adenomas (benign tumors of the liver) in their second to third decade of life, and these may bleed or become cancerous. Other complications include low white blood cell count with recurrent bacterial infections, mouth ulcers, and intestinal lesions that present as inflammatory bowel disease in type Ib. Type VI patients may have growth delay, motor delay, mild hepatitis, liver enlargement, and increased blood lipids in childhood, but show improvement with age. Muscle cramps and even acute rhadomyolysis with renal failure can occur in the muscle types V and VII.

Preventive medical needs

The goal of management for children with liver glycogen storage is to restore glucose supplies and prevent complications from low-blood sugar such as seizures, lactic acidosis, high uric acid and high blood lipids. Dietary treatment involves nocturnal tube feedings with glucose or corn starch and a high carbohydrate diet; precautions to ensure pump and tube function are important since interruptions may cause low blood sugar and death. Dietary therapy is accompanied by monitoring of growth, glucose levels, liver size, coagulation, metabolic, and liver function tests. Patients with type Ib will require complete blood counts and inspection for mouth ulcers. Regular assessments by gastroenterology and metabolic specialists are necessary, with options for liver transplantation in severe cases. Allopurinol for hyperuricemia, bleeding times before surgery, and daily checking of serum glucose is necessary. Management of older children should include monitoring of glucose, liver function, uric acid, renal function, and liver size. The occurrence of liver tumors should be monitored by abdominal examination and periodic abdominal ultrasound, with periodic α-fetoprotein measurements to check for transformations to liver cancer. If there is poor growth, referral to endocrinology may be considered, and women should be counseled about worsening symptoms that occur with pregnancy. The presence of liver cancers would constitute an immediate indication for liver transplant, and some patients have required kidney transplant because of chronic renal failure. Patients with aggressive dietary treatment have a good outlook for normal stature and regression of hepatic adenomas.

Family counseling

Medical counseling can be optimistic for glycogen storage diseases other than types II and IV. Emphasis on adherence to treatment regimens is important, since treatment is clearly related to the degree of short stature and adult complications. Families of patients with type II or type IV disease require psychosocial, pastoral, and hospice support appropriate for the early lethality of these disorders. The recurrence risk for parents of children with glycogen storage disease will be 25%, with type VIII families having the risk for affected sons rather than daughters. Type VIII carrier mothers do not have symptoms, so enzyme or DNA diagnosis is required to distinguish new mutations.

References

Abraham, E., Altiok, H. & Lubicky, J. P. (2004). Musculoskeletal manifestations of Russell–Silver syndrome. *Journal of Pediatric Orthopaedics* 24:552–64.

ACOG Committee on Genetics (2004). ACOG committee opinion. Prenatal and preconceptional carrier screening for genetic diseases in individuals of Eastern European Jewish descent. *Obstetrics and Gynecology* 104:425–8.

Adib, N., Davies, K., Grahame, R., Woo, P. & Murray, K. J. (2005). Joint hypermobility syndrome in childhood. A not so benign multisystem disorder? *Rheumatology* 44:744–50.

Agency for Health Care Policy and Research (1993). *Clinical Practice Guideline Development.* Washington DC: Government Printing Office, AHCPR #93–0023.

Aicardi, J. (2005). Aicardi syndrome. *Brain and Development* 27:164–71.

Aleck, K. (2004). Craniosynostosis syndromes in the genomic era. *Seminars in Pediatric Neurology* 11:256–61.

Allanson, J. E. & Hall, J. G. (1986). Obstetric and gynecologic problems in women with chondrodystrophies. *Obstetrics and Gynecology* 67:74–8.

Altschuler, E. L. (2004). Consideration of Rituximab for fibrodysplasia ossificans progressive. *Medical Hypotheses* 63:407–8.

American Cleft Palate-Craniofacial Association (1993). Parameters for evaluation and treatment of patients with cleft lip/palate or other craniofacial anomalies. *The Cleft Palate-Craniofacial Journal* 30:S1–8.

American College of Obstetricians and Gynecologists (2002). ACOG Committee Opinion: Number 281, December 2002. Rubella vaccination. *Obstetrics and Gynecology* 100:1417.

Ammann, R. A., Duppenthaler, A., Bux, J. & Aebi, C. (2004). Granulocyte colony-stimulating factor-responsive chronic neutropenia in cartilage-hair hypoplasia. *Journal of Pediatric Hematology Oncology* 26:379–81.

Anonymous (1985). Case history of a child with Williams syndrome. *Pediatrics* 75:962–8.

Apajasalo, M., Sintonen, H., Rautonen, J. & Kaitila, I. (1998). Health-related quality of life of patients with genetic skeletal dysplasias. *European Journal of Pediatrics* 157:114–21.

Arad, M., Maron, B. J., Gorham, J. M., et al. (2005). Glycogen storage diseases presenting as hypertrophic cardiomyopathy. *New England Journal of Medicine* 352:362–72.

Arbour, L., Rosenblatt, B., Clow, C. & Wilson, G. N. (1988). Post-operative dystonia in a female patient with homocystinuria. *Journal of Pediatrics* 113:863–4.

Armstrong, L., Abd El Moneim, A., Aleck, K., et al. (2005). Further delineation of Kabuki syndrome in 48 well-defined new individuals. *American Journal of Medical Genetics* 132A:265–72.

Axelrad, M. E., Glidden, R., Nicholson, L. & Gripp, K. W. (2004). Adaptive skills, cognitive, and behavioral characteristics of Costello syndrome. *American Journal of Medical Genetics* 128A:396–400.

Ayers, G. (1994). Statistical profile of special education in the United States. *Teaching Exceptional Child* 26(Suppl. 3):3–4.

Bachrach, S. J., Walter, R. S. & Trzcinski, K. (1998). Use of glycopyrrolate and other anticholinergic medications for sialorrhea in children with cerebral palsy. *Clinical Pediatrics* 37:485–90.

Balci, B., Uyanik, G., Dincer, P., et al. (2005). An autosomal recessive limb girdle muscular dystrophy (LGMD2) with mild mental retardation is allelic to Walker–Warburg syndrome (WWS) caused by a mutation in the POMT1 gene. *Neuromuscular Disorders* 15:271–5.

Balci, S., Oguz, K. K., Firat, M. M. & Boduroglu, K. (2002). Cervical diastematomyelia in cervico-oculo-acoustic (Wildervanck) syndrome: MRI findings. *Clinical Dysmorphology* 11:125–8.

Baldini, A. (2004). DiGeorge syndrome: an update. *Current Opinion in Cardiology* 19:201–4.

Bale, J. F. & Miner, L. J. (2005). Herpes simplex virus infections of the newborn. *Current Treatment Options in Neurology* 7:151–6.

Balmer, R., Cameron, A. C., Ades, L. & Aldred, M. J. (2004). Enamel defects and Lyonization in focal dermal hypoplasia. *Oral Surgery Oral Medicine Oral Pathology Oral Radiology and Endodontics* 98:686–91.

Barr Jr., M. & Cohen, M. M. (2000). Holoprosencephaly outcomes. *American Journal of Medical Genetics* 89C:116–20.

Baser, M. E., Friedman, J. M., Wallace, A. J., et al. (2002). Evaluation of clinical diagnostic criteria for neurofibromatosis-2. *Neurology* 59:1759–65.

Baspinar, O., Kininc, M., Balat, A., Celkan, M. A. & Coskun, Y. (2005). Long tortuous aorta in a child with Larsen syndrome. *Canadian Journal of Cardiology* 21:299–301.

Battaglia, A. & Carey, J. C. (1999). Health supervision and anticipatory guidance of individuals with Wolf–Hirschhorn syndrome. *American Journal of Medical Genetics* 89C:111–19.

Baty, B. J., Blackburn, B. L. & Carey, J. C. (1994a). Natural history of trisomy 18 and trisomy 13: I. Growth, physical assessment, medical histories, survival and recurrence risk. *American Journal of Medical Genetics* 49A:175–88.

Baty, B. J., Jorde, L. B., Blackburn, B. L. & Carey, J. C. (1994b). Natural history of trisomy 18 and trisomy 13: II. Psychomotor development. *American Journal of Medical Genetics* 49A:189–94.

Bauchner, H., Witzburg, R. & Jones, C. (1996). Early and Periodic Screening Diagnosis and Treatment. *Archives of Pediatrics and Adolescent Medicine* 150:1219.

Bauer, S. (1994). Urologic care of the child with spina bifida. *Spina Bifida Spotlight* July:1–4.

Bercovitch, L., Leroux, T., Terry, S. & Weinstock, M. A. (2004). Pregnancy and obstetrical outcomes in pseudoxanthoma elasticum. *British Journal of Dermatology* 151:1011–18.

Bernstein, R. M. (2002). Arthrogryposis and amyoplasia. *Journal of the American Academy of Orthopaedic and Surgery* 10:417–24.

Beutler, E. & Grabowski, G. A. (2001). Gaucher disease. In *The Metabolic and Molecular Bases of Inherited Disease*, 8th edn, eds C. R. Scriver, A. L. Beaudet, W. S. Sly & D. Valle, pp. 3635–68. New York: McGraw-Hill, Inc.

Biehl, R. F. (1996). Legislative mandates. In *Developmental Disabilities in Infancy and Childhood*, eds A. J. Capute & P. J. Accardo, pp. 513–24. Baltimore: Paul H. Brookes.

Binder, H., Conway, A., Hason, S., et al. (1993). Comprehensive rehabilitation of the child with osteogenesis imperfecta. *American Journal of Medical Genetics* 45:265–9.

Blair, S. N., Kohl III, H. W., Barlow, C. E., et al. (1995). Changes in physical fitness and all-cause mortality. *Journal of the American Medical Association* 273:1093–8.

Blake, K., Kirk, J. M. & Ur, E. (1993). Growth in CHARGE association. *Archives of Disease in Childhood* 68:508–9.

Blake, K. D., Russell-Eggitt, I. M., Morgan, D. W., Ratcliffe, J. M. & Wyse, R. K. H. (1990). Who's in charge? Multidisciplinary management of patients with CHARGE association. *Archives of Disease in Childhood* 65:217–23.

Blake, K. D., Davenport, S. L., Hall, B. D., et al. (1998). CHARGE association: an update and review for the primary pediatrician. *Clinical Pediatrics* 37:159–73.

Blasco, P. A. & Stansbury, J. C. (1996). Glycopyrrolate treatment of chronic drooling. *Archives of Pediatrics and Adolescent Medicine* 150:932–5.

Bocca, G., Weemaes, C. M., van der Burgt, I. & Otten, B. J. (2004). Growth hormone treatment in cartilage-hair hypoplasia: effects on growth and the immune system. *Journal of Pediatric Endocrinology and Metabolism* 17:47–54.

Bojesen, A., Juul, S. & Gravholt, C. H. (2003). Prenatal and postnatal prevalence of Klinefelter syndrome: a national registry study. *Journal of Clinical Endocrinology and Metabolism* 88:622–6.

Bojesen, A., Juul, S., Birkebaek, N. & Gravholt, C. H. (2004). Increased mortality in Klinefelter syndrome. *Journal of Clinical Endocrinology and Metabolism* 89:3830–4.

Bomalaski, M. D., Teague, J. L. & Brooks, B. (1995). The long-term impact of urological management on the quality of life of children with spina bifida. *Journal of Urology* 154:778–81.

Botvin, G. J., Baker, E., Dusenbury, L., Botvin, E. B. & Diaz, T. (1995). Long-term follow-up results of a randomized drug abuse prevention trial in a middle-class population. *Journal of the American Medical Association* 273:1106–12.

Boyce, H. W. & Bakheet, M. R. (2005). Sialorrhea: a review of a vexing, often unrecognized sign of oropharyngeal and esophageal disease. *Journal of Clinical Gastroenterology* 39:89–97.

Boyle, C., Decouflé, P. & Yeargin-Allsopp, M. (1994). Prevalence and health impact of developmental disabilities in US children. *Pediatrics* 93:399–403.

Brent, R. L. (2004). Environmental causes of human congenital malformations: the pediatrician's role in dealing with these complex clinical problems caused by a multiplicity of environmental and genetic factors. *Pediatrics* 113(Suppl. 4):957–68.

Briskin, H. & Liptak, G. S. (1995). Helping families with children with developmental disabilities. *Pediatric Annals* 24:262–6.

Bruandet, M., Molko, N., Cohen, L. & Dehaene, S. A. (2004). Cognitive characterization of dyscalculia in Turner syndrome. *Neuropsychology* 42:288–98.

Bruckner, A. L. (2004). Incontinentia pigmenti: a window to the role of NF-kappaB function. *Seminars in Cutaneous Medicine and Surgery* 23:116–24.

Bucciarelli, R. L. & Eitzman, D. V. (1988). Baby Doe: Where do we stand now? *Contemporary Pediatrics* January:116–28.

Buch, B., Noffke, C. & de Kock, S. (2001). Gardner's syndrome – the importance of early diagnosis: a case report and a review. *Journal of the South African Dental Association* 56:242–5.

Bugge, M., deLozier-Blanchet, C., Bak, M., et al. (2005). Trisomy 13 due to rea(13q;13q) is caused by i(13) and not rob(13;13)(q10;q10) in the majority of cases. *American Journal of Medical Genetics* 132A:310–13.

Buoni, S., Zannolli, R., Macucci, F., et al. (2004). The FBN1 (R2726W) mutation is not fully penetrant. *Annals of Human Genetics* 68:633–8.

Burstein, F. D. & Williams, J. K. (2005). Mandibular distraction osteogenesis in Pierre Robin sequence: application of a new internal single-stage resorbable device. *Plastic and Reconstructive Surgery* 115:61–9.

Butler, M. G., Brunschwig, A., Miller, L. K. & Hagerman, R. J. (1992). Standards for selected anthropometric measurements in males with the fragile X syndrome. *Pediatrics* 89:1059–62.

Cabana, M. D., Capone, G., Fritz, A. & Berkovitz, G. (1997). Nutritional rickets in a child with Down syndrome. *Clinical Pediatrics* 36:235–7.

Canadian task force on the periodic health examination (1994). *The Canadian Guide to Clinical Preventive Health Care*. Ottawa, Ontario: Canada Communication Group Publishing.

Capute, A. & Accardo, P. (1996). Cerebral palsy: the spectrum of motor dysfunction. In *Developmental Disabilities in Infancy and Childhood*, Vol. 2, 2nd edn, eds A. Capute & P. Accardo, pp. 81–94. Baltimore: Paul H Brookes.

Cardoso, C., Leventer, R. J., Ward, H. L., et al. (2003). Refinement of a 400-kb critical region allows genotypic differentiation between isolated lissencephaly, Miller–Dieker syndrome, and other phenotypes secondary to deletions of 17p13.3. *American Journal of Human Genetics* 72:918–30.

Cardoso, G., Daly, R., Haq, N. A., et al. (2004). Current and lifetime psychiatric illness in women with Turner syndrome. *Gynecological Endocrinology* 19:313–19.

Carey, J. C. (1992). Health supervision and anticipatory guidance for children with genetic disorders (including specific recommendations for trisomy 21, trisomy 18, and neurofibromatosis). *Pediatric Clinics of North America* 39:25–53.

Carlson, W. E., Vaughan, C. L., Damiano, D. L. & Abel, M. F. (1997). Orthotic management of gait in spastic diplegia. *American Journal of Physical Medicine and Rehabilitation* 76:219–25.

Casella, E. B., Bousso, A., Corvello, C. M., Fruchtengarten, L. V. & Diament, A. J. (2005). Episodic somnolence in an infant with Riley–Day syndrome. *Pediatric Neurology* 32:273–4.

Cassidy, S. B. (1987). Prader–Willi syndrome: characteristics, management, and etiology. *Alabama Journal of Medical Sciences* 24:169–75.

Cassidy, S. B., Pagon, R. A., Pepin, M. & Blumhagen, J. D. (1983). Family studies in tuberous sclerosis. Evaluation of apparently unaffected parents. *Journal of the American Medical Association* 249:1302–04.

Cecconi, M., Forzano, F. & Milani, D. (2005). Mutation analysis of the NSD1 gene in a group of 59 patients with congenital overgrowth. *American Journal of Medical Genetics* 134A:247–53.

Centers for Disease Control (1992). Spina bifida incidence at birth – United States, 1983–1990. *Morbidity and Mortality Weekly Report* 41:497–500.

Centers for Disease Control (1995). Health insurance coverage and receipt of preventive health services – United States, 1993. *Journal of the American Medical Association* 273:1083–4.

Cerniglia Jr., F. R. (1997). Frankie's story – spina bifida from the parents' perspective [editorial]. *Journal of Urology* 158:1291.

Chakravarthy, M. V. (2003). Inactivity and inaction: We can't afford either. *Archives of Pediatrics and Adolescent Medicine* 157:731–2.

Chalard, F., Ferey, S., Teinturier, C. & Kalifa, G. (2005). Aortic dilatation in Turner syndrome: the role of MRI in early recognition. *Pediatric Radiology* 35:323–6.

Chang, E. H., Menezes, M., Meyer, N. C., et al. (2004). Branchio-oto-renal syndrome: the mutation spectrum in EYA1 and its phenotypic consequences. *Human Mutation* 23:582–9.

Charney, E. B. (1990). Myelomeningocele. In *Pediatric Primary Care: A Problem-Oriented Approach*, ed. M. W. Schwartz, pp. 663. Chicago: Mosby-Year Book.

Chen, Y. T. (2001). Glycogen storage diseases. In *The Metabolic and Molecular Bases of Inherited Disease*, 8th edn, eds C. R. Scriver, A. L. Beaudet, W. S. Sly & D. Valle, pp. 1521–52. New York: McGraw-Hill, Inc.

Cheney, C. & Ramsdel, J. (1987). Effect of medical records' checklists on implementation of periodic health measures. *American Journal of Medicine* 83:129–36.

Cheng, T. L., Perrin, E. C., DeWitt, T. G. & O'Connor, K. G. (1996). Use of checklists in pediatric practice (letter). *Archives of Pediatrics and Adolescent Medicine* 150:768–9.

Cherniske, E. M., Carpenter, T. O., Klaiman, C., et al. (2004). Multisystem study of 20 older adults with Williams syndrome. *American Journal of Medical Genetics* 131A:255–64.

Chi-Lum, B. I. (1995). Putting more prevention into medical training. *Journal of the American Medical Association* 273:1402–03.

Chiriboga, C. A., Brust, J. C., Bateman, D. & Hauser, W. A. (1999). Dose-response effect of fetal cocaine exposure on newborn neurologic function. *Pediatrics* 103:79–85.

Chuang, D. T. & Shih, V. E. (2001). Maple syrup urine disease (branched chain ketoaciduria). In *The Metabolic and Molecular Bases of Inherited Disease*, 8th edn, eds C. R. Scriver, A. L. Beaudet, W. S. Sly & D. Valle, pp. 1971–2006. New York: McGraw-Hill, Inc.

Clark, D. & Wilson, G. N. (2003). Behavioral assessment of children with Down syndrome using the Reiss psychopathology scale. *American Journal of Medical Genetics* 118A:210–16.

Coberly, S., Lammer, E. & Alashari, M. (1996). Retinoic acid embryopathy: case report and review of literature. *Pediatric Pathology & Laboratory Medicine* 16:823–36.

Cohen Jr., M. M. (1987). The elephant man did not have neurofibromatosis. *Proceedings of the Greenwood Genetic Center* 6:187–92.

Cohen Jr., M. M. (1995). Craniosynostoses: phenotypic/molecular correlations. *American Journal of Medical Genetics* 56:334–9.

Cohen Jr., M. M. (2000). Klippel–Trenaunay syndrome (Editorial). *American Journal Medical Genetics* 93:171–5.

Cohen Jr., M. M. (2003). Mental deficiency, alterations in performance, and CNS abnormalities in overgrowth syndromes. *American Journal of Medical Genetics* 117C:49–56.

Cohen Jr., M. M. & Kreiborg, S. (1993). Growth pattern in Apert syndrome. *American Journal of Medical Genetics* 47:617–23.

Cohran, V. C. & Heubi, J. E. (2003). Treatment of pediatric cholestatic liver disease. *Current Treatment in Options and Gastroenterology* 6:403–15.

Cole, D. E. (1993). Psychosocial aspects of osteogenesis imperfecta: an update. *American Journal of Medical Genetics* 45:207–11.

Cole, T. R. & Hughes, H. E. (1994). Sotos syndrome: a study of the diagnostic criteria and natural history. *Journal of Medical Genetics* 31:20–32.

Committee on Children with Disabilities (2001). The pediatrician's role in the diagnosis and management of autistic spectrum disorder in children. *Pediatrics* 107:1221–6.

Committee on Genetics, American Academy of Pediatrics (1995a). Health supervision for children with achondroplasia. *Pediatrics* 95:443–51.

Committee on Genetics, American Academy of Pediatrics (1995b). Health supervision for children with neurofibromatosis. *Pediatrics* 96:368–71.

Committee on Genetics, American Academy of Pediatrics (1996a). Health supervision for children with Marfan syndrome. *Pediatrics* 98: 821–978.

Committee on Genetics, American Academy of Pediatrics (1996b). Health supervision for children with fragile X syndrome. *Pediatrics* 98:297–300.

Committee on Genetics, American Academy of Pediatrics (1996c). Health supervision for children with Turner syndrome. *Pediatrics* 96:1166–73.

Committee on Genetics, American Academy of Pediatrics (2001a). Health care supervision for children with Williams syndrome. *Pediatrics* 107:1192–204.

Committee on Genetics, American Academy of Pediatrics (2001b). Health supervision for children with Down syndrome. *Pediatrics* 107:442–9.

Committee on Sports Medicine and Fitness, American Academy of Pediatrics (1995). Atlantoaxial instability in Down syndrome: Subject review. *Pediatrics* 96:151–4.

Consensus Development Conference (2004). Management of Turner's syndrome. *Journal of Pediatric Endocrinology and Metabolism* (Suppl. 2):257–61.

Cook, S., Weitzman, M., Auinger, P., Nguyen, M. & Dietz, W. H. (2003). Prevalence of a metabolic syndrome phenotype in adolescents. *Archives of Pediatrics and Adolescent Medicine* 157:821–7.

Cooley, W. C. (1994a). The ecology of support for caregiving families. *Journal of Behavioral and Developmental Pediatrics* 15:117–19.

Cooley, W. C. (1994b). Changing care in private practice: management of chronic conditions in the primary care setting. In *Ross Roundtable on Management of Chronic Illness and Disability in the Primary Care Setting*. Washington DC: Ross Products Division, Abbott Laboratories.

Cooley, W. C. (1994c). Pediatric training and family-centered care. In *Families, Physicians, and Children with Special Health Care Needs: Collaborative Medical Education Models*, eds R. Darling & M. Peter. Southport, CT: Greenwood Press.

Cooley, W. C. (1999). Responding to the developmental consequences of genetic conditions: the importance of pediatric primary care. *American Journal of Medical Genetics* 89C:75–80.

Cooley, W. C. (2004). Redefining primary pediatric care for children with special health care needs: the primary care medical home. *Current Opinion in Pediatrics* 16:689–92.

Cooley, W. C. & Graham Jr., J. M. (1991). Down syndrome – an update and review for the primary pediatrician. *Clinical Pediatrics* 30:233–53.

Cooley, W. C. & McAllister, J. (2004): Building medical homes: improvement strategies in primary care for CSHCH. *Pediatrics* 113:1499–506.

Cooley, W. C. & The Committee on Children with Disabilities (2004). Providing a primary care medical home for children and youth with cerebral palsy. *Pediatrics* 114:1106–13.

Cooley, W. E., Rawnsley, G., Melkonian, C., et al. (1990). Autosomal dominant familial spastic paraplegia: report of a large New England family. *Clinical Genetics* 38:57–68.

Cornish, K. & Bramble, D. (2002). Cri-du-chat syndrome: genotype-phenotype correlations and recommendations for clinical management. *Developmental Medicine and Child Neurology* 44:494–7.

Couriel, J. M., Bisset, R., Miller, R., Thomas, A. & Clarke, M. (1993). Assessment of feeding problems in neurodevelopmental handicap: a team approach. *Archives of Disease in Childhood* 69:609–13.

Crocker, A. C. (1989). The spectrum of medical care for developmental disabilities. In *Developmental Disabilities: Delivery of Medical Care for Children and Adults*, eds I. L. Rubin & A. C. Crocker. Philadelphia: Lea and Febiger.

Cronk, C., Crocker, A. C., Pueschel, S. M., et al. (1988). Growth charts for children with Down syndrome: 1 month to 18 years of age. *Pediatrics* 81:102–10.

Cruickshank, W. (1976). The problem and its scope (cerebral palsy). In *Cerebral Palsy: A Developmental Disability*, 3rd revised edn, ed. W. Cruickshank, pp. 1–28. Syracuse: Syracuse University Press.

Cull, C. & Wyke, M. (1984). Memory function of children with spina bifida and shunted hydrocephalus. *Developmental Medicine and Child Neurology* 26:177–83.

Cunningham, C. C., Morgan, P. A. & McGucken, R. B. (1984). Down syndrome: is dissatisfaction with disclosure of diagnosis inevitable? *Developmental Medicine and Child Neurology* 26:33–9.

Da Costa, A. C., Savarirayan, R., Wrennall, J. A., et al. (2005). Neuropsychological diversity in Apert syndrome: a comparison of cognitive profiles. *Annals of Plastic Surgery* 54:450–5.

Dagoneau, N., Scheffer, D., Huber, C., et al. (2004). Null leukemia inhibitory factor receptor (LIFR) mutations in Stuve–Wiedemann/Schwartz–Jampel type 2 syndrome. *American Journal of Human Genetics* 74:298–305.

Davies, H. D., Leusink, G. L., McConnell, A., et al. (2003). Myeloid leukemia in Prader–Willi syndrome. *Journal of Pediatrics* 142:174–8.

De Bona, C., Zappella, M., Hayek, G., et al. (2000). Preserved speech variant is allelic of classic Rett syndrome. *European Journal of Human Genetics* 8:325–30.

de Heer, I. M., Hoogeboom, J., Vermeij-Keers, C., de Klein, A. & Vaandrager, J. M. (2004). Postnatal onset of craniosynostosis in a case of Saethre–Chotzen syndrome. *Journal of Craniofacial Surgery* 15:1048–52.

DeLuca, P. A. (1996). The musculoskeletal management of children with cerebral palsy. *Pediatric Clinics of North America* 43:1135–50.

Demirci, H., Shields, C. L. & Shields, J. A. (2005). New ophthalmic manifestations of branchio-oculo-facial syndrome. *American Journal of Ophthalmology* 139:362–4.

Denschlag, D., Tempfer, C., Kunze, M., Wolff, G. & Keck, C. (2004). Assisted reproductive techniques in patients with Klinefelter syndrome: a critical review. *Fertility and Sterility* 82:775–9.

Desnick, R. J., Ioannou, Y. A. & Eng, C. M. (2001). α-galactosidase A deficiency: Fabry disease. In *The Metabolic and Molecular Bases of Inherited Disease*, 8th edn, eds C. R. Scriver, A. L. Beaudet, W. S. Sly & D. Valle, pp. 3733–74. New York: McGraw-Hill, Inc.

Diab, M., Raff, M. & Gunther, D. F. (2003). Osseous fragility in Marshall-Smith syndrome. *American Journal of Medical Genetics* 119A:218–22.

Dimeglio, L. A., Ford, L., McClintock, C. & Peacock, M. (2005). A comparison of oral and intravenous bisphosphonate therapy for children with osteogenesis imperfecta. *Journal of Pediatric Endocrinology and Metabolism* 18:43–53.

Dise, J. E. & Lohr, M. E. (1998). Examination of deficits in conceptual reasoning abilities associated with spina bifida. *American Journal of Physical Medicine and Rehabilitation* 77:247–51.

Dobyns, W. (1987). Developmental aspects of lissencephaly and the lissencephaly syndromes. *Birth Defects: Original Article Series* 23:225–41.

Doerr, H. G., Bettendorf, M., Hauffa, B. P., et al. (2005). Uterine size in women with Turner syndrome after induction of puberty with estrogens and long-term growth hormone therapy: results of the German IGLU Follow-up Study 2001. *Human Reproduction* 20:1418–21.

Dworkin, P. H. (1989). British and American recommendations for developmental monitoring: the role of surveillance. *Pediatrics* 84:1000–10.

Ebara, S., Anwar, M. M., Okawa, A., Kajiura, I., Hiroshima, K. & Ono, K. (1996). The cervical spine in athetoid cerebral palsy. A radiological study of 180 patients. *Journal of Bone and Joint Surgery, Britain* 78:613–19.

Eissa, M. A. H. (2003). Overview of pediatric obesity: key points in the evaluation and therapy. *Consulting Pediatric* July/Aug: 293–6.

Ekinci, B., Apaydin, H., Vural, M. & Ozekmekci, S. (2004). Two siblings with homocystinuria presenting with dystonia and parkinsonism. *Movement Disorders* 19:962–4.

Elson, E., Perveen, R., Donnai, D., Wall, S. & Black, G. C. (2002). De novo GLI3 mutation in acro-callosal syndrome: broadening the phenotypic spectrum of GLI3 defects and overlap with murine models. *Journal of Medical Genetics* 39:804–6.

Elster, A. B. (1998). Comparison of recommendations for adolescent clinical preventive services developed by national organizations. *Archives of Pediatrics and Adolescent Medicine* 152:193–8.

Evans, C. A. (2004). Orthodontic treatment for patients with clefts. *Clinics in Plastic Surgery* 312:271–90.

Facher, J. J., Regier, E. J., Jacobs, G. H., et al. (2004). Cardiomyopathy in Coffin–Lowry syndrome. *American Journal of Medical Genetics* 128A:176–8.

Faivre, L., Le Merrer, M. & Lyonnet, S. (2002). Clinical and genetic heterogeneity of Seckel syndrome. *American Journal of Medical Genetics* 112A:379–83.

Fales, C. L., Knowlton, B. J., Holyoak, K. J., et al. (2003). Working memory and relational reasoning in Klinefelter syndrome. *Journal of the International Neuropsychological Society* 9:839–46.

Famy, C., Streissguth, A. P. & Unis, A. S. (1998). Mental illness in adults with fetal alcohol syndrome or fetal alcohol effects. *American Journal of Psychiatry* 155:552–4.

Fearon, J. A., Swift, D. M. & Bruce, D. A. (2001). New methods for the evaluation and treatment of craniofacial dysostosis-associated cerebellar tonsillar herniation. *Plastic and Reconstructive Surgery* 108:1855–61.

Fenton, W. A., Gravel, R. A. & Rosenblatt, D. S. (2001). Disorders of proprionate and methyl-malonate metabolism. In *The Metabolic and Molecular Bases of Inherited Disease*, 8th edn, eds C. R. Scriver, A. L. Beaudet, W. S. Sly & D. Valle, pp. 2165–94. New York: McGraw-Hill, Inc.

Feremback, D. (1963). Frequency of spina bifida occulta in prehistoric human skeletons. *Nature* 199:100.

Fleck, B. J., Pandya, A., Vanner, L., Kerkering, K. & Bodurtha, J. (2001). Coffin–Siris syndrome: review and presentation of new cases from a questionnaire study. *American Journal of Medical Genetics* A 99:1–7.

Fleischman, A. R. & Barondess, J. A. (2004). Adolescent suicide: vigilance and action to reduce the toll. *Contemporary Pediatrics* Dec:27–35.

Fletcher, J., Bohan, T., Brandt, M., et al. (1992). Cerebral white matter and cognition in hydro-cephalic children. *Archives of Neurology* 49:818–24.

Fletcher, J. M., McCauley, S. R., Brandt, M. E., et al. (1996). Regional brain tissue composition in children with hydrocephalus. Relationships with cognitive development. *Archives of Neurology* 53:549–57.

Fluck, C. E., Tajima, T., Pandey, A. V., et al. (2004). Mutant P450 oxidoreductase causes disor-dered steroidogenesis with and without Antley–Bixler syndrome. *Nature Genetics* 36:228–30.

Foran, J. R., Pyeritz, R. E., Dietz, H. C. & Sponseller, P. D. (2005). Characterization of the symp-toms associated with dural ectasia in the Marfan patient. *American Journal of Medical Genetics* 134A:58–65.

Frawley, P. A., Broughton, N. S. & Menelaus, M. B. (1996). Anterior release for fixed flexion defor-mity of the hip in spina bifida. *Journal of Bone and Joint Surgery-British Volume* 78:299–302.

Freed, G. L., Clark, S. J., Konrad, T. R. & Pathman, D. E. (1996). Variation in patient charges for vaccines and well-child care. *Archives of Pediatrics and Adolescent Medicine* 150:421–6.

Frerman, F. E. & Goodman, S. I. (2001). Defects of electron transfer flavoprotein and electron transfer flavoprotein-ubiquinone oxidoreductase: Glutaric acidemia type II. In *The Metabolic and Molecular Bases of Inherited Disease*, 8th edn, eds C. R. Scriver, A. L. Beaudet, W. S. Sly & D. Valle, pp. 2357–66. New York: McGraw-Hill, Inc.

Freud, S. (1897). Attempts at classification of various types of infantile cerebral paralysis. In *Infantile Cerebral Paralysis*, pp. 230–60. Coral Gables, FL: University of Miami Press.

Frías, J. L., Davenport, M. L. & Committee on Genetics and Section on Endocrinology (2003). Health supervision for children with Turner syndrome. *Pediatrics* 111:692–702.

Gabriel, R. & McComb, J. (1985). Malformations of the central nervous system. In *Textbook of Child Neurology*, 3rd edn, ed. J. Menkes, pp. 89–270. Philadelphia: Lea and Febiger.

Gaston, H. (1996). Patients with hydrocephalus should have regular eye checks [letter]. *British Medical Journal* 312:57.

Gath, A. & Gumley, D. (1984). Down syndrome and the family: follow-up of children first seen in infancy. *Developmental Medicine and Child Neurology* 26:500–8.

Geralis, E., ed. (1991). *Children with Cerebral Palsy – a Parents' Guide*, Baltimore: Woodbine Press.

Germain-Lee, E. L., Groman, J., Crane, J. L., Jan de Beur, S. M. & Levine, M. A. (2003). Growth hormone deficiency in pseudohypoparathyroidism type 1a: another manifestation of multi-hormone resistance. *Journal of Clinical Endocrinology and Metabolism* 88:4059–69.

Gerszten, P. C., Albright, A. L. & Johnstone, G. F. (1998). Intrathecal baclofen infusion and subsequent orthopedic surgery inpatients with spastic cerebral palsy. *Journal of Neurosurgery* 88:1009–13.

Ghosh, A. K., Smithson, S. F., Mumford, A., Patteril, M. & Amer, K. (2004). Klippel–Trenauney–Weber syndrome associated with hemoptysis. *Annals of Thoracic Surgery* 77:1843–5.

Giangreco, C. A., Steele, M. W., Aston, C. E., Cummins, J. H. & Wenger, S. L. (1996). A simplified six-item checklist for screening for fragile X syndrome in the pediatric population. *Journal of Pediatrics* 129:611–14.

Gill, T. M. & Feinstein, A. R. (1994). A critical appraisal of the quality of quality of life measurements. *Journal of the American Medical Association* 272:619–26.

Glascoe, F. P. & Dworkin, P. H. (1995). The role of parents in the detection of developmental and behavioral problems. *Pediatrics* 95:829–36.

Glascoe, F. P., Martin, E. D. & Humphrey, S. (1990). A comparative review of developmental screening tests. *Pediatrics* 86:547–54.

Golan, I., Barmert, U., Hrala, B. & Mussig, D. (2004). Dentomaxillofacial variability of cleidocranial dysplasia: clinicoradiological presentation and systematic review. *Dentomaxillofacial Radiology* 33:422.

Gold, M. A. (1999). Providing emergency contraception in the office. *Contemporary Pediatrics* Mar:53–74.

Golden, G. (1979). Neural tube defects. *Pediatrics in Review* 1:187–9.

Golden, N. H. (2000). Osteoporosis prevention: A pediatric challenge. *Archives of Pediatrics and Adolescent Medicine* 154:542–3.

Gooch, J. L. & Sandell, T. V. (1996). Botulinum toxin for spasticity and athetosis in children with cerebral palsy. *Archives of Physical Medicine and Rehabilitation* 77:508–11.

Goodrich, J. T. (2004). Craniofacial surgery: complications and their prevention *Seminars in Pediatric Neurology* 11:288–300.

Gorlin, R. J. (2004). Nevoid basal cell carcinoma (Gorlin) syndrome. *Genetics in Medicine* 6:530–9.

Gorlin, R. J., Cohen Jr., M. M. & Hennekam, R. (2001). *Syndromes of the Head and Neck*, 4th edn. New York: Oxford.

Gosain, A. K., McCarthy, J. G. & Pinto, R. S. (1994). Cervicovertebral anomalies and basilar impression in Goldenhar syndrome. *Plastic and Reconstructive Surgery* 93:498–506.

Gould, S. J. (1981). *The Mismeasure of Man*. New York: WW Norton and Company, Inc.

Gould, S. J., Raymond, G. V. & Valle, D. (2001). The peroxisome biogenesis disorders. In *The Metabolic and Molecular Bases of Inherited Disease*, 8th edn, eds C. R. Scriver, A. L. Beaudet, W. S. Sly & D. Valle, pp. 3181–218. New York: McGraw-Hill, Inc.

Graham, E. M., Bradley, S. M., Shirali, G. S., Hills, C. B. & Atz, A. M. (2004). Pediatric Cardiac Care Consortium effectiveness of cardiac surgery in trisomies 13 and 18 (from the Pediatric Cardiac Care Consortium). *American Journal of Cardiology* 93:801–3.

Graham Jr., J. M., Hennekam, R., Dobyns, W. B., Roeder, E. & Busch, D. (2004). MICRO syndrome: an entity distinct from COFS syndrome. *American Journal of Medical Genetics* 128A:235–45.

Greene, M., ed. (1994). *Bright Futures: Guidelines for Health Supervision of Infants, Children and Adolescents*. Arlington, VA: National Center for Education in Maternal and Child Health.

Griebel, M., Oakes, W. & Worley, G. (1991). The Chiari malformation associated with myelomeningocele. In *Comprehensive Management of Spina Bifida*, ed. H. Rekate, pp. 67–92, Boca Raton, FL: CRC Press.

Gururaj, A., Sztriha, L., Hertecant, J., et al. (2005). Magnetic resonance imaging findings and novel mutations in GM1 gangliosidosis. *Journal of Child Neurology* 20:57–60.

Haga, N. (2004). Management of disabilities associated with achondroplasia. *Journal of Orthopaedic Science* 9:103–7.

Hagerman, R. J. (1997). Fragile X syndrome. Molecular and clinical insights and treatment issues. *Western Journal of Medicine* 166:129–37.

Halac, I. & Zimmerman, D. (2004): Coordinating care for children with Turner syndrome. *Pediatric Annals* 33:189–96.

Hall, J. (1997). Arthrogryposis multiplex congenita: etiology, genetics, classification, diagnostic approach, and general aspects. *Journal of Pediatric Orthopaedics* 6:159–66.

Hall, J. G. (1988). Somatic mosaicism: observations related to clinical genetics. *American Journal of Human Genetics* 43:355–63.

Hall, J. G. (1990). Genomic imprinting: review and relevance to human diseases. *American Journal of Human Genetics* 46:857–3.

Hall, J. G. (1998). Overview of arthrogryposis. In *Arthrogryposis. A Text Atlas*, eds L. T. Staheli, J. G. Hall, K. M. Jaffe & D. O. Paholke, pp. 1–26. Cambridge UK: Cambridge University Press.

Halpern-Felsher, B. L., Ozer, E. M., Millstein, S. G., et al. (2000). Preventive services in a health maintenance organization. How well do pediatricians screen and educate adolescent patients. *Archives of Pediatrics and Adolescent Medicine* 154:173–9.

Happle, R. (2004). Gustav Schimmelpenning and the syndrome bearing his name. *Dermatology* 209:84–7.

Harris, M., Hofman, P. L. & Cutfield, W. S. (2004). Growth hormone treatment in children: review of safety and efficacy. *Paediatric Drugs* 6:93–106.

Harris, S. (1984). Predictive value of the movement assessment of infants. *Journal of Developmental and Behavioral Pediatrics* 5:336–41.

Hata, T. & Todd, M. M. (2005). Cervical spine considerations when anesthetizing patients with Down syndrome. *Anesthesiology* 102:680–5.

Hengge, U. R. (2005). Progress and prospects of skin gene therapy: a ten year history. *Clinics in Dermatology* 23:107–14.

Hennekam, R. C. M., Tilanus, M., Hamel, B. C. J., et al. (1993). Deletion at chromosome 16p13.3 as a cause of Rubinstein–Taybi syndrome: clinical aspects. *American Journal of Human Genetics* 52:255–62.

Hennessy, C. H., Moriarty, D. G., Zack, M. M., Scherr, P. A. & Brackbill, R. (1994). Measuring health-related quality of life for public health surveillance. *Public Health Reports* 109:665–72.

Herman-Staab, B. (1994). Screening, management, and appropriate referral for pediatric behavior problems. *Nurse Practitioner* 19:40–9.

Hersch, J. H. (1989). Toluene embryopathy: two new cases. *Journal of Medical Genetics* 26:333–7.

Hirschfelder, U., Piechot, E., Schulte, M. & Leher, A. (2004). Abnormalities of the TMJ and the musculature in the oculo-auriculo-vertebral spectrum (OAV). A CT study. *Journal of Orofacial Orthopedics* 65:204–16.

Ho, V. B., Bakalov, V. K., Cooley, M., et al. (2004). Major vascular anomalies in Turner syndrome: prevalence and magnetic resonance angiographic features. *Circulation* 110:1694–700.

Holm, V. A., Cassidy, S. B., Butler, M. G., et al. (1993). Prader–Willi syndrome: consensus diagnostic criteria. *Pediatrics* 91:398–402.

Holton, J. B., Walter, J. H. & Tyfield, L. A. (2001). Galactosemia. In *The Metabolic and Molecular Bases of Inherited Disease*, 8th edn, eds C. R. Scriver, A. L. Beaudet, W. S. Sly & D. Valle, pp.1553–88. New York: McGraw-Hill, Inc.

Holtzman, N. A. (1988). Recombinant DNA technology, genetic tests, and public policy. *American Journal of Human Genetics* 42:623–45.

Holtzman, N. A. (1989). *Proceed with Caution: The Use of Recombinant DNA Testing for Genetic Testing*. Baltimore: Johns Hopkins University Press.

Hopwood, J. J. & Ballabio, A. (2001). Multiple sulfatase deficiency and the nature of the sulfatase family. In *The Metabolic and Molecular Bases of Inherited Disease*, 8th edn, eds C. R. Scriver, A. L. Beaudet, W. S. Sly & D. Valle, pp. 3725–810. New York: McGraw-Hill, Inc.

Horton, W. A., Rotter, J. I., Rimoin, D. L., Scott, C. I. & Hall, J. G. (1978). Standard growth curves for achondroplasia. *Journal of Pediatrics* 93:435–8.

Horwitz, S. M., Leaf, P. J., Leventhal, J. M., Forsyth, B. & Speechley, K. N. (1992). Identification and management of psychosocial and developmental problems in community-based, primary care pediatric practices. *Pediatrics* 89:480–5.

Howlin, P., Karpf, J. & Turk, J. (2005). Behavioural characteristics and autistic features in individuals with Cohen Syndrome. *European Child and Adolescent Psychiatry* 14:57–64.

Hoybye, C., Hilding, A., Jacobsson, H. & Thoren, M. (2002). Metabolic profile and body composition in adults with Prader–Willi syndrome and severe obesity. *Journal of Clinical Endocrinology and Metabolism* 87:3590–7.

Hoyme, H. E., May, P. A., Kalberg, W. O., et al. (2005). A practical clinical approach to diagnosis of fetal alcohol spectrum disorders: clarification of the 1996 institute of medicine criteria. *Pediatrics* 115:39–47.

Humphreys, R. (1986). Tethering: theories of development and pathophysiology. In *Spina bifida: A Multidisciplinary Approach*, ed. R. McLaurin, pp. 215–20. New York: Praeger.

Hunt, J. A. & Hobar, P. C. (2002). Common craniofacial anomalies: the facial dysostoses. *Plastic and Reconstructive Surgery* 110:1714–25.

Hutchison, B. L., Hutchison, L. A., Thompson, J. M. & Mitchell, E. A. (2004). Plagiocephaly and brachycephaly in the first two years of life: a prospective cohort study. *Pediatrics* 114:970–80.

Hyman, S. L. (1996). A transdisciplinary approach to self-injurious behavior. In *Developmental Disabilities in Infancy and Childhood*, eds A. J. Capute & P. J. Accardo, pp. 317–36. Baltimore: Paul H. Brookes.

Ingram, T. (1984). A historical review of the definition and classification of the cerebral palsies. In *The Epidemiology of the Cerebral Palsies*, eds F. Stanley & E. Alberman, pp.1–11. Philadelphia: J. B. Lippencott.

Iskander, B. J., McLaughlin, C., Mapstone, T. B., Grabb, P. A. & Oakes, W. J. (1998). Pitfalls in the diagnosis of ventricular shunt dysfunction: radiology reports and ventricular size. *Pediatrics* 101:1031–6.

Issekutz, K. A., Graham Jr., J. M., Prasad, C., Smith, I. M. & Blake, K. D. (2005). An epidemiological analysis of CHARGE syndrome: preliminary results from a Canadian study. *American Journal of Medical Genetics* 133A:1–7.

Jackson, G. (1996). Checklists will help us stay SHARP [editorial]. *British Journal of Clinical Practice* 50:235–6.

Jackson, P. (1990). Primary care needs of children with hydrocephalus. *Journal of Pediatric Health Care* 4:59–71.

Jadeja, S., Smyth, I., Pitera, J. E., et al. (2005). Identification of a new gene mutated in Fraser syndrome and mouse myelencephalic blebs. *Nature Genetics* 23:12–15.

James, H. (1992). Hydrocephalus in infancy and childhood. *American Family Physician* 45:733–42.

Jenkins, R. R. & Saxena, S. B. (1995). Keeping adolescents healthy. *Contemporary Pediatrics* 12:76–89.

Jeret, J., Serur, D., Wisniewski, L. & Lubin, R. (1987). Clinicopathological findings associated with agenesis of the corpus callosum. *Brain and Develelopment* 9:255–64.

Jessop, D. J. & Stein, R. E. K. (1995). Consistent but not the same. Effect of method on chronic condition rates. *Archives of Pediatrics and Adolescent Medicine* 149:1105–10.

Jinnah, H. A. & Friedmann, T. (2001). Hypoxanthine-guanine phosphoribosyltransferase deficiency: Lesch–Nyhan disease and its variants. In *The Metabolic and Molecular Bases of Inherited Disease*, 8th edn, eds C. R. Scriver, A. L. Beaudet, W. S. Sly & D. Valle, pp. 2537–70. New York: McGraw-Hill, Inc.

Jmoudiak, M. & Futerman, A. H. (2005). Gaucher disease: pathological mechanisms and modern management. *British Journal of Haematology* 129:178–88.

Joffe, A. (2004). Women's health begins in pediatrics. *Archives of Pediatrics and Adolescent Medicine* 148:783–4.

Johns, M. B., Hovell, M. F., Drastal, C. A., Lamke, C. & Patrick, K. (1992). Promoting prevention services in primary care: a controlled trial. *American Journal of Preventive Medicine* 8:135–45.

Johnson, A., Palomaki, G. & Haddow, J. (1990). Maternal serum alpha-fetoprotein levels in pregnancies among black and white women with fetal open spina bifida: a United States collaborative study. *American Journal of Obstetrics and Gynecology* 67:1–16.

Johnston, L. B. & Borzyskowski, M. (1998). Bladder dysfunction and neurological disability at presentation inclosed spina bifida. *Archives of Disease in Childhood* 79:33–8.

Jones, J. L., Lane, J. E., Logan, J. J. & Vanegas, M. E. (2002). Beals–Hecht syndrome. *Southern Medical Journal* 95:753–5.

Jones, K. L. (1997). *Smith's Recognizable Patterns of Human Malformation*, 5th edn. Philadelphia: W.B. Saunders.

Jongmans, M., Sistermans, E. A. & Rikken, A. (2005). Genotypic and phenotypic characterization of Noonan syndrome: new data and review of the literature. *American Journal of Medical Genetics* 134A:165–70.

Kallen, K., Robert, E., Castilla, E. E., Mastroiacovo, P. & Kallen, B. (2004). Relation between oculo-auriculo-vertebral (OAV) dysplasia and three other non-random associations of malformations (VATER, CHARGE, and OEIS). *American Journal of Medical Genetics* 127A:26–34.

Kamata, S., Kamiyama, M., Sawai, T., et al. (2005). Assessment of obstructive apnea by using polysomnography and surgical treatment in patients with Beckwith–Wiedemann syndrome. *Journal of Pediatric Surgery* 40:E17–19.

Kamath, B. M., Spinner, N. B., Emerick, K. M., et al. (2004). Vascular anomalies in Alagille syndrome: a significant cause of morbidity and mortality. *Circulation* 109:1354–8.

Khosrotehrani, K., Bastuji-Garin, S., Riccardi, V. M., et al. (2005). Subcutaneous neurofibromas are associated with mortality in neurofibromatosis 1: a cohort study of 703 patients. *American Journal of Medical Genetics* 132A:49–53.

Kim, S. Y., Martin, N., Hsia, E. C., Pyeritz, R. E. & Albert, D. A. (2005). Management of aortic disease in Marfan syndrome: a decision analysis. *Archives of Internal Medicine* 165:749–55.

King, R. A., Hearing, V. J., Creel, D. J. & Oetting, W. S. (2001). Albinism. In *The Metabolic and Molecular Bases of Inherited Disease*, 8th edn, eds C. R. Scriver, A. L. Beaudet, W. S. Sly & D. Valle, pp. 5587–629. New York: McGraw-Hill, Inc.

Kinsman, S. (1996). Childhood-acquired hydrocephalus. In *Developmental Disabilities in Infancy and Childhood*, Vol. 2, 2nd edn, eds A. Capute & P. Accardo, pp. 189–97. Baltimore: Paul Brookes.

Kirby, D. (1999). Reducing adolescent pregnancy: approaches that work. *Contemporary Pediatrics* Jan:83–94.

Kline, A. D., Stanley, C., Belevich, J., et al. (1993b). Developmental data on individuals with the Brachmann–de Lange syndrome. *American Journal of Medical Genetics* 48A:1053–8.

Kohlhase, J. (2000). SALL1 mutations in Townes–Brocks syndrome and related disorders. *Human Mutation* 16:460–6.

Kosztolanyi, G. (1997). Leprechaunism/Donohue syndrome/insulin receptor gene mutations: a syndrome delineation story from clinicopathological description to molecular understanding. *European Journal of Pediatrics* 156:253–5.

Kottke, T. E., Brekke, M. L. & Solberg, L. I. (1993). Making 'time' for preventive services. *Mayo Clinic Proceedings* 68:785–91.

Kuban, K. C. K. & Leviton, A. (1994). Cerebral palsy. *New England Journal of Medicine* 330:188–95.

Kwittken, P. L., Sweinberg, S. K., Campbell, D. E. & Pawlowski, N. A. (1995). Latex hypersensitivity in children: clinical presentation and detection of latex-specific immunoglobulin E. *Pediatrics* 95:693–9.

Lalovic, A., Merkens, L., Russell, L., et al. (2004). Cholesterol metabolism and suicidality in Smith–Lemli–Opitz syndrome carriers. *American Journal of Psychiatry* 161:2123–6.

Lanfranco, F., Kamischke, A., Zitzmann, M. & Nieschlag, E. (2004). Klinefelter's syndrome. *Lancet* 364:273–83.

Leger, R. & Meeropol, E. (1992). Children at risk: latex allergy and spina bifida. *Journal of Pediatric Nursing* 7:373–6.

Lepage, C., Noreau, L. & Bernard, P. M. (1998). Association between characteristics of locomotion and accomplishment of life habits in children with cerebral palsy. *Physical Therapy* 78:458–69.

Lewis, C. E. (1988). Disease prevention and health promotion practices of primary care physicians in the United States. *American Journal of Preventive Medicine* 4(Suppl.):9–16.

Lin, A. E., Semina, E. V., Daack-Hirsch, S., et al. (2000). Exclusion of the branchio-oto-renal syndrome locus (EYA1) from patients with branchio-oculo-facial syndrome. *American Journal of Medical Genetics* 91:387–90.

Lipkin, P. H. (1991). Epidemiology of the developmental disabilities. In *Developmental Disabilities in Infancy and Childhood*, eds A. J. Capute & P. J. Accardo, pp. 43–67. Baltimore: Paul H. Brookes.

Liptak, G., Bloss, J., Briskin, H., et al. (1988). The management of children with spinal dysraphism. *Journal of Child Neurology* 3:3–20.

Liptak, G. S. & Revell, G. M. (1989). Community physician's role in the case management of children with chronic illness. *Pediatrics* 84:465–71.

Little, B. B., Wilson, G. N. & Jackson, G. (1996). Is there a cocaine syndrome? Dysmorphic and anthropometric assessment of infants exposed to cocaine. *Teratology* 54:145–9.

Little, W. (1862). On the influence of abnormal parturition, difficult labour, premature birth, and asphyxia neonatorum on the mental and physical condition of the child, especially in relation to deformities. *Transaction of the Obstetrical Society of London* 3:293–344.

Lopes, V. L., Guion-Almeida, M. L. & Giffoni, S. D. (2004). Frontonasal dysplasia, neuronal migration error and lymphoedema of limbs. *Clinical Dysmorphology* 13:35–7.

Lopez, A., Dietz, V. J., Wilson, M., Navin, T. R. & Jones, J. L. (2000). Preventing congenital toxoplasmosis. *Morbidity & Mortality Weekly Review, Recommendations & Reports.* 31(RR-2):59–68.

Lopponen, T., Saukkonen, A. L., Serlo, W., Lanning, P. & Knip, M. (1995). Slow prepubertal linear growth but early pubertal growth spurt in patients with shunted hydrocephalus. *Pediatrics* 95:917–23.

Lopponen, T., Saukkonen, A. L., Serlo, W., Tapanainen, P., Ruokonen, A. & Knip, M. (1996). Accelerated pubertal development in patients with shunted hydrocephalus. *Archives of Disease in Childhood* 74:490–6.

Lovell, C. M. & Saul, R. A. (1999). Down syndrome clinic in a semi-rural setting. *American Journal of Medical Genetics* 89C:100–10.

Ludecke, H.-J., Schaper, J., Meinecke, P., et al. (2001). Genotypic and phenotypic spectrum in tricho-rhino-phalangeal syndrome types I and III. *American Journal of Human Genetics* 68:81–91.

Lumley, M. A., Jordan, M., Rubenstein, R., Tsipouras, P. & Evans, M. I. (1994). Psychosocial functioning in the Ehlers–Danlos syndrome. *American Journal of Medical Genetics* 53:149–52.

Lurie, S., Manor, M. & Hagay, Z. J. (1998). The threat of type IV Ehlers–Danlos syndrome on maternal well-being during pregnancy: early delivery may make the difference. *Journal of Obstetrics and Gynaecology* 18:245–8.

Lyon, A. J., Preece, M. A. & Grant, D. B. (1985). Growth curve for girls with Turner syndrome. *Archives of Disease in Childhood* 60:932–6.

Maher, E. R. (2005). Imprinting and assisted reproductive technology. *Human Molecular Genetics* 14(Suppl. 1):R133–8.

Maiman, L. A., Becker, M. H., Liptak, G. S., Nazarian, L. F. & Rounds, K. A. (1988). Improving pediatricians' compliance-enhancing practices: a randomized trial. *American Journal of Diseases of Children* 142:773–9.

Majnemer, A. (1998). Benefits of early intervention for children with developmental disabilities. *Seminars in Pediatric Neurology* 5:62–9.

Makitie, O., Sulisalo, T., de la Chapelle, A. & Kaitila, I. (1995). Cartilage-hair hypoplasia. *Journal of Medical Genetics* 32:39–43.

Malfait, F., Coucke, P., Symoens, S., et al. (2005). The molecular basis of classic Ehlers–Danlos syndrome: a comprehensive study of biochemical and molecular findings in 48 unrelated patients. *Human Mutation* 25:28–37.

Manning, M. A. & Hoyme, H. E. (2002). Diagnosis and management of the adolescent boy with Klinefelter syndrome. *Adolescent Medicine* 13:367–74.

Marcus, C. L. (1996). Images in clinical medicine. Periodic breathing in an infant with hydrocephalus. *New England Journal of Medicine* 334:1577.

Marge, M. (1984). The prevention of communication disorders. *American Speech–Language–Hearing Association* August:29–33.

Margulis, A., Bauer, B. S. & Corcoran, J. F. (2003). Surgical management of the cutaneous manifestations of linear nevus sebaceus syndrome. *Plastic and Reconstructive Surgery* 111:1043–50.

Marinescu, R. C., Mainardi, P. C., Ross Collins, M., et al. (2000). Growth charts for cri-du-chat syndrome: an international collaborative study. *American Journal of Medical Genetics* 94:153–62.

Martin, J. W., Tselios, N. & Chambers, M. S. (2005). Treatment strategy for patients with ectodermal dysplasia: a case report. *Journal of Clinical Pediatric Dentistry* 29:113–18.

Martin, R. A., Grange, D. K., Zehnbauer, B. & Debaun, M. R. (2005). LIT1 and H19 methylation defects in isolated hemihyperplasia. *American Journal of Medical Genetics* 134A:129–31.

Martinez, M., Vazquez, E., García Silva, M. T., et al. (2000). Therapeutic effects of docosahexaenoic acid in patients with generalized peroxisomal disorders. *American Journal of Clinical Nutrition* 71:376S–85S.

Massa, G., Verlinde, F., De Schepper, J., et al. (2005). Trends in age at diagnosis of Turner syndrome. *Archives of Disease in Childhood* 90:267–8.

Massey, G. V. (2005). Transient leukemia in newborns with Down syndrome. *Pediatric Blood and Cancer* 44:29–32.

Mayfield, J. (1991). Comprehensive orthopedic management in myelomeningocele. In *Comprehensive Management of Spina Bifida*, ed. H. Rekate, pp. 113–63. Boca Raton, FL: CRC Press.

Mazzanti, L., Cacciari, E., Bergamaschi, R., et al. (1997). Pelvic ultrasonography in patients with Turner syndrome: age-related findings in different karyotypes. *Journal of Pediatrics* 131:135–40.

McClone, D., Czyzewski, D., Raimondi, A. & Sommers, R. (1982). Central nervous system infections as a limiting factor in the intelligence of children with myelomeningocele. *Pediatrics* 70:338–42.

McDonald-McGinn, D. M., Tonnesen, M. K., et al. (2001). Phenotype of the 22q11.2 deletion in individuals identified through an affected relative: cast a wide FISHing net! *Genetics in Medicine* 3:23–9.

McGinnis, J. M. & Lee, P. R. (1995). Healthy People 2000 at mid-decade. *Journal of the American Medical Association* 273:1123–9.

McMillan, J. A. (2002). Make the most of your last chance. *Contemporary Pediatrics* Aug:9.

McNeal, D., Hawtrey, C., Wolraich, M. & Mapel, J. (1983). Symptomatic neurogenic bladder in a cerebral palsied population. *Developmental Medicine and Child Neurology* 25:612–16.

Medley, J., Russo, P. & Tobias, J. D. (2005). Perioperative care of the patient with Williams syndrome. *Paediatric Anaesthesia* 15:243–7.

Meijboom, L. J., Vos, F. E., Timmermans, J., Boers, G. H., Zwinderman, A. H. & Mulder, B. J. (2005). Pregnancy and aortic root growth in the Marfan syndrome: a prospective study. *European Heart Journal* 26:914–20.

Meisels, S. J. (1989). Can developmental screening tests identify children who are developmentally at risk? *Pediatrics* 83:578–85.

Menezes, A. V., MacGregor, D. L. & Buncic, J. R. (1994). Aicardi syndrome: natural history and possible predictors of severity. *Pediatric Neurology* 11:313–18.

Merikangas, K. R. & Risch, N. (2003). Genomic priorities and public health. *Science* 302:599–601.

Metry, D. W., Dowd, C. F., Barkovich, A. J. & Frieden, I. J. (2001). The many faces of PHACE syndrome. *Journal of Pediatrics* 139:117–23.

Mignosa, C., Agati, S., Di Stefano, S., et al. (2004). Dysphagia: an unusual presentation of giant aneurysm of the right coronary artery and supravalvular aortic stenosis inWilliams syndrome. *Journal of Thoracic and Cardiovascular Surgery* 128:946–8.

Milani-Comparetti, A. & Gidoni, E. (1976). Routine developmental examination in normal and retarded infants. *Developmental Medicine and Child Neurology* 9:631–3.

Miller, F. & Bachrach, S. J. (1995). *Cerebral Palsy: A Complete Guide for Caregiving.* Baltimore: Johns Hopkins University Press.

Mittermayer, C., Lee, A. & Brugger, P. C. (2004). Prenatal diagnosis of the Meckel–Gruber syndrome from 11th to 20th gestational week. *Ultraschall In Der Medizin* 25:275–9.

Molnar, G. E. (1979). Cerebral palsy: prognosis and how to judge it. *Pediatric Annals* 8:596–605.

Moore, M. H. (1993). Upper airway obstruction in the syndromal craniosynostoses. *British Journal of Plastic Surgery* 46:355–62.

Moore, S. J., Turnpenny, P., Quinn, A., et al. (2000). A clinical study of 57 children with fetal anticonvulsant syndromes. *Journal of Medical Genetics* 37:489–97.

Msall, M. E. (1996). Functional assessment in neurodevelopmental disabilities. In *Developmental Disabilities in Infancy and Childhood*, eds A. J. Capute & P. J. Accardo, pp. 371–92. Baltimore: Paul H. Brookes.

Mudd, S. M., Levy, H. L. & Kraus, J. P. (2001). Disorders of transsulfuration. In *The Metabolic and Molecular Bases of Inherited Disease*, 8th edn, eds C. R. Scriver, A. L. Beaudet, W. S. Sly & D. Valle, pp. 2007–56. New York: McGraw-Hill, Inc.

Mulinare, J., Cordero, J. F., Erickson, J. D. & Berry, R. J. (1988). Periconceptional use of multivitamins and the occurrence of neural tube defects. *Journal of the American Medical Association* 260:3141–5.

Mulliken, R. F. (2004). The changing faces of children with cleft lip and palate. *New England Journal of Medicine* 351:745–7.

Munro, G. (1986). Epidemiology and the extent of mental retardation. *Psychiatric Clinics of North America* 9:591–602.

Nadel, A., Green, J. & Holmes, L. (1990). Absence of need for amniocentesis in patients with elevated levels of maternal serum alpha-feto-protein and normal ultrasonographic examinations. *New England Journal of Medicine* 323:557–61.

Naessens, A., Casteels, A., Decatte, L. & Foulon, W. A. (2005). Serologic strategy for detecting neonates at risk for congenital cytomegalovirus infection. *Journal of Pediatrics* 146:194–7.

Naeye, R. L., Peters, E. C., Bartholomew, M. & Landis, J. R. (1989). Origins of cerebral palsy. *American Journal of Diseases of Children* 143:1154–61.

Nargozian, C. (2004). The airway in patients with craniofacial abnormalities. *Paediatric Anaesthesia* 14:53–9.

Neff, J. M. & Anderson, G. (1995). Protecting children with chronic illness in a competitive marketplace. *Journal of the American Medical Association* 274:1866–9.

Nellhaus, G. (1986). Head circumference from birth to eighteen years. *Pediatrics* 41:106–14.

Nelson, K. & Ellenberg, J. (1986). Antecedents of cerebral palsy: multivariate analysis of risk. *New England Journal of Medicine* 315:81–6.

Neufeld, E. F. & Meunzer, J. (2001). The mucopolysaccharidoses. In *The Metabolic and Molecular Bases of Inherited Disease*, 8th edn, eds C. R. Scriver, A. L. Beaudet, W. S. Sly & D. Valle, pp. 3421–52. New York: McGraw-Hill, Inc.

Nitahara, J., Dozor, A. J., Schroeder, S. A. & Rifkinson-Mann, S. (1996). Apnea as a presenting sign of hydrocephalus. *Pediatrics* 97:587–9.

Nold, J. L. & Georgieff, M. K. (2004). Infants of diabetic mothers. *Pediatric Clinics of North America* 51:619–37.

Oliveri, B., Mastaglia, S. R., Mautalen, C., et al. (2004). Long-term control of hypercalcaemia in an infant with Williams–Beuren syndrome after a single infusion of biphosphonate (Pamidronate). *Acta Paediatrica* 93:1002–3.

Olson, A. & Cooley, W. (1996). The role of medical professionals in supporting child self-competence. In *Making Our Way: Building Self-Competence Among Youth With Disabilities*, eds L. Powers & G. Singer. Baltimore: Paul Brookes.

Opitz, J. M. & Wilson, G. N. (1997). Terminology and causes of birth defects. In *Pathology of the Fetus and Infant*, ed. E. Gilbert-Barness, pp. 44–64. Philadelphia: Mosby Year Book.

Opitz, J. M., Weaver, D. W. & Reynolds Jr., J. F. (1998). The syndromes of Sotos and Weaver: reports and review. *American Journal of Medical Genetics* 79A:294–304.

Orrico, A., Galli, L., Cavaliere, M. L., et al. (2004). Phenotypic and molecular characterisation of the Aarskog–Scott syndrome: a survey of the clinical variability in light of FGD1 mutation analysis in 46 patients. *European Journal of Human Genetics* 12:16–23.

Ostberg, J. E., Brookes, J. A., McCarthy, C., Halcox, J. & Conway, G. S. A. (2004). Comparison of echocardiography and magnetic resonance imaging in cardiovascular screening of adults with Turner syndrome. *Journal of Clinical Endocrinology and Metabolism* 89:5966–71.

Palfrey, J. S., Singer, J. D., Walker, D. K. & Butler, J. A. (1987). Early identification of children's special needs: a study of five metropolitan communities. *Journal of Pediatrics* 111:651–9.

Paller, A. S. (2004). Piecing together the puzzle of cutaneous mosaicism. *Journal of Clinical Investigation* 114:1407–9.

Palmer, F. & Hoon, A. (1995). Cerebral palsy. In *Developmental and Behavioral Pediatric*, eds S. Parker & B. Zuckerman, pp. 88–94. Boston: Little, Brown, and Company.

Paltiel, A. D., Weinstein, M. C., Kimmel, A. D., et al. (2005). Expanded screening for HIV in the United States – an analysis of cost-effectiveness. *New England Journal of Medicine* 352:586–95.

Parvin, M., Roche, E., Costigan, C. & Hoey, H. M. (2004). Treatment outcome in Turner syndrome. *Irish Medical Journal* 97:14–15.

Pauli, R. M., Horton, V. K., Glinski, L. P. & Reiser, C. A. (1995). Prospective assessment of risks for cervicomedullary-junction compression in infants with achondroplasia. *American Journal of Human Genetics* 56:732–44.

Peeling, R. W. & Ye, H. (2004). Diagnostic tools for preventing and managing maternal and congenital syphilis: an overview. *Bulletin of the World Health Organisation* 82:439–46.

Pennell, P. B. (2003). The importance of monotherapy in pregnancy. *Neurology* 60(11 Suppl. 4):S31–8.

Pharoah, P. O., Cooke, T., Johnson, M. A., King, R. & Mutch, L. (1998). Epidemiology of cerebral palsy in England and Scotland, 1984–9. *Archives of Disease in Childhood* 79:F21–5.

Pollex, R. L. & Hegele, R. A. (2004). Hutchinson–Gilford progeria syndrome. *Clinical Genetics* 66:375–81.

Porter, F. D. (2003). Human malformation syndromes due to inborn errors of cholesterol synthesis. *Current Opinion in Pediatrics* 15:607–13.

Posnick, J. C. (1997). Treacher Collins syndrome: perspectives in evaluation and treatment. *Journal of Oral and Maxillofacial Surgery* 55:1120–33.

Pyeritz, R. E., Murphy, E. A., Lin, S. J. & Rosell, E. M. (1985). Growth and antrhopometrics in the Marfan syndrome. In *Endocrine Genetics and the Genetics of Growth*, eds C. J. Papadatos & C. S. Bartsocas, pp. 355–66. New York: Alan R. Liss.

Raffin, T. A. (1991). Withholding and withdrawing life support. *Hospital Practice* March:133–55.

Rahlin, M. (2005). TAMO therapy as a major component of physical therapy intervention for an infant with congenital muscular torticollis: a case report. *Pediatric Physical Therapy* 17:209–18.

Ray, A. K., Marazita, M. L., Pathak, R., et al. (2004). TP63 mutation and clefting modifier genes in an EEC syndrome family. *Clinical Genetics* 66:217–22.

Reilly, S., Skuse, D. & Poblete, X. (1996). Prevalence of feeding problems and oral motor dysfunction in children with cerebral palsy: a community survey. *Journal of Pediatrics* 129:877–82.

Richards, A. J., Baguley, D. M., Yates, J. R. W., et al. (2000). Variation in the vitreous phenotype of Stickler syndrome can be caused by different amino acid substitutions in the X position of the type II collagen Gly-X-Y triple helix. *American Journal of Human Genetics* 67:1083–94.

Ringpfeil, F. (2005). Selected disorders of connective tissue: pseudoxanthoma elasticum, cutis laxa, and lipoid proteinosis. *Clinics in Dermatology* 23:41–6.

Rios, A., Furdon, S. A., Adams, D. & Clark, D. A. (2004) Recognizing the clinical features of Trisomy 13 syndrome. *Advances in Neonatal Care* 4:332–43.

Roach, E. S. & Miller, V. S., eds (2004). *Neurocutaneous Disorders*. Cambridge UK: Cambridge University Press.

Roach, E. S. & Sparagana, S. P. (2004). Diagnosis of tuberous sclerosis complex. *Journal of Child Neurology* 19:643–9.

Roberts, J. E., Schaaf, J. M., Skinner, M., et al. (2005). Academic skills of boys with fragile X syndrome: profiles and predictors. *American Journal of Mental Retardation* 110:107–20.

Robinson, B. H. (2001). Lactic academia: disorders of pyruvate carboxylase and pyruvate dehydrogenase. In *The Metabolic and Molecular Bases of Inherited Disease*, 8th edn, eds C. R. Scriver, A. L. Beaudet, W. S. Sly & D. Valle, pp. 2275–96. New York: McGraw-Hill, Inc.

Roodman, S., Bothwell, M. & Tobias, J. D. (2003). Bradycardia with sevoflurane induction in patients with trisomy 21. *Paediatric Anaesthesia* 13:538–40.

Ropers, H. H. & Hamel, B. C. (2005). X-linked mental retardation. *Nature Reviews Genetics* 6:46–57.

Rose, G. (1992). *The Strategy of Preventive Medicine*. Oxford: Oxford University Press.

Rosenbloom, L. (1995). Diagnosis and management of cerebral palsy. *Archives of Disease in Childhood* 72:350–4.

Ross, J. L., Roeltgen, D., Feuillan, P., Kushner, H. & Cutler Jr., G. B. (1998). Effects of estrogen on nonverbal processing speed and motor function in girls with Turner's syndrome. *Journal of Clinical Endocrinology and Metabolism* 83:3198–204.

Rubinstein, W. & Lopez-Soler, R. I. (2001). The genetics of sudden death. *Journal of the American Medical Association* 28:1636.

Ryan, A. K., Goodship, J. A., Wilson, D. I., et al. (1997). Spectrum of clinical features associated with interstitial chromosome 22q11 deletions: a European collaborative study. *Journal of Medical Genetics* 34:798–804.

Sabatini, D. D. & Adesnik, M. B. (2001). The biogenesis of membranes and organelles. In *The Metabolic and Molecular Bases of Inherited Disease*, 8th edn, eds C. R. Scriver, A. L. Beaudet, W. S. Sly & D. Valle, pp. 433–520. New York: McGraw-Hill, Inc.

Santer, R., Rischewski, J., von Weihe, M., et al. (2005). The spectrum of aldolase B (ALDOB) mutations and the prevalence of hereditary fructose intolerance in Central Europe. *Human Mutation* 25:594–9.

Sarwark, J. F. (1996). Spina bifida. *Pediatric Clinics of North America* 43:1151–8.

Saudubray, J.-M. & Carpentier, C. (2001). Clinical phenotypes; diagnoses, algorithms. In *The Metabolic and Molecular Bases of Inherited Disease*, 8th edn, eds C. R. Scriver, A. L. Beaudet, W. S. Sly & D. Valle, pp. 1327–406. New York: McGraw-Hill, Inc.

Sawin, P. D. & Menezes, A. H. (1997). Basilar invagination in osteogenesis imperfecta and related osteochondrodysplasias: medical and surgical management. *Journal of Neurosurgery* 86:950–60.

Schaffer, S. J. & Campbell, J. R. (1994). The new CDC and AAP lead poisoning prevention recommendations: consensus versus controversy. *Pediatric Annals* 23:592–9.

Schardein, J. L. (2000). *Chemically Induced Birth Defects*, 3rd edn. New York: Marcel Dekker, Inc.

Schinzel, A. (2001). *Catalogue of Unbalanced Chromosome Aberrations in Man*. Berlin: de Gruyter.

Schleiss, M. R. & McVoy, M. A. (2004). Overview of congenitally and perinatally acquired cytomegalovirus infections: recent advances in antiviral therapy. *Expert Review of Anti-Infective Therapy* 2:389–403.

Schlictemeier, T. L., Tomlinson, G. E., Kamen, B. A., Waber, L. J. & Wilson, G. N. (1994). Multiple coagulation defects and the Cohen syndrome. *Clinical Genetics* 45:212–16.

Schmickel, R. D. (1986). Contiguous gene syndromes. A component of recognizable syndromes. *Journal of Pediatrics* 109:231–41.

Schrander-Stumpel, C. (1999). "Preconception care" challenge of the millennium? *American Journal of Medical Genetics* 89C:58–61.

Schrander-Stumpel, C., Gerver, W. J., Meyer, H., et al. (1994). Prader–Willi-like phenotype in fragile X syndrome. *Clinical Genetics* 45:175–80.

Schreibman, I. R., Baker, M., Amos, C. & McGarrity, T. J. (2005). The hamartomatous polyposis syndromes: a clinical and molecular review. *American Journal of Gastroenterology* 100:476–90.

Scott, C. S., Neighbor, W. E. & Brock, D. M. (1992). Physicians' attitudes toward preventive care services: a seven-year prospective cohort study. *American Journal of Preventive Medicine* 8:241–8.

Scriver, C. R. (2001). Hyperphenylalaninemia: Phenylalanine hydroxylase deficiency. In *The Metabolic and Molecular Bases of Inherited Disease*, 8th edn, eds C. R. Scriver, A. L. Beaudet, W. S. Sly & D. Valle, pp. 1667–724. New York: McGraw-Hill, Inc.

Scriver, C. R., Beaudet, A. L., Sly, W. S. & Valle, D. eds (2001). *The Metabolic and Molecular Bases of Inherited Diseases*. 8th edn. New York: McGraw-Hill, Inc.

Scrutton, D. & Baird, G. (1997). Surveillance measures of the hips of children with bilateral cerebral palsy. *Archives of Disease in Childhood* 76:381–4.

Seller, M. (1994). Risks in spina bifida. *Developmental Medicine and Child Neurology* 36:1021–5.

Sells, J. M., Jaffe, K. M. & Hall, J. G. (1996). Amyoplasia, the most common type of arthrogryposis: the potential for good outcome. *Pediatrics* 97:225–31.

Semprini, A. E. & Fiore, S. (2004). HIV and pregnancy: is the outlook for mother and baby transformed? *Current Opinion in Obstetric and Gynecology* 16:471–5.

Sgouros, S. (2005). Skull vault growth in craniosynostosis. *Childs Nervous System* 14:200–02.

Shapiro, B. J. (1983). Down syndrome – a disorder of homeostasis. *American Journal of Medical Genetics* 14:241–69.

Shofner, J. M. (2001). Oxidative phosphorylation diseases. In *The Metabolic and Molecular Bases of Inherited Disease*, 8th edn, eds C. R. Scriver, A. L. Beaudet, W. S. Sly & D. Valle, pp. 2367–424. New York: McGraw-Hill, Inc.

Shprintzen, R. J. (2000). Velo-cardio-facial syndrome: a distinctive behavioral phenotype. *Mental Retardation and Developmental Disabilities Research Reviews* 6:142–7.

Shurtleff, D. (1986). Selection process for infants. In *Myelodysplasias and Exotrophies: Significance, Prevention, and Treatment*, ed. D. Shurtleff, pp. 89–115. Orlando, Florida: Grune and Stratton.

Shurtleff, D., Lemire, R. & Warkany, J. (1986). Embryology, etiology, and epidemiology. In *Myelodysplasias and Exotrophies: Significance, Prevention, and Treatment*, ed. D. Shurtleff, pp. 39–64. Orlando, Florida: Grune and Stratton.

Sikora, D. M., Ruggiero, M., Petit-Kekel, K., et al. (2004). Cholesterol supplementation does not improve developmental progress in Smith–Lemli–Opitz syndrome. *Journal of Pediatrics* 144:783–91.

Simpson, J. L. (2005). Choosing the best prenatal screening protocol. *New England Journal of Medicine* 353:2068–70.

Simpson, J. L., de la Cruz, F., Swerdloff, R. S., et al. (2003). Klinefelter syndrome: expanding the phenotype and identifying new research directions. *Genetics in Medicine* 5:460–8.

Singer, G. H. S. (1991). The evolution of models of family adaptation to disability. Unpublished manuscript. Hood Center for Family. Dartmouth Medical School, Lebanon, NH.

Singer, G. H. S. & Irvin, L. K. (1991). Supporting families of persons with severe disabilities: emerging findings, practices, and questions. In *Critical Issues in the Lives of People with Severe Disabilities*, eds L. H. Meyer, C. A. Peck & L. Brown, pp. 271–312. Baltimore: Paul Brookes.

Sirotnak, J., Brodsky, L. & Pizzuto, M. (1995). Airway obstruction in the Crouzon syndrome: case report and review of the literature. *International Journal of Pediatrics Otorhinolaryngology* 31:235–46.

Slavotinek, A., Poyser, L., Wallace, A., et al. (2003). Two unique patients with trisomy 18 mosaicism and molecular marker studies. *American Journal of Medical Genetics* 117A:282–8.

Slavotinek, A. M., Schauer, G. & Machin, G. (2005). Fryns syndrome: report of eight new cases. *Genetics in Medicine* 7:74–6.

Sleesman, J. B. & Tobias, J. D. (2003). Anaesthetic implications of the child with Robinow syndrome. *Paediatric Anaesthesia* 13:629–32.

Spadoni, E., Colapietro, P., Bozzola, M., et al. (2004). Smith–Magenis syndrome and growth hormone deficiency. *European Journal of Pediatrics* 163:353–8.

Spahis, J. (1994). Sleepless nights. Obstructive sleep apnea in the pediatric patient. *Pediatric Nursing* 20:469–72.

Spahis, J. & Wilson, G. N. (1999). Down syndrome: perinatal complications and counseling experiences in 216 patients. *American Journal of Medical Genetics* 89C:96–9.

Srivastava, V. K. (1995). Wound healing in trophic ulcers in spina bifida patients. *Journal of Neurosurgery* 82:40–3.

Staheli, L. T., Hall, J. G., Jaffe, K. M. & Paholke, D. O., eds (1998). *Arthrogryposis. A Text Atlas.* Cambridge UK: Cambridge University Press.

Steinmann, B., Royce, P. M. & Superti-Furga, A. (1993). The Ehlers–Danlos syndrome. In *Connective Tissue and its Heritable Disorders*, eds P. M. Royce, B. Steinmann, pp. 351–407. New York: Wiley-Liss.

Steinmann, B., Gitzelmann, R. & Van den Berghe, G. (2001). Disorders of fructose metabolism. In *The Metabolic and Molecular Bases of Inherited Disease*, 8th edn, eds C. R. Scriver, A. L. Beaudet, W. S. Sly & D. Valle, pp. 1489–520. New York: McGraw-Hill, Inc.

Stiehm, E. R. (1995). Now is the time for routine voluntary HIV testing of pregnant women. *Archives of Pediatrics and Adolescent Medicine* 149:484–5.

Stoler, J. M. & Holmes, L. B. (2004). Recognition of facial features of fetal alcohol syndrome in the newborn. *American Journal of Medical Genetics* 127C:21–7.

Strickland, B., McPherson, M., Cooley, W. C., et al. (2004). Access to the medical home: results of the National Survey of Children with Special Health Care Needs. *Pediatrics* 113:1485–98.

Summers, J. A., Behr, S. K. & Turnbull, A. P. (1989). Positive adaptation and coping strengths of families who have children with disabilities. In *Support for Caregiving Families*, eds G. H. S. Singer & L. K. Irvin, pp. 27–40. Baltimore: Paul Brookes.

Swartz, K. R., Resnick, D. K., Iskandar, B. J., et al. (2003). Craniocervical anomalies in Dubowitz syndrome. Three cases and a literature review. *Pediatric Neurosurgery* 38:238–43.

Sybert, V. P. (1994). Hypomelanosis of Ito: a description, not a diagnosis. *Journal of Investigative Dermatology* 103(Suppl. 5):141S–3S.

Sybert, V. P. & McCauley, E. (2004). Turner's syndrome. *New England Journal of Medcine* 351:1227–38.

Taylor, G. A. & Madsen, J. R. (1996). Neonatal hydrocephalus: hemodynamic response to fontanelle compression – correlation with intracranial pressure and need for shunt placement. *Radiology* 201:685–9.

Thomas, G. H. (2001). Disorders of glycoprotein degradation: α-mannosidosis, β-mannosidosis, fucosidosis, and sialidosis. In *The Metabolic and Molecular Bases of Inherited Disease*, 8th edn, eds C. R. Scriver, A. L. Beaudet, W. S. Sly & D. Valle, pp. 3507–34. New York: McGraw-Hill, Inc.

Thompson, R. S., Taplin, S. H., McAfee, T. A., Mandelson, M. T. & Smith, A. E. (1995). Primary and secondary prevention services in clinical practice. *Journal of the American Medical Association* 271:1130–5.

Tian, X.-L., Kadaba, R. & You, S.-A. (2004). Identification of an angiogenic factor that when mutated causes susceptibility to Klippel–Trenaunay syndrome. *Nature* 427:640–5.

Tolar, J., Teitelbaum, S. L. & Orchard, P. J. (2004). Osteopetrosis. *New England Journal of Medicine* 351:2839–49.

Tomita, Y. & Suzuki, T. (2004). Genetics of pigmentary disorders. *American Journal of Medical Genetics* 131C:75–81.

Tonkin, E. T., Wang, T.-J., Lisgo, S., Bamshad, M. J. & Strachan, T. (2004). NIPBL, encoding a homolog of fungal Scc2-type sister chromatid cohesion proteins and fly *Nipped-B*, is mutated in Cornelia de Lange syndrome. *Nature Genetics* 36:636–41.

Tsang, V. T., Pawade, A., Karl, T. R. & Mee, R. B. (1994). Surgical management of Marfan syndrome in children. *Journal of Cardiac Surgery* 9:50–4.

Tyler, C. & Edman, J. C. (2004). Down syndrome, Turner syndrome, and Klinefelter syndrome: primary care throughout the life span. *Primary Care* 31:627–48.

US Department of Health and Human Services (1987) Surgeon general's report on children with special health care needs. DHHS publication #HRS/D?MC87-2, Rockville, MD.

US Public Health Service (1991). *Healthy People 2000: National Health Promotion and Disease Prevention Objectives*, 91–50212. Washington DC: US Government Printing Office, PHS.

US Public Health Service (1994). *Put Prevention Into Practice Education and Action Kit.* Washington DC: US Government Printing Office, #017-001-00492-8.

Udwin, O., Howlin, P., Davies, M. & Mannion, E. (1998). Community care for adults with Williams syndrome: how families cope and the availability of support networks. *Journal of Intellectual Disability Research* 42:238–45.

Valdez, B. C., Henning, D., So, R. B., Dixon, J. & Dixon, M. J. (2004). The Treacher Collins syndrome (TCOF1) gene product is involved in ribosomal DNA gene transcription by interacting with upstream binding factor. *Proceedings of the National Academy Science of the United States of America* 101:10709–14.

Van Allen, M. I., Fung, J. & Jurenka, S. B. (1999). Health care concerns and guidelines for adults with Down syndrome. *American Journal of Medical Genetics* 89C:100–10.

Varkey, J. J. & Jones, R. A. (2004). Perinatally lethal, short-limbed dwarfism with distinct features – Schneckenbecken dysplasia. *Ultrasound in Obstetrics and Gynecology* 24:575–7.

Vega, H., Waisfisz, Q., Gordillo, M., et al. (2005). Roberts syndrome is caused by mutations in ESCO2, a human homolog of yeast ECO1 that is essential for the establishment of sister chromatid cohesion. *Nature Genetics* 37:468–70.

Verkh, Z., Russell, M. & Miller, C. A. (1995). Osteogenesis imperfecta type II: microvascular changes in the CNS. *Clinical Neuropathology* 14:154–8.

Verzijl, H. T., van Es, N., Berger, H. J., Padberg, G. W. & van Spaendonck, K. P. (2005). Cognitive evaluation in adult patients with Mobius syndrome. *Journal of Neurology* 252:202–7.

Visootsak, J., Aylstock, M. & Graham Jr., J. M. (2001). Klinefelter syndrome and its variants: an update and review for the primary pediatrician. *Clinical Pediatrics* 40:639–51.

Vits, L., van Camp, G., Coucke, P., et al. (1994). MASA syndrome is allelic to X-linked hydrocephalus at the L1CAM locus. *Nature Genetics* 7:108–13.

Vogels, A., De Hert, M. & Descheemaeker, M. J. (2004). Psychotic disorders in Prader–Willi syndrome. *American Journal of Medical Genetics* 127A:238–43.

Waite, K. A. & Eng, C. (2002). Protean PTEN: form and function. *American Journal of Human Genetics* 70:829–44.

Wallace, D. C., Lott, M. T., Brown, M. D. & Kerstann, K. (2001). Mitochondria and neuro-ophthalmological diseases. In *The Metabolic and Molecular Bases of Inherited Disease*, 8th edn, eds C. R. Scriver, A. L. Beaudet, W. S. Sly & D. Valle, pp. 2425–512. New York: McGraw-Hill, Inc.

Ward, B. A. & Gutmann, D. H. (2005). Neurofibromatosis 1: from lab bench to clinic. *Pediatric Neurology* 32:221–8.

Weiskop, S., Richdale, A. & Matthews, J. (2005). Behavioural treatment to reduce sleep problems in children with autism or fragile X syndrome. *Developmental Medicine and Child Neurology* 47:94–104.

Weng, E. Y., Mortier, G. R. & Graham Jr., J. M. (1995). Beckwith–Wiedemann syndrome. An update and review for the primary pediatrician. *Clinical Pediatrics* 34:317–32.

Wessel, A., Gravenhorst, V., Buchhorn, R., et al. (2004). Risk of sudden death in the Williams–Beuren syndrome. *American Journal of Medical Genetics* 127A:234–7.

Whitaker, R. C. (2003). Obesity prevention in pediatric primary care. *Archives of Pediatrics and Adolescent Medicine* 157:725–6.

White, C. C., Koplan, J. P. & Orenstein, W. A. (1985). Benefits, risks and costs of immunization for measles, mumps and rubella. *American Journal of Public Health* 75:739–44.

Whittington, J., Holland, A., Webb, T., et al. (2002). Relationship between clinical and genetic diagnosis of Prader–Willi syndrome (Letter). *Journal of Medical Genetics* 39:926–32.

Whyte, M. P., Kurtzberg, J., McAlister, W. H., et al. (2003). Marrow cell transplantation for infantile hypophosphatasia. *Journal of Bone and Mineral Research* 18:624–36.

Wide, K., Winbladh, B. & Kallen, B. (2004). Major malformations in infants exposed to antiepileptic drugs in utero, with emphasis on carbamazepine and valproic acid: a nationwide, population-based register study. *Acta Paediatrica* 93:174–6.

Wiesner, G. L., Cassidy, S. B., Grimes, S. J., Matthews, A. L. & Acheson, L. S. (2004). Clinical consult: developmental delay/fragile X syndrome. *Primary Care* 31:621–5.

Wiktor, A. & Van Dyke, D. L. (2004). FISH analysis helps identify low-level mosaicism in Ullrich–Turner syndrome patients. *Genetics in Medicine* 6:132–5.

Wilkin, D., Hallam, L. & Doggett, M.-A. (1993). *Measures of Need and Outcome for Primary Health Care*. Oxford: Oxford University Press.

Williams, C. A. (2005). Neurological aspects of the Angelman syndrome. *Brain and Development* 27:88–94.

Wills, K. (1993). Neuropsychological functioning in children with spina bifida and/or hydrocephalus. *Journal of Clinical Child Psychology* 22:247–65.

Wills, K., Holmbeck, G., Dillon, K. & McClone, D. (1990). Intelligence and achievement in children with myelomeningocele. *Journal of Pediatric Psychology* 15:161–76.

Wilmshurst, S., Ward, K., Adams, J. E., Langton, C. M. & Mughal, M. Z. (1996). Mobility status and bone density in cerebral palsy. *Archives of Disease in Childhood* 75:164–5.

Wilson, G. N. (1983). Cranial defects in the Goldenhar syndrome. *American Journal of Medical Genetics* 14:435–43.

Wilson, G. N. (1986). What is Zellweger syndrome? *Journal of Pediatrics* 109:398.

Wilson, G. N. (1987). Heterochrony and human malformation. *American Journal of Medical Genetics* 29A:311–21.

Wilson, G. N. (1990). Office approach to the genetics patient. *Pediatric Annals* 19:79–91.

Wilson, G. N. (1992). Genomics of human dysmorphogenesis. *American Journal of Medical Genetics* 42:187–196.

Wilson, G. N. (1998). Thirteen cases of Niikawa–Kuroki syndrome: report and review with emphasis on medical complications and preventive management. *American Journal of Medical Genetics* 79A:112–20.

Wilson, G. N. (2000). *Clinical Genetics: A Short Course*. New York: Wiley-Liss.

Wilson, G. N. & Barr Jr., M. (1983). Trisomy 9 mosaicism: another etiology for the manifestations of Goldenhar syndrome. *Journal of Craniofacial Genetics and Developmental Biology* 3:313–16.

Wilson, G. N., Holmes, R. D., Custer, J., et al. (1986). Zellweger syndrome: diagnostic assays, syndrome delineation, and potential therapy. *American Journal of Medical Genetics* 24:69–82.

Wilson, G. N., Holmes, R. D. & Hajra, A. K. (1988). Chondrodysplasia punctatas and the peroxisomopathies: overlapping syndrome communities. *Pathology and Immunopathology Research* 7:113–18.

Wilson, G. N., de Chadarévian, J.-P., Kaplan, P., et al. (1989). Glutaric aciduria type II: review of the phenotype and report of an unusual glomerulopathy. *American Journal of Medical Genetics* 32:395–401.

Wilson, M. E. H. (1995). Assumptions, prevention, and the need for research. *Archives of Pediatrics and Adolescent Medicine* 149:356.

Witt, D. R., Keena, B. A., Hall, J. G. & Allanson, J. E. (1986). Growth curves for height in Noonan syndrome. *Clinical Genetics* 30:150–3.

Wraith, E. J., Hopwood, J. J., Fuller, M., Meikle, P. J. & Brooks, D. A. (2005). Laronidase treatment of mucopolysaccharidosis I. *BioDrugs* 19:1–7.

Wyatt, D. (2004). Lessons from the national cooperative growth study. *European Journal of Endocrinology* 151(Suppl. 1):S55–S59.

Yen, I., Khoury, M., Erickson, J., et al. (1992). The changing epidemiology of neural tube defects: United States, 1968–1989. *American Journal of Diseases of Children* 146:857–61.

Yetman, A. T., Bornemeier, R. A. & McCrindle, B. W. (2005). Usefulness of enalapril versus propranolol or atenolol for prevention of aortic dilation in patients with the Marfan syndrome. *American Journal of Cardiology* 95:1125–7.

Yoon, P. W., Olney, R. S., Khoury, M. J., et al. (1996). Contribution of birth defects and genetic diseases to pediatric hospitalizations. A population-based study. *Archives Pediatrics and Adolescent Medicine* 151:1096–103.

Young, P. C., Shyr, V. & Schork, M. (1994). The role of the primary care physician in the care of children with serious heart disease. *Pediatrics* 94:3, 284–90.

Zaffanello, M., Zamboni, G., Schadewaldt, P., Borgiani, P. & Novelli, G. (2005). Neonatal screening, clinical features and genetic testing for galactosemia. *Genetics in Medicine* 7:211–12.

Zoghbi, H. Y. & Francke, U. (2001). Rett syndrome. In *The Metabolic and Molecular Bases of Inherited Disease*, 8th edn, eds C. R. Scriver, A. L. Beaudet, W. S. Sly & D. Valle, pp. 6329–38. New York: McGraw-Hill, Inc.

Index

α-galactosidase, 481, 483
β-glucosidase gene, 482
β-glucosidase, 481, 511

abdominal CT scan, 492
abdominal ultrasound, 329, 354
absent corpus callosum, 461
absent lacrimal glands, 440
acanthosis nigricans, 268, 269
accelerated aging, 451
accelerated growth, 487
acetaldehyde, 128
achondrogenesis, 300
achondroplasia, complications, 308
achondroplasia, definition, 307
achondroplasia, genetic counseling, 308
achondroplasia, preventive management, 309
acid phosphatase, 304
acidosis, 10, 490, 506, 516
acrocallosal syndrome, 398
acrocephaly, 378
acrocyanosis, 424
activities of daily living, 54
acute monocytic leukemia, 284
acyclovir, 121
ADL scale, 54
adrenal carcinomas, 359
adrenal insufficiency, 498
AFP, 75
agenesis of corpus callosum, 466, 500
aggressive behaviors, 363
Aicardi syndrome, 460
airway obstruction, 381, 391, 488
alanine, 518
Albers–Schonberg syndrome, 304
albinism, 441
alcohol, 131

alcoholic persons, 129
alkaline phosphatase, 303
Alzheimer disease, 179
ambiguous genitalia, 500
amblyopia, 393
American Academy of Pediatrics, 46, 48
amino acid metabolism, 514
amino acid profile, 17
aminoacidopathies, 514
amnion rupture sequence, 92
amniotic bands, 90, 462
amyoplasia, 463
anesthesia, 271, 364, 459
aneurysm, 421
angiofibromas, 361
angiography, 421
angioid streaks, 419, 424
angiokeratoma, 480
angiokeratoma corporis diffusum universale, 481
angiomyolipomas, 363
angiosarcoma, 354
ankylosis, 462
anophthalmia, 396
anosmia, 305
anticipatory guidance, 3
anticoagulant therapy, 421
anticonvulsant therapy, 132
anticonvulsants, 460
antipyretics, 439
antithrombin III, 499
Antley–Bixler syndrome, 377
aortic aneurysm, 427
aortic regurgitation, 413
aortic root dilatation, 312, 415
Apert syndrome, 378
arachidonic acid, 135
arachnodactyly, 427

Arnold–Chiari malformation, 70, 445
arrhinencephaly, 461
arthralgia, 428
arthritis, 309, 416
arthrochalasis multiplex congenita, 422
arthrogryposes, 455
arthrogryposis, 466
arthrogryposis multiplex congenita, 462
arthrogryposis syndromes, definition, 467
arthrogryposis syndromes, diagnosis, 468
arthrogryposis syndromes, genetic counseling, 468
arthrogryposis syndromes, incidence, 467
arthrogryposis syndromes, preventive
    management, 469
ascorbate, 494
aspartylglucosaminuria, 480
aspirin therapy, 421
associations, 14, 99
ataxia, 452
atelosteogenesis, 300
atlantoaxial instability, 179, 306, 383, 394, 398, 488
atrial septal defect, 329
atrophic rhinitis, 439
audiology screening, 46
Austin syndrome, 483
autism, 23, 216
autoimmune disorders, 180
autoimmune thryoiditis, 280
Autosomal aneuploidy syndromes, 151
autosomal dominant inheritance, 10
avascular necrosis, 481

Baby Doe, 42
"baby on back", 95
baclofen, 69
Baller–Gerold syndrome, 379
Bannayan–Riley–Ruvalcaba syndrome, 347
Barr body, 197
basal cell carcinomas, 267
basal cell nevus syndrome, 350
basal ganglia, 305
basilar impression, 397
basilar skull invagination, 312
Bayley Scales of Infant Development, 65
beaked nose, 454
Beals syndrome, 425
Beckwith–Wiedemann syndrome, 326
Beckwith–Wiedemann syndrome,
    complications, 333
Beckwith–Wiedemann syndrome, counseling, 333
Beckwith–Wiedemann syndrome, definition, 332

Beckwith–Wiedemann syndrome, differential, 332
Beckwith–Wiedemann syndrome, genetic
    counseling, 333
Beckwith–Wiedemann syndrome, preventive
    management, 334
behavioral screening instruments, 45
Bendectin, 116
beneficence, 52
beta-adrenergic blockade, 428
beta-blocker therapy, 427
betaine, 417
bicornuate uterus, 405, 468
biopterin, 515
biotin, 517
biotinidase, 518
biotinidase deficiency, 518
biotinylation, 518
biphosphonates, 313, 325
BKM gene, 268
blastomere analysis before implantation
    (BABI), 215
bleeding diathesis, 280
blepharitis, 180, 401
blepharophimosis, 416, 464
blindness, 304, 483
Bloch–Sulzberger syndrome, 446
Bloom syndrome, 267
blue sclerae, 310, 424
bone crises, 482
bone fragility, 310
bone marrow transplantation, 304, 489
Bonnevie–Ullrich syndrome, 194
Börjeson–Forssman–Lehmann syndrome, 326
botulinum toxin, 69
Brachmann–de Lange syndrome,
    complications, 283
Brachmann–de Lange syndrome, definition, 281
Brachmann–de Lange syndrome, diagnosis, 282
Brachmann–de Lange syndrome, incidence, 281
brain imaging, 360
branched chain α-keto acid dehydrogenase, 516
branched chain amino acids, 516
branchial arches, 388
branchial clefts, 388
branchial cysts, 390
branchio-oculo-facial syndrome, 388
branchio-oto-renal syndrome, 395
breasts, absent, 439
breech presentation, 459
broad thumbs, 404
bronchiectasis, 416

bruisability, 312, 423
Brushfield spots, 175
burden of suffering, 34
burning pain, 481

café-au-lait spots, 357
camptodactyly, 415
carbamazapine, 481
carbohydrate-deficient glycoprotein syndrome, 498
carbohydrate metabolism, disorders, 507
cardiac arrhythmias, 494
cardiac arrythmia, 513
cardiac valves, 489
cardiomyopathy, 268, 279, 498, 511, 517
carnitine, 492, 517
carnitine supplementation, 517
carotid arteries, 416
Carpenter syndrome, 380
cartilage-hair hypoplasia, 297
cataracts, 127, 271, 299, 305, 337, 405, 462, 468
catastrophic illness, 16
caudal regression sequence, 101
celiac arteries, 419
celiac disease, 180
cerebellar anomalies, 123
cerebellar hypoplasia, 466
cerebral aneurysm, 312
cerebral dysgenesis, 61
cerebral palsy, 22, 61
cerebral palsy, choreoathetoid, 62
cerebral palsy, coping by families, 69
cerebral palsy, familial, 66
cerebral palsy, implications of diagnosis, 66
cerebral palsy, natural history, 67
cerebral palsy, outcomes, 63
cerebral palsy, parent support group, 66
cerebral palsy, prevalence, 62
cerebral palsy, preventive checklist, 69
cerebral palsy, risk factors, 63
cerebral palsy, services, 67
cerebral palsy, spastic, 67
Cerezyme, 482
cervical spinal cord, 301
cervical spine, 381
cervical spine compression, 306
cervical spine fusion, 378
Cervical vertebral fusion, 394
CHARGE association, cardiac anomalies, 106
CHARGE association, complications, 106
CHARGE association, definition, 103
CHARGE association, diagnosis, 105

CHARGE association, differential, 104
CHARGE association, genetic counseling, 106
CHARGE association, incidence, 104
CHARGE association, preventive management, 106
CHARGE syndrome, 104
Charles Darwin, 439
Charlie M syndrome, 402
checklists, compliance, 53
cherry red spot, 480
cherry red spots, 480
cherubism, 280
chest pain, 428
child development clinic, 28
children with special health care needs, 31
choanal atresia, 96, 127, 329, 377, 393
cholesterol metabolism, 499
cholesterol screening, 454
chondrodysplasia, 463
chondrodysplasia punctata, 298, 495
chondrodystrophic myotonia, 463
choreoathetosis, 460
chorioretinal degeneration, 420
chorioretinitis, 119
chorioretinopathy, 327
choristomas, 346
choroidal angioma, 353
choroidemia, 494
chromosomal analysis, 18
chromosomal imbalance, 156
chromosomal inheritance, 12
chromosome 11p15 region, 332
chromosome 15 region, 443
chromosome analysis, 28
chromosome disorders, parent support groups, 161
chromosome region 7p13, 402
chromosome region Xq26–28, 404
Chronic Condition Management, 29, 30
chronic otitis, 93, 95, 200, 281, 283, 301, 337, 400
chronic rhinorrea, 484
cigarette paper scars, 424
claudication, 419
clavicles, absent, 299
cleft lip and palate, 405
cleft lip/cleft palate, 93
cleft lip/palate, 440
cleft palate, 123, 380, 418, 420
cleft palate team, 93
cleft palate, U-shaped, 98
cleidocranial dysplasia, 299
clinodactyly, 175
club feet, 418

coagulation disorder, 327
coarctation of the aorta, 198
cocaine, 118
Cockayne syndrome, 451, 466
coenzyme Q, 493
Coffin–Siris syndrome, 133, 400
cognitive disability, 194
Cohen syndrome, 327
collision sports, 421
coloboma, 97
colobomata, 445
colon perforation, 421
conductive hearing loss, 380, 398
cone-shaped epiphyses, 392
congenital contractural arachnodactyly, 415
congenital contractures, 457, 467, 468
congenital heart disease, 301
congenital hip dislocation, 134, 488
congenital rubella infection, 123
congenital syphilis, 125
congenital toxoplasmosis, 126
congenital toxoplasmosis infection, 126
conjunctival aneurysms, 481
connective tissue dysplasia, 413
connective tissue laxity, 418
connective tissue weakness, 413
consanguinity, 10
constipation, 178, 274
contractures, 451
corneal abrasions, 459
corneal clouding, 483, 486
corneal reflex, 459
coronal synostosis, 382
coronary disease, 417
corpus callosum, 337
cortical atrophy, 400
cost-effectiveness, 56
Costello syndrome, 268
costovertebral defects, 461
cranial nerve paralysis, 304
craniofacial surgery team, 375
craniosynostosis, 277
craniosynostosis syndromes, 375
"crippled children's services", 62
cryptophthalmos, 400
Cryptophthalmos syndrome, 400
cryptorchidism, 172, 280, 302, 327, 380, 391, 392, 402, 441, 445, 448, 465, 499
curare paralysis, 462
cutis laxa syndromes, 415
cystathionine-β-synthase, 417

cystic hygroma, 278
cystic kidneys, 330, 389, 500
cystic medial necrosis, 413
cytochrome c, 492
cytogenetic notation, 18
cytomegalovirus, 119

7-dehydrocholesterol, 499
Dandy–Walker cyst, 401
Dandy–Walker malformation, 461
Dandy–Walker syndrome, 70
deafness, 106
deep plantar crease, 176
degenerative course, 466
del(22q11), 104
demyelination, 496, 517
dental anomalies, 178, 424
dental decay, 459
dental hypoplasia, 439
dentinogenesis imperfecta, 312
dermatitis, 452
developmental delay, 10, 28
developmental differences, 21
developmental disabilities, allied health professionals, 28
developmental disabilities, causes, 23
developmental disabilities, early intervention services, 26
developmental disabilities, epidemiology, 22
developmental disabilities, parental adaptation, 30
developmental disabilities, parental support, 25
developmental disabilities, people-first language, 31
developmental disabilities, prenatal diagnosis, 25
developmental disabilities, recognition, 24
developmental disabilities, team approach, 43
developmental pediatrician, 28
developmental regression, 28
developmental screening, 21, 27
dextrocardia, 172
diabetes mellitus, 135, 452
diabetic embryopathy, complications, 136
diabetic embryopathy, counseling, 136
diabetic embryopathy, definition, 135, 148
diabetic embryopathy, diagnosis, 135
diabetic embryopathy, history, 135
diabetic embryopathy, incidence, 135
diaphragmatic hernia, 330
diastrophic dwarfism, 300
dichloroacetate, 493
dietary treatment, 506

DiGeorge anomaly, 96, 105, 130
DiGeorge anomaly, preventive management, 96
dihydroxyacetone phosphate acyltransferase, 496
dimpling, 463
diphenylhydantion, 481
dipyridamol, 417
disability, definition, 54
dislocation of the radial head, 418
disruptions, 92
diverticulae, 416
DNA diagnosis, 18
dolichostenomelia, 415
Donohue syndrome, 269
dorsal rhizotomy, 68
double-jointed, 413
Down syndrome, complications, 178
Down syndrome, definition, 175
Down syndrome, diagnosis, 176
Down syndrome, genetic counseling, 176
Down syndrome, history, 175
Down syndrome, incidence, 175
Down syndrome, preventive management, 179
Duane syndrome, 394
Dubowitz syndrome, 270
dwarfism, 293
dwarfism, neonatal lethal, 295
dysarthric speech, 460
dysmorphology, 8, 12
dysphagia, 459
dysphonia, 439
dyspnea, 428
dystonia, 460

ear pits, 333
early intervention, 44
early intervention services, 26
ectodermal dysplasia, 481
ectodermal dysplasias, 437
ectomesenchyme, 388
ectopia lentis, 415, 425
ectrodactyly, 440
ectrodactyly–ectodermal dysplasia-clefting (EEC)
    syndrome, 440
ectropion, 391
eczematoid rash, 447
Ehlers–Danlos syndrome, 420
Ehlers–Danlos syndrome, type VII, 422
Ehlers–Danlos syndrome, types I–III,
    complications, 424
Ehlers–Danlos syndrome, types I–III, genetic
    counseling, 423

Ehlers–Danlos syndrome, types I–III, preventive
    management, 424
Ehlers–Danlos syndrome, type IV, 421
Ehlers–Danlos syndrome, type VI, 422
Ehlers–Danlos syndrome, types I–III, definition,
    422
Ehlers–Danlos syndrome, types I–III, incidence,
    422
elastin fibers, 419
electron transfer flavoprotein, 490
Elephant Man, 357
Ellis–van Crevald syndrome, 301
emphysema, 416
enamel hypoplasia, 277, 305, 383
encephalocele, 74, 396
enchondroma, 354
enlarged penis, 405
enzyme assay, 17
enzyme therapy, 482
eosinophilia, 447
epibulbar dermoid, 97
epibulbar dermoid cysts, 394
epicanthal folds, 175
epidermal nevus syndrome, 348
epilepsy, 132
epinephrine response, 459
epiphyseal dysplasia, 326
erythrocyte plasmalogens, 498
estrogen treatment, 200
ETF, 490
exclude spinal stenosis, 305
exposure keratitis, 381
external ophthalmoplegia, 494

5-fluorouracil, 351
Fabry disease, 481
facial angiofibromas, 363
facial asymmetry, 349
facioauriculovertebral spectrum, 395
factor IX, 499
FAE, 128
false teeth, 439
familial dysautonomia, 458
Fanconi syndrome, 512
FAP gene, 350
FAS, 128
fatty acid oxidation, 517
fatty acid oxidation disorders, 517
fatty liver, 512
fetal akinesia sequence, 466
fetal alcohol effects, 128

fetal alcohol syndrome, 128

fetal alcohol syndrome, animal models, 128

fetal alcohol syndrome, complications, 130

fetal alcohol syndrome, diagnosis, 128

fetal alcohol syndrome, family support, 130

fetal alcohol syndrome, growth hormone
    secretion, 131

fetal alcohol syndrome, history, 128

fetal alcohol syndrome, incidence, 128

fetal alcohol syndrome, preventive
    management, 131

fetal anticonvulsant associations, preventive
    management, 134

fetal cocaine syndrome, 118

fetal HIV infection, 121

fetal hydantoin syndrome, 400

fetal hydantoin syndrome, animal models, 133

fetal hydantoin syndrome, history, 132

fetal hydrops, 295, 466, 486

fetal immobility, 462

fetal movement, 467

fibrillin-1 locus, 425

fibrillin-2 gene, 415

fibroblast growth factor receptor 2 (FGFR2)
    gene, 376

fibroblast growth factor-3 receptor, 309

fibrodysplasia ossificans progressiva, 302

fibroma, 351

fibrosarcomas, 351

financial issues, 44

first and second branchial arch syndrome, 395

flat feet, 217, 268, 332

"fleur-de-lys" nose, 127

flexion contractures, 283

fluorescent DNA probes, 19

fluorescent *in situ* hybridization (FISH)
    technology, 19

focal dermal hypoplasia, 445

folate deficiency, 417, 460

folic acid, 75

foramen magnum, 309

foveal hypoplasia, 441

fractures, 459

fragile X DNA testing, 215

fragile X syndrome, complications, 216

fragile X syndrome, diagnosis, 215

fragile X syndrome, genetic counseling, 215

fragile X syndrome, preventive management, 217

fragile X testing, 28

Franceschetti–Klein syndrome, 392

Fraser syndrome, 400

Freeman–Sheldon syndrome, 466

frontonasal dysplasia, 96, 396

frontonasal malformation, 96

Fryns syndrome, 401

fucosidosis, 480

full mutation, 216

functional screening, 47

G protein, 357

Gardner syndrome, 346, 349

gastric carcinoma, 349

gastroesophageal reflux, 216, 282

gastrointestinal anomalies, 179

Gaucher disease, 481

genetic diseases, presentations, 8

genitourinary anomalies, 301

genitourinary defects, 441

genu recurvatum, 424

germinal mosaicism, 310, 383

giant cell astrocytomas, 363

gibbus, 487

glabellar hemangioma, 333, 463

globe rupture, 423

glomerular lesions, 390

glucocerebroside, 481

glucose-6-phosphatase, 513

glucose-6-phosphate, 512

glutaric acid, 490

glutaric acidemia type II, 490

glycogen storage diseases, 17

glycogen storage diseases, definition, 510

glycogen storage diseases, diagnosis, 511

glycogen storage diseases, genetic counseling, 511

glycogenoses, 512

glycolipid deposition, 481

glycolysis, 512

glycoprotein degradation disorders, 480

glycopyrrolate, 69

glycosaminoglycans, 484

glypican 3 gene, 330

G_{M1} gangliosidosis, 483

G_{M2} gangliosidosis, 479

Goldenhar syndrome, 388

Goldenhar syndrome, complications, 397

Goldenhar syndrome, description, 394

Goldenhar syndrome, diagnosis, 396

Goldenhar syndrome, genetic counseling, 396

Goldenhar syndrome, incidence, 395

Goldenhar syndrome, preventive management,
    397

Goltz–Gorlin syndrome, 445

gonadoblastoma, 401
Gorlin sign, 423
Gorlin syndrome, 350
Greig syndrome, 402
growth failure, 266
growth failure, disproportionate, 265
growth failure, proportionate, 265
growth hormone deficiency, 305
growth hormone therapy, 200, 310, 451
Gs alpha gene, 305
gynecomastia, 327

hair-bulb assay, 442
Hallermann–Streiff syndrome, 271
hamartoma, 346
hamartomas, 354
hamartosis syndromes, 346
handicap, definition, 54
Hanhart syndrome, 402
HARD-E syndrome, 461
Hay–Wells syndrome, 440
Head circumference monitoring, 73
head sparing, 265
health care resources, 1
health outcome, 53
health supervision, 179
healthcare "carve-outs", 57
Healthy People 2000, 48
hearing loss, 284, 483
helmets, 95
hemangiomas, 329, 351
hemangiomatous disorders, 439
hematochezia, 364
hemifacial microsomia, 394
hemifacial microsomia/Goldenhar complex, 101
hemihyperplasia, 328, 334, 349
hemihypertrophy, 276
hemiplegia, 61
hepatic adenomas, 512
hepatic cholestasis, 269
hepatic transaminase, 492
hepatocarcinoma, 514
hepatocellular carcinoma, 337
hepatosplenomegaly, 486
hereditary sensory and autonomic
    neuropathies, 458
hernia, 428
hernias, 416, 424, 464
herpes virus, 120
heteroplasmy, 490
heterotopia, 497

heterotopias, 362
heterozygotes, 217
hexokinase deficiency, 511
high TSH form of hypothyroidism, 180
Himalayan mice, 442
hip dislocation, 131, 500
histamine, 459
HIV testing, 50
Hodgkin disease, 298
holocarboxylase synthetase deficiency, 518
holoprosencephaly, 174, 397
homeostasis, 156
homocystinuria, 417
horseshoe kidney, 445
HSAN, 458
human immunodeficiency virus-1 (HIV-1), 121
human teratogen, criteria, 116
Hunter syndrome, 485
Hurler-like syndrome, 480
Hurler syndrome, 487
Hutchinson–Gilford syndrome, 454
hydrocephalus, 97, 127, 308, 379, 484, 487, 500
hydrocephalus, arrested, 70
hydrocephalus, communicating, 312
hydrocephalus, compensated, 70
hydrocephalus, complications, 73
hydrocephalus, definition, 70
hydrocephalus, diagnosis, 71
hydrocephalus, family support, 72
hydrocephalus, incidence, 70
hydrocephalus, non-communicating, 70
hydrocephalus, parent groups, 72
hydronephrosis, 276, 380, 445
hyperactivity, 129, 217, 363
hyperammonemia, 506, 518
hypercalcemia, 303
hyperinsulinism, 269
hyperlipidemia, 512
hyperphagia, 326
hyperphenylalaninemia, 514
hyperphosphatemia, 305
hyperpigmented lesions, 445
hyperpyrexia, 440
hypertonia, 460
hypertrophic cardiomyopathy, 490
hyperuricemia, 460, 512
hypochondrogenesis, 306
hypochondroplasia, 307
hypoglossia–hypodactylia syndrome, 402
hypoglycemia, 10, 333, 506, 513
hypogonadism, 267, 284

hypohidrosis, 481
hypohidrotic ectodermal dysplasia, 439
hypomelanosis of Ito syndrome, 446
hypophosphatasia, 303
hypopigmented macules, 361
hypoplastic nails, 301
hypoplastic teeth, 440
hypospadias, 270, 490, 499
hypothyroidism, 175, 305
hypotonia, 27

I-cell disease, 486
ichthyosis, 299, 483
imaging studies, 47
impairment, definition, 54
imperforate anus, 377, 379, 397
imprinting, 332
inborn errors of metabolism, 9, 475
incontinentia pigmenti, 446
incontinentia pigmenti achromians, 446
increased intracranial pressure, 379
Individual Family Service Plan (IFSP), 26
Individuals with Disabilities Education Act
        (IDEA), 44
infantile reflexes, persistence, 64
infantile spasms, 363
infants of diabetic mothers (IDM), 134
infertility, 451
inflammatory bowel disease, 513
inheritance mechanisms, 10
integument, 437
integumentary glands, 439
intestinal atresias, 401
intestinal malrotation, 330
intestinal polyps, 348
intestinal rupture, 421
intracranial bleeding, 283
intracranial calcifications, 119, 353, 363
intracranial hypertension, 363
intracranial pressure, 71
intrauterine growth retardation, symmetrical,
        265
isochromosome Xp, 195
isotretinoin, 123, 351

Jackson–Weiss syndrome, 381
joint contractures, 462, 463
joint deterioration, 482
joint fusions, 383
joint hypermobility, 422
joint laxity, 312, 348, 400, 419, 420, 423

Joseph Merrick, 357
juvenile rheumatoid arthritis, 29

Kabuki theater, 272
Kearns–Sayre syndrome, 494
keratitis, 180, 380, 401
keratosis, 453
kernicterus, 62
ketogenic diet, 493
Klinefelter syndrome, definition, 201
Klinefelter syndrome, history, 201
Klinefelter syndrome, incidence, 202
Klippel–Feil anomaly, 97, 131, 394
Klippel–Trenaunay–Weber syndrome, 351
Krabbe disease, 479
kyphoscoliosis, 415, 427, 467
kyphosis, 308, 355

lactate/pyruvate ratio, 493
lactic acidosis, 492, 512
large anterior fontanelle, 300, 490, 497
Larsen syndrome, 418
laryngeal hypoplasia, 301
laryngeal stenosis, 401
laryngomalacia, 96, 329, 418
latex allergy, 79
laxatives, 421
learning disabilities, 129
Leber hereditary optic neuropathy
        (LHON), 493
Leigh disease, 492
LEOPARD syndrome, 279, 448
Leprechaunism, 269
Lesch–Nyhan syndrome, 459
leukemia, 270, 298
limb anomalies, 377
limb bowing, 310
lipodystrophy, 498
lipomas, 348
lipophoresis, 454
Lisch spots, 358
lissencephaly, 61
Little People of America, 296
Little's disease, 61
live viral vaccines, 123
lobster-claw deformity, 440
long philtrum, 282
loose skin, 415
loss of heterozygosity, 357
lower extremity paralysis, 79
lymphangiomas, 355

lymphoma, 298
lysosomal enzyme deficiencies, 478
lysosomal enzymes, 477
lysosome, 478
lysyl oxidase deficiency, 416

macrocephaly, 27, 300, 309, 312, 329, 348, 357, 487, 490
macroglossia, 330, 335
Mafucci syndrome, 353
Major anomalies, 12
malignant hyperthermia, 281, 288
malocclusion, 459, 469
mandibular hypoplasia, 98
mandibular prognathism, 335, 381
mandibulofacial dysostosis, 391, 392
mannose-6-phosphate, 484
mannosidoses, 480
maple syrup urine disease, 516
Marden–Walker syndrome, 463
Marfan syndrome, diagnosis, 426
Marfan syndrome, genetic counseling, 427
Marfan syndrome, incidence, 425
Marfan syndrome, preventive management, 428
Marfanoid habitus, 419, 420
Maroteaux–Lamy disease, 486
Marshall–Smith syndrome, 329
Marshall syndrome, 419
maternal inheritance, 490
maternal PKU, 516
maternal serum alpha-fetoprotein (MSAFP), 75
maternal vasculopathy, 135
Meckel syndrome, 402
medicaid benefits, 45
medium chain coenzyme A dehydrogenase deficiency, 517
medulloblastomas, 351
megaloblastic anemia, 460
megalocornea, 427
melanin pigment, 442
melanin-regulating genes, 441
MELAS, 494
melena, 354
Mendelian inheritance, 7
meningomeylocele, 74
mental retardation, 23
MERRF, 494
mesomelic shortening, 273
metabolic disorders, 8
metabolic disorders, categories, 16

metabolic disorders, large molecule, 14
metabolic disorders, small molecule, 14
metabolic dysplasias, 475
metachromatic leukodystrophy, 479, 483
Meténier sign, 423
microcephaly, 27, 123, 265, 299, 326, 398, 452, 468, 499
microcornea, 380, 424
microdeletion, chromosome, 22, 96, 104
microdontia, 451
micrognathia, 403, 454
microgyria, 379
micropenis, 274, 402
microphthalmia, 446, 466
microstomia, 467
Miller–Dieker syndrome, 461
Miller syndrome, 391
minor anomalies, 8, 12
mitochondrial disease, 492
mitochondrial disorders, 493
mitochondrial DNA deletions, 494
mitochondrial encephalopathy with lactic acidemia and strokes, 494
mitochondrial encephalopathy with ragged red fibers, 494
mitochondrial genome, 490
mitochondrial membranes, 489
mitochondrial myopathy, 492
mitochondrial proteins, 489
mitochondrial respiratory function, 490
mitral regurgitation, 427
mitral valve prolapse, 217, 293, 416, 427, 464
Moebius syndrome, 402
monosomy X, 197
Morquio disease, 486
mosaicism, 197
Movement Assessment of Infants (MAI), 65
moya moya disease, 280
MRI scan, 72
mucolipidoses, 480
mucopolysaccharidoses, 480
mucopolysaccharidoses, complications, 487
mucopolysaccharidoses, definition, 485
mucopolysaccharidoses, genetic counseling, 487
mucopolysaccharidoses, incidence, 485
mucopolysaccharidoses, preventive management, 488
multiple congenital anomalies, 9
multiple miscarriages, 8
multiple sulfatase deficiency, 483

myasthenia gravis, 462
myeloid malignancy, 174
myelodysplasia, 74
myelomeningocele, 103
myocardial infarction, 421
myoclonic seizures, 363, 401
myopathies, 462
myopia, 284, 420

NADH dehydrogenase, 492
Naegeli syndrome, 447
Nager syndrome, 391
nasal saline drops, 180
nasal septum, 381
natural history, 54
neonatal HIV Infection, 121
neonatal polycythemia, 332
neonatal seizures, 63
neonatal vesicles, 121
nephroblastosis, 330
nephrolithiasis, 460
nephromegaly, 334
nephrotic syndrome, 306
neural crest, 441
neural tube defects, causes, 74
neural tube defects, incidence, 74
neurectoderm, 441
neuroblastoma, 131, 270, 337
neurodegeneration, 477
neurofibromas, 357
neurofibromatosis-2, 355
neurofibromin, 357
neuronopathic, 482
neurosensory damage, 130
neutropenia, 513
nevoid basal cell carcinoma syndrome, 350
nevus flammeus, 353
NF-1, definition, 357
NF-1, diagnosis, 358
NF-1, genetic counseling, 359
NF-1, incidence, 357
NF-1, preventive management, 358
Niemann–Pick disease, 479
Niikawa–Kuroki syndrome, 272
nocturnal glucose feeding, 513
Noonan syndrome, 448
Noonan syndrome, complications, 280
Noonan syndrome, definition, 278
Noonan syndrome, diagnosis, 279
Noonan syndrome, differential, 279, 288
Noonan syndrome, genetic counseling, 279

Noonan syndrome, history, 278
Noonan syndrome, incidence, 278
normal variants, 12
Norplant, 180
nystagmus, 441, 444, 446, 492

obesity, 310, 327
obstructive hydrocephalus, 119
obstructive sleep apnea, 271, 378
occipital horn disease, 420
occult blood, 419
ocular albinism, 443
ocular proptosis, 382
oculoauriculovertebral dysplasia, 395
oculocutaneous albinism, 441
odontoid hypoplasia, 488
oligosaccharidoses, 480
omphalocele, 329, 334, 401
opisthotonic posturing, 460
optic atropy, 380
optic disc anomalies, 97
optic gliomas, 359
optic nerve hypoplasia, 462
oral–facial–digital syndromes, 403
orange-peel skin, 419
organellar diseases, 477
organic acid profile, 17
organic acidemias, 517
oromandibular-limb hypogenesis
        syndromes, 402
oromandibular-limb syndromes, 403
orthopedic treatment, 425
osteodysplastic primordial dwarfism, 277
osteogenesis imperfecta, definition, 310
osteogenesis imperfecta, diagnosis, 310
osteogenesis imperfecta, genetic
        counseling, 311
osteogenesis imperfecta, incidence, 310
osteogenesis imperfecta, preventive
        management, 312
osteomyelitis, 459
osteopenia, 310, 469
osteopetrosis, 304
osteoporosis, 417
otopalatodigital syndrome, 404
outcome criteria, 53
outcome studies, 56
outcome, interval, 55
outcome, ordinal, 55
outcomes, functional, 54
ovarian failure, 327

overbite, 217
overgrowth disorders, 326
oxygen radicals, 135

p, 18
P gene, 443
pain insensitivity, 457
palpitations, 428
pamidronate, 313, 325
pancytopenia, 304
papilledema, 71
papillomas, 268
paradoxical growth retardation, 135
parathormone, 305
parenteral nutrition, 517
paresthesias, 481
parietal foramina, 401
partial chromosome aneuploidies, 159
peau d'orange, 419, 498
pectus deformity, 427
pectus excavatum, 217, 416, 448
pedigree, 10
Pena–Shokeir type I syndrome, 465
Pena–Shokeir type II syndrome, 465
penicillin, 125
penicillin prophylaxis, 482
people-first language, 31, 176
perinatal complications, 21
periventricular leukomalacia, 63
Perlman syndrome, 330
peroxisomal disorders, definition, 495
peroxisomal disorders, diagnosis, 497
peroxisomal disorders, genetic counseling, 497
peroxisomal disorders, incidence, 496
peroxisomes, 299, 494
persistent hyperplastic primary vitreous, 461
Peutz–Jeghers syndrome, 354
pharyngeal muscle hypoplasia, 388
phenylalanine, 514
phenylalanine hydroxylase, 514
phenylketonuria, 514
phosphenolpyruvate carboxykinase, 493
photophobia, 453
physical restraints, 460
phytanic acid, 496
Pierre Robin sequence, 98
pigmentary disorders, 437
pigmentary lesions, 174
pilocarpine, 459
piracetam, 180
PKU, 514

PKU diet, 516
plagiocephaly, 95
plasmalogen, 299
plasmalogens, 496
plastic surgery, 181
platybasia, 293
platyspondyly, 452
plexiform neuroma, 358
Pneumocystis, 122
Poland sequence, 403
policeman's tip, 468
polydactyly, 295, 329, 334
polyhydramnios, 295, 334
Pompe disease, 511
poor impulse control, 129
popliteal pterygium syndrome, 465
porencephaly, 61
postaxial polydactyly, 402
potassium bromide, 132
Potter sequence, 90, 390
precocious puberty, 73, 360, 363
preconceptional supplementation, 75
prematurity, 424
premutation, 215
prevention, cost-effectiveness, 52
prevention, costs, 48
prevention, disease incidence, 50
prevention, guidelines, 46
prevention, health care systems, 52
prevention, high-risk population, 51
prevention, justification, 34
prevention, physician compliance, 52
prevention, population strategies, 50
prevention, rationale, 34
prevention, scope of disease, 49
prevention, secondary, 49
prevention, tertiary, 49
preventive care checklists, 53
preventive checklist, 48
preventive medical checklists, 46, 179
primordial growth failure syndromes, 265
procollagen, 311
Progeria, 454
prolapse of the uterus, 424
proprionyl coenzyme A carboxylase, 517
proptosis, 381
protein-losing enteropathy, 352
proteins S and C, 499
Proteus syndrome, 346, 355, 358
pseudoarthrosis, 358
pseudohermaphroditism, 194

pseudo-Hurler polydystrophy, 483
pseudo-hypoparathyroidism, 305
pseudothalidomide syndrome, 404
pseudotumor cerebri, 71
pseudoxanthoma elasticum, 419
psychosocial problems, 42, 423
pterygia, 464
pterygium colli, 97
ptosis, 280, 464
puckered lips, 467
pulmonary hypertension, 131
pulmonary hypoplasia, 390, 401, 402, 466, 469
pulmonary stenosis, 416
pulmonic stenosis, 268, 423, 448
punctate calcifications, 298
pyloric stenosis, 497
pyrimethamine, 127
pyruvate, 493
pyruvate carboxylase, 493, 517
pyruvate dehydrogenase deficiency, 492, 516

q, 18
quadriparesis, 313
quality of life measures, 55

rachischisis, 73
radial aplasia, 451
radial ray, 379
radiohumeral synostosis, 377
radioulnar synostosis, 392
ragged red fibers, 492
Rapp–Hodgkin syndrome, 440
rectal prolapse, 423
recurrence risks, 10
recurrent pneumonias, 465
reflux nephropathy, 424
Refsum syndrome, 495
renal agenesis, 90, 389, 390, 401, 497
renal cysts, 490
renal duplication, 441
renal failure, 494
renal sonography, 398, 403
renal tubular acidosis, 494
renal ultrasound, 389
renovascular hypertension, 419
respiratory complex I, 492
respiratory complex IV, 492
retinal detachment, 419, 423, 424, 462
retinal lattice degeneration, 428
retinal pigmentation, 498
retinitis pigmentosa, 452, 494

retinoic acid, 123
rib fractures, 311
riboflavin, 492, 493
Riley–Day syndrome, 458
Roberts syndrome, 405
Robertsonian translocation, 176
Robin sequence, 98, 420
Robinow syndrome, 273
Rothmund–Thomson syndrome, 450
rubella embryopathy, 123
Rubinstein–Taybi syndrome, 274
Russell–Silver phenotype, 275, 276

sacrococcygeal dysgenesis, 101
Saethre–Chotzen syndrome, 382
salivary gland hypoplasia, 396
Sandhoff disease, 479
Sandifer syndrome, 94
sarcomas, 451
Scheie syndrome, 488
school issues, 44
Schwartz–Jampel syndrome, 463
scoliosis, 131, 269, 299, 329, 422, 424, 445, 459, 461,
    463, 464
screening by history, 47
Seckel syndrome, 277
see-saw winking, 403
seizures, 28, 217, 273, 312, 353, 362, 398, 494,
    506, 518
self esteem, 200
self-mutilation, 458, 460
sensorineural deafness, 302, 308, 313, 398,
    418, 444
sensorineural hearing loss, 131, 356, 390, 392, 394
sensory impairments, 29
septum pellucidum, 331
sequence, 13, 90
serum alpha-fetoprotein, 334
sex chromosome aneuploidies, 194
Sex chromosome imbalance, 194
sexually transmitted diseases, 125
shagreen patch, 361
"shaken baby syndrome", 65
short limbs, 299
short nose, 299
short stature, 310
Shprintzen syndrome, 105
sialidoses, 480
Siamese cats, 442
simplified pinna, 397
Simpson–Golabi–Behmel syndrome, 330

Single anomalies, 12, 90
single palmar creases, 175
sinusitis, 180, 439
skeletal dysplasias, 293
skeletal myopathy, 517
skin fragility, 413, 423
skin rashes, 515
sleep apnea, 94, 180, 381, 459
sleep difficulties, 337
Smith–Lemli–Opitz syndrome, 499
social security law, 45
somatic chromosomal mosaicism, 447
Sotos syndrome, complications, 336
Sotos syndrome, definition, 335
Sotos syndrome, genetic counseling, 336
Sotos syndrome, incidence, 335
Sotos syndrome, preventive management, 337
sparse hair, 439
spastic quadriplegia, 68
spatial visualization, 198
special education services, 22
spina bifida, 445
Spina Bifida Association of America, 78
spina bifida occulta, 300
spina bifida, cognitive abilities, 80
spina bifida, complications, 78
spina bifida, definition, 73
spina bifida, family support, 76
spina bifida, foster care, 77
spina bifida, history, 74
spina bifida, intellectual outcomes, 79
spina bifida, level of lesion, 75
spina bifida, management, 76
spina bifida, prenatal diagnosis, 75
spina bifida, preventive checklist, 80
spina bifida, school performance, 80
spina bifida, selection of cases for surgery, 74
spinal compression, 309
spinal cord lipomas, 75
spinal fusion, 337, 425
spiramycin, 126
splenectomy, 482
split hand, 440
spondyloepiphyseal dysplasia congenita, 305
stapedial foot plate, 378
Stickler syndrome, 98, 419
stippled epiphyses, 131, 298
stool guaiac, 450
storage diseases, 17, 477
strabismus, 127, 178, 271, 280, 337, 355, 393, 424,
    427, 441, 446, 464, 492

stretch marks, 413
Strudwick spondylometaphyseal dysplasia, 306
Sturge–Weber syndrome, 352
subacute necrotizing encephalomyelopathy, 492
subependymal nodules, 361
subluxation, 422
submucous cleft palate, 270
sudden death, 427
sulfate transporter, 300
sulfatide lipidosis, 483
sunscreen, 443
"sunset sign", 70
supernumerary bones, 418
supernumerary teeth, 382, 451
Supplemental Security Income (SSI), 65
supraorbital ridges, 393
sweat pores, 439
sweat testing, 439
syndactyly, 376
syndromes, 12, 14
synophrys, 282
syphilis IgM antibodies, 125
syringomyelia, 300, 396
systolic click, 427

tactile defensiveness, 216
Tay–Sachs disease, 479
Taybi syndrome, 404
telangiectases, 445
telangiectasia, 267
telangiectasias, 481
temporomandibular joint, 424
teratogens, 116
testicular atrophy, 460
tethered cord, 64, 79, 136
tethered cord, spinal dysraphism, 103
tetralogy of Fallot, 106, 172, 380, 396, 500
thalidomide, 117
thanatophoric dwarfism, 295
thanatophoric dysplasia, 307
thiamine, 517
thoracic dysplasia, 303
thrombocytopenia, 405
thromboembolism, 418
thrombotic complications, 417
thumb anomalies, 302
thyroxine-binding globulin, 334
Title V, 44
Title XIX, 45
toluene, 126
toluene embryopathy, 126

tongue hypoplasia, 397, 403
TORCH acronym, 117
torticollis, 94, 330
Townes–Brocks syndrome, 392
tracheo-esophageal fistula, 395
tracheomalacia, 301
transferrin, 499
transient myeloid proliferation, 178
translocation, 173
Treacher–Collins syndrome, 391, 392
triangular facies, 275
triglyceride synthesis, 512
triphalangeal thumbs, 392
triplet repeat expansion, 19
triplet repeats, 215
trisomy 13/18, complications, 171, 173
trisomy 13/18, definitions, 171
trisomy 13/18, diagnosis, 172
trisomy 13/18, genetic counseling, 173
trisomy 13/18, preventive management, 174
TSC1 gene, 361
tuberous sclerosis, definition, 360
tuberous sclerosis, diagnosis, 361
tuberous sclerosis, genetic counseling, 362
tuberous sclerosis, preventive management, 363
Turner syndrome, complications, 198
Turner syndrome, definition, 195
Turner syndrome, diagnosis, 197
Turner syndrome, genetic counseling, 197
Turner syndrome, history, 195
Turner syndrome, incidence, 196
Turner syndrome, preventive management, 200
type I collagen, 422
type II collagen gene, 306
tyrosinase gene, 441
tyrosine, 515

Ullrich–Turner syndrome, 194
ultrasound screening, 335
ungual fibromas, 361
unusual distribution of body fat, 498
unusual movements, 28
upslanting palpebral fissures, 175
urinary tract anomalies, 174
urine mucopolysaccharide screen, 486
urogenital anomalies, 469
uterine fibroids, 309

VACTERL association, 100
vaginal atresia, 377
vascular accidents, 92

vascular fragility, 420
VATER association, 136
VATER association, complications, 103
VATER association, definition, 100
VATER association, diagnosis, 102
VATER association, differential, 101
VATER association, etiology, 101
VATER association, genetic counseling, 102
VATER association, history, 101
VATER association, incidence, 101
VATER association, preventive management, 103
velopalatine insufficiency, 420
ventricular septal defect, 391
ventriculomegaly, 72
ventriculoperitoneal (VP) shunt, 72
vestibular schwannomas, 356
vidarabine, 121
visceromegaly, 10, 332, 482, 483
vitamin A (retinol), 123
vitamin D-deficient rickets, 303
vitamin K_3, 493
vitamin supplements, 181
vitreoretinal degeneration, 419

Wagner syndrome, 419
Walker–Warburg syndrome, 461
Warfarin, 299
Warfarin embryopathy, 127
Watson syndrome, 279
webbed neck, 464
WeeFIM scale, 55
Weissenbacher–Zweymüller syndrome, 419
Werdnig–Hoffman disease, 467
whistling face syndrome, 466
Wildervanck syndrome, 97, 394
Wilms tumor, 284, 349, 359
windvane fingers, 467
Wood's lamp, 362
Wormian bones, 300
WT-1 Wilms tumor gene, 333

X chromosome, 194
X-linked adrenoleukodystrophy, 495
X-linked inheritance, 10
xeroderma pigmentosum, 452

Y chromosome, 194

Zellweger syndrome, 495
zinc, 135
zygomatic process, 393